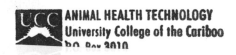

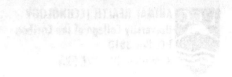

Georgis'
Parasitology
FOR
Veterinarians

PROPERTY OF

_____

_____

_____

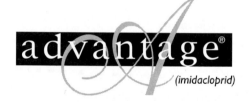

Georgis' Parasitology
FOR
Veterinarians

DWIGHT D. BOWMAN, MS, PhD
Associate Professor of Parasitology
Department of Microbiology and Immunology
College of Veterinary Medicine
Cornell University College of Veterinary Medicine
Ithaca, New York

RANDY CARL LYNN, MS, DVM
Diplomate, American College of Veterinary Clinical Pharmacology
Director of Product Development
Blue Ridge Pharmaceuticals
Greensboro, North Carolina

MARK L. EBERHARD, PhD
Chief, Biology and Diagnostics Branch
Division of Parasitic Diseases
National Center for Infectious Diseases
Centers for Disease Control
Atlanta, Georgia

EIGHTH EDITION

SAUNDERS
An Imprint of Elsevier Science

SAUNDERS
An Imprint of Elsevier Science

11830 Westline Industrial Drive
St. Louis, Missouri 63146

GEORGIS' PARASITOLOGY FOR VETERINARIANS   ISBN 0-7216-9283-4
Copyright © 2003, Elsevier Science (USA). All rights reserved.

NOTICE

Veterinary medicine is an ever-changing field. Standard safety precautions must be followed, but as new research and clinical experience broaden our knowledge, changes in treatment and drug therapy may become necessary or appropriate. Readers are advised to check the most current product information provided by the manufacturer of each drug to be administered to verify the recommended dose, the method and duration of administration, and contraindications. It is the responsibility of the licensed prescriber, relying on experience and knowledge of the patient, to determine dosages and the best treatment for each individual patient. Neither the publisher nor the author assumes any liability for any injury and/or damage to persons or property arising from this publication.

Previous editions copyrighted 1969, 1974, 1980, 1985, 1990, 1995, 1999

International Standard Book Number 0-7216-9283-4

Acquisitions Editor: Raymond R. Kersey
Developmental Editor: Denise LeMelledo
Publishing Services Manager: Patricia Tannian
Design Manager: Gail Morey Hudson
Cover Design: Liz Rhone Rodder

Printed in the United Sates of America

Last digit is the print number: 9   8   7   6   5   4   3   2   1

PREFACE

The text for the eighth edition of *Parasitology for Veterinarians* is very similar to the seventh edition. The text is divided into four chapters on arthropods, protozoans, helminths, and antiparasitic drugs. In this edition, the last chapter has been divided into two parts: Chapter 5 on diagnostic parasitology and Chapter 6 on histopathological parasitology. New to this edition is a table on Greek and Latin roots on the inside front and back covers. This table was compiled with the help of Dr. Hanna Roisman of the Classics Department of Colby College. Knowing these roots may make it easier for the student to learn the many names that appear in the text.

Plans had been originally made to add an additional chapter on veterinary vaccines for parasites, but there were fewer on the market at the time we finished the chapters than there were at the time that the eighth edition was planned. I am not sure what this says about the feasibility of vaccines in the world of veterinary parasitology. Vaccines are available for giardiasis, trichomoniasis, equine protozoal myeloencephalitis (EPM), and neosporosis, but there have been few new additions to the market in the United States. Several of the overseas vaccines, such as those for ticks and larval tapeworms, have not proved to be commercially viable entities. Perhaps such a chapter will be forthcoming in the next edition; only time will tell.

The text has been updated to present new and appropriate material for each topic. Dr. Randy Lynn has once again updated the section on veterinary pharmaceutical products for animal parasites, and he also decided to add tables to his chapter. Also, several new tables now appear in Chapter 3, Helminths, with the goal being to assist students in rapidly gaining details relative to some of the life stages and times associated with helminth parasites, dipterans, lice, and fleas. Chapter 6, Histopathological Diagnosis, was prepared by Dr. Mark Eberhard of the Division of Parasitic Diseases at the Centers for Disease Control. Dr. Eberhard is an expert in the identification of parasites in histological sections and presents a chapter that should prove helpful to those needing to identify parasites in this type of material.

Very little material relative to the parasites of large animals was found for inclusion in the text. Although several new products have been introduced to the market and different efficacy trials have been published, there has been very little presented that is new relative to the basic biology of the parasites of these hosts. It is hard to tell if this is due to the feeling that everything is currently known or because funds are being directed toward areas of protective immunity and molecular biology. These latter topics have yet to provide a great deal of practical information that can be applied to routine veterinary practice. However, it is expected that as these studies progress, one area where marked changes will be seen is the arena of diagnostics. There is every reason to believe that in the next several years marked improvements will be made in the methodologies for the specific diagnosis and detection of infections through either fecal or blood examination and the application of these techniques will become more available to diagnostic laboratories and clinics. In the future it may be possible to differentiate more rapidly the various trichostrongylid and strongylid parasites in large animals solely by analysis of fecal material for either DNA or RNA of parasites present, but currently such work is still very much in the realm of research arena.

Relative to the parasites of the horse, several things have happened of note in the past few years. The excellent work done on Potomac Horse Fever has elucidated a rather confusing life cycle through a combination of excellent work in molecular epidemiology and basic parasitology; this has been a great melding of different fields and methodologies to produce valuable findings that will ultimately improve the health of horses. EPM continues to be markedly frustrating. It would seem that a disease of such magnitude where so much is known would be easy to define parasitologically, but the important detail as to the routine natural host still remains a mystery. Although overshadowed now by the events of September 11, 2001, the introduction of West Nile virus is a threat to horses that is now firmly entrenched on our continent. Fortunately for veterinary medicine, the West Nile virus will be handled through vaccination (although humans will not be so lucky). The West Nile virus outbreak once again underscores the need to maintain surveillance for foreign animal diseases (kudos to Dr. Tracey

McNamara of the Bronx Zoo for a job extremely well done) and to maintain adequate mosquito control throughout the nation.

Dog and cat parasites are under constant attack from the great preventives currently on the market and routinely and wisely prescribed by veterinarians. The reality is that well-cared-for pets should probably have as little to worry about from worms as we do. However, it does not work out that way in reality. There are still many dogs treated each year for adult heartworms and many dogs and cats are still infected routinely with hookworms and roundworms. The typical disease produced by these infections is not as common as 20 years ago, but the parasites persist in spite of our intentions. Fleas have been given a severe hit through the various new products that target their destruction, but they continue to thrive. The concern is that resistance may develop and the heyday of flea-free pets may pass. Best to enjoy it while it is available.

I have a bit in this edition on a truly exotic host, the honeybee. In the world of interdependencies, it is amazing how much of our existence depends on this European colonizer of the New World. I am not expecting veterinarians to flock to the world of entomological medicine, but on the other hand, they are the group responsible for protecting farmers and the public from threats to animal agriculture. When the different diseases were destroying the honeybee population of the United States, it fell to the USDA laboratories and the Center for Veterinary Medicine at the FDA to come up with the means of protecting bees while still having honey remain a safe commodity for the consumer. All of a sudden, veterinarians were placed in positions where they had to learn something about bees. They rose well to the task, but a little preparedness and awareness never hurt.

I want to pay homage here to my father, Lawrence Lincoln Bowman, who fostered my initial interest in biology. My father was a field biologist type with a long-term interest in ornithology. When working on his master's degree in ornithology from the University of Michigan during summers at Douglas Lake, Michigan, he had his initial encounter with the field of parasitology. All he ever said about parasitologists still rings true today: if you want to enjoy lunch or dinner, do not eat with the parasitologists. I am certain that many veterinary students have ruined the dinners of friends or family as they have recounted parasite stories from class to those who have been foolish enough to eat with them while they are in the middle of their parasitology course. Likewise, I am certain that many parasitologists have has been invited to present their work to nonparasitologists over a meal of some sort and have had to work their way through aspects of the topic that are best not presented over food.

My father was also an avid photographer. He tried to capture beauty in all his images and was entranced by birds and flowers along with the majestic scenery of the United States. Thus he developed a large collection of Kodachromes on many different species of birds and flowers from around the United States and many images of the national parks that he visited before World War II (I had the good fortune of visiting almost all these parks with him as a child during summer camping trips). Out of all of these Kodachromes, there is very little related to parasitology or anything close. He was also an avid entomologist, but macrophotography in the 1930s and 1940s was a lot of work (mainly because of the need for bright light when film speeds were a lot slower), so most of the images are close-ups of various flowers and fungi that did not move. The only image that seemed at all fitting to pay tribute to his large collection is this image of a dung beetle. This is probably as close as my father ever wanted to get to feces, although he was very good about cleaning up after my sisters' pet Basenjis. My father passed away just as I completed my PhD, and I moved away to Wisconsin to start my postdoctoral position and my introduction to the wonderful world of veterinary medicine, veterinarians, and veterinary students. He has been sorely missed all these years, and I hope that this representation of a scarab moving the world will serve as a small tribute to his artistic endeavors.

I did not think I would have a poem in this book, but I recently discovered a copy of a silly poem written by my father for a camp newspaper in WWII. It deals with parasites, although the signature on the poem, "LL Bowman, a victim," indicates that my father was acting as a host rather than as a biologist. It does not deal with veterinary medicine, but it is close.

ODE TO A CHIGGER
O Chigger!
Who loves to burrow in my figger.
Thou mighty mite
Whose love of me is now my plight.
Where com'st thou from so stealthily and subtle?
I never see thee and my search is futile.
In my anatomy you happily reside
While I in hapless misery abide.
Get thou from me lest I lose my wits
And scratch you out in fiendish frenzied fits!
Let me alone I beg you, O thou pest
And on thy mitey head my blessings rest.

Many people need to be thanked for assistance with this book. Close to home, I need to thank once again the Drs. Jay and Marion Georgi, who can

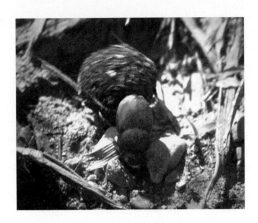

always be reached by phone when I have a serious parasitology question that needs answering or just a simple pick-me-up. The people in the clinics who provide my major assistance in matters parasitological are Drs. Hornbuckle and Barr, who keep me straight as to what is realistic in the world of small animals, and Dr. Divers, who keeps me in line relative to the world of large animals. Dr. Frongillo is always helpful in diagnosis and always has good material on hand for examination and teaching. Again, the membership of the American Association of Veterinary Parasitologists needs commendation for being a great group of people with whom to associate, work, and share ideas. Also, the members of the diagnostic and pharmaceutical industry continue their steadfast work to improve the lives of pets and domestic animals through better testing and products. I also want to thank my editor, Ray Kersey, and his assistants, Denise Lemelledo and Cass Stamato, without whom the book would never have happened. Finally, I need to thank my family for putting up with the long hours I spend away from home.

Dwight D. Bowman

CONTENTS

CHAPTER 1

ARTHROPODS

The body of a typical arthropod is composed of a series of segments, some of which bear jointed legs. Not all arthropods display these characteristics. Thus body segmentation has all but disappeared with the evolution of the mites and ticks, and many insect larvae have no legs. Adaptation to parasitism has led to extreme deviation in body form in certain cases. For example, mites of the genus *Demodex* have evolved into tiny cigar-shaped organisms that fit comfortably into the hair follicles and sebaceous glands of the skin. An even more extreme example is provided by *Sacculina,* a relative of barnacles that grows like a plant's root system in the body of its crab host. However, most parasitic arthropods resemble their free-living relatives morphologically but differ from them in quite remarkable physiological and behavioral adaptations to the parasitic mode of life. For example, the bloodsucking stable fly, horn fly, and tsetse strongly resemble their scavenging cousin the common house fly, and there is no obvious morphological difference between the many species of maggots that thrive in decaying plant and animal matter and the "screwworm" that completes its larval development in living flesh. The resemblance of certain parasites to their free-living relatives creates a diagnostic pitfall. Even their presence at the scene of the crime is not sufficient proof of guilt. Fly maggots and coprophilic beetles are frequently found in fecal specimens. In almost every such case, these insects have invaded the fecal mass after defecation and never were parasites at all.

Unfortunately, even when we restrict our consideration to unambiguously parasitic arthropods, we still have too big a chore on our hands. Medical entomology is a formidable subject, and the selection of appropriate information is not always an easy task because certain topics that at first appear to bear directly on current problems of veterinary practice actually lie within the responsibilities of very few veterinarians. For example,

information on mosquitoes may occupy half of a textbook of medical entomology, and mosquitoes serve as vectors of such important diseases as equine encephalomyelitis and canine heartworm infection. However, few veterinarians invest the time and effort necessary to acquire a detailed knowledge of mosquitoes because control of these pests is usually the responsibility of the medical entomologist. Of more direct interest to veterinarians are the kinds of parasitic arthropods that live in more prolonged and intimate association with domestic animals. In this book, considerably more attention is therefore devoted to lice, fleas, ticks, and mites than to mosquitoes.

The arthropods of veterinary importance belong to the classes Insecta, Arachnida, Pentastomida, Crustacea, and Diplopoda. Insects and arachnids compose the bulk of this chapter. The class Pentastomida, or "tongue worms," comprises a small group of parasites of the respiratory systems of predacious reptiles, birds, and mammals and is considered only briefly. The class Crustacea (copepods, crabs, crayfish, and sowbugs) contains many taxa that serve as intermediate hosts of helminth parasites, but only the copepods are discussed because they tend to be a little less familiar to the average person. The class Diplopoda (millipedes), which contains at least one genus, *Narceus,* that serves as intermediate host of *Macracanthorhynchus ingens,* a very large acanthocephalan parasite of the raccoon and domestic dog, is mentioned only in passing in this book.

■ CLASS INSECTA
Structure

The body of adult insects consists of the **head, thorax,** and **abdomen.** The head consists of a variable number of fused segments and bears two eyes, two antennae, and a complex set of mouthparts. The thorax consists of three segments, the prothorax, mesothorax, and metathorax, and bears six jointed legs and four, two, or no wings, depending on the zoological order to which the insect in question belongs. Thus roaches (Dictyoptera), beetles (Coleoptera), and certain bugs (Hemiptera) have four wings, most flies (Diptera) have two, and the lice (Mallophaga and Anoplura) and fleas (Siphonaptera) are wingless. When four wings are present, one pair arises from the mesothorax and the second pair from the metathorax. The functional wings of Diptera arise from the mesothorax. The abdomen consists of 11 or fewer segments, of which the terminal ones are modified for copulation or egg laying. As typical arthropods, insects have a **chitinous cuticle** secreted by the **hypodermis,** a single layer of columnar epithelial cells of ectodermal origin, which is cast off or **molted** at intervals to permit growth and metamorphosis. The chitinous cuticle serves as an **exoskeleton,** thus as both a body covering and a place for attachment of muscles. Heavily chitinized areas or plates of cuticle are connected by thinner, lightly chitinized areas, thus permitting movement and some degree of expansion as, for example, when the abdomen of a feeding female mosquito fills with blood. Insect muscles are striated and often capable of extraordinarily rapid contraction. The cuticle is overlain by a thin lipoidal surface layer, the **epicuticle,** which is impermeable to water but freely permeable to lipids and lipid-soluble substances. Disruption of the epicuticle by silica aerogel insecticides results in death of the insect by dehydration; such insecticides are thus physically rather than chemically active.

When a developing insect has grown too large for its cuticle, the hypodermis lays down a new, thin, elastic cuticle under the old one. The old cuticle then splits, and the insect emerges from it. This process, termed **molting** or **ecdysis,** divides the life of the individual insect into a series of **stages,** or **instars.** All instars of cockroaches, bugs, and lice resemble their parents except for being smaller, whereas a newly hatched fly, beetle, or flea looks more like a worm than an insect. The former situation is called **simple metamorphosis** and the series of juvenile instars are called **nymphs,** whereas the latter situation is called **complex metamorphosis** and the juvenile instars are called **larvae.** In complex metamorphosis, the complete restructuring necessary for the transformation of the wormlike larva into the adult insect takes place during the **pupal** stage, and all related events are referred to as **pupation.**

Order Trichoptera, Caddisflies

Trichoptera is a very large group of flies (some 7000+ species) that is better known to fly fishermen than to medical entomologists. These flies have four wings and short mouth parts that are used for consuming water and nectar (Figure 1-1).

In species that occur in temperate climates, the adult population is often limited to one generation per year, and they may occur in large blooms. The larvae are aquatic in fresh water and feed on microorganisms or as predators on other insects. The larvae will often construct a portable case in which they live, with only their legs and head protruding. Ultimately the larva will form a cocoon from which the adult emerges. The males swarm over bodies of water, and females fly into the swarms to be fertilized. The females lay their eggs near water so the larvae that hatch can make their way into this environment. A good guide to the species of caddisflies has been produced for the fly-fishing enthusiast (Pobst and Richards, 1999).

The flies became important in veterinary medicine only recently. Work by Madigan and others at the University of California–Davis has shown that they serve as vectors of Potomac horse fever's causative agent, *Ehrlichia risticii*. It seems that the caddisflies are intermediate hosts of the metacercarial stage of trematode parasites of bats (trematodes of the family Lecithodenriidae) or trout, *Deropegus* sp., *Crepidostomum* sp. and *Creptotrema* sp. (Pusterla et al, 2000). Unfortunately, these trematodes are often, as in the case of the rickettsial disease of salmon poisoning in dogs, infected with a rickettsia, *E. risticii*. Horses fed mature caddisflies *(Dicosmoecus gilvipes)* developed the clinical and hematological disease of Potomac horse fever (Madigan et al, 2000). Thus when the horse digests the caddisfly containing the trematode metacercaria, it releases the *E. risticii* that causes the disease in the horse. The finding is important because control can be as simple as providing horses with waterers that are covered in some fashion to prevent the bodies of these flies from contaminating the horse's drinking water.

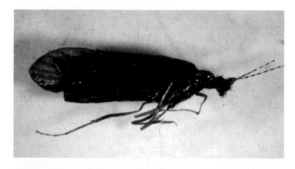

FIGURE 1-1   Caddisfly adult. The larvae of these flies become infected with the metacercariae of trematodes harboring the causative agent of Potomac horse fever.
(Courtesy Dr. John E. Madigan, School of Veterinary Medicine, University of California, Davis, California.)

Order Diptera, Flies

Adult flies, except certain specialized groups such as the parasites of the family Hippoboscidae, have one pair of functional mesothoracic wings. The metathoracic pair are represented by club-shaped balancing organs called **halteres** (Figure 1-2), which are present even in the wingless hippoboscids. Metamorphosis is complex. Although most flies produce eggs or are **oviparous,** a few deposit larvae that have already hatched, and the females producing larvae in this manner are said to be **ovoviviparous.** Hippoboscids and tsetses retain their larvae within their abdomens through the third larval instar, and these pupate almost immediately upon being born.

There are three main groups of flies: the gnats and mosquitoes of the Nematocera, the horse flies and deer flies of the Brachycera, and the more highly evolved flies of the Cyclorrhapha (Table 1-1). All three contain bloodsucking species, many of which serve as disease vectors. In the Nematocera and Brachycera, only the females take blood meals, and usually, larval development occurs in aquatic environments. Larvae of muscid, sarcophagid, calliphorid, and oestrid cyclorrhaphans can invade living tissues to produce a pathological condition called **myiasis.**

TABLE 1-1 ■ Classification of the Diptera

Nematocera	Brachycera	Cyclorrhapha
Culicidae, mosquitoes	Horse and deer flies	Muscidae, house flies
Simulidae, black flies		Sarcophagidae, flesh flies
Ceratopogonidae, midges		Calliphoridae, blow flies
Psychodidae, sand flies		Oestridae and other bot flies

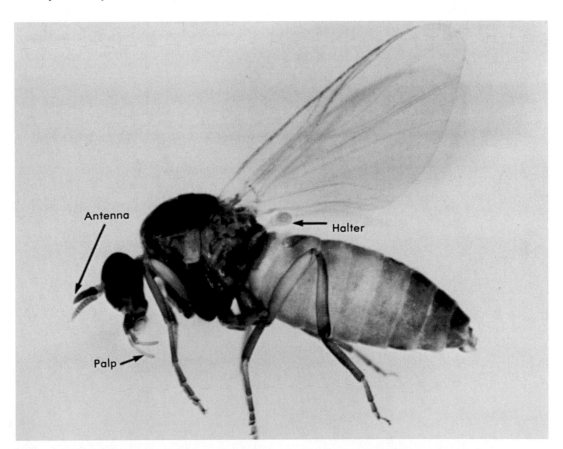

FIGURE 1-2 *Simulium* (Nematocera: Simuliidae), a black fly (×24). The halteres (singular, halter) are balancing organs that have evolved in Diptera in place of the metathoracic wings. The maxillary palpi are sensory structures associated with the mouthparts. The antennae of black flies consist of 11 similar segments.

Nematocera

Nematocerans are typically small and relatively delicate. The antennae are long and many-segmented, and the individual segments resemble one another like beads on a string. Nematocerans generally breed in aquatic or semiaquatic habitats, and their larvae are suitably endowed with appendages for swimming, breathing, and gathering food in water. Only female nematocerans suck blood; the males never do and subsist instead on nectar.

Family Culicidae, Mosquitoes

Identification

Mosquitoes have long, 14- or 15-segmented antennae, an elongated proboscis consisting of a bundle of stylets loosely encased in a sheath formed by the labium, and fringes of scales on the wings (Figure 1-3). These anatomical details are sufficient **taxonomic characters** to reliably distinguish the **taxon** that we recognize as mosquitoes from other insects with which they might be confused.

Life History

Mosquitoes lay their eggs on water or in dry places that tend to flood seasonally. Eggs laid on water hatch in less than a week. Larvae (Figure 1-4) are air breathers and die within hours if their air supply is shut off by an oil film on the water's surface. The larvae molt four times, usually within the space of 2 weeks, and then pupate. As is characteristic of all nematocerans and brachycerans, the pupa emerges through a T-shaped hole in the back of the last larval skin. Culicid pupae are elaborate, free-swimming organisms with a large cephalothorax. As development proceeds, the structures of the adult mosquito become apparent (Figure 1-5). The pupal stage ordinarily lasts from 2 days to a week, but a few hours suffice for certain dry climate species. The adult mosquito emerges through a hole in the back of the pupal case as it floats at the water's surface. After about 24 hours, the wings have expanded and hardened, and the mosquito is able to fly. Only female mosquitoes suck blood, the protein of which is necessary for the maturation

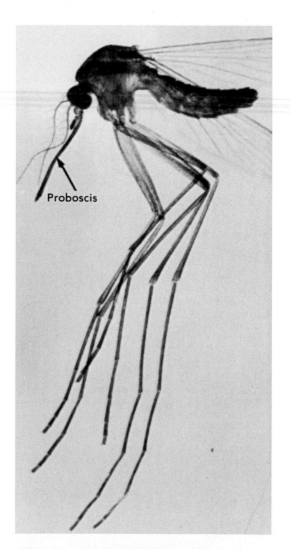

FIGURE 1-3   A mosquito (Nematocera: Culicidae) (×13). Note the long antennae and long mouthparts (proboscis).

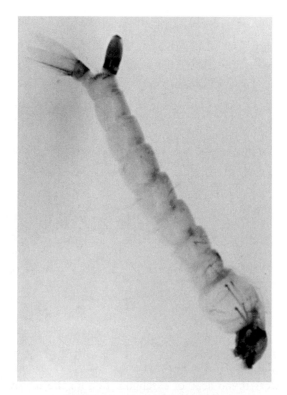

FIGURE 1-4   Mosquito larva (×15).

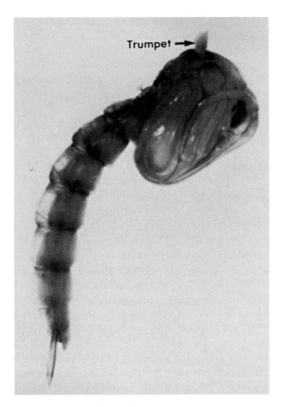

Trumpet →

FIGURE 1-5 Mosquito pupa (×16). The "trumpets" on the cephalothorax are pupal respiratory structures. The eyes, legs, thorax, and abdomen of the developing adult mosquito can be seen through the pupal cuticle.

of the ovaries. Males and nonreproductive females get by on nectar and plant juices. The females of some species that normally feed on blood are sometimes capable of ovarian maturation without a blood meal (i.e., the females are **autogenous**). Other species of mosquitoes feed only on plants, and therefore these species are of little interest as pests or disease vectors. Mammals and birds are preferred hosts (or victims) both of blood-feeding mosquitoes and of the various disease organisms that they transmit.

Injury
Under ordinary circumstances, the amount of blood lost to mosquito attack is entirely trivial. Sometimes, however, circumstances favor the simultaneous emergence of enormous swarms of mosquitoes that by their concerted attacks can actually bleed cattle to death. For example, 7 days after Hurricane Allen (August 10, 1980) brought a prolonged drought to an abrupt end and flooded 5000 acres of a Texas ranch, cattle were observed to be visibly distressed by swarms of *Aedes sollicitans* mosquitoes. The next morning, 15 cattle were found dead of exsanguination manifested by extreme pallor of the mucous membranes and

postmortal evidence of severe anemia. The interval of 7 days between flooding of the pastures and the sudden death of the cattle corresponded exactly to the time required for *Ae. sollicitans* to develop from egg to biting adult once its dormancy had been ended by high water. The flood led to the synchronous development of vast numbers of eggs that had accumulated during the prolonged drought, thus producing the enormous swarms of mosquitoes capable of exsanguinating mature cattle overnight. Abbitt and Abbitt, who obtained and thoughtfully analyzed the evidence in this outbreak, estimated that 3.8 million mosquito bites (5300 bites per minute for 12 hours) would be required to remove half of the total blood volume from a 366-kg cow, assuming that a mosquito removes 0.0039 ml per blood meal (Abbitt and Abbitt, 1981). Cats will sometimes develop allergies to flea bites that will present as large pruritic and erythremic lesions on the nose or other parts of the face (Clare and Medleau, 1997).

Disease Transmission
A **vector** is an animal, often an arthropod, that transmits an infective organism from one host to another. A vector that transmits infective organisms directly (and necessarily, promptly) to a recipient host without development or multiplication of the organisms having occurred is called a **mechanical vector.** A **biological vector,** by contrast, is one in which the infective organisms either undergo development or multiply or do both before being transmitted to the recipient host. Thus a biological vector is a true host of the disease organism. In the case of sexually reproducing disease organisms such as protozoans and helminths, vectors that host developing or asexually reproducing stages of the organism are termed **intermediate** hosts, whereas vectors that host sexually mature stages are termed **definitive hosts.** *Culex, Aedes, Anopheles,* and other genera of mosquitos serve as biological vectors (intermediate hosts) of filariid worms such as *Dirofilaria immitis,* the canine heartworm, and *Wuchereria bancrofti,* the cause of human lymphatic filariasis. Mosquitoes of the genus *Anopheles* serve as biological vectors (definitive hosts) of the blood-inhabiting protozoon genus *Plasmodium* that causes malaria in birds, rodents, and primates. Mosquitoes also serve as biological vectors of viral encephalitides (e.g., equine encephalomyelitis), West Nile virus, and the viruses of rabbit myxomatosis, fowl pox, and yellow, dengue, and Rift Valley fevers. In the case of viruses, bacteria, and the like, the terms "intermediate" and "definitive" are redundant inasmuch as sexual reproduction does not occur in these groups.

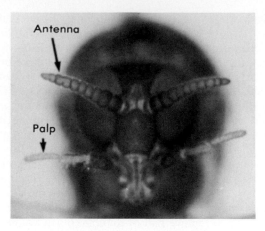

FIGURE 1-6 Head of a black fly (Nematocera: Simuliidae) (×27).

Family Simuliidae, Black Flies

Identification

Black flies (see Figure 1-2) are small, stout-bodied, black, gray, or yellowish-brown flies with relatively short antennae consisting of nine to 12 (usually 11) similar segments, and short mouthparts with prominent maxillary palps (Figure 1-6).

Life History

Black flies breed only in running water. Although mountain torrents and temporary upland streams are favored breeding sites of many species, some particularly important species breed in large rivers. Eggs are deposited on the water's surface or on partly submerged stones, twigs, or vegetation. In species that produce several broods per year (**multivoltine** species), larvae hatch from these eggs a few days later, but in species that produce only one brood per year (**univoltine** species), the eggs remain in a protracted state of metabolic quiescence, or **diapause,** and do not hatch until the following year. Black fly larvae manage to cling to the surfaces of stones in rapidly moving, turbulent streams partly by means of little hooks on their posteriors and on a short **proleg** near the anterior end of their bodies (Figure 1-7). By flexing their bodies, the larvae are able to move from place to place like inchworms. Black fly larvae also spin silken strands to help anchor themselves and later to form cocoons, by means of which the pupae continue to cling to the rocks. Adults emerge from these pupae and are carried to the surface in a bubble of air.

Injury

The female black fly is a vicious biter. Her mouthparts comprise a bundle of flattened, serrated, bladelike stylets loosely ensheathed by the labium, which itself terminates in a pair of labella. Instead of piercing a blood vessel and feeding from the lumen as a mosquito, bed bug, or sucking louse does, the female black fly lacerates tissues until a pool of blood forms, and then she imbibes the blood from the pool.

Susceptibility to and severity of host reaction to the bites of many arthropods vary remarkably among individuals. With continued exposure to bites, initially susceptible individuals may become relatively immune so that they are less frequently bitten or suffer less reaction to the bites. Or, less fortunately, they may become hypersensitive so that continued attack excites a more severe and sometimes even fatal reaction. Sensitivity to the bites of black flies is a common phenomenon, and the reactive wheal may continue to itch for many days and tends to be aggravated by scratching. In a hypersensitive person, a single bite may evoke sufficient edematous reaction to force the eyelids shut. Burghardt, Whitlock, and McEnerney (1951) described a dermatitis in cattle due to *Simulium.* The lesions consisted of blisters, welts, and scabs affecting the head, thorax, and ears, and acute exudative lesions along the midabdominal line. Heavy swarms of black flies have been known to kill grazing livestock by the thousands. However, the exact cause of death, whether it be anemia, hypersensitivity reactions, or toxin absorbed from fly saliva injected into the bite, remains problematical. During black fly season, dogs and cats can present with small pruritic bloody spots on the ears, face, or body. Prevention of such bites is best done using repellents.

Disease Transmission

Black flies transmit leucocytozoonosis, a disease of poultry and wild birds caused by several species of the haemosporidian protozoan genus *Leucocytozoon.* Black flies also serve as obligate intermediate hosts of the filariid nematode *Onchocerca gutterosa,* an apparently innocuous parasite of cattle. In the black fly, the worm develops from the skin-dwelling microfilarial stage ingested by the fly to the third-stage larval nematode that is infective to the next host. Black flies also serve as vectors of the related nematode parasite *Onchocerca volvulus* that causes human onchocerciasis, which is manifested by the formation of dermal nodules and leads, predominantly in the African form of the disease, to blindness. Because the vectors are riverine breeders, the disease tends to be concentrated along valleys, and the ensuing blindness is thus called "river blindness."

Control

Black flies attack in swarms during daylight hours and when the air is relatively still. Smoke repels them and, although chemical repellents afford a

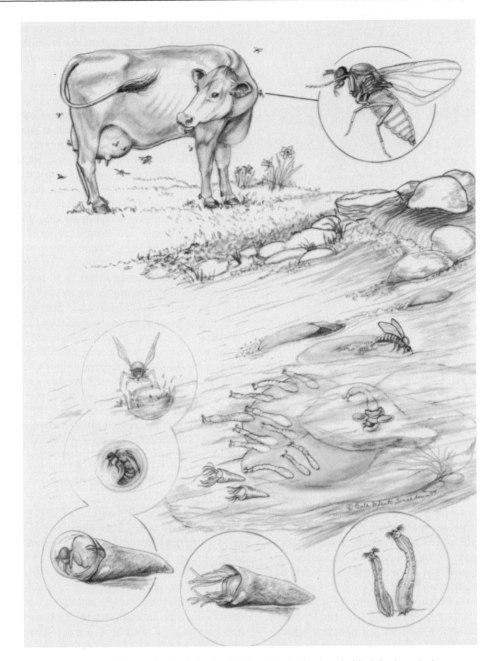

FIGURE 1-7 Life history of a black fly (family Simuliidae). The female black fly deposits her eggs on partly submerged objects in rapidly flowing streams. The larvae that hatch from these eggs cling to the stones and feed on organic matter carried by the current. When ready to pupate, the larvae spin silken cocoons that secure them to the substrate. Adults that emerge from these pupal cases are carried to the surface in a bubble of air and fly off in search of a blood meal.

degree of protection, campers, gardeners, and livestock usually find their surest relief in the lee of a smudge pot. Livestock should be stabled until sundown during seasons of particularly heavy black fly attack. Black flies can be discouraged from attacking horses' ears by applying petroleum jelly to the inner surface of the pinna.

Family Ceratopogonidae (Heleidae), Biting Midges, "No-See-Ums"

Identification

Ceratopogonids are tiny (less than 2 mm), relatively glabrous flies. Their antennae are long and slender, and their mouthparts are relatively short (Figure 1-8).

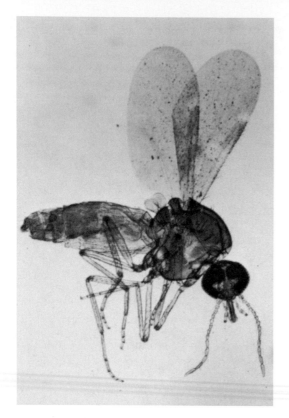

FIGURE 1-8 *Culicoides* (Nematocera: Heleidae), a "no-see-um" (×37). *Culicoides* differs from Culicidae mosquitoes in being smaller and having a shorter proboscis.

Life History

Life histories of various species differ in detail, some requiring freshwater and others saltwater habitats. Some breed in water-filled holes in trees, others in decaying vegetation, sandy and silt soils, and the like. Adults are crepuscular and nocturnal. Only females suck blood and, although they are fairly strong flyers, tend to remain close to their breeding grounds. A few, however, may venture forth as far as a half mile when the air is still. Most important species belong to the genera *Culicoides* and *Leptoconops*.

Injury

The bites of *Culicoides* inflict pain far out of proportion to the size of the fly. In fact, people victimized by these tiny terrors frequently do not realize that they are being tormented by insects, sometimes mistaking them for a bit of cigarette ash because of their small size. *Culicoides* easily pass through standard window screening and make themselves obnoxious to sleepers. In sensitized individuals, the bites last longer and are more painful than mosquito bites.

"Queensland itch," demonstrated by Riek (1953a) as representing allergic dermatitis caused by the development of hypersensitivity to the bites of *Culicoides robertsi,* afflicts only certain horses. Other horses pastured with the sufferers never show any signs of disease. Initial lesions are discrete papules confined to the dorsal surfaces. Later, the hair mats and crusts form and eventually fall off, leaving hairless areas that, in severe cases, become confluent. Pruritus is intense, and horses may injure themselves by scratching and rolling to relieve the itching. The attacks of *C. robertsi* and associated allergic dermatitis were prevented by stabling the affected horses from 4:00 in the afternoon until 7:00 the next morning or by spraying them weekly with dichlorodiphenyltrichloroethane (DDT). Antihistamine therapy accelerated regression of the lesions (Riek, 1953b).

Disease Transmission

Culicoides spp. transmit the viruses of bluetongue, African horse sickness, and possibly bovine ephemeral fever. *Onchocerca cervicalis* of horses, *Onchocerca gibsoni* of cattle, and three relatively innocuous filariid parasites of man (*Dipetalonema perstans, Dipetalonema streptocerca,* and *Mansonella ozzardi*) all develop from microfilaria to infective third-stage larva in the bodies of *Culicoides.* Protozoans transmitted by *Culicoides* include *Hepatocystis* of Old World monkeys and *Haemoproteus* and *Leucocytozoon* of wild and domestic birds.

Family Psychodidae, Sand Flies
Identification

Psychodids are small, dull-colored, slender flies with long antennae. The wing veins radiate in nearly straight lines from the base to the tip of the wing (Figure 1-9).

Life History

Psychodids lay their eggs in cracks, crevices, or burrows where moderate temperatures, darkness, and nearly 100% humidity prevail. They spend at least 2 months as egg, larva, and pupa but are short-lived as adults. Adult psychodids are weak flyers and nocturnal in habit. Important species belong to the genera *Phlebotomus* and *Lutzomyia. Phlebotomus* occurs in the Old World and *Lutzomyia* in the New World; all species are tropical or subtropical in distribution.

Disease Transmission

Psychodids transmit *Leishmania* spp., hemoflagellate parasites of dogs, rodents, and primates, including humans (Table 1-2). It appears that molecules in the salivary gland secretions of the ceratopogonid vector modulate to some extent the course of *Leishmania* development in the host that

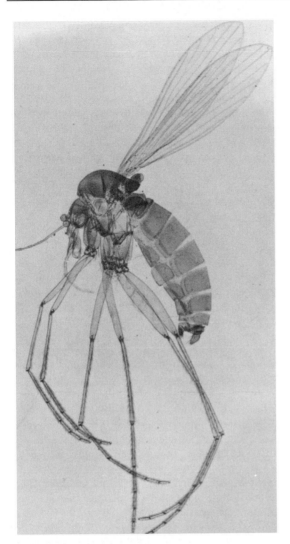

FIGURE 1-9 *Phlebotomus* (Nematocera: Psychodidae) (×29). The wing veins radiate in nearly straight lines from the base to the tip of the wing.

TABLE 1-2 ■ Some Pathogens Vectored by Nematoceran Flies

Vector	Some transmitted pathogens
Culicidae (mosquitos)	Filariids *Setaria:* horses, cattle, deer Heartworm: dogs and cats *Wuchereria* and *Brugia:* humans and cats Protozoa Malaria *(Plasmodium):* birds and primates Viruses Equine encephalitis West Nile virus Rift Valley fever
Simulidae (black flies)	Filariids *Onchocerca:* horses, cattle, sheep, humans Protozoa Malaria *(Leucocytozoon):* birds
Ceratopogonidae (biting midges)	Filariids *Onchocerca*: horses *Dipetalonema*: primates Protozoa Malaria *(Leucocytozoon):* birds Viruses Blue tongue African horse sickness
Pychodidae (sand flies)	Protozoa *Leishmania* spp. Rickettsia *Bartonella* Viruses 3-day fever virus

is bitten (Warburg et al, 1994). Also transmitted are the 3-day fever virus and *Bartonella bacilliformis* infection of humans.

Brachycera

Family Tabanidae, Horse Flies and Deer Flies
Identification
Tabanids are stout-bodied flies varying from about the size of a house fly to as large as a hummingbird. The short, stout, anteriorly projecting antennae consist of three markedly different segments (Figures 1-10 and 1-11). The first segment is small, the second may be expanded, and the third is marked by annulations that make tabanid antennae appear to have many more than three units.

Life History
Female tabanids require a blood meal for maturation of their eggs and obtain it from mammals, reptiles, and, occasionally, birds. Male tabanids are not blood feeders but subsist on nectar, sap, and aphid feces; the females also require these sources of carbohydrate in addition to blood (Mally and Kutzer, 1984). With the exception of a few xerophilic species, tabanids tend to be concentrated along water courses. Eggs are neatly glued in masses of 400 to 1000 to foliage overhanging water. Larvae hatch in a week or so, depending on temperature and relative humidity, and drop into the water. First- and second-stage larvae do not feed, but the third and later stages are aggressively carnivorous or saprophagic and feed on insect larvae, crustaceans, snails, earthworms, young

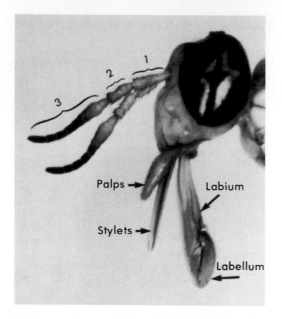

FIGURE 1-10 *Chrysops* (Brachycera: Tabanidae), a deer fly (×19). Because the distal segment of the tabanid antenna is annulated, it gives the impression that the antenna consists of many segments; however, there are only three.

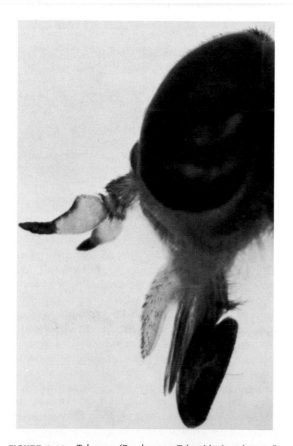

FIGURE 1-11 *Tabanus* (Brachycera: Tabanidae), a horse fly (×20).

frogs, plant tissues, and dead organic matter, depending on the species of tabanid and the availability of food (Mally and Kutzer, 1984). In temperate regions, larvae overwinter by burying themselves in soil or dead vegetation and pupate the following spring. Thus usually only one generation is produced each year. Adult tabanids are strong flyers and very difficult to discourage. In Michigan, *Hybomitra* spp. were found to reach maximum abundance in early summer (May to June), whereas *Chrysops* spp. and *Tabanus* spp. were most abundant in late summer (early to late July; Strickler and Walker, 1993). In the salt marshes of Cape Cod, Massachusetts, the greenhead flies, *Tabanus nigrovittatus and Tabanus conterminus,* were found to be most active in the afternoon (Hayes et al, 1993). In Florida, peak *Chrysops* activity occurred in the morning and evening, with a correlation to relative humidity rather than to temperature and light intensity (Cilek and Schreiber, 1996). Konstantinov (1993) showed that masking the visibility of a cow by placing it in a wooded area did not reduce the number of *Hybomitra* flies that found the cow when they were released 150 meters from the host animal.

Injury

All arthropod attacks cause some annoyance to the host and exact some expenditure of energy in efforts to avoid or relieve their effects. When flies are particularly numerous, pastured livestock may be driven frantic by incessant attacks and can spend so much time and energy combating the onslaught that they cannot rest or graze adequately. The resultant exhaustion always interferes with production and sometimes proves fatal. Certain insects are particularly feared by livestock. Some horse flies are as large as hummingbirds and inflict an excruciating bite. When one of these monsters attacks, horses are likely to bolt, and it behooves the rider or driver to come promptly to their aid. In biting, the mandibles and maxillae of tabanids lacerate the blood vessels and the labella lap up the blood that flows freely from the wound. Repeated attacks in the skin folds about a cow's udder and in the groove between the udder halves lead to extensive weeping eczematous lesions that may become secondarily infected with bacteria. After a tabanid has finished feeding, the bite wound tends to bleed for many minutes, thus attracting opportunists such as *Musca.* In fact, *Musca* and other flies can often be seen clustered about a feeding tabanid, exploiting the bounty afforded by its sloppy manner of taking a meal. Vicious daylight bloodsuckers, tabanids do not usually attack indoors, but if already feeding when the host enters a building, they will continue to feed until replete. The most efficient solution to tabanid attack is to stable the animals during the hours of peak fly activity.

Disease Transmission

The pain that a tabanid inflicts when it bites tends to increase its efficiency as a mechanical vector of disease organisms. The fly, driven away by its victim's defenses before it has had time to feed to repletion, soon alights on a second host to finish its meal and perhaps to contaminate the wound with fresh, mechanically borne bacteria (e.g., anthrax), viruses (e.g., equine infectious anemia), and the like. The large volume of blood imbibed by each tabanid (up to four times the weight of the fly; Krinsky, 1976) also contributes to its efficiency as a mechanical vector by helping to compensate for the low concentration of microorganisms usually found in blood, and for their failure to multiply in the body of the intermediate host.

Tabanids have been incriminated in the mechanical transmission of anaplasmosis (*Anaplasma* spp.), anthrax *(Bacillus anthracis),* tularemia ("deer fly fever," *Francisella tularensis*), and equine infectious anemia virus. Mechanical transmission of equine infectious anemia virus from acutely infected ponies to susceptible ponies occurred after as few as 10 bites by contaminated *Tabanus fuscicostatus,* but all attempts at transmission from a chronically infected pony failed (Hawkins et al, 1973). Mammalian trypanosomes (hemoflagellate protozoans) may be transmitted mechanically or biologically by tabanids, depending on the species involved. Surra *(Trypanosoma evansi),* a fatal disease of horses, camels, elephants, and dogs in Asia, is transmitted mechanically, and the flies lose their ability to transmit the infection a few hours after feeding on an animal infected with surra (Table 1-3). *Trypanosoma theileri,* on the other hand, must multiply in the body of the tabanid because it is so scarce in the blood of cattle that one must usually resort to culture techniques to demonstrate its presence there. Otherwise, *T. theileri* would not be distributed throughout the world as a parasite of cattle and their near relatives. A vector in which

such parasitic organisms multiply is sometimes referred to as a **cyclopropagative host** to distinguish it from a **cyclodevelopmental host,** in which the parasite actually undergoes ontogenetic development. An example of the latter is *Elaeophora schneideri,* the arterial worm of deer, elk, and domestic sheep in the southwestern United States, which develops from the microfilarial stage in the blood to the infective third stage within the body of the tabanid (Hibler and Adcock, 1971). More details concerning disease transmission by tabanids are to be found in the review by Krinsky (1976).

Control

Horse flies and deer flies are most difficult to kill or repel; often the best solution is to stable livestock during the hours of peak fly activity. These flies can use blood from wild animals as food and have larval habitats independent of domestic livestock. Thus unlike flies more directly dependent on their hosts, such as *Stomoxys* and *Haematobia*, these flies can be controlled chemically by repellents alone (Foil and Hogsette, 1994). Konstantinov (1992) showed that only 3% of flies attacking a cow are killed by the cows during their attacks. McMahan and Gaugler (1993) suggested that the draining of salt marsh areas to decrease mosquito populations may inadvertently have actually increased habitats preferred by larval tabanids and hence increased the numbers of these biting flies.

Cyclorrhapha

The Cyclorrhapha represents the apex of dipteran evolution, and the common house fly, *Musca domestica,* is a typical example. Instead of the aquatic habitats favored by nematocerans and brachycerans, cyclorrhaphans tend to breed in decaying plant and animal tissues, manure, carrion, and the like. The three larval instars are more or less conical animals with a mouth, usually armed with hooks, at the apex and a pair of prominent respiratory openings called **spiracles** or **stigmata** at the base. Slender larvae of the families Muscidae, Sarcophagidae, and Calliphoridae are usually referred to as **maggots** (Figure 1-12), whereas the rather stout larvae of the family Oestridae and its relatives are called **bots** or grubs (compare with Figure 1-27). When the third instar larva enters the pupal stage, its integument hardens to form a **puparium,** or pupal case. Pupae of most cyclorraphan flies are found in decaying organic material or soil. A few species have specialized pupation sites. For example, pupae of the sheep ked *Melophagus ovinus* are found attached to the wool of their host. The adult fly emerges through a circular hole in the anterior end of the puparium. Cyclorrhaphan antennae consist of three dissimilar

---

TABLE 1-3 ■ **Some Pathogens Vectored by Brachyceran Flies**

Mechanically vectored	Biologically vectored
Anthrax	Filariids
Tularemia	*Elaeophora:* elk, sheep
Protozoa *Trypanosoma evansi*	Protozoa *Trypanosoma theileri:* cattle

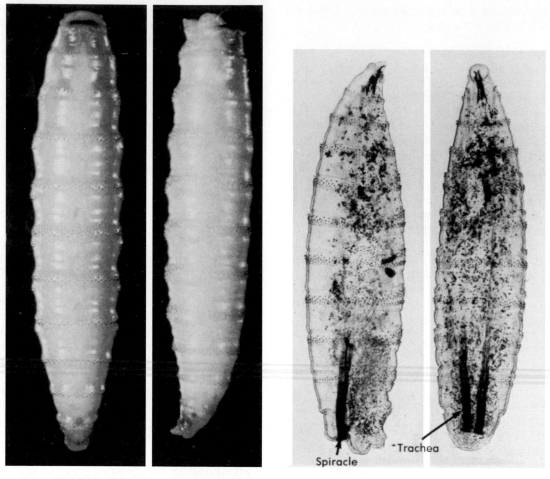

FIGURE 1-12 Muscoid third-stage larva or maggot of the family Calliphoridae (×10). Note the pigmented tracheal trunks leading from the posterior spiracles. Pigmented tracheae are a specific character of *Cochliomyia hominivorax*, the American screwworm. (Specimens courtesy R.J. Gagné.)

segments, the third and largest of which bears a frondlike structure called an **arista** near its proximal end. The antennae are directed ventrally, but the aristae project anteriorly (Figure 1-13). Parasitic specialization has proceeded in two directions in the Cyclorrhapha. In the families Muscidae and Hippoboscidae there has been specialization from a type adapted to lapping up liquids (e.g., *Musca*) (Figure 1-13) toward a bayonet-like proboscis for piercing the skin and sucking blood (e.g., *Stomoxys*) and thus toward parasitism in the adult stage. In the families Calliphoridae and Sarcophagidae and certain members of the family Muscidae, the adult flies have retained their lapping mouthparts and remained scavengers; instead, it is in the larval stages that parasitism has evolved. The botflies (e.g., *Hypoderma* and *Gasterophilus*) have proceeded even further in this direction. Their larvae have become highly specialized host- and site-specific parasites,

whereas the mouthparts of the adult flies have become vestigial and nonfunctional. Parasitism by fly larvae is termed **myiasis** and is of worldwide economic importance.

Family Muscidae
Musca

IDENTIFICATION. The genus *Musca* contains 26 species of which three, *M. domestica,* the common house fly, *Musca autumnalis,* the face fly, and *Musca vetustissima,* the Australian bush fly, may serve as examples. These three species resemble each other closely enough to require an expert to distinguish specimens on morphological grounds but differ sufficiently in behavior to make their identities obvious to anyone familiar with their habits. The mouthparts of these all too familiar flies consist of a fleshy, retractable proboscis terminating in a pair of corrugated spongy organs, the **labella** (see Figure 1-13).

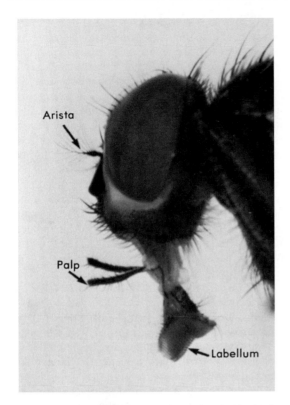

Arista

Palp

Labellum

FIGURE 1-13 Head of *Musca domestica* (Cyclorrhapha: Muscidae), the common house fly (×29). The proboscis is retractable into the head.

LIFE HISTORY AND DISEASE TRANSMISSION. *M. domestica* lays its eggs on animal manure or almost any kind of decaying organic material. A female *M. domestica* may deposit 2000 eggs in an average lifetime of 6 to 8 weeks. A tiny, white, first-stage larva (maggot) hatches from the egg in a day or less at summer temperatures. This larva grows, molts twice, and in a few days becomes a fully developed third-stage larva. When ready to pupate, the third-

stage larva migrates into a drier medium, shortens, thickens, and becomes darker in color as a result of hardening and tanning of the third-stage cuticle in forming the puparium. The adult fly emerges in 2 or 3 weeks by forcing off the end of the puparium with its **ptilinum,** a bladderlike structure inflated with hemolymph. The ptilinum projects from the **frontal suture** and is withdrawn into the head after the fly has emerged from the puparium. Like the umbilicus of mammals, it is of no further service to the animal. The adult fly then makes its way to the surface of the medium in which the pupa lies buried, expands its wings by pumping hemolymph into the wing veins, and flies away in search of food. The house fly feeds on feces, syrup, milk, decaying fruit, and other dissolved and soluble materials. House flies will feed on secretions around the eyes, nostrils, and mouth and on blood that continues to ooze from wounds made by tabanids. *Musca* species annoy horses and cattle to distraction on warm, sunny days. Bacteria, protozoan cysts, helminth eggs, and other disease organisms may be transported from filth to food, body openings, and wounds by way of the feces, vomit spots, sticky feet, and body hairs of house flies. The house fly also serves as a biological vector of *Draschia megastoma* and *Habronema muscae,* nematode parasites of the stomach of the horse (Table 1-4).

M. autumnalis (face fly) was introduced into North America from Europe, Asia, or Africa in the early 1950s. These flies crawl about the faces of horses and cattle, feeding on the ocular and nasal discharges induced by their presence, and are extremely annoying to pastured animals. Eggs are deposited in fresh cattle dung, and the larvae pupate in the dried dung of nearby soil. The adult flies overwinter in buildings. These hibernating adults, like those of the cluster fly, *Pollenia rudis*

TABLE 1-4 ■ Some Pathogens Vectored by Flies of the Family Muscidae

Fly	Mechanically vectored	Biologically vectored
Musca domestica	Suspected of transmitting many agents but seldom shown conclusively	Spirurid nematodes *Draschia megastoma:* horses *Habronema muscae:* horses
Musca autumnalis	Keratoconjunctivitis	Spirurid nematodes *Thelazia* spp.: cattle
Fannia	Unknown	Spirurid nematodes *Thelazia* spp.: dogs
Stomoxys	Suspected	Spirurid nematodes *Habronema microstoma:* horses
Haematobia	Suspected	Filariid nematodes *Stephanofilaria*

(a calliphorid fly that as a maggot parasitizes earthworms and whose adults cluster together inside dwellings in winter to hibernate), cause considerable annoyance to the human occupants when, aroused by a spell of warmish weather, they go buzzing and blundering about the house, falling into drinks and making themselves generally disagreeable. Curiously, the active adult face fly of summer appears loath to enter buildings and may be observed to swarm off dairy cows as they enter the stable to be milked. They wait outside during milking and swarm back on the cows as they emerge from the stable. This, of course, contrasts with the behavior of *M. domestica,* so appropriately called the house fly. Grazing cattle afflicted with face fly infestations have been shown to increase their herbage dry matter intake as they graze deeper in the sward by taking heavier bites as they try to dislodge the flies from their muzzles (Dougherty et al, 1993). Face flies serve as biological vectors of *Thelazia* spp. (eyeworm), a genus of nematode worms that infect the conjunctival sacs of horses and cattle (Chitwood and Stoffolano, 1971). *M. autumnalis* also serves as mechanical vector of infectious bovine keratoconjunctivitis organisms (*Moraxella bovis),* which can survive for up to 3 days on the legs of the fly (Steve and Lilly, 1965). Cattle protected from face flies had less keratoconjunctivitis and yielded fewer isolates of hemolytic *M. bovis* than did unprotected cattle. "Infection first began to spread from herd to herd after face fly populations exceeded 10/animal for 1 month" (Gerhardt et al, 1981).

M. vetustissima, the Australian bush fly, resembles *M. autumnalis* in preferring to remain out-of-doors, by breeding in livestock manures, and in crawling about on the faces of livestock. However, *M. vetustissima* differs in displaying an exasperating affinity for the faces of human beings as well as livestock, by involvement of its larvae in wound myiasis, and by an inability to hibernate. Instead of hibernating, *M. vetustissima* reinvades southeastern Australia each spring from the more tropical regions to the north.

In South Africa, *Musca lusoria, Musca fasciata,* and *Musca nevilli* have been identified as vectors of a filariid worm *Parafilaria bovicola* that lives in the subcutis, bores a hole to the surface, and discharges its eggs in the bloody fluid that weeps from the lesion (Nevill, 1975, 1985; Kleynhans, 1987).

CONTROL. Selection and manner of applying insecticide must conform to regulations that are subject to change. Read the label carefully before applying any insecticide to premises or to domestic animals. Regular spraying of animal sheds, stables, and kennels with residual insecticides should provide good control of flies and other flying insects if reasonable effort is expended to minimize the extent of breeding sites available to these insects. Space sprays, insecticidal baits, and insecticidal resin strips offer additional control. Fenthion, diazinon, dimethoate, tetrachlorvinphos, and dichlorvos have excellent residual activity against house flies, face flies, horn flies, stable flies, and mosquitoes for from 1 to 4 weeks after application. Spraying resting and breeding areas is often effective. Dichlorvos, naled, pyrethrins, and pyrethroids are used as space sprays for feedlots and sheds. These insecticides may be misted over the backs of animals every 3 to 7 days. Fly baits containing dichlorvos and naled may be sprayed or sprinkled on fly-roosting areas. The sugar fly bait New Improved Golden Malrin contains methomyl and muscalure, a fly-attracting pheromone. The bait is sprinkled around barns. Muscalure attracts and keeps the flies around the bait, thus achieving an increased kill by the insecticide.

Fly control in dairy barns and milk rooms may be achieved with dichlorvos resin strips, baits, foggers, and sprays. Tetrachlorvinphos and coumaphos are used as sprays or in dust bags and may be applied after milking.

The application of insecticides to lactating cows producing milk for human consumption demands extreme caution because there must not be any pesticide in the milk. READ THE LABEL BEFORE USING ANY PESTICIDE. It is against the law to use a pesticide in any manner not specified on the label, and violations with respect to dairy cows are particularly serious.

The control of face flies and house flies on beef cattle and dry dairy cattle may be achieved by regular application of insecticides to animals and fly-breeding sites. Dichlorvos in mineral oil may be smeared daily on the faces of cattle for face fly control. Coumaphos, malathion, or tetrachlorvinphos may be applied to cattle as a free-flowing dust 2 or 3 times a week or self-applied by means of self-treatment dust bags. Pyrethrin or pyrethroid sprays may also be used. Pyrethroid-containing ear tags and similar devices that can be attached to animals allow a continuous, controlled release of insecticides to aid in the control of flies attacking cattle. Tetrachlorvinphos, a larvicidal organophosphate, prevents the growth of larvae of coprophilic flies in the manure of cattle fed this compound and may be given to lactating dairy cows.

Face fly control on horses may be attempted by application of coumaphos, pyrethrins, or pyrethroids to the entire horse, and elimination or insecticidal treatment of breeding sites (i.e., cow manure) when feasible. Face flies do not pursue their victims indoors, so stabling horses during hours of peak fly activity often proves to be the best solution.

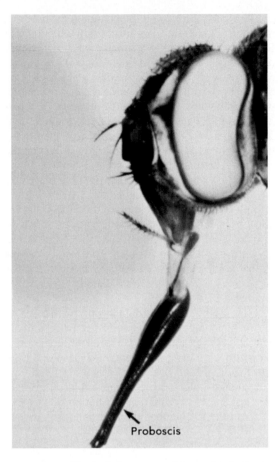

FIGURE 1-14 Head of *Stomoxys calcitrans* (Cyclorrhapha: Muscidae), the stable fly (×24). In feeding, the entire proboscis is thrust into the skin of the host.

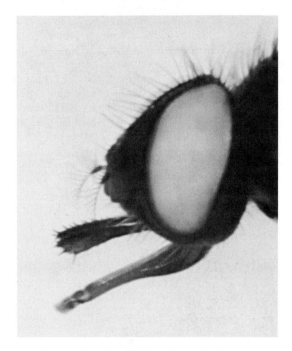

FIGURE 1-15 Head of *Haematobia irritans* (Cyclorrhapha: Muscidae), the horn fly (×65). *Haematobia* somewhat resembles *Stomoxys* but is only half as large and has palps almost as long as its proboscis (compare with Figure 1-13).

Biological control methods using parasitoid wasps have been developed and commercialized for the control of *Musca* spp. The larvae of the wasps develop in the maggots of these flies, causing their death. It is possible to purchase parasitized fly pupae from which the adult wasps will emerge, and these can be used to release the wasps on farms. The use of these wasps has proved to be of some benefit when incorporated into integrated fly management programs.

Stomoxys

IDENTIFICATION. The stable fly, *Stomoxys calcitrans*, resembles *Musca* spp. but has a long, pointed proboscis with which it inflicts painful bites instead of the vacuum cleaner affair with which *Musca* sucks up liquids from little puddles. The palpi of *Stomoxys* are shorter than the proboscis (Figure 1-14; compare with *Haematobia,* Figure 1-15). The third-stage larvae resemble those of *Musca* and have posterior spiracles with sinuous slits, but the spiracles are set farther apart than those of *Musca* (see Figure 1-19).

LIFE HISTORY. Stable flies have a life history similar to that of face flies but differ in preferring decaying organic materials, such as piles of lawn clippings, damp hay, grain, or animal manure for egg laying. Stable flies of both sexes feed on blood once or twice a day, depending on the ambient temperature, and suspend operations entirely during cold spells.

INJURY AND DISEASE TRANSMISSION. The presence of *Stomoxys* on grazing cattle will cause increased head and ear movement, skin twitches, and tail swishes. Interestingly, the annoyed cattle will increase their herbage dry matter intake and bite masses (Dougherty et al, 1994). The bite of the stable fly is painful and results in the interrupted feeding patterns observed with tabanids. The stable fly serves as biological vector of *Habronema microstoma,* a nematode parasite of the stomach of the horse.

CONTROL. Stable flies attack cattle, horses, most other domestic animals, and humans on warm days throughout the summer. Regular application of pyrethrins, synergized pyrethrins, pyrethroids, coumaphos, or dichlorvos is indicated. Efforts to control *S. calcitrans* should include elimination of breeding sites (e.g., lawn clippings, green chop, damp bedding) and application of insecticides to areas where they habitually rest. Repellents in the form of sprays or smears may afford relief for several hours. These flies, with their piercing mouthparts, can theoretically be controlled with systemic and topical insecticides. Chlorpyrifos, coumaphos, malathion, phosmet, methoxychlor, or tetrachlorvinphos are applied either by spray or with self-treatment dust bags or backrubbers. The biological control of *S. calcitrans* by the release of parasitoid wasps seems to require further refinement before routine success occurs in the field (Andress and Campbell, 1994).

Haematobia

IDENTIFICATION. The horn fly, *Haematobia irritans*, found on the backs of cattle and to a lesser extent on horses, is about half the size of *Stomoxys* and has a relatively shorter proboscis. The palps are nearly long enough to reach the tip of the proboscis, in contrast to those of *Stomoxys* (compare Figures 1-14 and 1-15). Horn flies were first reported in the United States in the fall of 1887 when they were found in Camden, New Jersey. They spread rapidly throughout the United States, appeared in Hawaii in 1897, and have spread though Mexico, Central America, and northern South America (e.g., Guyana) (Craig, 1976). The horn fly was also discovered in Argentina, and it has rapidly spread throughout that country (Anziani et al, 1993).

LIFE HISTORY. Horn flies remain on cattle during the warmer seasons of the year, periodically biting their hosts and sucking blood. They are most obvious on the backs of their hosts but take refuge on the ventral abdomen during rain or on particularly hot, sunny days. When a cow defecates, a number of her horn flies swarm to the dropping to lay their eggs and then return to the cow. Larvae hatch in less than a day and crawl into the dropping to feed. Pupation occurs in 4 days, and emergence of the adult follows in 6 more days. In ideal warm, humid weather, the entire cycle from egg to egg requires 2 weeks or less but may require a month or longer in dryer, cooler weather. In temperate climates, the horn fly overwinters in the pupal stage, diapause occurring principally during September (Thomas, Hall, and Berry, 1987).

INJURY AND DISEASE TRANSMISSION. When sufficiently numerous, horn flies can impair milk production and weight gains. Cattle protected from horn fly attack by ear tags impregnated with fenvalerate achieved 18% greater live weight gains than did untreated controls (Foil, DeRoven, and Morrison, 1996; Haufe, 1982). *H. irritans* serves as a biological vector of *Stephanofilaria stilesi,* a filarioid nematode parasite of North American cattle and etiological agent of stephanofilariasis, a dermatitis usually confined to the midventral region of the abdomen.

CONTROL. Because they remain on the host most of their lives, adult horn flies are vulnerable to effective insecticides applied to cattle by means of sprays, dusts, backrubbers, stock oilers, and insecticide-impregnated plastic ear tags. In fact, horn fly control has depended almost exclusively on insecticides with the unfortunate development of resistance on the part of the fly to many of them (e.g., DDT, methoxychlor, toxaphene, fenchlorphos, stirofos, permethrin, and fenvalerate) (Marchionado, 1987). The insecticide tetrachlorvinphos or the synthetic juvenile hormone methoprene may be fed to cattle to render the manure unfit for development and pupation, thus interrupting the life history of *H. irritans*. Treatment of cattle with eprinomectin produced efficacy against horn flies for at least 2 weeks with good efficacy for longer periods, whereas ivermectin in a pour-on form is effective for at least 4 weeks (Arrioja-Dechert, 1997; Shoop et al, 1996).

The Bruce walk-through horn fly trap affords 50% reduction in horn fly numbers mechanically. Cattle walking through the 10-foot trap contact strips of canvas or carpeting, which dislodge the horn flies on their backs and sides. The host leaves some of its flies behind in the trap and, provided the process is repeated often enough, the population of horn flies in the herd is significantly reduced (Hall, Doisy, and Teasley, 1987).

Glossina

IDENTIFICATION. Tsetses (*Glossina* spp.) are localized to Africa but are included here because of their great importance to human and animal health, to the preservation of African wildlife, and to the economy of Africa and the world at large. Each antenna of *Glossina* has a long arista that is "feathered" along one edge. The palps and long slender proboscis are equal in length, the palps forming a sheath for the proboscis at rest (Figure 1-16).

LIFE HISTORY. The female tsetse bears only one larva at a time. Larval development is completed in the abdomen of the mother, with all three stages feeding on fluids from special uterine glands. It is interesting that milk secretion has evolved independently among both the highest vertebrates and the highest invertebrates. Several blood meals at regular intervals are required to support the larva during its developmental period of roughly 1 to 4 weeks. When extruded by the female tsetse, the fully developed third-stage larva almost immediately burrows into the soil and prepares to enter the pupal stage. A fourth larval stage occurs within the puparium before metamorphosis to the adult stage at last takes place.

DISEASE TRANSMISSION. The great importance of the tsetse is its role as biological vector of

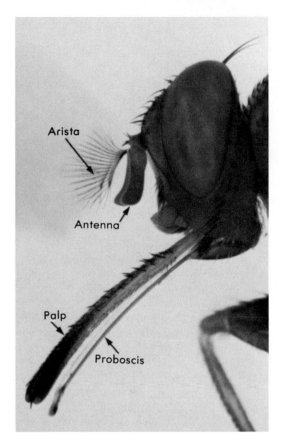

FIGURE 1-16 Head of *Glossina* (Cyclorrhapha: Muscidae), a fly (×22).

Labels on figure: Arista, Antenna, Palp, Proboscis

various trypanosomiases of humans and their domestic animals. African sleeping sickness of humans and "nagana" and related diseases of domestic animals are briefly considered in Chapter 2.

Family Hippoboscidae, Keds
Identification
Hippoboscids are dorsoventrally flattened, sometimes wingless flies with piercing mouthparts. The antennae are embedded in pits in the sides of the head. *Melophagus ovinus,* the sheep ked; *Hippobosca equina,* the horse louse fly; and *Lipoptena cervi,* the deer ked, are examples (Figure 1-17). *Melophagus* is wingless; the wings of *Hippobosca* remain well developed and functional throughout life; and *Lipoptena* have wings when they emerge from the pupal case. However, the wings of *Lipoptena* break off near the base (see Figure 1-17) once the fly has alighted on a host. *Lipoptena* may attack horses and other domestic animals in addition to deer, and casual observation suggests that their attacks are particularly obnoxious to horses.

LIFE HISTORY. Like tsetses, hippoboscids retain their larvae in their abdomens until they are ready to pupate, nourishing them during development with uterine gland secretions. In the case of *M. ovinus,* larval development requires about a week, and the extruded larva pupates within a few hours. The chestnut-brown pupal cases remain glued to the wool of the host sheep throughout metamorphosis of the adult fly, which emerges in 3 to 6 weeks, depending on the ambient temperature. The entire life of the sheep ked is thus spent on the host. Shearing and organophosphorus insecticides make life very uncertain for these parasites.

Dealate *L. cervi* males and females remain on their normal North American hosts, white-tailed deer *(Odocoileus virginianus)* and wapiti *(Cervus canadensis),* through most of the year. In spring, larvae are deposited in the hair coat, where they pupate and fall to the ground. Adult *L. cervi* flies emerge from the puparia from September to early December and fly off in search of a host. As soon as the ked alights on a deer, its wings break off and the ked begins to feed. The bite of *L. cervi* is relatively painless to humans but may be followed in several days by a pruriginous welt that may remain intensely pruritic for 2 to 3 weeks (Bequaert, 1942).

DISEASE TRANSMISSION. *M. ovinus* is host to *Trypanosoma melophagium,* which it transmits to sheep. If all keds are removed, the trypanosomes rapidly disappear from the sheep's blood, so it is the ked and not the sheep that represents the true reservoir of infection. Like *T. theileri* of cattle, *T. melophagium* appears to be totally nonpathogenic to its vertebrate host.

CONTROL. Coumaphos, diazinon, malathion, and methoxychlor as dips or sprays provide excellent control of *M. ovinus* when applied after shearing. In small flocks, diazinon can be applied most conveniently with a garden sprinkling can. Groups of about 20 sheep should be crowded in a small pen so there is just room enough left for one person to move among them. Waterproof overalls and boots should be worn while sprinkling the insecticide over the backs of the sheep. Ivermectin at 200 μg/kg given subcutaneously in sheep controls *M. ovinus* (Molina and Euzeby, 1982). *L. cervi* has been controlled also in red deer and roe deer by the administration of ivermectin (Kutzer, 1988).

What to do about attacks of *L. cervi* on horses short of keeping them indoors until the alate hippoboscids find their proper hosts is problematical.

Family Sarcophagidae, Flesh Flies
An adult sarcophagid is about twice as large as a house fly. The thorax is gray with dark, longitudinal stripes, and the abdomen is checkered gray and black (Figure 1-18). Third-stage sarcophagid larvae resemble house fly maggots but are larger. The

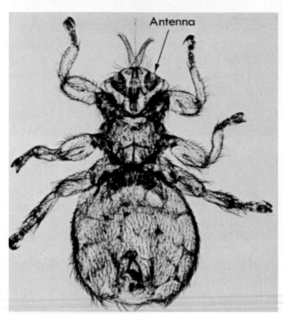

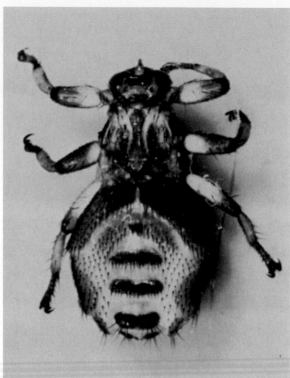

FIGURE 1-17 Examples of family Hippoboscidae. *Left, Melophagus ovinus*, the sheep ked (×12); *right, Lipoptena cervi* (×11.5) from a horse.

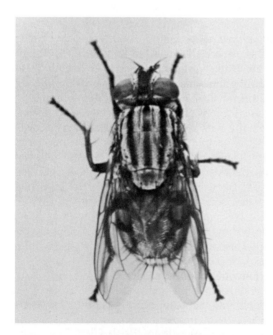

FIGURE 1-18 *Sarcophaga* (Cyclorrhapha: Sarcophagidae), a flesh fly (×5). About twice as large as a house fly, *Sarcophaga* is gray, with longitudinal dark stripes on the thorax and a checkered gray and black abdomen.

posterior spiracles are deeply sunken in a rounded concavity; the inner slit of each spiracle is directed down and away from the median line (Figure 1-19, *3*). Differentiation of *Sarcophaga* and *Wohlfahrtia* larvae requires that adult flies be reared from them. Place the larvae in question and a piece of liver on 3 to 5 cm of sand or loamy soil in a canning jar. When, after a day or so, the larvae have entered the substrate to pupate, remove the liver to avoid obnoxious odors and cover the mouth of the jar with a layer of cheesecloth secured with a rubber band to provide air yet prevent the escape of flies after they have emerged from the pupal cases. The arista of *Wohlfahrtia* bears only very short hairs, whereas the arista of *Sarcophaga* is covered nearly to its tip with long hairs. These rearing instructions serve equally well for calliphorids, but best results are obtained with larvae that are almost ready to pupate, especially when obligate parasitic species are involved.

Family Calliphoridae, Blow Flies
Identification
Adult calliphorids (Gr. *kallos* beauty, plus *phoros* bearing) are usually intermediate in size between *Musca* and *Sarcophaga* and typically display brilliant metallic blue, green, copper, or black hues.

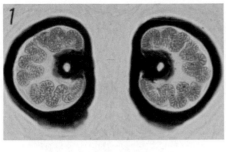

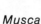
Musca

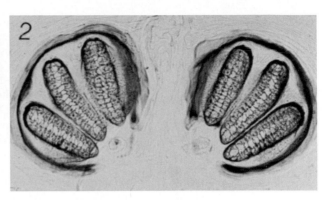

Calliphoridae

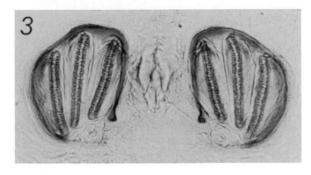

Sarcophagidae

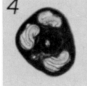

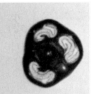

Stomoxys

FIGURE 1-19   Muscoid spiracles (*1, 2,* and *4,* ×108; *3,* ×70).

The common names "bluebottle" and "greenbottle" fly refer to the coloration of these flies, which are also called "blow flies" because they "blow" (i.e., deposit) their eggs or larvae in meat. Particular species differ in their preferences regarding the freshness of the meat, from living flesh to carrion in an advanced state of decomposition. Most calliphorids are scavengers or facultative parasites, but a few (e.g., *Cochliomyia hominivorax,* the American screwworm) are obligate parasites. Third-stage larvae of Calliphoridae are muscoid maggots differing from those of Sarcophagidae in having posterior spiracles that lie flush with the posterior face of the larva (or, less commonly, are sunken in a shallow, slitlike concavity); the inner slits of the spiracles are directed obliquely downward and toward the median line (see Figure 1-19, *2*). Larvae of the very important species *C. hominivorax* may be identified by the dark pigmentation of their tracheal trunks through the last three or four segments (see Figure 1-12).

Life History and Injury (Myiasis)
Females of the American screwworm fly *C. hominivorax* lay their eggs on fresh, uninfected wounds of all kinds. About 200 eggs are deposited in tidy rows. The eggs hatch within a day, and the obligate parasitic maggots commence feeding on living flesh and, in so doing, produce a foul-smelling, brownish-red discharge. The larvae leave the host in 5 to 7 days and enter the soil to pupate. Adult flies emerge from the pupal cases one to several weeks later. Wherever it occurs, *C. hominivorax* is a serious menace to man and beast alike. Unconscious victims of accidents or alcohol intoxication lying helplessly exposed have been fatally infected or have had their facial bones completely eaten away by screwworm maggots. Docking and castrating wounds, wire cuts, the navels of newborn animals, tick-bite wounds, shear cuts, needle grass wounds, and even fresh brands may attract the attentions of *C. hominivorax*. A nationwide control program based on treating wounds of all infected animals with insecticidal smears and releasing billions of sterilized flies has succeeded in eliminating screwworm myiasis from the United States. The adult flies are sterilized by gamma radiation, which induces dominant lethal mutations in the sperm. Because the female screwworm mates only once and because the wild population of the fly is relatively small, adding hordes of sexually competent but sterile males

reduces the probability of successful fertilization to nil. By the use of sterile males produced in Mexico, the American screwworm was eradicated from Libya where it had been accidentally introduced, probably on imported livestock, in 1988 (Linquist, Abusowa, and Hall, 1992).

Facultatively parasitic calliphorids are drawn to such attractions as suppurating wounds, skin soiled with urine, vomitus, or feces, and bacterial decomposition products that tend to accumulate in the fleece of a wet sheep. Once established in exudate or necrotic tissue, some kinds of these facultative parasites may later invade living tissue, whereas others do not. For example, the "surgical maggots" of *Phaenicia sericata* and *Phormia regina* are still used occasionally in the treatment of osteomyelitis and other refractory suppurative lesions to clear away necrotic debris and promote healing. Ideally, the surgical maggots do not invade healthy tissue, but strains vary and some of them do not know where to stop. A brave and resourceful gentleman of Dr. Georgi's acquaintance applied this technique in treating his own wounds when a prisoner of war in Vietnam. Once the maggots had done their work to his satisfaction, he flushed them away with his urine.

Wool strike is a common and serious problem in many sheep-raising regions of the world (Figure 1-20). Adult calliphorids are attracted to areas of fleece that have become soiled by feces or urine or were kept damp long enough for bacterial growth to occur and generate odors that lure flies to feed and lay their eggs. The areas involved in wool strike thus include the perineum, prepuce, and, during periods of considerable rainfall, water-soaked wool of the flanks, withers, and ventral neck region. Fleece rot, caused by *Pseudomonas aeruginosa,* and dermatophilosis, caused by *Dermatophilus congolense,* predispose sheep to wool strike by *Lucilia cuprina,* and a significantly greater incidence of body strikes was observed in lambs infected with both of these bacteria than with either bacterium alone (Gherardi et al, 1983). Several genera of calliphorid flies are commonly involved, and each geographical region has its particular scourge among the general assemblage of facultative parasites and scavengers. In Australia, one species, *L. cuprina,* stands out as a specialist in wool strike. This fly, although still a facultative parasite in that it is able to develop in carrion, has become so adept at locating suitable sheep on which to deposit its eggs that it has become the culprit responsible for initiating most cases of wool strike in Australia. The maggots feed on scales and exudate at the surface of the skin, occasionally penetrating the underlying tissues. When ready to pupate, the larvae of *L. cuprina* wait until night to leave the carcass (Smith et al, 1981). In this way, the pupae and emerging adults of this highly specialized parasite tend to become concentrated around the preferred resting sites, or **camps,** of their host species. Once *L. cuprina* has initiated a strike, other species of flies are attracted to feed and lay their eggs in the developing lesions. As the morbid process advances, these less-specialized newcomers tend to replace *L. cuprina.* Toxins absorbed from the myiasis lesion rapidly incapacitate the sheep and lead to its death in a matter of days. Eventually, scavenger species take over the carcass and reduce it to hair and bone. Financial loss caused by wool strike is reckoned in terms of outright death losses, loss of wool, decreased quality of wool, loss of weight, and costs of treatment and preventive measures.

A condition analogous to wool strike occurs in old, weakened, or paretic dogs with urine-soaked haircoats. As such an unfortunate animal lies in the "healing rays of the sun," the blow flies are busy laying eggs in its haircoat and, in a few days, maggots will be skinning it alive. Frequently, owners who present long-haired dogs suffering from advanced cases of cutaneous myiasis are totally unaware of the mayhem taking place underneath the haircoat. The condition of the patient can be evaluated accurately and effective treatment undertaken only after the hair has been clipped away and all affected areas bathed. Most of the maggots will be removed in the process; any remaining may be routed by judicious local application of an insecticidal solution such as a pyrethroid or an organophosphate. A really vigorous application of insecticide might easily kill the debilitated and denuded host.

Weakened or defective calves born at pasture are also fair game for members of the family Calliphoridae. It is amazing how quickly the shiny flies appear seemingly out of nowhere and how rapidly their egg masses accumulate about the umbilicus of a newborn calf with cerebellar hypoplasia or muscle contracture. The possibility of myiasis must always be considered in the case of animals incapacitated during warm weather, especially if they are forced to remain outdoors.

Wild animals and birds may suffer serious losses to myiasis. For example, Arendt (1985) estimated that infection with larvae of *Philornis deceptivus* (family Muscidae) were responsible for 97% of the mortality observed among pearly-eyed thrasher nestlings *(Margarops fuscatus)* in Puerto Rico. In North America, major causes of avian myiasis are maggots of the genus *Protocalliphora* (Sabrosky, Bennett, and Whitworth, 1989). Larvae of the sarcophagid fly *Neobellieria citellivora* causes lethal myiasis in ground squirrels *(Spermophilus columbianus)* in Canada (Michener, 1993). Larvae of sarcophagid flies, genus *Cistudinomyia,* are capable of causing lethal myiasis in geckos (DeMarmels, 1994).

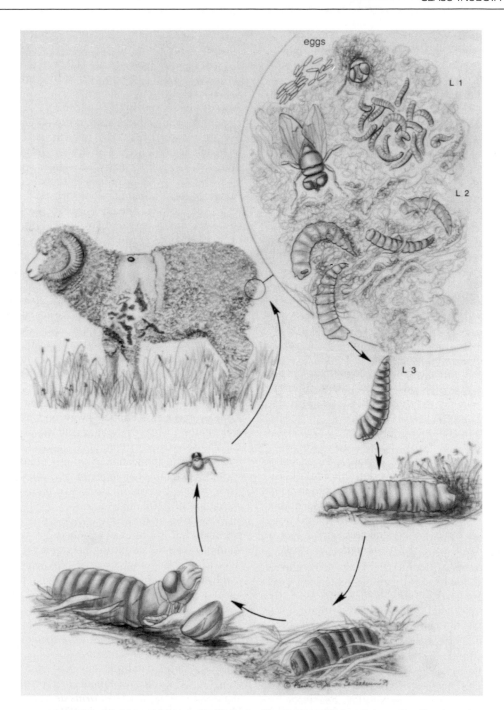

FIGURE 1-20 Life history of the wool strike fly, *Lucilia cuprina*. Adult female L. cuprina flies deposit their eggs in moist and soiled wool. Larvae hatch from these eggs, feed on scales and exudate at the surface of the skin, and undergo two molts before falling to the ground to pupate. The adult fly pushes off the end of the puparium by inflating its baglike ptilinum with hemolymph. Having emerged from the puparium, the fly inflates its wings by pumping hemolymph into the wing veins, retracts its ptilinum into the head once and for all, and flies off in search of suitably smelly sheep. The Australian Merino wether in the picture has suffered fly strike in three stages. The flies first attacked a spot between his shoulders that had collected rainwater and supported bacterial growth. The exudate from this lesion flowed over the wether's shoulders and brisket and greatly extended the area susceptible to fly attack. The shepherd has clipped all of the wool from both shoulders and brisket and treated the lesions with an insecticide, but now the flies are attracted to the breech area, which is soiled with feces, so this area too must be clipped and medicated or the wether will likely die of "crutch strike."

Treatment

Coumaphos is widely employed in the treatment of cutaneous myiasis. This agent may be applied to the cattle by dipping, but most commonly it is sprayed or smeared directly on the maggot-infested lesions. Ivermectin and doramectin administered subcutaneously to cattle can serve as a prophylactic against infestation by larvae of *C. hominivorax* and appear to be useful aids in the prevention of umbilical myiasis and fly strike associated with castration (Anziani and Loreficce, 1993; Muniz et al, 1995).

For treatment of wool strike in sheep, coumaphos and diazinon are recommended as sprays, dips, or local applications to affected areas. All wool soiled or underrun by maggots should first be clipped away. Ivermectin when applied as a jetting fluid appears to aid against blow fly strike of sheep in Australia (Eagleson et al, 1993). Subcutaneous injections of infested sheep in Hungary with either ivermectin or moxidectin failed to cause rapid-acting treatment of the infested sheep, and 7 days after treatment, the majority of treated sheep were still severely infested (Farkas et al, 1996). Also used in Australia with good success is a jetting fluid with cyromazine, an insect growth regulator, that can be mixed with diazinon (Levot and Sales, 1998).

The extent of measures taken to prevent flystrike in sheep should be proportional to the degree of risk. Clipping the wool of the breech and area around the prepuce greatly reduces the amount of moisture and filth that can be retained in those regions of the fleece. Amputating the tails of lambs represents about the minimum of effort that ought to be expended on flystrike control, but in some parts of the world lambs manage to grow up with their tails intact. In the **Mules' operation,** widely practiced in Australia, with perhaps up to 30 million lambs treated each year, redundant folds of skin from the posterior aspects of the thighs and the tail head are removed with a pair of sharp "dagging" shears. When the resultant wounds heal, the skin of the breech is drawn taut, thus extending the relatively hairless area immediately surrounding the anus and vulva and thereby reducing the moisture- and filth-carrying capacity of the breech. This operation, carried out in a minute or so without surgical preparation, anesthesia, or aftercare, seems brutal until one has had an opportunity to compare its effects on the patient with those inflicted by *L. cuprina.*

Families Oestridae, Hypodermatidae, Gasterophilidae, and Cuterebridae; the Bot Flies

The bot flies are highly host-specific and site-specific parasites in the larval (i.e., bot) stage and total slaves to reproduction in the adult stage. The adults have vestigial mouthparts and must carry on their courtship rituals and egg laying on energy stored away when they were larvae. Fully developed bots are larger and stouter than are muscid, sarcophagid, and calliphorid maggots, from which they can readily be distinguished by their posterior spiracles (Figures 1-19 and 1-21). In fact, when found in their accustomed locations in their normal hosts, bots present very little in the way of a diagnostic challenge; a bot in a sheep's nasal passages is an *Oestrus;* a bot in a cow's dorsal subcutis is a *Hypoderma;* a bot in a horse's stomach is a *Gasterophilus;* and there is hardly any sense in making more an exercise of it than that. However, the earlier stages of bots are more difficult to distinguish from maggots and, if found migrating in other than its normal host, will require the services of an expert entomologist for identification. First-stage *Hypoderma* larvae have been found migrating aberrantly through the brain of horses, and *Cuterebra* larvae, normally parasites of rodents and lagomorphs, have been found in the brains of cats and dogs and much more commonly in their subcutaneous tissues. *Hypoderma* and *Cuterebra* also occasionally invade humans and migrate subcutaneously. *Oestrus ovis* may larviposit in the eyes of shepherds and thus cause a temporary but painful ocular myiasis.

Oestrus ovis

Oe. ovis, the "sheep nasal bot fly," somewhat resembles a honeybee. It is a stout, grayish-brown fly, about 1 cm long and covered with short hairs; the mouthparts are vestigial. The flies are most active during the warmer hours of the day, especially during intervals of bright sunshine. In early morning and late afternoon, they are more likely to be found resting on buildings, tree trunks, water tanks, and the like. It is interesting to watch a mob of Australian Merino sheep on a warm, sunny day with a few scattered clouds. While in the shadow of a cloud, the sheep tend to distribute themselves more or less at random over the paddock, but as the sun emerges from behind the cloud, the sheep immediately huddle together and continue to graze with their heads toward the center of the huddle, only to disperse again with the arrival of the next cloud. This behavior may represent a defensive adaptation to the attack of the larvipositing female *Oe. ovis;* it seems plausible, at least. While *Oe. ovis* females are actively depositing their larvae in sheep's nostrils, the sheep hold their noses close to the ground or in each other's fleeces, stamp their feet as if annoyed, and occasionally bolt away. The tiny first-stage larvae may be demonstrated postmortem by sawing the skull in half longitudinally, rinsing the nasoturbinates and nasal sinuses with water, and examining the collected rinsings with a hand lens or stereoscopic microscope. The fully developed third-stage bots can hardly escape notice in the frontal sinuses.

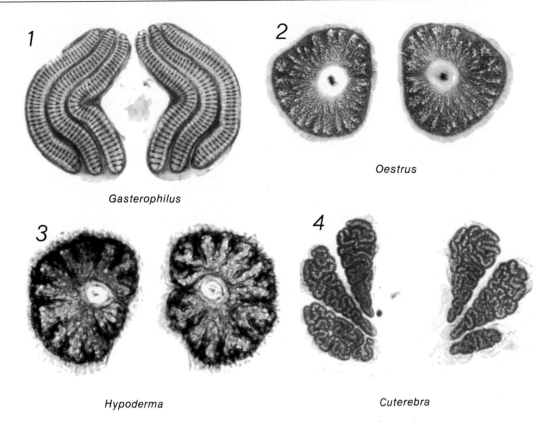

FIGURE 1-21   Bot spiracles (*1* and *2*, ×27; *3*, ×55; and *4*, ×65).

LIFE HISTORY. On being deposited in the nostril of a sheep, the larva crawls onto the mucous membrane of the nasal passage, where it will remain for at least 2 weeks anchored to the mucous membrane by its mouth hooks. Larvae arriving late in the season remain arrested in the first stage throughout the winter, and development proceeds only with the return of warm weather. After a sojourn in the nasal cavity, the larvae proceed to the frontal sinuses, where development to the third stage is completed. On reaching full development, the third-stage larvae crawl down into the nasal passages, are expelled by the sheep's sneezing, and enter the soil to pupate. Adults may emerge in about 4 weeks in summer but require considerably longer in cool weather. When pupation occurs in autumn, adult flies do not emerge until the following spring. Thus *Oe. ovis* overwinters both as arrested first-stage larvae in the nasal cavities of sheep and as pupae in soil.

PATHOLOGICAL SIGNIFICANCE. Although moderate numbers of *Oe. ovis* larvae in the nasal and paranasal sinuses do no apparent harm, heavy infections cause sneezing, nasal discharge, and partial blockage of the nasal passages.

TREATMENT. The larva of *Oe. ovis* is very susceptible to ivermectin at the standard dosage rate of 0.2 mg/kg (Roncalli, 1984). Dichlorvos or Fenthion may be sprayed directly into the nostrils for the control of nasal bots.

Other Nasal Bots

Rhinoestrus purpureus infects horses in parts of Europe, Asia, and Africa; *Cephalopsis titillator* infects camels and dromedaries in Africa; and *Cephenomyia* spp. infect deer, elk, caribou, and other cervids in the Northern Hemisphere. Their life histories generally resemble that of *Oe. ovis.* However, the third-stage larvae of *R. purpureus* and *C. titillator* are found in the nasal and paranasal sinuses, pharynx, and even larynx, and those of *Cephenomyia* spp. are found in the pharyngeal pouches.

Hypoderma

IDENTIFICATION. *Hypoderma bovis* and *Hypoderma lineatum,* or "heel flies," occur in cattle-raising areas of the Northern Hemisphere between 25° and 60° North latitude. The adult fly is about 15 mm long and looks rather like a bumblebee. Although these flies have no functional mouthparts for biting, and the process of oviposition on the hairs is presumably painless, cattle tend to become apprehensive and excited at their approach and gallop off aimlessly with their tails held high over their backs. Such behavior, termed "gadding about," tends to involve the whole herd simultaneously in needless, hysterical exertion and distracts it from the more profitable business of grazing. (Agricultural research administrators, practiced in the art of extracting financial support for their institutions from legislative bodies, can tell you exactly how much this form of bovine entomophobia costs the American stockman each year.) The fully developed third-stage *Hypoderma* larva or "cattle grub" is found in walnut-sized lumps, or **warbles,** on the backs of cattle in spring. Each warble has a small hole at its summit to which the posterior spiracles of the larva are pressed to obtain air. When it emerges or is extracted from the warble, the larva (sometimes also called a warble) is about 25 mm long and whitish to light brown.

LIFE HISTORY AND PATHOGENESIS. *H. lineatum* and *H. bovis* females glue their eggs to the hairs on the legs of cattle. *H. lineatum* appears with the advent of warm weather and remains active for about 2 months. Then *H. bovis* takes over and persists into summer. The eggs hatch spontaneously in less than a week, and the larvae burrow through the skin and set off on prolonged migrations through the connective tissues of their host. Larvae of *H. lineatum* accumulate in the tissues of the esophagus 5 months later and remain there for about 3 months. Finally, they migrate to the subcutaneous tissues of the back, cut breathing holes in the skin to which they appose their spiracles, and, molting twice, grow larger. The larvae spend about 2 months in warbles in the backs of the infested cows (Pruett and Kunz, 1996). When fully developed, the larvae enlarge their breathing holes, emerge through them, and fall to the ground to pupate. Adult flies emerge from pupal cases about 1 month later and immediately set about their reproductive duties. *H. bovis* larvae tend to accumulate in the spinal canal instead of the esophagus and appear in the subcutaneous tissues of the back about 2 months later than *H. lineatum.*

Hypoderma larvae occasionally invade horses and render them useless for equitation by warble formation in the saddle area or even cause fatal neurological disease by migrating in the brain (Olander, 1967). In humans, *Hypoderma* larvae tend to produce bouts of creeping subcutaneous myiasis ("migrating lumps") as the confused larvae try to find the top of the cow in which they "think" they are migrating. Local paralysis may result from invasion of the spinal cord, and blindness may result from invasion of the eye. These fortunately are rare accidents.

TREATMENT AND CONTROL. *Hypoderma* infection is usually treated with systemic ivermectin, doramectin, or moxidectin. Organophosphate insecticides, coumaphos and Fenthion are also widely used as sprays, pour-ons, or spot-ons to kill the larvae in the early stages of their migration. The "safe periods" for applying these insecticides vary for different localities because of differences in fly activity. The insecticides must be applied immediately after adult *Hypoderma* activity ceases for the season. Host-parasite reactions manifested clinically by bloat, salivation, ataxia, and posterior paralysis may occur when cattle are treated with larvicidal insecticides while *H. lineatum* larvae are in the esophagus or while *H. bovis* larvae are in the spinal canal. The host-parasite reaction was once thought to be an anaphylactoid reaction caused by antibodies produced by cattle in response to *Hypoderma* larval antigens. However, experimental evidence indicates that this reaction is caused by a toxin liberated from the dead *Hypoderma* larvae. Injection of phenylbutazone at a dosage rate of 20 mg/kg body weight 20 minutes before injection of larval toxin protected calves against both systemic shock and local inflammatory reactions (Eyre, Boulard, and Deline, 1981). The host-parasite reaction is best treated with sympathomimetic drugs (e.g., adrenaline) and steroids to alleviate local inflammatory reactions. Atropine, the antidote for cholinesterase-inhibiting agents, is contraindicated; host-parasite reaction is not a manifestation of organophosphate toxicity even though it may be precipitated by organophosphate medication. In cases in which preventive treatment has been neglected, late second-stage and third-stage *Hypoderma* larvae can be safely and quickly removed from the backs of cattle by slowly injecting 1 ml of 3% hydrogen peroxide solution into the breathing hole using a blunt canula or needle shank of the syringe and taking care not to pierce the grub. Most grubs will emerge within 15 seconds after the foaming action of the hydrogen peroxide begins and leaves behind a cleansed cavity (Scholl and Barrett, 1986).

National eradication efforts directed against *Hypoderma* spp. have met with success in Denmark, the Federal Republic of Germany, the Netherlands, and the Republic of Ireland, and the incidence in Great Britain has been reduced from 38% in 1978 to 0.01% in 1985 (Wilson, 1986). Surveillance against reintroduction of *Hypoderma* spp. in imported cattle is critical as evidenced by 19% of tested cattle entering Great Britain in 1993 being seropositive for *Hypoderma* (Sinclair, 1995). In parts of Great Britain where the ox warble has persisted or reappeared, all cattle over 12 weeks old are required to undergo treatment within specific dates, and cattle are routinely inspected at livestock sales and on farms.

RELATED SPECIES. *Hypoderma diana* occurs in deer and occasionally in man in Europe. Other species of *Hypoderma* and genera of warble flies parasitize sheep, goats, and deer in Mediterranean countries and India. *Oedemagena tarandi* is a serious enough pest of reindeer, musk oxen, and caribou in the subarctic regions to require prophylactic medication of these wild or semiwild hosts. In one study, 70% of untreated reindeer harbored more than 100 *Oe. tarandi* larvae (Washburn et al, 1980). Both ivermectin and doramectin have proven highly effective in the treatment of infections with this parasite.

Gasterophilus

IDENTIFICATION. The adult fly superficially resembles a honeybee, with a long, curved ovipositor carried beneath the abdomen. The females may be observed on warm, sunny days hovering near horses and darting very rapidly to attach an egg to a hair.

Eggs are deposited by *Gasterophilus nasalis* females on the hairs of the intermandibular space, by *Gasterophilus hemorrhoidalis* on the short hairs that adjoin the lips, and by *Gasterophilus intestinalis* on the hairs of the forelegs and shoulders (Figure 1-22). An illustrated key for identifying the eggs of the eight species of *Gasterophilus* that occur around the world has been prepared by Cogley (1991).

First-stage larvae of *G. intestinalis* can be found in tunnels in the epithelium covering the dorsal surface of the rostral two thirds of the tongue and in pockets between the molar teeth. Second-stage larvae are found in interdental pockets, attached to the root of the tongue, and attached to the wall of the stomach (Cogley, Anderson, and Cogley, 1982). Less is known regarding the initial migrations of other species of *Gasterophilus*. First- and second-stage larvae of *G. nasalis* are usually completely hidden well below the gum line in interdental pus pockets extending into the root sockets of molar teeth (Schroeder, 1940).

The third-stage larva of *G. nasalis* is yellowish and has one row of spines on each segment (Figure 1-23); it is usually found in the first ampulla of the duodenum. All of the following species of *Gasterophilus* have two rows of spines per segment: The *G. intestinalis* third-stage larva is red, has coarse spines that are blunted at their tips, and attaches in clusters in the nonglandular part of the stomach either near the *margo plicatus* or in the *saccus cecus*. The following species have small spines that taper to a fine point: *G. hemorrhoidalis,* which is reddish and found in the duodenum and rectum of horses in the North-Central United States and Canada; and *Gasterophilus inermis,* which is

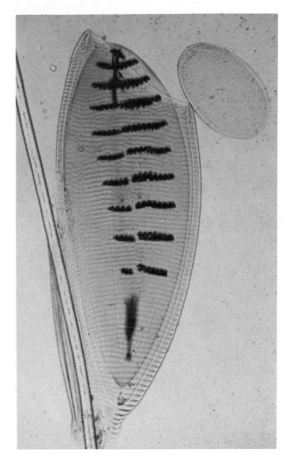

FIGURE 1-22 Egg of *Gasterophilus intestinalis* (Cyclorrhapha: Gasterophilidae) on a horse hair (×63). The eggshell contains a first-stage larva, and the operculum has become dislodged.

light yellow and found in the rectum of European horses. Individual larvae of all species may occasionally be found in atypical locations in the alimentary tract.

LIFE HISTORY. *G. nasalis* females deposit their eggs on the hairs of the intermandibular space. These eggs hatch spontaneously in 5 or 6 days, and the larvae crawl downward toward the chin until they arrive at a point opposite the commissures of the lips, whereupon they proceed directly toward the mouth and pass between the lips. The black eggs of *G. hemorrhoidalis* on the hairs adjoining the lips hatch after 2 to 4 days on contact with moisture, penetrate the epidermis of the lips, and burrow toward the mucous membrane of the mouth (Wells and Knipling, 1938).

The eggs of *G. intestinalis* on the hairs of the front legs are far removed from their destination and depend on direct assistance from the horse to find their way into the mouth (Figure 1-24). Five days after being laid, these eggs contain first-stage

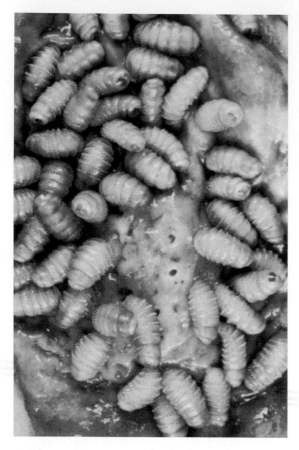

FIGURE 1-23 *Gasterophilus nasalis* (Cyclorrhapha: Gasterophilidae) third-stage larvae attached to the gastric mucosa of a horse. This appears to be an exceptional location for *G. nasalis*, which usually is found in the dorsally directed first ampulla of the duodenum (Price and Stromberg, 1987). Former attachment sites are visible as shallow, rounded ulcers in the lower center (approximate natural size).

larvae that are prepared to hatch rapidly in response to the sudden rise in ambient temperature that occurs when the horse brings its warm muzzle and breath in contact with them; they do not respond to gradual warming (Knipling and Wells, 1935). The larvae then enter the horse's mouth and burrow into the stratified squamous epithelium on the dorsal surface of the tongue. The first- and second-stage larvae of *G. intestinalis* spend about one month in the oral cavity. The white first-stage larvae drill burrows up to 13 cm long in the mucosa of the tongue, with "air holes" at an average interval of 4.2 mm to which they apply their caudal spiracles to breathe (Cogley, Anderson, and Cogley, 1982). The burrows typically extend in a rostral to caudal direction, but all terminate several centimeters rostral to the vallate papillae. Having approximately doubled in size during their sojourn in the tongue, the first-stage larvae now enter pockets in the interdental spaces predominantly of the upper

molar teeth, where they molt from first to second stage. The second-stage larvae develop a red color as a result of synthesis of the insect's own hemoglobin, an adaptation to the low oxygen tension environment they will presently encounter in the stomach. At last, the second-stage larvae leave the interdental spaces, attach briefly to the root of the tongue, and then proceed to the stomach where they molt to the third larval stage, or full-grown "bot" (Cogley, Anderson, and Cogley, 1982). The oral migrations of other species of *Gasterophilus* have not yet been elucidated in such detail as they have been for *G. intestinalis*. However, migration within tissues affords protection from the host's teeth and a source of nourishment and is probably a key feature of the oral migrations of other *Gasterophilus* species as well.

The third-stage larvae remain attached by their mouth hooks to the wall of the stomach *(G. intestinalis)* or duodenum *(G. nasalis)* for up to 12 months (farthest from the intestine—*intestinalis;* farthest from the nose—*nasalis*). The predilection sites of both species are located above the fluid level in the alimentary tract. In these locations, the bots are surrounded by gas pockets that apparently supply these air-breathing animals with sufficient oxygen (Figure 1-25; Price and Stromberg, 1987). From late spring onward, the larvae release their grip on the mucosa and pass out with the feces to pupate in the soil. Adult bot flies emerge from the pupal cases in 3 to 9 weeks, depending on the ambient temperature. Bot fly activity continues through summer and fall but ceases completely when cold weather sets in.

IMPORTANCE. In spite of the rather impressive oral lesions produced by first- and second-stage larvae and the chronic lesions in gastric and intestinal mucosae caused by attachment of the second and third stages, there is remarkably little pathological or experimental evidence associating *Gasterophilus* infection with clinical illness. In fact, many horses support substantial populations of these parasites without apparent ill effect. However, disease is not a simple subject, and *Gasterophilus* infection has been held to etiological account in cases of stomach rupture, subserosal abscess, splenic abscess, ulceration, and peritonitis (Underwood and Dikmans, 1943; Rainey, 1948; Rooney, 1964; Waddell, 1972). Principato (1988) described, classified, and superbly illustrated the main macroscopic lesions produced by larvae of *G. intestinalis, G. nasalis, G. hemorrhoidalis, G. inermis,* and *Gasterophilus pecorum* in freely ranging horses in Italy.

TREATMENT. The common treatment is now a macrolide. In the southern United States, bot flies are active most of the year (Craig, 1984), and in the

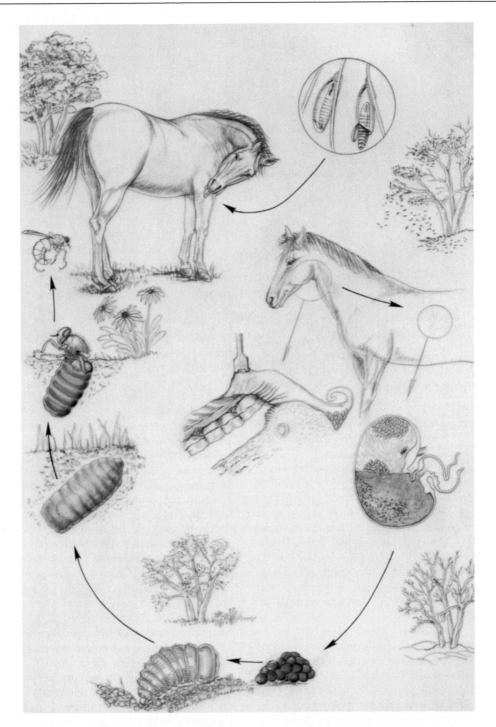

FIGURE 1-24 Life history of the equine stomach bot *Gasterophilus intestinalis*. The female bot fly attaches fertilized eggs on the hair shafts of the forelegs and shoulders of horses. First-stage larvae develop in 5 days and stand ready to literally pop out of their shells in response to the warm breath of the horse. Having landed on the horse's face and entered its mouth, the larvae first tunnel quite extensively in the mucous epithelium of the dorsum and sides of the tongue, then enter pockets between the upper molar teeth, where they molt to the second stage. One month after infection, the larvae emerge from the interdental spaces, attach temporarily to the wall of the pharynx, then pass to the stomach, where they molt to the third stage. The third stage larvae remain attached in the saccus cecus or along the margo plicatus for almost a year. From late spring onward, they let go, pass out in the feces, and pupate in the soil. Adult *G. intestinalis* flies emerge from their pupal cases 3 to 9 weeks later and fly off in search of a horse.

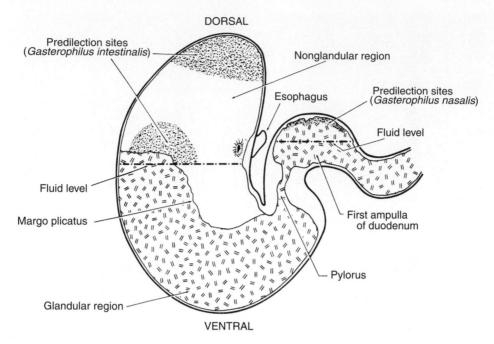

FIGURE 1-25 Predilection sites of *Gasterophilus intestinalis* and *Gasterophilus nasalis* in the stomach and duodenum of the horse.
(From Price RE, Stromberg PC: *Am J Vet Res* 48:1230, 1987.)

case of *G. intestinalis,* the eggs glued to the hairs of the forelegs remain infective long after adult fly activity has ceased. The eggs may be removed from the haircoat with a special fine-tooth comb available from saddlery shops, but the process is rather slow and laborious. If more than a very few horses are involved, the larvae can be lured out of their egg cases by copious sponging with water at 40° to 48° C (104° to 118° F) (Knipling and Wells, 1935); the addition of 0.06% coumaphos ensures rapid destruction of these larvae as they emerge. The eggs of *G. nasalis* and *G. hemorrhoidalis* hatch spontaneously when development of the larva is complete.

Cuterebra

IDENTIFICATION. The rarely seen (or noticed) adult fly somewhat resembles a bumblebee and has vestigial mouthparts (Figure 1-26). The fully developed third-stage larva is large (up to 45 mm) and dark-brown to black, the color being due to the stout black spines that cover the body (Figure 1-27). The posterior spiracles consist of groups of elegantly curved openings (see Figure 1-21, *4*). Earlier stages are much paler or even white and the posterior spiracles are quite different from those of the third stage, but the dark spines covering the body furnish evidence of the larva's identity as *Cuterebra*. At the present state of knowledge, it is impossible to differentiate species of even fully developed third-stage larvae of *Cuterebra*, except

in the few cases in which their life histories have been worked out in detail.

LIFE HISTORY AND PATHOGENESIS. *Cuterebra* spp. infect rabbits, squirrels, chipmunks, mice, cats, dogs, and occasionally humans (Baird, Podgore, and Sabrosky, 1982). Female *Cuterebra* flies lay their eggs along rabbit runs and near rodent burrows. As the host brushes past, the first-stage larvae hatch instantaneously and crawl immediately into the host's fur. These larvae enter the host through its natural body openings (Baird, 1971, 1972; Timm and Lee, 1981). *Cuterebra* larvae are usually found in the cervical subcutaneous connective tissue of cats and dogs during August, September, and October. *Cuterebra* larvae may also locate in the nasal and oral regions and sometimes migrate through the brains of cats and dogs, with fatal results. The migration of the larva in the brain of cats is believed to cause infarction and be responsible for feline ischemic encephalopathy (Williams, Summers, and de Lahunta, 1998).

Although no data is available, cats on avermectin heartworm preventative might be protected from Cuterebra infection. Similarly, the topically applied flea and tick products, imidacloprid and fipronil, may kill the young maggots on the hair coats of cats. None of these products are, however, approved for preventing cuterebriasis.

A *Cuterebra* larva can be removed by enlarging its breathing hole in the skin sufficiently to allow it

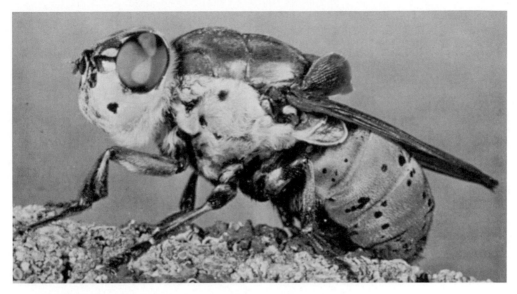

FIGURE 1-26 *Cuterebra jellisoni* (Cyclorrhapha: Cuterebridae), a bot fly (approximately ×8). The mouthparts of bot flies are vestigial. (From Baird CR: *J Med Entomol* 8:616, 1971.)

to be extracted with forceps, with care being taken not to crush the larva in the process. Tranquilization or sedation facilitates restraint but is rarely necessary. The wound heals rather slowly and sometimes

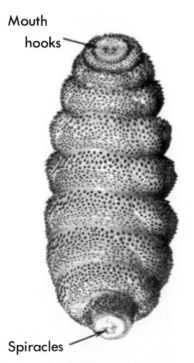

Mouth
hooks

Spiracles

FIGURE 1-27 A *Cuterebra jellisoni* (Cyclorrhapha: Cuterebridae) bot, or third-stage bot fly larva (×2). The bot flies belong to the families Cuterebridae, Oestridae, Hypodermatidae, and Gasterophilidae.
(From Baird CR: *J Med Entomol* 8:616, 1971.)

suppurates or even sloughs; this may be due to secondary bacterial infection or leakage of *Cuterebra* antigens into the surrounding tissues during extraction.

Dermatobia

IDENTIFICATION. The adult of *Dermatobia hominis*, another member of the family Cuterebridae, somewhat resembles a brilliant blue calliphorid fly but, like all bot flies, has vestigial mouthparts. The fully developed third-stage larva is pear-shaped and has posterior spiracles with straight slits deeply sunken in a concavity.

LIFE HISTORY AND PATHOGENESIS. The *D. hominis* female uses a slave to carry her eggs to a prospective host. She captures another fly, usually a bloodsucker such as a mosquito or a stable fly, and glues her eggs to its abdomen. The eggs develop in a week or two, and the larvae inside them stand ready to disembark when the slave fly alights on the skin of a warm-blooded animal to feed. Each *D. hominis* larva that succeeds in penetrating the skin develops at or near the site of penetration in a separate warble. The larva emerges through the breathing hole to pupate about 6 weeks later. The *D. hominis* larva is a serious pest of humans, cattle, sheep, dogs, and other mammals in Central and South America. The adult flies tend to concentrate at the edges of large forests.

Expert Identification of Myiasis Larvae

The major taxa of fully developed myiasis larvae can be identified by means of the criteria set forth earlier. More detailed information can be found in James (1948). However, identification of all three larval stages of even the more common species is a chore for a taxonomic specialist. If preliminary findings are inconclusive, intriguing, or of great practical importance, larvae can be cleaned by shaking them vigorously in water, fixing them in 70% ethyl alcohol or 10% formalin, and submitting these specimens for expert identification. Precise identification in certain cases requires rearing the adult fly; instructions are provided under Sarcophagidae in an earlier section. Living larvae also may be submitted for expert identification in addition to but not in lieu of fixed specimens; include these in a separate jar loosely packed in moist cotton.

Orders Anoplura, Bloodsucking Lice, and Mallophaga, Chewing Lice

There are two main kinds of lice, represented by the orders Anoplura, or bloodsucking lice, and Mal-lophaga, or chewing lice (Table 1-5). Anoplurans have piercing mouthparts consisting of three stylets that, in fixed specimens, are usually concealed within the relatively narrow head (Figure 1-28). Anoplurans are parasites of placental animals only. Mallophagans have stout mandibles on the ventral side of their relatively broad heads (Figure 1-29), and these lice feed on epidermal scales, feathers, and sebaceous secretions of birds and mammals. Both anoplurans and mallophagans spend their entire lives among the hairs or feathers of their hosts and display a high order of host specificity. Even the eggs are securely attached to the hairs or feathers of the host (see Figure 1-37). The lice that hatch from these eggs are tiny replicas of the adults; they molt several times but undergo only minor changes in appearance (i.e., **simple metamorphosis**). The cycle from egg to egg requires several weeks, and only one or two eggs may be found developing within the abdomen of a female louse at any one time, but enormous populations may develop notwithstanding. The hatching process itself is of passing interest. The

TABLE 1-5 ■ Lice Found on Domestic Animals and Humans

Host	Anoplura	Mallophaga
Dog	*Linognathus setosus*	*Trichodectes canis* *Heterodoxus spiniger*
Cat	None	*Felicola subrostratus*
Cow	*Haematopinus eurysternus* *Haematopinus quadripertusus* *Haematopinus tuberculatus* *Linognathus vituli* *Solenopotes capillatus*	*Damalinia bovis*
Horse	*Haematopinus asini*	*Damalinia equi*
Pig	*Haematopinus suis*	None
Sheep	*Linognathus ovillus* *Linognathus pedalis* *Linognathus africanus*	*Damalinia ovis*
Goat	*Linognathus africanus* *Linognathus stenopsis*	*Damalinia caprae* *Damalinia crassipes* *Damalinia limbata*
Rat	*Polyplax spinulosa*	None
Mouse	*Polyplax serrata*	None
Guinea pig	None	*Gliricola porcelli* *Gyropus ovalis* *Trimenopon hisidum*
Humans	*Pediculus humanus capitus* *Pediculus humanus humanus* *Pthirus pubis*	None

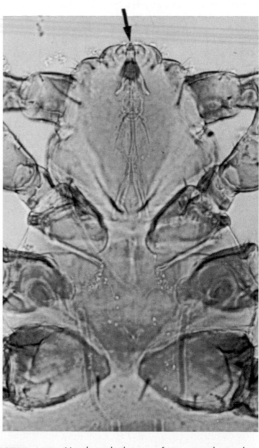

FIGURE 1-28 Head and thorax of an anopluran louse (×312). The bloodsucking stylets occupy the median plane of the head; mouth at arrow.

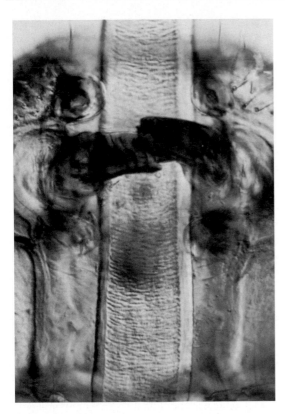

FIGURE 1-29 Mandibles of a mallophagan louse grasping a goat hair (×210).

entiation. Occasionally a few lice are collected from sources other than their normal host. For example, *Pthirus pubis*, the human crab louse, has been reported now and again on dogs. In such cases, it is necessary to note the obvious morphological differences displayed by *L. setosus*, the anopluran normally found on dogs, and *P. pubis,* denizen of the human pubic hairs, to avoid misdiagnosis.

Lice are well-adapted parasites and are usually more a nuisance than a threat to their hosts. The role of the human body louse in the spread of *Rickettsia prowazekii,* the etiological agent of epidemic typhus, is an outstanding exception, and a few other examples of lice serving in the role of vectors and intermediate hosts can be cited. However, it takes a large population of lice to drain the vitality of their host directly, and usually contributory conditions such as stress of inclement weather, crowding, poor nutrition, and individual diathesis can be demonstrated in cases of clinical illness related to louse infestation. If a very large number of lice is found on cattle, on a puppy, or on a stock of laboratory rats, there is something wrong in the way the animals are kept, and merely spraying insecticide to kill the lice falls far short of full clinical management of the case.

Order Anoplura

Anoplurans, about 400 some species, have pincerlike tarsal claws for clinging to the hairs of their hosts. The size of these claws is related to the diameter of the hair shaft and is probably an important factor in establishing host specificity and site specificity. Without hair, these lice are helpless; they pass from host to host most efficiently when a "bridge" of hair exists between host individuals. This is why *P. pubis* is frequently transmitted during sexual intercourse. According to Chandler and Read (1961), the French call this parasite "papillon d'amour."

Haematopinus

All tarsal claws are of equal size, and the lateral margins of the abdomen are heavily sclerotized (Figure 1-30). The two other anopluran genera found on cattle, *Linognathus* and *Solenopotes*, differ in having smaller claws on their first pair of legs. Species of *Haematopinus* that infest domestic animals include *Haematopinus asini* of horses, *Haematopinus suis* of swine (Figure 1-31), and *Haematopinus eurysternus, Haematopinus quadripertussus,* and *Haematopinus tuberculatus* of cattle. *H. eurysternus* is a common parasite of domestic cattle *(B. taurus)* in North America and tends to concentrate on the neck, poll, brisket, and tail, but in heavy infestation it may be generally distributed over the body. *H. quadripertussus,* normally a

young louse swallows air and ejects it through its anus to form a cushion of compressed air that forces the animal against the operculum (i.e., lid) of the eggshell until it pops open. Thus it may be said (with due application of etymology and low humor) that "every louse is hoisted by its own petard."

Because of the sedentary habits of lice, one searches for them by carefully examining the hair coat or plumage of the host. The one exception to this generalization, the human body louse *Pediculus humanus humanus*, clings to the fibers of the clothing instead of body hairs while it feeds on its host. With a little practice, bloodsucking lice and chewing lice can be distinguished by inspection. This plus high host specificity simplifies identification, especially for hosts that have only one species of louse (e.g., *Haematopinus suis* on *Sus scrofa* and *Felicola subrostratus* on *Felis catus*). The next simplest case involves one anopluran and one mallophagan species per host species (e.g., *Haematopinus asini* plus *Damalinia equi* on *Equus caballus* and *Linognathus setosus* plus *Trichodectes canis* on *Canis familiaris*). Cattle (*Bos taurus*) present a more complex case; they are infested by three anoplurans and one mallophagan, and attention to generic morphological characteristics is required for their differ-

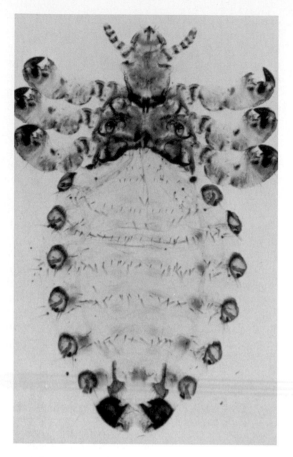

FIGURE 1-30 *Haematopinus eurysternus* (Anoplura) of cattle (×31). All tarsal claws are of equal size.

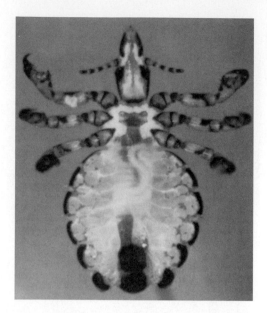

FIGURE 1-31 *Haematopinus suis* (Anoplura) of swine (×20).

tropical and subtropical parasite of *Bos indicus* and indicus-taurus hybrids, lays its eggs in the tail switch but may be found around the eyes and long hairs of the ears (Roberts, 1952). *H. tuberculatus* is an Old World parasite of water buffalo *(Bubalus bubalus)* and of domestic cattle associated with them (Meleney and Kim, 1974).

Heavy infestations of *H. eurysternus* are capable of causing severe anemia in adult range cattle (Peterson et al, 1953). Certain individuals are predisposed to the growth of large populations of lice, whereas other members of the same herd support only light infestations. These "louse breeders," as they are called, are likely to perish during winter storms, weakened as they are by their louse burdens. Such animals may be saved by insecticide applications. The rate of increase in hematocrit is, however, considerably slower than one would expect in a simple blood loss anemia.

Linognathus

Unlike *Haematopinus,* the first pair of tarsal claws of *Linognathus* is smaller than the second and third

pairs, and the lateral margins of the abdomen are not heavily sclerotized (Figure 1-32). *Linognathus* differs from *Solenopotes* in having more than one row of setae per abdominal segment and in lacking a sternal plate and protuberant abdominal spiracles. Species of *Linognathus* infesting domestic animals include *Linognathus vituli* of cattle, *Linognathus ovillus, Linognathus pedalis,* and *Linognathus africanus* of sheep, *Linognathus stenopsis* and *L. africanus* of goats, and *L. setosus* of dogs and foxes (Figure 1-33).

Solenopotes

Solenopotes capillatus, the "little blue louse" of cattle, is distinguished from *Linognathus* in having only one row of setae per abdominal segment, a sternal plate at least half as wide as it is long, and protuberant abdominal spiracles (Figure 1-34).

Polyplax

Polyplax spinulosa is a parasite of the rat, and *Polyplax serrata* is a parasite of the mouse (Figure 1-35). Both of these anoplurans may develop into serious nuisances in laboratory animal colonies and, when sufficiently abundant, may even bleed animals to death (Figure 1-36).

Pthirus

The large tarsal claws of *P. pubis* (Figure 1-37) are adapted to the coarse hairs of the pubic and perianal regions, armpits, mustache, beard, and, particularly in young children, the eyebrows and eyelashes, these latter two furnishing the nearest approximation to a pubic hair that a child has to offer. Pruritus

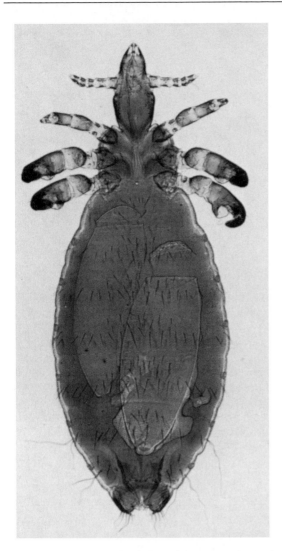

FIGURE 1-32 *Linognathus vituli* (Anoplura) of cattle (×45). The first pair of tarsal claws is smaller than the second and third pairs. Spiracles are flush with the surface of the abdomen, and there is more than one row of setae per abdominal segment.

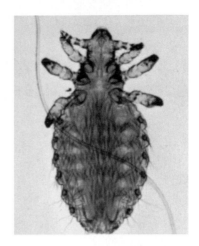

FIGURE 1-33 *Linognathus setosus* (Anoplura) of dogs and foxes (×38).

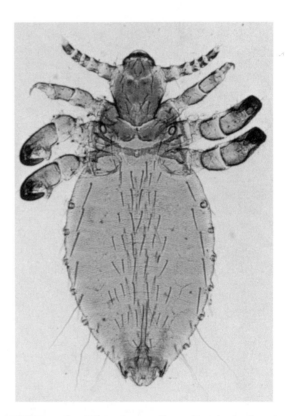

FIGURE 1-34 *Solenopotes capillatus* (Anoplura) of cattle (×60). The first pair of tarsal claws is smaller than the second and third pairs. Spiracles protrude above the surface of the abdomen, and there is only one row of setae per abdominal segment.

is intense, and a papular dermatitis with discoloration of the skin develops. Once feeding, these lice display a marked disinclination to move and tend to remain fixed at one point for days while their feces accumulate about them. The life cycle requires about 1 month from egg to egg, so that considerable time may elapse between acquisition and awareness of infestation. Although sexual contact is the principal means of transmission between individuals, towels, clothing, and bedding used by an infested person are to be avoided. Entire families, children and family dog included, may become infested through fomites such as these. During crises of this sort, the dog may be presented to the veterinarian for euthanasia in the mistaken belief that the dog is the culprit and reservoir of pestilence. Dealing with a family outbreak of crab lice and falsely incriminated dog requires considerable tact.

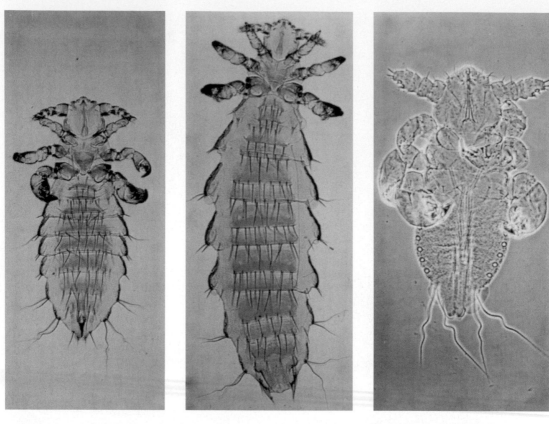

FIGURE 1-35 *Polyplax serrata* (Anoplura) of the mouse. *Left,* Male (×70); *center,* female (×70); *right,* nymph (×168).

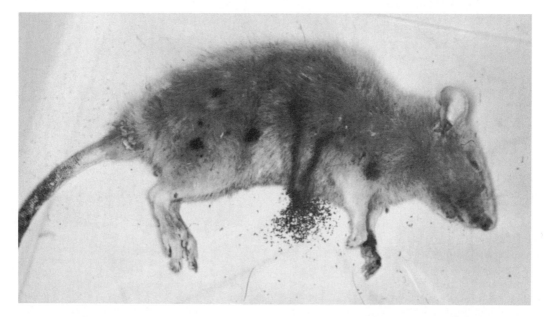

FIGURE 1-36 *Polyplax spinulosa* leaving a rat that died of the effects of its louse population. Urged on by the heat of an incandescent bulb, these lice are emulating their host's legendary tendency to flee from unpromising situations. This is a general phenomenon among the more mobile ectoparasites and can be exploited to advantage in diagnosis. However, if it is necessary to euthanize the host, do not use chloroform, ether, or other agents that will surely kill the parasites, as well as their hosts.

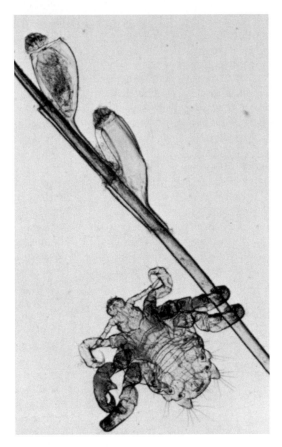

FIGURE 1-37 *Pthirus pubis* (Anoplura), the human crab louse and two of its eggs on a pubic hair (×25). Dogs occasionally acquire *P. pubis* by contact with infested humans or their clothing.

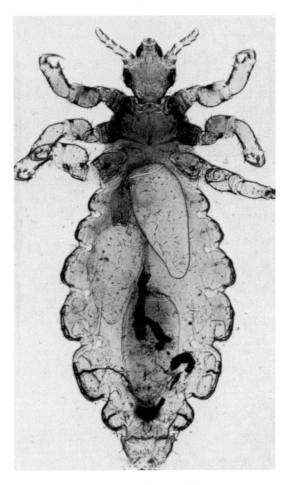

FIGURE 1-38 *Pediculus humanus capitis* (Anoplura), the human head louse (×34).

Lindane is the treatment of choice for *P. pubis* infestation and is available in pharmacies as a cream, a lotion, and a shampoo. Usually one application suffices, but treatment may need to be repeated in heavy infestations. Lice and their eggs are killed by exposure to a temperature of 50° C for 30 minutes, so sufficiently rigorous laundering can be an effective adjunct in control (Kraus and Glassman, 1976).

Another species in this genus is *Pthirus gorillae* of *Gorilla gorilla*.

Pediculus

The human head louse, *Pediculus humanus capitis,* stays mainly on the human head, especially around the ears and nape of the neck (Figure 1-38). Dogs are rarely infested. Eggs are attached firmly to the hairs and hatch within a week. Infestation spreads rapidly because of the ease with which hairs are shed and wafted about. Outbreaks of head lice may occur under the best conditions of sanitation and personal deportment. The human body louse, *Pediculus h. humanus,* does not cling to hair.

Instead, this louse clings to the fibers and deposits its eggs in the seams of clothing. Except in very heavy infestations, all people need do to be rid of body lice is to remove their clothing. When people are unable to bathe and change clothing for extended periods, as, for example, during wars and natural disasters, body louse populations are likely to expand rapidly. Under such circumstances, epidemic typhus *(R. prowazekii),* which is transmitted by the body louse, is likely to break out, and it is not for mere comfort's sake that vigorous delousing measures must be adopted.

Order Mallophaga

Some 4000 species of mallophagans, or chewing lice, are parasites of birds and mammals. All bird lice are biting lice, and there are many species of them. Mallophagans ingest a variety of epidermal materials. Some readily ingest feather keratin and can be cultured on this substance in vitro. A few, such as *Heterodoxus spiniger* of the dog and related amblyceran parasites of birds, are blood feeders (Agarwal, Chandra, and Saxena, 1982).

Because their hosts are insectivorous and very fastidious, bird lice are in constant danger of being eaten by their host instead of vice versa. However, they tend to be far less sluggish than their relatives that parasitize mammals; many have long legs to help them keep "one step ahead," and they frequently develop enormous populations. Mallophagans may cause their hosts considerable irritation when present in large numbers, especially in situations in which it is difficult for the animals to groom themselves, as in the case of stanchioned cattle. There are three suborders of chewing lice: Ischnocera, Amblycera, and Rhynchophthirina.

Suborder Ischnocera

Ischnocerans have salient antennae that are three-jointed in species infesting mammals (Figure 1-39)

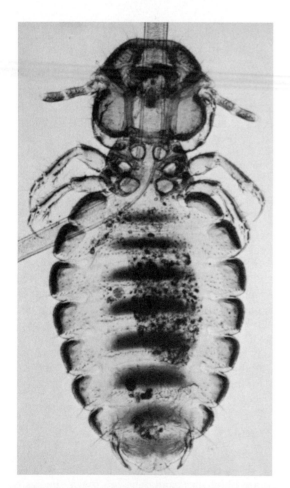

FIGURE 1-39   *Damalinia (Holokartikos) crassipes* (Mallophaga: Ischnocera) of the goat (×33). Typical of ischnocerans parasitizing mammals, *D. crassipes* has three-segmented antennae.

and five-jointed in species infesting birds; all lack maxillary palps (Figure 1-40).

Damalinia (Bovicola)

Species infesting domestic mammals include *Damalinia bovis* on cattle, *Damalinia equi* on horses, *Damalinia ovis* on sheep, and *Damalinia caprae, Damalinia limbata,* and *Damalinia Holokartikos* crassipes on goats.

Trichodectes

Trichodectes canis, the canine chewing louse (Figures 1-41 and 1-42), may serve as intermediate host (cyclodevelopmental vector) of the tapeworm *Dipylidium caninum,* although the flea *Ctenocephalides* is far more important in this respect. *T. canis* must be differentiated from the anopluran *L. setosus* and from the warm-climate amblyceran, *Heterodoxus spiniger.*

Felicola

Felicola subrostratus is the only louse found on cats (Figure 1-43).

Suborder Amblycera

Amblycerans have club-shaped antennae that lie in grooves in the head and four-segmented maxillary palpi (Figure 1-44). Many amblycerans are parasites of birds, but one species, *H. spinger,* is a parasite of dogs in warm climates, and three species, *Gliricola porcelli, Gyropus ovalis,* and *Trimenopon hispidum,* are parasites of the guinea pig (Figure 1-45).

Suborder Rhynchophtherina

Haematomyzus spp. are parasites of both Asian and African elephants and of wart hogs (Figure 1-46). The preferred location on elephants is the posterior

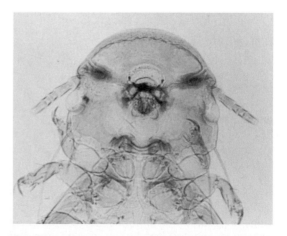

FIGURE 1-40   *Goniocotes* sp. (Mallophaga: Ischnocera) of the chicken (×79). Typical of ischnocerans parasitizing birds, *Goniocotes* has five-segmented antennae.

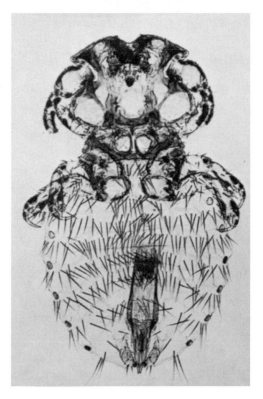

FIGURE 1-41 *Trichodectes canis* (Mallophaga: Ischnocera), male, of the dog (×51).

aspect of the ears and adjacent areas of the head and neck.

Treatment of Louse Infestations
Dogs and Cats

Lice are readily controlled with carbaryl-containing shampoo, spray, or dip. Usually two treatments are adequate when applied at an interval of 1 week.

Beef and Nonlactating Dairy Cattle

Most cases of louse infestation in cattle are mild and manifested only by occasional scratching and restlessness on the part of the animals. However, as populations increase through the winter and early spring, the degree of irritation to the animals (and to any sympathetic observer) verges on the unbearable, and treatment must be carried out. Coumaphos, chlorpyrifos, Fenthion, methoxychlor, and tetrachlorvinphos as sprays, dips, or pour-ons provide excellent control of lice. The macrolides administered subcutaneously are highly effective against anopluran infestations in cattle. The pour-on formulations of the macrolides also provide good efficacy against *D. bovis*. It has been shown in New York State that calves housed in outdoor

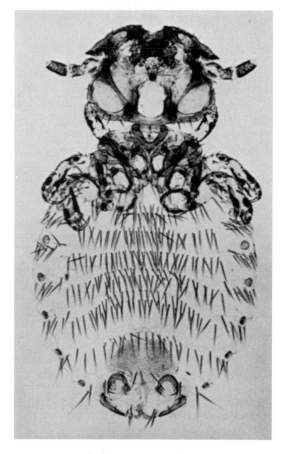

FIGURE 1-42 *Trichodectes canis* (Mallophaga: Ischnocera), female, of the dog (×51).

hutches have markedly lower louse infestation rates than calves held in collective stalls or pens in barns (Geden, Rutz, and Bishop, 1990).

Dairy Cattle

Tetrachlorvinphos, synergized pyrethrins, methoxychlor, and coumaphos are applied to lactating dairy cows as sprays, in dust bags, in backrubbers, and as sprinkle-on dusts. Two applications should provide good control. Eprinomectin is efficacious against louse infestations of lactating cows.

Swine

Coumaphos, methoxychlor, and tetrachlorovinphos provide good control of lice when applied as sprays or poured on the topline from shoulders to hips. It is good practice when treating swine to apply insecticide also to the bedding of the holding pens. Usually two applications are adequate. Ivermectin, doramectin, and moxidectin all have excellent efficacy against *H. suis*.

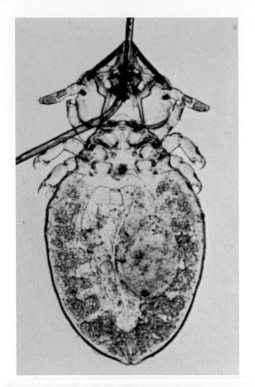

FIGURE 1-43 *Felicola subrostratus* (Mallophaga: Ischnocera) of the cat (×70).

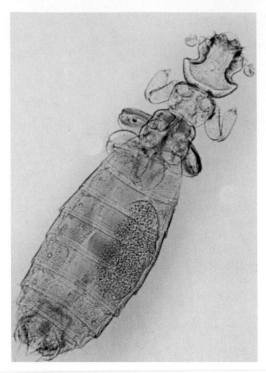

FIGURE 1-45 *Gliricola porcelli* (Mallophaga: Amblycera) of the guinea pig (×90).

Horses

Lice are found on horses principally during winter and spring. Two spray applications of coumaphos 2 weeks apart should provide adequate control. In cold weather, dusting horses with a mixture of rotenone and synergized pyrethrins is a less stressful procedure.

Elephants

Treatment of *Haematomyzus elephantus* infestations with oral administration of ivermectin at

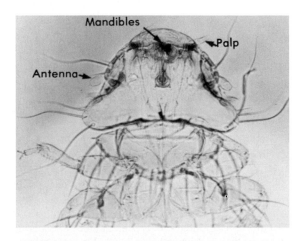

FIGURE 1-44 *Menopon* sp. (Mallophaga: Amblycera) of the chicken (×75).

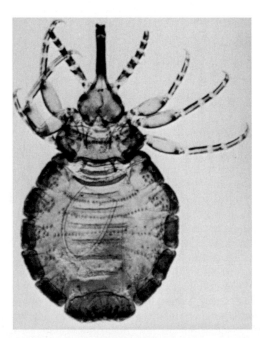

FIGURE 1-46 *Haematomyzus elephantis* (Mallophaga: Rhynchophthirina) of the elephant (×34).

dosages in the range 0.059 to 0.087 mg/kg body weight was found to be highly effective (Karesh and Robinson, 1985).

Order Siphonaptera, Fleas

Adult fleas are wingless, laterally flattened insects that feed on the blood of such animals as dogs, cats, pigs, humans, rodents, and birds. Metamorphosis is complex, with three caterpillar-like larval stages and an enduring pupal stage enclosed in a silken cocoon. Certain hosts develop hypersensitive reactions to flea bites characterized by intense pruritus. A hypersensitive dog or human suffers intolerably from the bites of a small number of fleas that a normal individual would scarcely notice. Various species of fleas transmit plague *(Yersinia pestis),* murine typhus *(Rickettsia typhi),* rabbit myxomatosis virus, and feline parvovirus (Torres, 1941) and serve as intermediate hosts of the tapeworm *Dipylidium caninum* and the filariid nematode *Dipetalonema reconditum.*

Ctenocephalides

Identification

The ubiquitous *Ctenocephalides felis* and the relatively rare *Ctenocephalides canis* are parasites of a very wide range of domestic and wild mammals, including cats, dogs, cattle, and humans. *Ctenocephalides* have both genal and pronotal combs (Figure 1-47), which easily distinguishes them from *Echidnophaga* (Figure 1-48), *Xenopsylla* (Figure 1-49), and *Pulex* (Figure 1-50), which have neither genal nor pronotal combs, and from certain rodent fleas that have only pronotal combs. *Cediopsylla* (Figure 1-51), a rabbit flea, resembles *Ctenocephalides* in having both genal and pronotal combs but can be distinguished as follows. If a line drawn along the bases of the genal teeth runs parallel to the long axis of the head, the specimen is *Ctenocephalides*, whereas if it runs at an appreciable angle, it is *Cediopsylla*. Do not fail to recognize the eggs and larvae of fleas as such (Figures 1-52 and 1-53). *Ctenocephalides* lay their eggs on the host. Many of these 0.5-mm-long, glistening, white eggs remain on the host long enough to hatch, so not only adults but eggs and larvae of *Ctenocephalides* are found in the haircoat of infested dogs and cats.

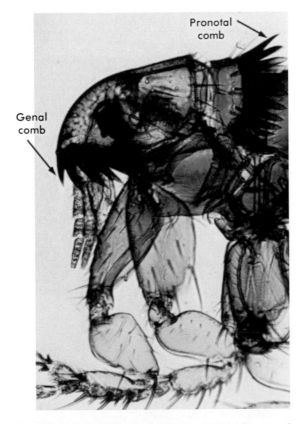

FIGURE 1-47 *Ctenocephalides* (Siphonaptera) of the cat and dog (×88). The bases of the genal teeth of *Ctenocephalides* lie on a line running parallel to the long axis of the head, thus serving to distinguish this genus from certain rodent and leporid fleas that have both genal and pronotal combs.

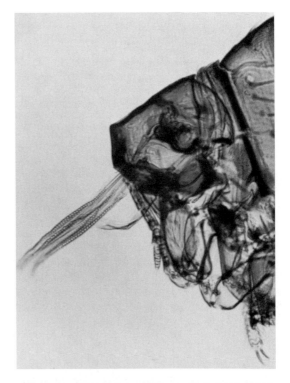

FIGURE 1-48 *Echidnophaga* (Siphonaptera) (×87). *Echidnophaga gallinacea*, the poultry sticktight flea, may be found firmly attached in clusters on chickens' heads and on the eyelids or in the ear canals of dogs, cats, and other animals.

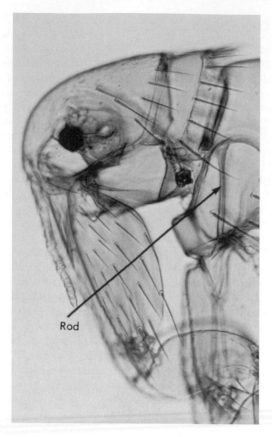

Rod

FIGURE 1-49 *Xenopsylla* (Siphonaptera), a rat flea and biological vector of plague (*Yersinia pestis*) and endemic typhus (*Rickettsia typhi*) (×82). The vertical rod on the mesothorax distinguishes this genus from *Pulex*.

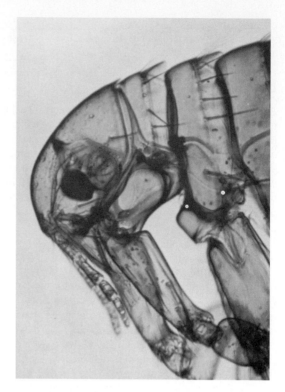

FIGURE 1-50   *Pulex* (Siphonaptera) (×81). *Pulex irritans*, the human flea, attacks a wide range of hosts.

Diagnosis of dog and cat flea infestation is sometimes difficult because only a few fleas are required to cause great misery, especially in a sensitized individual. Flea feces are essentially tiny particles of dried blood. The larval fleas eat their parents' feces, as well as other organic debris. Flea feces may be detected in the haircoat of a dog or cat by a sort of paper chromatography. Suspect detritus may be placed on filter paper or other absorbent material that has been dampened with dilute soap or detergent solution. Hemoglobin will diffuse out of flea feces in a few minutes and form a red halo around the speck of debris, or a similarly dampened pledget of absorbent cotton may be rubbed over the haircoat and skin to pick up particles of flea feces; little red spots appear on the cotton.

Life History

Metamorphosis of fleas is complex, with life stages consisting of egg, larval stages one, two, and three, pupa, and adult (Figure 1-54). The adult *Ctenocephalides* displays little tendency to leave its dog or cat host unless the population approaches about 200.

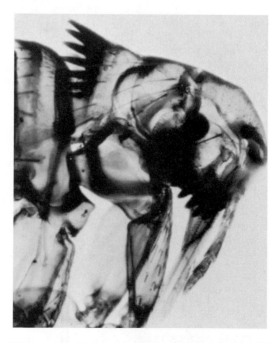

FIGURE 1-51   *Cediopsylla* (Siphonaptera) of the rabbit (×71). The bases of the genal teeth lie on a line running at an angle to the long axis of the head, thus serving to distinguish this genus from *Ctenocephalides*.

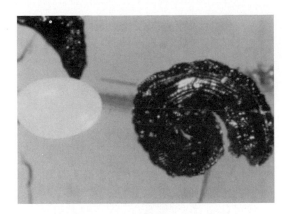

FIGURE 1-52 Egg of *Ctenocephalides* and two masses of flea feces (×50). Flea feces consists essentially of dried host's blood and serves as food for the flea larvae, which have chewing mouthparts.

Then, a few fleas may get off occasionally, especially when their host comes in contact with another, possibly less parasitized individual. A common misconception exists that *Ctenocephalides* fleas constantly jump on and off their hosts and find new hosts in this manner. In fact, most of the fleas a dog or cat acquires are brand new ones straight out of their pupal cases, and it is most

important to remember this fact in connection with control efforts (Figure 1-55). For every flea on the host, there are many eggs, larvae, pupae, and newly emerged adults in the environment, and these tend to be concentrated wherever the host habitually rests. The longer the host stays in one place, the more eggs and adult flea feces will be deposited there. Flea feces serve as the principal food of the three larval stages. Development of *C. felis* from egg to adult occurs within the ranges 13° to 32° C and 50% to 92% relative humidity and requires from 14 to 140 days at the extremes of temperature. Temperatures above 35° C are lethal to larvae and pupae. Unfed adults may survive for many weeks under cool, humid conditions but probably cannot long withstand the low relative humidities associated with subfreezing conditions (Silverman, Rust, and Reierson, 1981). Unfed *Ctenocephalides* adults can survive for about 2 months waiting for a host to happen by. People returning home after an absence of several weeks may be greeted by hordes of bloodthirsty fleas that, although preferring to feed on dogs, are quite willing to make do with humans when no dog is available. One of Dr. Georgi's mentors used to deal with this situation as follows. On arriving back in town, he would go directly to the kennel where his dog had been housed during his absence and take the dog home to collect the hungry fleas that were sure to be lying in wait there. After a brief tour of the house, the dog was immediately taken back to the kennel for a flea bath while the rest of the family retook possession of the house.

Disease Transmission

C. canis and *C. felis* are true intermediate hosts (biological vectors) of the tapeworm *D. caninum* and the filariid nematode *D. reconditum*. Fleas acquire *D. caninum* infection as larvae, since these are the stages with chewing mouthparts suitable for ingesting solid material such as the eggs of this tapeworm. The cysticercoid that develops from the egg is passed along through metamorphosis to the adult flea and infects the dog or cat that chances to ingest that particular flea. Microfilariae of *D. reconditum* are ingested by the blood-feeding adult flea and develop into third-stage larvae capable of infecting a dog. Feline parvovirus, the etiological agent of feline panleukopenia, can be transmitted from infected to susceptible cats by *C. felis* (Torres, 1941).

Treatment

Flea control has changed dramatically over the past few years owing to the introduction of several products designed to be administered to dogs and cats on a monthly basis. The impact of these products has been so dramatic that pest control operatives in

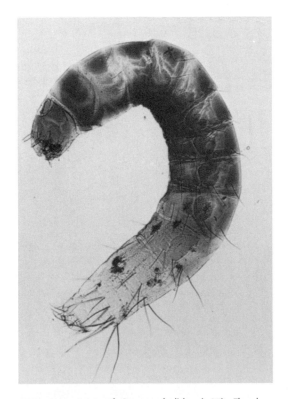

FIGURE 1-53 Larva of *Ctenocephalides* (×67). Flea larvae are frequently overlooked or misidentified.

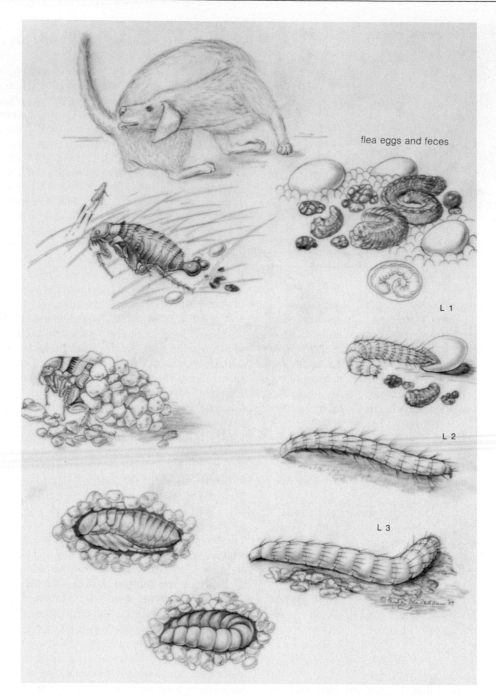

flea eggs and feces

L 1

L 2

L 3

FIGURE 1-54 Life history of *Ctenocephalides felis*. Eggs appear 2 days after male and female fleas arrive on a cat or dog. Most eggs fall out of the pelage and tend to accumulate where the host habitually rests, and first-stage larvae *(L1)* begin to hatch out of them on day 4. Larvae feed on adult flea feces, which, like the eggs, continuously rain down from the coat of an infested dog or cat, and pass through two molts. In about 2 weeks of warm, moist conditions, the third-stage larvae begin to spin cocoons and metamorphose into adult fleas (i.e., pupate). The cocoons are sticky so that fine debris, such as the sand grains in the picture, tends to accumulate on their surfaces. Adults begin to emerge from cocoons at 3 to 4 weeks, females preceding males by several days. Having found a dog or cat, the adult *C. felis* remains aboard feeding repeatedly and reproducing until it is exhausted and dies or is nipped and swallowed by the host. *C. felis* rarely leaves a suitable host of its own accord.

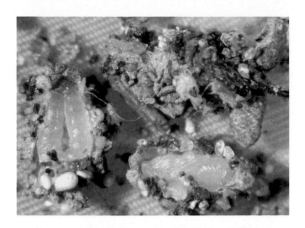

FIGURE 1-55 Cocoons of *Ctenocephalides felis. Left,* The cocoon has been opened to reveal the larva within; *bottom right,* the cocoon shows a flea that has almost completed metamorphosis.

the United States are seeing a decline in their flea-control contracts. It has been recommended that for fiscal reasons they should enter into local agreements with veterinarians over the sale of flea-control products (Fehrenbach, 1996). Three products have had this major effect on the science of flea control: lufenuron, an insect developmental inhibitor; fipronil, which blocks the passage of chloride ions in the gamma-aminobutyric acid (GABA)-mediated chloride channel of invertebrates; and imidacloprid, which binds to and blocks the nicotinic acetylcholine receptor of the flea. These three products are administered as a tablet, suspension, or injectable formulation (lufenuron), as a "spot-on" solution (imidacloprid and fipronil), or as an alcohol-based spray (fipronil). Lufenuron is also available in combination with milbemycin oxime in the form of a tablet designed for monthly administration to dogs for the regular interruption of the flea life cycle coupled with prophylaxis against canine heartworm infection. The three products either prevent the development of the larval fleas (lufenuron) or have direct effects against the adult fleas (imidacloprid and fipronil). Only one of the products, fipronil, is also active against ticks that may be found on dogs and cats.

A fourth product that has more recently entered the veterinarian's pharmacopeia is selamectin. Selamectin is an avermectin analog that, after becoming systematized after topical administration, is sequestered in the sebaceous glands of the cat or dog. From this site, the product acts to kill adult fleas and to prevent the development of flea eggs. The product is designed to be given monthly (Kwochka et al, 2000). Selamectin has the additional effect of preventing heartworm infection in the host to which it is applied. The product will also treat ear mites and sarcoptic mange. In cats,

selamectin also treats hookworm and roundworm infections. The product also has efficacy against the tick *Dermacentor variabilis.*

In the case of lufenuron, the female flea, which is the stage that ingests the majority of blood from a dog or cat, must take a blood meal. Then the larvae within the eggs of the flea are damaged by the insect developmental inhibitor that has been ingested by the female flea, and the eggs never hatch (Blagburn et al, 1994). Thus when a control program using lufenuron is initiated, additional products should be applied to both the pet and the household to reduce existing flea populations on the pet and in the environment. If such control does not accompany the initiation of this approach, the presence of fleas may be perceived by the clients as product failure. Like most people, clients want to see dead fleas as proof that control is occurring. Tablets containing nitenpyram, a neonicotinoid, will cause the very rapid death of adult fleas on dogs and cats. These tablets can be given daily, and fleas will begin to die within 30 minutes of administration (Dobson et al, 2000). In the case of fipronil and imidacloprid, the adult fleas on the dog or cat are killed. Thus there will be an initial decrease in the number of adult fleas. Because the majority of all fleas are to be found as eggs, larvae, and pupae in the environment, it is still highly beneficial to perform environmental treatments at the start of control programs using these products.

Environmental control is still a major means of controlling fleas, and it does not necessarily require chemicals. The vacuum cleaner is virtually indispensable in reducing the number of eggs, larvae, pupae, and unfed adult fleas in the environment. Remove, close, and dispose of the bag after vacuuming to prevent fleas from escaping back into the cleaned areas. Efforts to control fleas should be concentrated on the places where the dog or cat habitually rests, because here is where eggs and flea feces, the provender of larvae, are most likely to be deposited, and the development of adults fleas is likely to follow. One simple measure that affords 100% control of fleas is to keep the dogs or cats in wire-bottom cages elevated at least 13 inches (33 cm) above the ground or floor. In a commercial beagle-breeding establishment housing several thousand dogs and employing no chemical flea control, there were no fleas at all because the dogs in the colony were beyond the range of the staunchest jump that *C. felis,* champion jumper of the universe, can put forth (i.e., 33 cm) (Rothschild et al, 1973). Application of this latter environmental control method is clearly limited to strictly confined animals.

There are still numerous products designed for topical application to both animals and premises that will continue to be useful in flea control. Products that contain pyrethrins, carbaryl, phosmet, tetrachlorvinphos, and methoprene are usually effective and suitable for application to both animals and their surroundings. Chlorinated hydrocarbons are contraindicated for cats. Resistance to carbaryl and some organophosphates is on the rise, however, and this possibility must be taken into account in cases of apparent insecticide failure. Clients may treat pets with several different preparations and the premises with additional preparations, but if the labels are examined, it might be discovered that all preparations contain the same active ingredient. On the market are various dog and cat flea collars impregnated with various insecticidal compounds: chlorpyrifos, tetrachlorvinphos, naled, diazinon, amitraz. Some also are impregnated with the insect growth regulator, methoprene. These products do produce a certain level of control and when combined with careful premise management can produce rather successful treatment programs.

There are other available methods for the control of fleas that differ widely in their apparent effect on flea populations under various conditions. There are several traps commercially available for the capture of adult fleas. Some of these traps will collect more than 85% of released fleas, whereas others collect only slightly more than 10% (Dryden and Bruce, 1993). A citrus oil, D-limonene, appears to possess some activity against the various stages in the life cycle of the flea (Hink and Fee, 1986), and dips or shampoos containing this "natural" chemical may be a helpful adjunct to other flea control methods. Brewer's yeast failed as a repellent to fleas on dogs when fed as a dietary supplement at the rate of 14 g/day (Baker and Farver, 1983). Ultrasonic flea collars appear also not to repel fleas from dogs, at least under certain laboratory conditions (Dryden, Long, and Gaafar, 1989). Powdered boric acid, granular boric acid, and disodium octaborate tetrahydrate produced much less than 90% mortality of flea larvae when the larvae were exposed for 4 days in carpets at an application rate of 0.2 g/cm^2 (Hinkle, Koehler, and Patterson, 1995).

Fipronil, both the spray and the spot-on formulations, has been found to cause severe toxic reactions in rabbits treated for flea control. Thus the nonapproved use of fipronil on rabbits should be suspended for the time being.

It is important to remember that all insecticides are toxicants, not only to the insects but to the animal on which they are applied and to the person who applies them. Frequently the chore of bathing and treating dogs and cats falls on one or two members of a veterinary hospital staff, and by the nature of their work, such persons repeatedly become soaked with water containing insecticides. Unless great care is exercised to limit contact with these toxic chemicals, such persons are in considerable danger of suffering acute intoxication, and some degree of chronic intoxication is almost inevitable. It is the responsibility of veterinarians in charge to enforce procedures designed to minimize exposure of their employees to toxic chemicals.

Echidnophaga

Echidnophaga gallinacea, the "sticktight flea" of poultry, attacks all kinds of domestic birds, as well as dogs, cats, rabbits, horses, and humans, in subtropical America. Dr. Georgi once found several embedded in the eyelids of a cat recently arrived in New York from Alabama. On birds, *E. gallinacea* embeds itself in the skin around the eyes and cloaca and on the combs, wattles, and other glabrous areas. These are small fleas with angular heads devoid of genal and pronotal combs; the thoracic tergites (dorsal sclerites of the thorax) are very narrow (see Figure 1-48).

Tunga

Tunga penetrans, the "jigger" or "chigoe," is a small (1 mm) flea of tropical America and Africa that somewhat resembles *Echidnophaga* in having an angular head and narrow thoracic segments and in lacking combs. The impregnated *Tunga* female embeds in the skin of the ankles, instep, and between the toes, with only the last few abdominal segments protruding. Eggs are retained in the abdomen, and the flea swells to the size of a pea. Lesions caused by this flea are painful and subject to secondary infection and are supposedly the inspiration for the sailor's oath, "I'll be jiggered" (Chandler and Read, 1961).

Xenopsylla

Xenopsylla is a widely distributed genus of rat fleas that also attack humans and are an important vector of plague *(Yersinia pestis)* and murine (endemic) typhus *(Rickettsia typhi)*. Combs are absent, and the head is smoothly rounded, thus distinguishing *Xenopsylla* from the foregoing genera; it differs from *Pulex* in having a vertical rod on the mesothorax (see Figure 1-49).

Disease Transmission

Plague is normally a disease of rodents caused by the bacterium *Y. pestis* and transmitted by various fleas, of which *Xenopsylla cheopis* stands out, especially in relation to human infection. The great plague pandemics that decimated civilization during the Middle Ages may have been precipitated

TABLE 1-6 ■ Some Details on the Times Required for the Life Cycle Stages of Various Diptera, Fleas, and Lice*

Group	Egg (persistence and time to hatching)	Larva	Pupa	Adult Life Span Male	Female
NEMATOCERA					
Mosquito	Days to years	7 days	2–3 days	1 wk	4–5 mo; can hibernate
Black fly	3–7 days Diapause	7–12 days Weeks to months	2–6 days	2–10 wk	
Tabanid	5–7 days	1 year 6 mo–3 yr	1–3 wk	Few days	Months
	1 generation/year in temperate climates				
CYCLORRHAPHA					
Musca	8–12 hr	5 days	4–5 days	<Females	2–10 wk; can hibernate
	10 to 12 generations/summer				
Stomoxys	1–3 days	9–60 days	4–9 days		Weeks
Haematobia	1 day	4–8 days	6–8 days (overwintering stage)		Weeks
Calliphorid	6–48 hr	3–9 days	5–10 days		35 days
Cochliomyia	11–21 hr	3.5–4.5 days	7 days		Weeks
Sarcophagid	Often skipped	14 days			Weeks
Melophagus	Skipped	Hours (10–12/female)	3 wk		4 mo (1 mo to mature)
Gasterophilus	5 days	9–11 mo	3–5 wk		Weeks (early spring)
Hypoderma	5–7 days	8–11 mo	4–5 wk		Weeks
Oestrus	Skipped	25–35 days or 8–10 mo	Hibernation or 3–6 wk		4 weeks
FLEAS: SIPHONAPTERA					
Ctenocephalides	2–21 days	9–15 days	7 days–1 yr		Weeks (can be kept alive a long time in laboratory)

LICE (SIMPLE METAMORPHOSIS)

Group	Egg	(Nymph—no larvae or pupae)	Adult
Pediculus	7–9 days	9–11 days	30 days
Haematopinus	11 days	11–22 days	14 days
Felicola	10–20 days	14–21 days	14–21 days
Trichodectes	7–14 days	14 days	20 days

*These represent generalities.

by large-scale plague mortality among humans' rodent cohabitants, resulting in the vector turning to humans for its blood meals and communicating *Y. pestis* to them in the process.

Pulex

Pulex irritans, the human flea, is widely distributed and attacks a wide range of hosts, including humans, swine, and dogs. *Pulex* resembles *Xenopsylla* but lacks the mesothoracic rod (see Figure 1-50).

The developmental times of various flies, fleas, and lice are presented in Table 1-6.

Order Hemiptera, Bugs

Hemipterans have two pairs of wings (which may be vestigial), a triangular shield between the wing bases, four-segmented antennae, and a three-segmented beak that is directed caudally beneath the head when not in use (see Figure 1-55; Figure 1-56).

Metamorphosis is simple. Some hemipterans feed on plants; some kill insects and suck their juices; and some are bloodsuckers and pests of rodents and humans, occasionally attacking other animals. Predacious reduviids (assassin bugs) inflict painful bites, and many such species have been reported to attack humans, but the bites of the more specialized parasitic reduviids (cone-nose bugs) and cimicids (bed bugs) are painless.

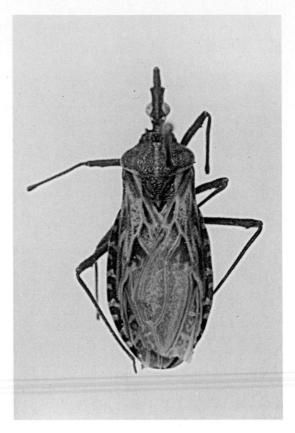

FIGURE 1-56 *Triatoma protracta* (Hemiptera: Reduviidae), an assassin bug. Vector of *Trypanosoma cruzi* in North America. (Courtesy Dr. Stephen C. Barr.)

Family Reduviidae, Assassin Bugs, and Kissing- or Cone-Nose Bugs

The reduviids (see Figure 1-56) have wings and a characteristic three-segmented beak. The parasitic species of the subfamily Triatominae, which feed exclusively on the blood of vertebrates, have a more slender beak than the predatory species and are able to feed painlessly enough so as not to awaken a sleeping host. They hide in crevices by day and attack their sleeping hosts by night in the manner of bed bugs, argasid ticks, and some species of mesostigmatid mites. Triatomids of the genera *Triatoma, Rhodnius,* and *Panstrongylus* transmit American trypanosomiasis or Chagas' disease *(Trypanosoma cruzi). Triatoma sanguisuga* may play a minor role in the transmission of equine encephalomyelitis.

Family Cimicidae, Bed Bugs

Bed bugs (Figure 1-57) have oval, dorsoventrally flattened bodies, vestigial wings, three-segmented beaks, and a disagreeable odor. They are nocturnal and secretive bloodsucking parasites of humans, chickens, bats, and nesting birds. Like triatomids,

bed bugs hide in crevices by day and attack their sleeping host at night. They lay their eggs in their hiding places and molt 5 times at approximately weekly intervals, taking one blood meal between each molt and another before egg laying. Bed bugs can endure starvation for several months. Although such a blood-feeding pattern as this would seem ideally suited to the transmission of disease organisms, bed bugs, though frequently indicted, have yet to be convicted on any such counts.

Order Blattaria, Cockroaches

Cockroaches are important as intermediate hosts of certain parasitic worms such as the spirurid nematodes *Spirura, Oxyspirura,* and *Gongylonema,* the acanthocephalans *Moniliformis, Prosthenorchis,* and *Homorhynchus,* and the pentastomid *Raillietiella.* They also serve as mechanical vectors of filth-borne diseases of humans. Inspection of premises where food is prepared is often a veterinary function. Presence or absence of cockroaches is an

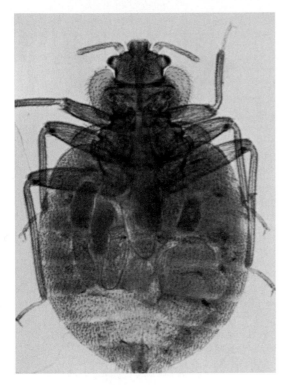

FIGURE 1-57 *Cimex lectularius* (Hemiptera: Cimicidae), the bed bug (×15).

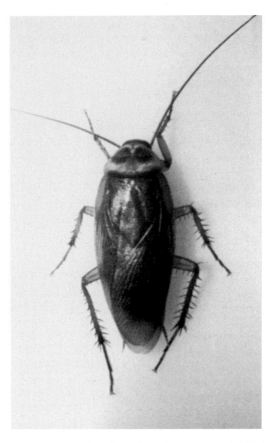

FIGURE 1-58 A cockroach, *Periplaneta americana* (Blattaria) (×1.5).

important criterion of the adequacy of food sanitation (Figure 1-58).

Order Coleoptera, Beetles

Beetles have hard, shell-like outer wing covers called **elytra** that lack venation (Figure 1-59). Metamorphosis is complete; the larvae are grubs.

Beetles, like cockroaches, are important as intermediate hosts of parasitic worms that infect domestic animals and humans. The spirurid nematodes *Gongylonema* and *Physocephalus,* the acanthocephalans *Macracanthorhynchus* and *Moniliformis,* and the cestodes *Hymenolepis* and *Raillietina* (not to be confused with the pentastomid *Raillietiella* or, for that matter, with the mesostigmatid *Raillietia*), all develop in beetles to the stage infective for the vertebrate host.

Some species of beetles are also extremely toxic. For example, blister beetles (*Epicauta* spp.) (Figure 1-60) release an irritant and vesicant chemical (**cantharidin**) when crushed during single-operation mowing and crimping of alfalfa hay. Hay containing these crushed beetles is lethal for horses and may remain so even after years of storage. Clinical signs of cantharidin toxicosis include abdominal pain, fever, depression, frequent urination, shock, and occasionally, synchronous diaphragmatic flutter

and mortality may exceed 70% of affected individuals. Hematological findings included hemoconcentration, neutrophilic leukocytosis, and hypocalcemia. As in all clinical poisonings, locating the source of the toxic agent is essential both to reaching a definitive diagnosis and to preventing further losses; the beetles should be sought in hay fed to the affected horses (Schoeb and Panciera, 1978, 1979). The lethal dose of cantharidin for the horse is probably less than 1 mg/kg body weight (Beasley et al, 1983).

Dung beetles (some 14,000 species of the family Scarabaeidae) are very important in the grazing ecology because they break up, remove, and bury manure. Without their services, ruminant and horse dung tends to accumulate on the pasture, where it breeds flies, physically interferes with the growth of grass, and discourages grazing in the immediate vicinity. Besides simply clearing the surface of pastures, dung beetles enhance fertility and tilth by burrowing in the soil and carrying their little balls of dung down into the burrows, where it is attacked by bacteria and fungi and the nutrients therein are made available to plants. Australia has gone so far as to import dung beetles from Africa in a

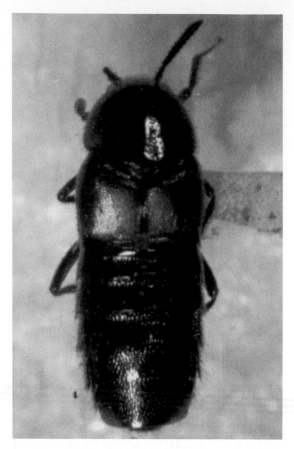

FIGURE 1-59 A beetle, *Aleochara bimaculata* (Coleoptera; Staphylinidae). This beetle is an ectoparasite on horn fly and face fly pupae as a larva and feeds on fly eggs as an adult (×22). The elytra of this beetle cover only the anterior portion of the abdomen.

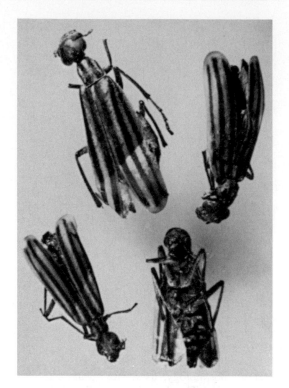

FIGURE 1-60 *Epicauta* sp. striped blister beetles (approximately ×2). Consumption of alfalfa hay containing dead striped blister beetles causes acute cantharidin toxicosis in horses. (Specimens courtesy Dr. R.J. Panciera.)

successful effort to reduce accumulations of cattle dung on pasture and the fly populations that breed therein. Administration of ivermectin to grazing cattle suppressed not only target organisms but dung beetle populations as well. This unforeseen effect of anthelmintic medication may have potentially disastrous effects on dung removal and soil nutrient cycling, at least under some environmental conditions and dosage regimens (Coe, 1987; Wall and Strong, 1987).

The small hive beetle, *Aethina tumida,* was introduced into the United States sometime around 1998 (Elzen et al, 1999). The beetle is now known to be in Florida, Georgia, South Carolina, Pennsylvania, Ohio, Minnesota, and Michigan. The beetles enter the hives of the European honeybee *(Apis mellifera),* and the beetle larvae feed upon honey in the combs and cause the bees to flee the hive. This is one of several recently introduced arthropod pathogens of honeybees that have caused severe damage to these important pollinators throughout the United States.

■ CLASS ARACHNIDA

Although the class Arachnida includes spiders, scorpions, whip scorpions, and other forms that are of occasional interest to veterinarians, the following exposition is restricted to the ticks and mites. Larval stages of both ticks and mites normally have three pairs of legs, and the nymphs and adults have four pairs. The head, thorax, and abdomen are fused; antennae and mandibles are absent. The mouthparts (**palps, chelicerae,** and **hypostome**) together with the **basis capituli,** form a capitulum, or gnathosome (Figure 1-61).

Suborder Metastigmata, Ticks

All ticks are bloodsucking parasites. The hypostome is armed with backward-projecting teeth, and the chelicerae are armed with movable denticles (see Figure 1-61). The lateral stigmata are caudodorsal to the fourth coxae (Figure 1-62) and lack the sinuous peritremes characteristic of the somewhat similar suborder Mesostigmata.

The greatest importance of ticks attaches to the large number and variety of microbial diseases that they transmit among domestic animals. These

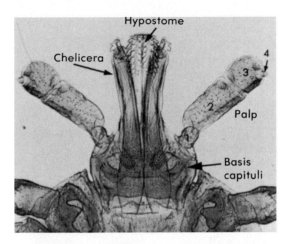

FIGURE 1-61 Capitulum of *Amblyomma* (×40).

diseases are listed later in the discussion on the particular genera involved as vectors. Other injuries inflicted by ticks include toxicosis, the bite wound, worry, and blood loss. There are two major families of ticks, the Argasidae, or **soft ticks,** and the Ixodidae, or **hard ticks.** Besides markedly different morphology, these ticks vary greatly in their behavior. The Argasidae family tends to be composed of species that live in nests or burrows from where they surreptitiously feed quickly on unsuspecting hosts. Ixodid ticks tend to spend most of their lives in fields or scrub areas where they await passing hosts. These ixodid ticks then attach

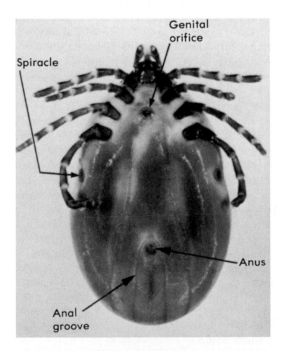

FIGURE 1-62 Ventral aspect of *Ixodes* (×11). The anal groove of *Ixodes* curves anteriorly around the anus.

and remain attached to their hosts for up to several days before they release and drop to the ground.

Family Argasidae

The family Argasidae, or **soft ticks,** is small, consisting of 140 species belonging to four genera, *Argas, Ornithodoros, Otobius,* and *Antricola.* Antricola spp. are limited to bats and will not be considered further here. Argasids live in nests, burrows, buildings, and sleeping places of their host animals and are distributed mostly in arid regions or in drier habitats in moist regions. The life stages consist of the egg (laid in several batches of hundreds), larva, two or more nymphal stages, and adult male and female. Unlike ixodid nymphs and adults, which require several days to complete engorgement and feed only once during each stage, argasid nymphs and adults feed to repletion on their sleeping hosts in minutes or hours and feed repeatedly. Females lay a clutch of eggs after each blood meal. Argasid larvae, on the other hand, feed for several days, and *Otobius* nymphs may remain in the external ear canal of cattle for several weeks.

Argas
Identification
Argas spp. are 5 to 10 mm, flattened, ovoid, and yellow to reddish-brown ticks with leathery, mammillated, and wrinkled dorsal and ventral surfaces meeting at a sharp lateral margin. The mouthparts are on the ventral surface and thus hidden when the tick is viewed from above (Figure 1-63). *Argas* is rarely found on the host. Search cracks and crannies in the hen house for this parasite. In the United States, *Argas* is distributed along the Gulf of Mexico and Mexican border.

Life History
Female *Argas* ticks deposit their eggs in clutches of 25 to 100 in the crevices that serve as hiding places during the day. Several clutches are laid, each preceded by a blood meal lasting 45 minutes or less. The six-legged larva hatches in 1 to 4 weeks, attaches to a host, and feeds for about 5 days; the larva is thus active day and night. When replete, the larva leaves the host and finds a hiding place in which to spend a week or so molting into a nymph. The eight-legged nymph feeds at night and undergoes a second molt to a second nymphal stage, which again feeds and undergoes a third molt into an adult male or female. Although development from egg to adult may be completed in as few as 30 days, lack of suitable hosts may prolong the process. Larvae and nymphs may survive for months and adults for more than 2 years without a blood meal. Trying to starve them out does not pay.

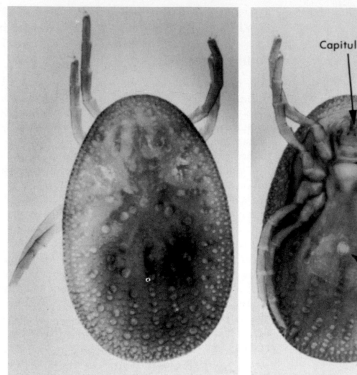
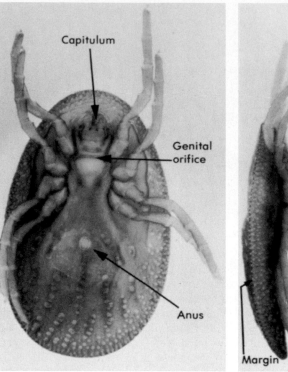

FIGURE 1-63 *Argas. Left,* Dorsal aspect; *center,* ventral aspect; *right,* lateral aspect (×10).

Disease Transmission

In South America, *Argas* spp. transmit fowl spirochetosis *(Borrelia anserina),* via tick fecal contamination, to domestic-poultry, grouse, canaries, guinea fowl, and pigeons. Ticks may remain infective for 6 months or more and transmit the spirochetes to their offspring via the ovaries (transovarial transmission). *Argas* spp. also transmit a rickettsial agent, *Aegyptianella pullorum,* to chickens and geese in the tropics and subtropics of the Old World.

TICK PARALYSIS. Infestation with larvae of *Argas persicus* can result in fatal flaccid paralysis of young chickens (Rosenstein, 1976).

Ornithodoros
Identification

Ornithodoros differs from *Argas* in being more globular, in lacking a sharp lateral margin, and in not appearing distinctly ovoid when viewed from above. The body is flattened in unfed specimens but strongly convex dorsally when distended with blood. These ticks (Figure 1-64) are found in cracks and crannies of avian roosts and nests, rodent burrows, and the resting places of large mammals.

Life History

Species of *Ornithodoros* differ with respect to whether the larvae feed, to the number of nymphal instars (three to five), and to host and lair preferences. *Ornithodoros hermsi* is a rodent parasite in the Rocky Mountain and Pacific Coast states, breeding in rodent burrows and rodent-infested buildings, whereas *Ornithodoros coriaceus* of California and Oregon attacks deer and cattle from the soil of their bedding areas. As typical argasids, *Ornithodoros* spp. can survive unfed for months or even years.

Disease Transmission

Ornithodoros spp. are most important as vectors and reservoirs of relapsing fever spirochetes *(Borrelia recurrentis)* of humans. Infection may be maintained in tick populations for many years by transovarial transmission of the spirochetes from female ticks to their offspring and tends to remain endemic in wild rodent populations. Tick-borne relapsing fever typically involves an individual or small group of campers who have slept in a tick-infested cabin out in the wilderness. Because the *Ornithodoros* ticks involved in transmission are nocturnal and surreptitious, relapsing fever victims are frequently unaware of recent tick exposure.

Otobius
Identification

Larvae and two nymphal stages of *Otobius megnini,* the spinose ear tick, parasitize the ear canals of

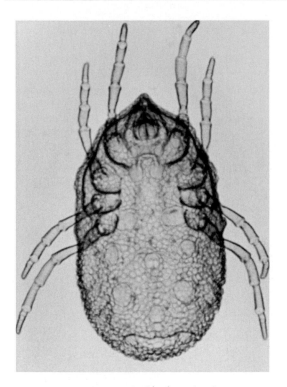

FIGURE 1-64 *Ornithodoros* (×14).

cattle, remaining in a particular host for as long as 4 months. Other domestic animals and humans also sometimes serve as hosts. One of Dr. Georgi's former students reported that he had suffered several painful attacks by *Otobius*. As implied by the common name, the cuticle of *Otobius* is covered by spines. The second nymphal stage is particularly distinctive (Figure 1-65).

Life History

Larvae feed in the ear canal and molt into the first nymphal stage, which in turn feeds in the same host's ear canal and molts into the second nymphal stage, which again feeds but leaves the ear canal and drops to the ground to molt to the adult stage. Adult *Otobius* have vestigial hypostomes and do not feed; they copulate within a day or two after emergence, and the females oviposit in the soil. Larvae survive unfed for as long as 2 months. Thus *Otobius* differs from *Argas* and *Ornithodorus* in being a one-host tick and in laying only one clutch of eggs.

Family Ixodidae

Members of the family Ixodidae, or **hard ticks,** have a shield, or **scutum,** that covers the entire dorsal surface of the male but only part of the dorsal surface of the female (Figure 1-66). The size of the scutum remains constant during engorgement of a female and consequently covers a progressively smaller proportion of her dorsum. Eggs are laid in a single clutch of thousands. Ixodid larvae, nymphs, and adults each feed only once, and several days are usually required for complete engorgement. Ixodids usually live outdoors and attach to passing host animals. There are two molts: the first from larva to

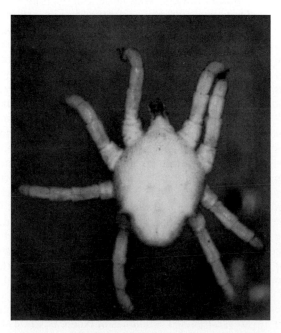
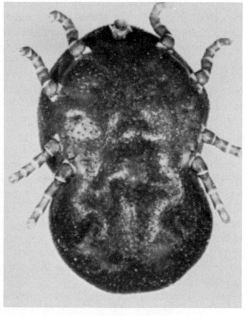

FIGURE 1-65 *Otobius megnini. Left,* First nymph (×12); *right,* second nymph (×8).

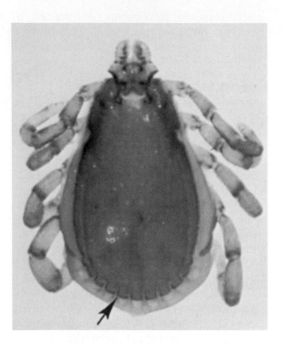 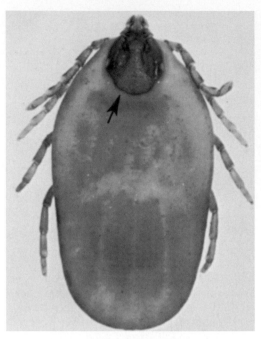

FIGURE 1-66 *Rhipicephalus* male (*left*, ×23) and female (*right*, ×12). The scutum *(arrows)* covers the entire dorsal surface of male ixodid ticks but only a portion of the dorsal surface of females. As the female engorges, the scutum remains constant in size and, at last, covers only a small proportion of the fully engorged female.

nymph and the second from nymph to adult. Species that complete both molts without leaving the host are called **one-host ticks;** species whose engorged nymphs drop off to molt are called **two-host ticks;** and those whose nymphs and larvae drop off to molt are called **three-host ticks.** *Dermacentor variabilis* is a three-host tick whose larvae and nymphs engorge on small mammals and whose adults engorge on dogs. *Rhipicephalus sanguinius* is a three-host tick whose larvae, nymphs, and adults all engorge on dogs. The individual or species identity of the host has no bearing on the use of these terms. What is important relative to these terms is that a one-host tick or a three-host tick that feeds on only one host is often easier to control through the management of the single host than a three-host tick that has different hosts throughout the environment. For example, if cattle are hosts to a one-host tick, dipping and other applications of chemotherapeutic agents or vaccination of the cattle will have effects on all life stages of the tick. If three hosts were involved, the first host might be a rodent, the second a rabbit or bird, and the third cattle. Thus it would be more difficult to manage these two- or three-host systems because it would be difficult to manage or treat all three hosts involved.

Two- and three-host ticks can transmit disease organisms **interstadially;** that is, infection acquired by a larval tick is carried through the molt to the

nymphal stage and then conveyed to the host on which the nymph feeds, or infection acquired by a nymph is carried through the molt and conveyed to the host on which the adult tick feeds. Thus three-host ticks can transmit disease organisms interstadially through both larva to nymph and nymph to adult transitions, whereas two-host ticks are limited to the latter. In **transovarial transmission,** the disease organisms are passed from the adult female tick to her larvae through infection of her ovaries. *Babesia bigemina* is transmitted from the adult female *Boophilus* tick to her progeny by way of her ovaries. Transovarial transmission of disease organisms is the only mechanism that allows one-host ticks, such as *Boophilus,* to serve as vectors.

Ixodid ticks found attached to domestic animals may be removed individually by cautious traction with thumb forceps. The long hypostomes of *Ixodes, Amblyomma,* and *Hyalomma* are effective anchors. *Dermacentor, Rhipicephalus, Boophilus,* and *Haemaphysalis* compensate for their shorter hypostomes by secreting a cement in which the mouthparts are embedded and that attaches them securely to the skin (Moorhouse and Tatchell, 1966; Moorhouse, 1973). Therefore unless reasonable care is exercised, the capitulum may be torn away and remain embedded as a foreign body in the skin of the host. Outdoor areas suspected as sources of ixodid tick infestation may be surveyed with a drag made by attaching one

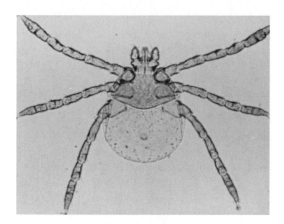

FIGURE 1-67   Six-legged *Rhipicephalus* larva (×40).

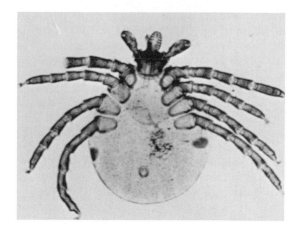

FIGURE 1-68   Eight-legged *Ixodes* nymph (×20). Although difficult to discern in this figure, an anterior anal groove can be found in the nymphal and larval stages of ticks of the genus *Ixodes*.

edge of a square yard of flannel to a stick and drawing it slowly over the vegetation. Hungry ticks will climb aboard the passing drag and can then be removed at intervals and placed in specimen bottles.

Veterinarians should carefully examine the ticks they encounter in practice. If a specimen is found that looks different from normal ticks, it should be sent to a diagnostic laboratory for expert identification. However, many practical problems can be solved by generic identification of adult ixodid ticks, and criteria for accomplishing that goal are presented here. No attempt is made here to identify larvae and nymphs beyond the family level; larvae have six legs (Figure 1-67) and nymphs have eight legs and a scutum of the female type, but the genital aperture is absent (Figure 1-68). A key to the nymphs of ixodid ticks that may be helpful to veterinarians has been presented elsewhere (Bowman and Giovengo, 1991).

In the following outline of genera of ixodid ticks, the **character in bold type** is either sufficient or nearly sufficient to represent the genus alone, provided, of course, that the corresponding morphological feature of the specimen is seen and correctly interpreted. Any ixodid tick must have one or another of these characters, and they serve as convenient starting points for identifying specimens; however, to be on the safe side, check each subsidiary character as well. Further details may be found in *Ticks of Veterinary Importance,* Animal and Plant Health Inspection Service (APHIS), United States Department of Agriculture (USDA), Agriculture Handbook No. 485.

Genera Found in North America

Ixodes
Identification
The anal groove forms an arch anterior to the anus; this can be seen with oblique illumination of

uncleared specimens (see Figure 1-62). Other genera have a groove posterior to the anus or no groove at all. *Ixodes* spp. have no eyes, festoons, or scutal ornamentation; their palpi are broadest at the junction of segments two and three (Figure 1-69). A tick's eye, by the way, is a mere roundish lucent area at the margin of the scutum about opposite the second coxa.

Life History and Disease Transmission
In Europe, species of *Ixodes* are vectors of bovine piroplasmosis and various vital diseases, including louping ill. *Ixodes holocyclus* of Australia is the most virulent tick paralysis producer known. *Ixodes pacificus* is known to cause tick paralysis in North America. Species of *Ixodes* are the major vectors of Lyme disease in North America and Europe.

Nymphs of *Ixodes dammini*, a three-host tick that normally feeds on mice and voles as larva and nymph

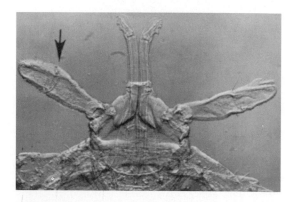

FIGURE 1-69   Capitulum of *Ixodes* (×40). The palps of *Ixodes* are broadest at the junction of the second and third segments *(arrow).*

and on deer as adult, transmits both microtine piroplasmosis *(Babesia microti),* Lyme disease *(Borrelia burgdorferi),* and human granulocytic ehrlichiosis to humans (Spielman, 1976; Burgdorfer et al, 1982), dogs (Lissman et al, 1984, Hinrichsen et al, 2001), and other animals. In the northeastern United States, the white-footed mouse, *Peromyscus leucopus,* is the principal reservoir host for *B. burgdorferi* and serves as host for larvae and nymphs of *I. dammini,* and the white-tailed deer, *Odocoileus virginianus,* serves as host to the adult tick, transmitting the spirochete both transovarially and transstadially (Lane and Burgdorfer, 1987). *Ixodes scapularis* and *Amblyomma americanum* may also occasionally transmit Lyme disease to humans (Matushka and Spielman, 1986). *I. pacificus* is a major vector of Lyme disease and human granulocytic ehrlichiosis in the western United States (Piesman, 1991). The incidence of human Lyme disease in May and June coincides with the activity of nymphs that were infected as larvae the previous summer. Thus nymphs feed in each transmission season before the larvae do. The white-tailed deer plays a dominant role as principal host of the adult *I. dammini* ticks, which feed on this host from late fall through winter (Matushka and Spielman, 1986).

Haemaphysalis
Identification
The palpi have laterally flared second segments (Figure 1-70). Avoid confusing these structures with the hexagonal basis capituli of *Rhipicephalus* and *Boophilus.* Like *Ixodes,* these ticks have neither eyes nor scutal ornamentation, but they differ in having festoons and a posterior anal groove.

Life History
Larvae and nymphs of *Haemaphysalis leporispalustris,* the rabbit tick, feed on ground-nesting birds and small mammals, and the adults attach to rabbits, especially to the ears and around the eyes. Occasional specimens are collected from cats.

Rhipicephalus
Identification
The basis capituli is hexagonal (Figure 1-71); eyes and festoons are present but the scutum is unornamented; males have salient adanal and accessory shields (Figure 1-72).

Life History and Disease Transmission
Larvae, nymphs, and adults of *Rhipicephalus sanguineus,* the brown dog tick, all feed on dogs and sometimes on humans (Figure 1-73). Originally a tropical species, *R. sanguineus* has taken advantage of central heating to spread into the temperate zones, where it often generates enormous populations in homes, kennels, and veterinary hospitals; it cannot survive the winter outdoors in the North. Dogs living in temperate regions frequently acquire their *R. sanguineus* ticks in such infested premises, but during summer, infestation may occur out-of-doors. Therefore if enduring results are to be achieved, elimination of these ticks must include acaricidal treatment of both the dog and the home or kennel. The latter procedure is a job for a professional exterminator. Development from egg to egg may be completed in slightly more than 2 months under favorable conditions; unfed adults may survive for well over a year. A household, including two dogs and the client's wife and

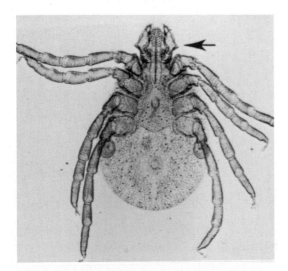

FIGURE 1-70 *Haemaphysalis* (×20). The second palpal segment *(arrow)* is flared laterally.

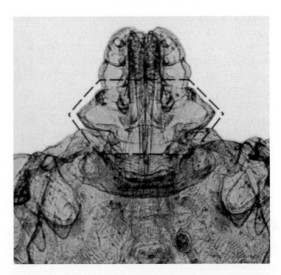

FIGURE 1-71 Capitulum of *Rhipicephalus* (×40). The basis capituli is hexagonal.

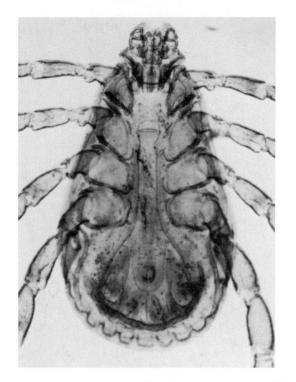 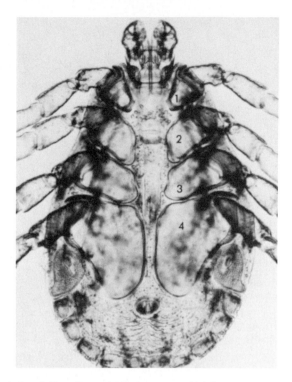

FIGURE 1-72 Ventral aspects of a male *Rhipicephalus (left)* and a male *Dermacentor (right)* (×21). Coxae of male *Dermacentor* progress in size from the first to fourth coxa.

mother-in-law who never left England, apparently acquired infestations with *R. sanguineus* through the introduction of the ticks into the client's car when he gave rides to a neighbor's dogs while at his summer home in France (Jagger, Banks, and Walker, 1996). He brought the ticks home to England from France in his car, thus indicating just how mobile ticks of this species can be.

R. sanguineus transmits canine piroplasmosis *(Babesia canis)* transovarially and tropical canine pancytopenia *(Ehrlichia canis)* interstadially.

African species of *Rhipicephalus* serve as vectors of the devastating East Coast fever *(Theileria parva)* and other forms of bovine theileriosis, bovine piroplasmosis *(Babesia bigemina)*, and the virus of Nairobi sheep disease.

Boophilus
Identification
The palps are ridged dorsally and laterally (Figure 1-74). Like *Rhipicephalus*, these ticks have a hexagonal basis capituli, eyes, and an unornamented scutum, and the males have adanal and accessory shields. However, *Boophilus* differs from *Rhipicephalus* in that it has ridged palpi and lacks festoons. *Boophilus* specimens encountered in the field should be immediately reported to state or federal authorities because *Boophilus* transmits bovine piroplasmosis, *B. bigemina*.

Life History and Disease Transmission
Boophilus annulatus, the transovarial vector of bovine piroplasmosis, was eradicated from the United States through 40 long years of dipping cattle that began in 1906. Losses from piroplasmosis were estimated then at 40 to 100 million dollars per year at a time when cattle were selling at 2 to 4 cents a pound. Eradication was favored by the affinity of this tick species for cattle and by its one-host life history, which made it possible to destroy a substantial proportion of the tick population each time the cattle were dipped. Comparable efforts to eradicate any species with broader host preferences, especially those feeding on wildlife, would have been much more difficult. *Boophilus microplus,* also a piroplasmosis vector, has a broader host range that includes horses, goats, sheep, and deer.

Dermacentor
Identification
The basis capituli is rectangular as viewed from above (Figure 1-75). Coxae of males progress in size from the first to the fourth (see Figure 1-72). *Dermacentor* resembles *Rhipicephalus* in having eyes and 11 festoons, but the basis capituli is rectangular, the scutum is ornamented (Figure 1-76), and the males lack adanal shields. *Dermacentor (Anocentor) nitens*, the tropical horse tick, has only seven festoons.

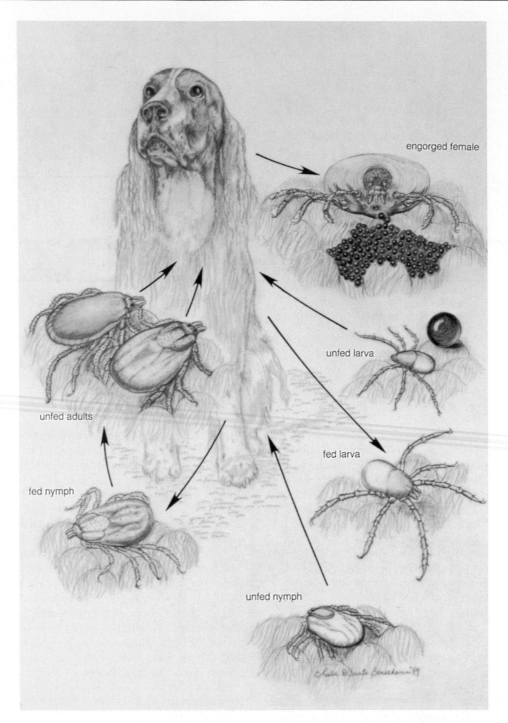

FIGURE 1-73 Life history of the brown dog tick, *Rhipicephalus sanguineus*. Six-legged larvae feed on the dog for a few days, drop off, and molt to the eight-legged nymphal stage. Nymphs feed on the dog for about a week, drop off, and molt into male and female adults. Females are fertilized on the dog and feed for 1 to 3 weeks and become greatly engorged with blood before dropping to the floor to lay their clutches of 2000 to 4000 eggs several weeks later. Eggs emerge from the genital opening one at a time and accumulate in front of the female tick over a period of several more weeks. The complete cycle requires 2 to 3 months, which is fast compared with that of most tick species.

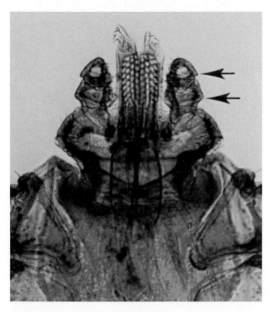

FIGURE 1-74 Capitulum of *Boophilus* (×60). The basis capituli is hexagonal, and the palpi are ridged dorsally and laterally (*arrows*).

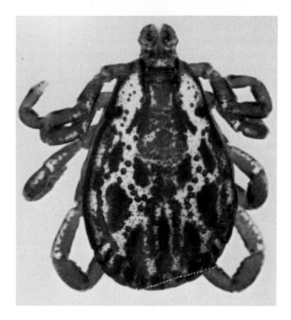

FIGURE 1-76 *Dermacentor* male (×14). Notice the ornamented scutum.

Life History and Disease Transmission

Dermacentor variabilis, the American dog tick, is widely but discontinuously distributed over the eastern half and West Coast of the United States and parts of Canada and Mexico. Larvae and nymphs engorge on small rodents; adults engorge on humans, dogs, horses, cattle, and wildlife. *D.*

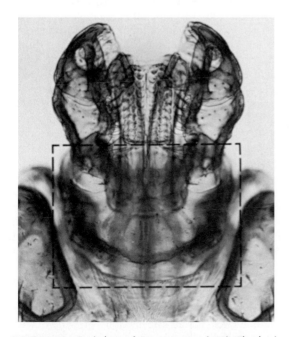

FIGURE 1-75 Capitulum of *Dermacentor* (×55). The basis capituli is rectangular.

variabilis transmits Rocky Mountain spotted fever *(Rickettsia rickettsi)* and tularemia *(Francisella tularensis)* and causes tick paralysis.

Dermacentor andersoni, the Rocky Mountain wood tick, requires 1 to 3 years to complete its life history, depending on the latitude, altitude, and abundance of small mammals on which it feeds as larva and as nymph. *D. andersoni* transmits Rocky Mountain spotted fever, tularemia, Colorado tick fever, and Q fever and causes tick paralysis.

D. nitens, the tropical horse tick, is limited, in the United States, to the southern portions of Florida and Texas. Preferring the external ear canals of horses but also found on other sites and other hosts such as cattle, sheep, goats, and deer, *D. nitens* is the vector of equine piroplasmosis *(Babesia caballi).* Other North American species of *Dermacentor* include *Dermacentor albipictus,* the winter tick that causes heavy losses among deer, elk, and moose; *Dermacentor nigrolineatus,* the brown winter tick; and *Dermacentor occidentalis,* the Pacific Coast tick.

In moose *Alces alces,* infestation with *D. albipictus* causes hair loss, which progresses rapidly from February to April and may amount to as much as 44% of the hair coat. McLaughlin and Addison (1986) estimated that loss of 30% of its hair in a winter environment of −20° C would double the daily energy requirements of an otherwise normal 230-kg yearling moose. The increased catabolic rate imposed by hair loss then leads to reduction in body fat stores and to lowered resistance to disease and predation.

Amblyomma

Identification

The mouthparts are much longer than the basis capituli; the second palpal segment is at least twice as long as the third (see Figure 1-61). Eyes and festoons are present, scutum is ornamented, and adanal shields are absent. *Aponomma elaphensis* resembles *Amblyomma* but is smaller and lacks eyes; it is a parasite of a rat snake in Texas.

Disease Transmission

In the United States, species of *Amblyomma* that attack humans, livestock, dogs, and cats (e.g., *A. americanum*, *Amblyomma maculatum*, *Amblyomma cajennense*, and *Amblyomma imitator*) are distributed mainly in the southeastern coastal states, Missouri, Oklahoma, and Texas, but specimens may occasionally be found as far north as Ithaca, New York. These species have been incriminated in the transmission of Rocky Mountain spotted fever, *Ehrlichia chaffeensis, Ehrlichia ewingi,* and tularemia, and in the causation of tick paralysis. African species of *Amblyomma* transmit heartwater *(Cowdria ruminatium)* of cattle, sheep, and goats, as well as the virus of Nairobi sheep disease. *Amblyomma dissimili,* the iguana tick, and *Amblyomma tuberculatum,* the gopher tortoise tick, are parasites of reptiles and amphibians; the latter is the largest ixodid tick, with engorged females reaching a length of 25 mm.

Genera Not Found in North America

Hyalomma

Hyalomma resembles *Amblyomma* in having mouthparts much larger than the basis capituli but differs in that the second and third palpal segments are approximately the same length (Figure 1-77). Eyes are present, festoons are irregularly coalesced; the male has adanal and accessory shields.

Margaropus

Margaropus resembles *Boophilus,* but the palps are not ridged and the legs of the male progress in size from the first to the fourth.

Rhipicentor

Rhipicentor resembles *Rhipicephalus* dorsally, and *Dermacentor* ventrally; eyes and festoons are present, adanal and accessory shields are absent, and fourth coxae are greatly enlarged.

Direct Effects of Ixodid Ticks on the Host

Tick Toxicosis

In North America, the species most frequently involved in tick paralysis are *D. andersoni, D.*

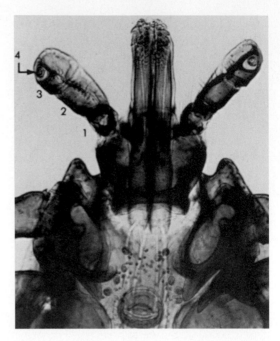

FIGURE 1-77   Capitulum of *Hyalomma* (×70). Palpal segments two and three of *Hyalomma* are approximately the same length, whereas the second palpal segment of *Amblyomma* is about twice as long as the third.

variabilis, A. americanum, and *A. maculatum.* Tick paralysis is an ascending paralysis caused by absorption of toxins from the saliva of engorging female ticks. The tick injects a considerable volume of saliva into the wound partly as an aid to digestion and partly as a means of disposing of surplus water extracted from the blood meal. A single female tick can produce paralysis in humans, dogs, or cats, especially if the site of attachment is near or on the head, but paralysis does not invariably occur even if many ticks of a suitable species are present. Usually, heavy infestations are required to produce tick paralysis in cattle. The first clinical sign is incoordination of the hindquarters that rapidly proceeds to complete paralysis and spreads to the forequarters, neck, and finally to the respiratory muscles, with fatal consequences. Removal of engorging ticks usually leads to gratifyingly rapid recovery. In Australia, *Ixodes holocyclus,* a parasite of the bandicoot and other marsupials, causes a particularly severe form of tick paralysis in domestic animals. Of 577 Australian dogs affected and seen by veterinarians in 1998, 5% of the dogs died from the disease (Atwell, Campbell, and Evans, 2001). Effective treatment of paralysis caused by *I. holocyclus* requires administration of specific antitoxin and general supportive treatment as well as removal of all ticks from the victim. Even larvae and nymphs of *I. holocyclus* are potentially capable of inducing paralysis when present in sufficient numbers. However, as is the case with other tick paralysis species, the engorging female of *I. holocyclus* is usually responsible. The surest prevention of tick paralysis lies in careful daily examination of exposed animals and removal of ticks. Because clinical signs of paralysis do not begin to appear until the ticks have been feeding for at least 4 days, they should be large enough to be found relatively easily before clinical signs develop. In areas of heavy exposure, weekly acaricidal dipping is necessary.

The Bite Wound

Ixodes, Amblyomma, and other genera with long mouthparts produce deep, painful bite wounds that tend to become inflamed, secondarily infected with bacteria, and flyblown. In Great Britain, secondary infection of *Ixodes ricinus* bites with *Staphylococcus* results in both local and metastatic abscessation (tick pyemia) in lambs. In the Gulf Coast states, *A. maculatum,* which prefers to attach to the ears of larger mammals, causes such pain and swelling that cattle are unable or at least reluctant to flick their ears and thus ward off flies. Before screwworm control, such ears were prone to invasion by larvae of *C. hominivorax,* frequently with the loss of the external ear or death.

Blood Loss and Worry

Sir Arnold Theiler once collected *half* of the *Boophilus decoloratus* ticks from a horse that had died of acute anemia. His collection weighed 14 lb (Theiler, 1911). That horse's tick burden must have contained about 13 L of blood. This example may appear extreme to those of us who dwell in temperate zones and experience only an occasional mosquito or black fly bite, but there are places in the tropics where light-colored cattle are so totally covered by the dark bodies of engorging ticks that they appear from a distance to be black. Loss of blood, pain from and swelling of bite wounds, secondary infection, myiasis, and absorption of toxins, in moderate and varying proportions, result in a form of ill thrift referred to as "tick worry." Because tick worry is the most common practical consequence of tick infestation, it may be even more important than the more dramatic ones.

Treatment and Control of Tick Infestations

Ticks on dogs and cats are now most easily treated by prevention with the topical application of fipronil. The application of this pesticide has been found to be an excellent means of preventing tick infestations of dogs and cats. Other topical products included pyrethrins and permethrins (permethrin should not be used on cats). Another approach is to use collars containing amitraz, chlorpyriphos, diazinon, methylcarbamate, naled, or tetrachlorvinphos. Control of *R. sanguineus* in buildings may be achieved by spraying with diazinon and could require the use of professional exterminators.

For lactating dairy cattle, coumaphos and dichlorvos are applied as sprays or in backrubbers for the control of ticks. There are no restrictions when used as recommended.

For beef cattle and nonlactating dairy cattle, coumaphos, dichlorvos, and malathion may be used as dips and sprays in the control of ticks. *Otobius megnini* ear ticks are treated with insecticidal dusts or emulsion concentrates instilled into the ear canal from squeeze bottles or an oil can. Ivermectin, doramectin, and moxidectin all provide some level of protection against ticks, but none of these products are currently labeled for tick control.

In horses particularly, tick-attachment sites may become markedly irritated and lead to an itch-scratch cycle marked by serious self-mutilation. Coumaphos is effective as a spray or dust when applied to the horse's entire body. Always wear rubber gloves and wash skin thoroughly after handling organophosphate and carbamate insecticides.

There are attempts, mainly driven by the fear people have of becoming infected with Lyme disease by tick bite, to develop means of controlling ticks within the environment. One means used is removal of an essential host. This has been tried for *I. dammini* by eliminating all deer in an area (Wilson et al, 1988). Such a drastic method may produce significant tick reductions, although alternative hosts may be found that allow the ticks to persist in the environment at lower numbers. Methods also have been examined for reducing the numbers of ticks on deer by the use of ivermectin-treated feed bait (Pound et al, 1996); this method also shows some potential for control. Another approach has been to attack the larvae of ticks by using acaricidal-impregnated baits or nesting material containing ectoparasiticides, which mice and rats carry to their nesting areas (Mather, Ribiero, and Spielman, 1987); again, this method can be quite successful in controlling ticks in isolated areas. Work is also underway to produce vaccines against ticks causing the host to produce antibodies that the tick ingests while feeding and that damage the gut of the feeding tick (Willadsen et al, 1995); such vaccines are likely to be used more and more widely as they become available for use in cattle, dogs, and cats.

Suborder Mesostigmata, Mesostigmatid Mites

Mesostigmatids, as the name implies, have **stigmata** (respiratory pores) in the middle of their bodies. A stigma lies between the third and fourth coxae on each side of the body and is connected to a sinuous **peritreme.** The coxae are evenly spaced and crowded into the anterior half of the body; the tarsi are generally armed with claws; and the ventrum is armored with sclerotized plates (Figure 1-78).

Families Dermanyssidae and Macronyssidae

Bloodsucking mesostigmatid mites that parasitize birds (e.g., *Dermanyssus gallinae, Ornithonyssus sylviarum*) and rodents (e.g., *Ornithonyssus bacoti, Liponyssoides sanguineus*) frequently turn on the human inhabitants of a building when deprived of their normal hosts, as may occur when fledglings leave their nests or after rodents have been exter-

minated. Generic or even familial identification of these mites is sufficient to establish the general nature of the epidemiological situation, but specific identification sometimes provides a very helpful lead in the search for nests. For example, a hospital administrator submitted a specimen of a mite that was causing great consternation by its abundance in the hospital's linens. Dr. Georgi identified the specimen as a dermanyssid mite and advised the gentleman to hunt for bird or rodent nests. A few days later, he reported no success in finding nests of either kind. However, by that time the specimen had been shown to an expert acarologist who identified it as *Dermanyssus hirundinus,* a relatively host-specific parasite of swallows. Thus advised, the hospital administrator knew just where to look, and the problem was quickly solved.

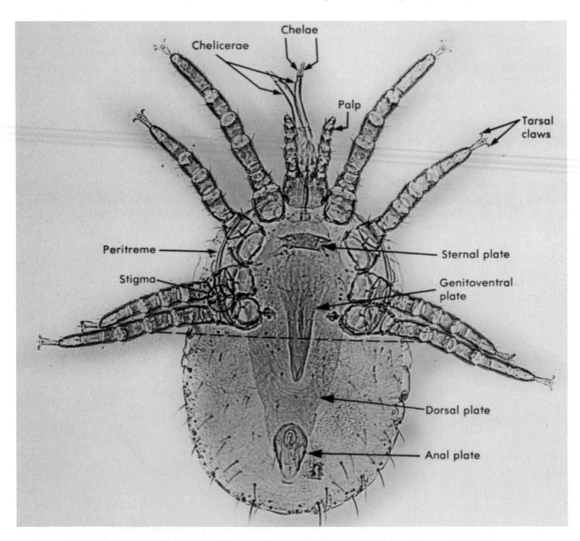

FIGURE 1-78 *Ornithonyssus sylviarum,* a bloodsucking mesostigmatid mite (×110). The legs are confined to the anterior half of the body of mesostigmatid mites; the stigma is located between the third and fourth coxae and has a peritreme. The chelae of *Ornithonyssus* are much larger than those of *Dermanyssus.*

Dermanyssids and macronyssids all look very much alike on casual inspection, but because they vary significantly in habits and host preferences, accurate identification is a prerequisite to effective control. The **chelicerae** (piercing mouthparts), **chelae** (scissorlike structures on the end of the chelicerae), and form and septation of various sclerotized plates provide the main taxonomic characters used in differentiating these mites.

Dermanyssus (Dermanyssidae)

The chelicerae are long and slender and the chelae minute (Figure 1-79). There is a single dorsal plate; the sternal plate has two pairs of setae; and the anus is in the posterior half of the anal plate. *Dermanyssus* mites are infrequently found on the bird because these mites hide in nests, roosts, and the like during the day and attack the sleeping bird at night. Life stages include the egg, which is deposited in the diurnal hiding places of the mites; the six-legged, nonfeeding larva; and the bloodfeeding protonymph, deutonymph, and adult male or female. A generation can be completed in as little as a week, and large populations may build up in chicken houses or birds' nests. The adults can survive starvation for months. *Dermanyssus* mites remove enough blood to kill nestlings and reduce egg production. Ramsay and Mason (1975) reported a case in a dog that was so severe that the mites crawling through the hair resembled the "walking dandruff" usually associated with *Cheyletiella* infestations. Their importance as disease vectors is unclear.

Liponyssoides (Dermanyssidae)

The chelicerae are long and slender and the chelae minute. There are two dorsal plates, the anterior plate 10 times as large as the posterior; the sternal plate has three pairs of setae. *Liponyssoides (Allodermanyssus) sanguineus,* a parasite of the house mouse, *Mus musculus,* and other small rodents, is the vector of rickettsial pox *(Rickettsia akari)* of humans.

Ornithonyssus (Macronyssidae)

The chelicerae are much stouter than those of *Dermanyssus,* and the chelae are easily visible under ordinary magnification. There is a single dorsal plate, and the anus is in the anterior half of the anal plate (see Figure 1-78). When the mite is alive, the

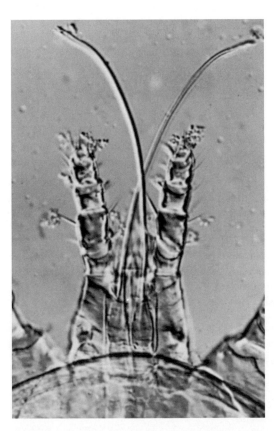

FIGURE 1-79 Gnathosome of *Dermanyssus gallinae* (×280). The chelicerae of *Dermanyssus* are slender and whiplike, and the chelae are very small.

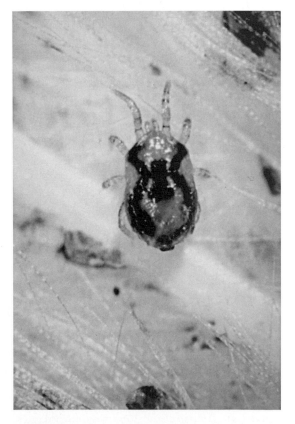

FIGURE 1-80 Living *Ornithonyssus sylviarum* (×52) crawling on a chicken feather collected from litter. Note the dark X-shaped gut.

gut often appears black or dark red (Figure 1-80). Common species include *O. sylviarum,* the northern fowl mite; *Ornithonyssus bursa,* the tropical fowl mite; and *O. bacoti,* the tropical rat mite. *Ornithonyssus* spp. remain on the host much of the time and cause considerable loss of blood. Persons handling eggs from laying flocks heavily infested with *O. sylviarum* may experience annoyance and serious discomfort from the bites of these mites. *O. bacoti* is an important pest in laboratory rodent stocks and serves as intermediate host for *Litmosoides carinii,* a filariid parasite of the cotton rat, *Sigmodon hispidus. L. carinii* is a favorite laboratory model for testing antifilarial drugs.

Ophionyssus (Macronyssidae)

Ophionyssus natricis, the snake mite, is a formidable bloodsucking pest that tends to thrive on captive snakes. Treatment of snakes has been performed using injectable ivermectin (Stanchi and Grisolia, 1986).

Family Raillietidae

Raillietia

Raillietia auris (Figure 1-81), long considered a harmless parasite of the ears of cattle, has been shown to cause ulceration and blockage of the auditory canals by pus with resultant loss of hearing (Heffner and Heffner, 1983). Jubb, Vasallo, and Wroth (1993) reported that infestations with this mite were associated with calves circling, ataxia, and unilateral facial paralysis. In their work, calves were cleared of their infestations with the application of flumethrin to the ear canal, whereas

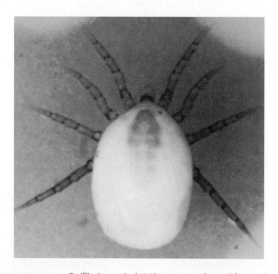

FIGURE 1-81 *Raillietia auris* (×30), a mesostigmatid parasite of the ear canal of cattle. In this reflected light photomacrograph, the specimen appears as it would under a stereoscopic microscope or powerful hand lens.

the topical application of flumethrin or subcutaneous ivermectin was unsuccessful.

Family Halarachnidae

Pneumonyssus

Groups of *Pneumonyssus simicola* mites may be found in the lung parenchyma of most if not all *Macaca mulatta* monkeys. The lesions are pinhead or larger, whitish or yellow foci that have soft or empty centers and contain mites and a black pigment. These lesions are scattered throughout the lungs and may be mistaken for those of tuberculosis. It is difficult to correlate clinical signs of pulmonary acariasis with the degree of pathological change in the lungs, and antemortem diagnosis is difficult. Monkeys can be reared free of *Pneumonyssus* infection if they are separated from their mothers at birth and reared in isolation from adult monkeys. The histopathological diagnosis of *P. simicola* infection is discussed in Chapter 5.

Pneumonyssoides

A parasite of the nasal and paranasal sinuses of dogs, *Pneumonyssoides caninum* sometimes causes chronic sneezing and epistaxis. Occasionally, nasal discharge has been reported in dogs with this infestation (King, 1988). Rhinoscopy and nasal swabbing are aids to diagnosis. Treatment of *P. caninum* is easily induced by the subcutaneous administration of ivermectin (Mundell and Ihrke, 1990).

Family Rhinonyssidae

Sternostoma

Sternostoma tracheacolum is a bloodsucking mite of the respiratory passages, including the abdominal air sacs, of canaries, finches, and a wide range of other wild and domestic birds. S. *tracheacolum* infection may not be apparent clinically or may cause chronic respiratory illness manifested by loss of voice, shaking of the head, and sneezing. Diagnosis in the living bird is facilitated by moistening and parting the feathers in the neck region and transilluminating the trachea with a strong light; the mites appear as shadowy spots in the trachea. On necropsy examination, these mites appear to the unaided eye as black spots in the posterior nares, trachea, air sacs, lung tissues, and abdominal cavity (Kummerfeld and Hinz, 1982).

Family Varroidae

Varroa

Varroa jacobsoni is a parasite of honey bees that was introduced into the United States sometime in the 1980s. Mites and other parasites of bees are a serious threat to U.S. agriculture. All one has to do is visit a local lawn with clover and notice that there are either no honeybees or very few honeybees present; some have estimated that greater than 95% of the wild honeybees in the United States have been eliminated by these parasites. Wild honeybees are no longer considered effective as providers of pollination for farmers. Within commercial hives, in the winter of 1995, losses ranged from 40% in Delaware to 80% in Maine. Although bees produce honey valued at some $125 million, more importantly, they are responsible for pollinating nearly $15 billion worth of crops in the United States each year (Doebler, 2000). *V. jacobsoni* is an external parasite of honeybees and is very large; females are 1 to 1.5 mm in diameter, reddish to dark brown, and easy to observe on bees with the naked eye. The mites suck hemolymph from both adult bees and the brood, preferring the blood of drones. A female mite enters a brood cell about 1 day before capping and becomes sealed in the brood capsule with the larval bee. The female then lays eggs, and the developing larval mites feed off the developing bee. When the adult bee emerges from the brood cell, the mites in the cell will have developed to adulthood and mated, and the females will be ready to enter a new cell. The disease is spread between hives by mites attached to worker bees. Untreated infestations of hives destroy colonies. Treatment of infested colonies is performed using strips that contain the miticides flumethrin or fluvalinate. It should not be forgotten that bees are food animals, and the strips should not be used during honey flow or when honey is present that may be removed for human consumption. Veterinarians need to be aware that pesticides may be used in manners that can lead to honey contamination (Harman, 1998). The development of resistance to these agents in mites is also problematic because the fact that bees are also arthropods makes it difficult to increase treatment levels because bees are usually killed through the same pharmacological pathway.

Suborder Astigmata, Astigmatid Mites

In contrast to mesostigmatids, astigmatid mites lack stigmata, and respiration is integumental; the first and second coxae are widely separated from the third and fourth, the ventrum is devoid of conspicuous plates, and the tarsi are equipped with suckers (sarcoptiform pretarsi). Astigmatids include the mange mites, certain hair-clasping mites, two internal parasites of chickens, and the "grain mites."

Mange mites (families Sarcoptidae, Knemidokoptidae, and Psoroptidae) cause mange or scabies, a dermatitis characterized by pruritus, alopecia, and epidermal hyperplasia with desquamation. Rubbing and scratching by the host frequently results in deeper wounds that ooze serum and blood. These coagulate, gluing hair, epidermal debris, and foreign matter together to form crusts and scabs. Secondary bacterial infection may complicate the situation.

The typical distribution and manner of spread of mange lesions vary with the host and parasite species and are often characteristic enough to permit accurate diagnosis by an experienced observer. However, recovery and identification of mites are necessary for positive diagnosis. Negative scrapings are inconclusive. Therefore typical mange lesions should be subjected to persistent examination until mites are found or until further scraping would do excessive injury to the patient. For lesions with minimal epidermal hyperplasia and lesions caused by deeply burrowing mites (e.g., *Sarcoptes* and *Demodex*), dip a scalpel blade into glycerin or mineral oil, pinch a fold of skin firmly between thumb and forefinger and, holding the blade at right angles to the skin, scrape until blood begins to seep from the abrasion. Much of the detritus will adhere to the layer of mineral oil on the scalpel blade and may be transferred to a microscope slide and searched for mites. For lesions with marked epidermal hyperplasia and exfoliation and lesions caused by superficially dwelling mites (e.g., *Chorioptes*) and lice, scrape the detritus into an ointment tin using the cover as a scraper. Examine the scrapings under a stereomicroscope or hand lens to find the mites crawling about. If no mites are observed directly, recourse may be had to digestion of the skin scrapings in potassium hydroxide as described in Chapter 5.

Generic differentiation of mange mites likely to be encountered in routine veterinary practice requires little more than examination of their **pretarsi** (Figures 1-82 and 1-83). If the pretarsus has a long, unsegmented **pedicel** (stalk), the specimen is most likely *Sarcoptes* or *Notoedres*. If the pretarsus has a long, three-segmented pedicel, it is bound to be *Psoroptes*. Pretarsi with short pedicels are found on *Chorioptes* from ungulates and *Otodectes* from dogs; the species identity of the host is a sufficiently reliable differential criterion in this case. *Knemidokoptes* females lack pretarsi, but the males have pretarsi resembling those of *Sarcoptes*. Certain particularly destructive manges, such as psoroptic mange in sheep and cattle and sarcoptic mange in cattle, should be reported to state animal disease control authorities.

Family Sarcoptidae

Sarcoptes
The pretarsi have long, unsegmented pedicels, and the anus is at the posterior edge of the body

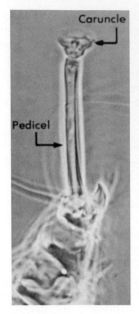
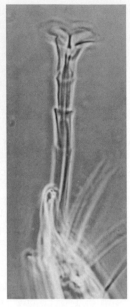

FIGURE 1-82 Pretarsi of *Sarcoptes* (*left*, ×830) and *Psoroptes* (*right*, ×870). Both have long pedicels; that of *Psoroptes* is jointed.

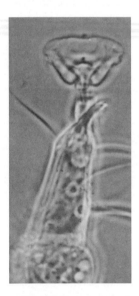
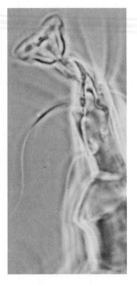

FIGURE 1-83 Pretarsi of *Otodectes* (*left*, ×810) and *Chorioptes* (*right*, ×710). Both have short pedicels. *Otodectes* is a parasite of the ear canal of carnivorans; *Chorioptes* is a parasite of the epidermis of ungulates.

(Figure 1-84). *Sarcoptes scabiei* causes sarcoptic mange or scabies of humans, dogs, foxes, horses, cattle, and others. Sarcoptic mange of cattle is reportable. Although *S. scabiei* infests a wide range of hosts, a considerable degree of host specificity has arisen among populations of this parasite so that scabies of pigs tends to spread more readily among pigs, scabies of humans tends to spread more readily among humans, and when interspecific transmission does occur, the resulting dermatitis tends to be atypical and transient. In fair-skinned human subjects suffering relatively mild infestations, it is possible to see the tiny serpentine tunnels that trace the wanderings of the egg-laying female mite as she burrows through the epidermis. Along the course of the burrow, dark areas representing eggs and accumulations of feces may be observed and, at the end of the tunnel, the mite may be found and lifted out with the point of a needle. Hair obscures such lesions on domestic animals, and it may be that many relatively mild cases of sarcoptic mange are overlooked. As few as 10 to 15 mites constitute a case of ordinary (but nonetheless unendurable) human scabies, but thousands to millions may be found on a mangy pig or fox. Curiously, however, *Sarcoptes* mites are frequently difficult to find on dogs, even those exhibiting advanced lesions.

Sarcoptic mange of domestic animals usually starts on relatively hairless areas of skin and may later generalize. In dogs, the lateral aspect of the elbow and pinna of the ear are favorite starting places; the lesions consist of follicular papules, areas of erythema, crusts of dried serum and blood, and excoriations from scratching to relieve the intense pruritus. Secondary bacterial infection is a frequent complication. In swine, sarcoptic mange usually starts around the eyes and on the nose, back, sides, and inner surface of the thighs; lesions may progress to hyperkeratosis and exfoliation of epidermal debris. The red fox, *Vulpes fulva*, suffers a lethal form of sarcoptic mange in which the epidermis may undergo a tenfold increase in thickness and contain countless hordes of mites.

Notoedres

A parasite of cats, rats, rabbits, and occasionally and temporarily of humans, *Notoedres* much resembles *Sarcoptes* but is smaller, and its anus is on the dorsal surface instead of on the posterior margin of the body (Figures 1-85 and 1-86). Face mange of cats caused by *Notoedres cati* starts on the medial edge of the pinna of the ears and then spreads over the ears, face, paws, and hindquarters by contiguity and contact. The lesions of notoedric mange consist principally of alopecia and marked hyperkeratosis with abundant epidermal flakes; mites are easily demonstrated. An epizootic of notoedric mange has been reported in the Florida Keys where over 500 cats were examined (Foley, 1991a). Major signs included pruritus, self-mutilation dermatitis, gray crusts on the skin, secondary pyoderma, and hypertrophied skin.

Not all cases of cat mange are caused by *Notoedres,* however, especially as regards exotic

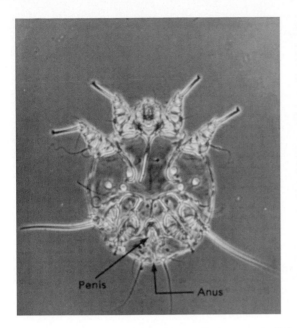
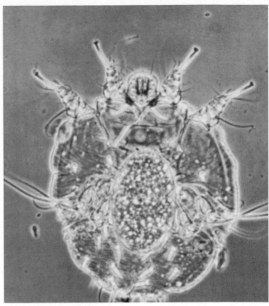

FIGURE 1-84 *Sarcoptes* male (*left*, ×140) and female (*right*, ×140).

cats. For example, a half dollar-sized area of dermatitis on the top of a pet ocelot's head was tentatively diagnosed as notoedric mange. However, a scraping revealed that the villain was *Sarcoptes* and raised the possibility of an infested human contact. In fact, the owner had been suffering from a severe itch below her breasts but had not connected her discomfort with her ocelot's skin lesion. In this particular case, it was not at all clear who had harbored the mites first, but that, after all, is an academic question. What is important is that correct generic identification of the parasite led to effective control through appropriate medication of both infested individuals.

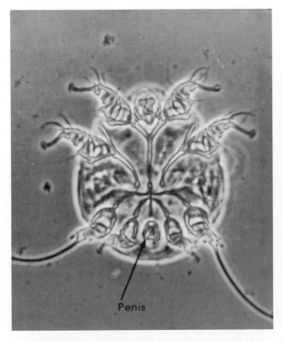
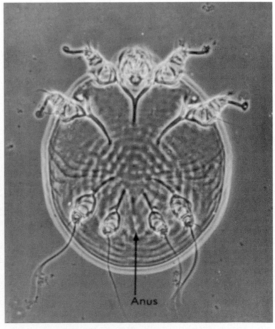

FIGURE 1-85 *Notoedres* male (*left*, ×250) and female (*right*, ×290).

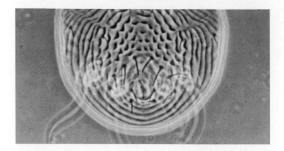

FIGURE 1-86 Same as Figure 1-83 *right*, but with dorsal anus in focus (×290).

Cosarcoptes, Prosarcoptes, Pithesarcoptes, and Kutzerocoptes

The first three genera are parasites of Old World monkeys (Cercopithecidae), and the last one is a parasite of New World monkeys (Cebidae). All resemble *Sarcoptes* morphologically, biologically, and pathogenetically. Mange of monkeys, at least that caused by *Cosarcoptes scanloni*, may be transmissible to humans (Smiley and O'Connor, 1980).

Trixacarus caviae

A parasite of the guinea pig, *T. caviae* closely resembles *Sarcoptes* scabiei but is only half as large; the anus is on the dorsal surface of the female and on the posterior margin of the body of the male. *Trixacarus* causes pruritus so intense that affected guinea pigs are subject to fits and seizures brought on by vigorous scratching or manipulation of the skin (Kummel, Estes, and Arlian, 1980). Mange in guinea pigs has been successfully treated with ivermectin administered subcutaneously (Mandigers, van der Hage, and Dorrstein, 1993).

Family Knemidokoptidae

Knemidokoptes

Knemidokoptes mutans causes scaly leg in chickens, turkeys, pheasants, and other gallinaceous birds. The mites burrow in the epidermis of the legs, causing the scales to lift and become loosened and the legs to become thickened and deformed. To demonstrate mites, simply remove a loose leg scale and examine the underside of it with a hand lens. The female *K. mutans* is about 0.5 mm in diameter; the legs are very short and lack pretarsi (Figure 1-87). The males are much smaller and have longer legs equipped with pretarsi resembling those of *Sarcoptes*.

Knemidokoptes pilae and *Knemidokoptes jamaicensis* cause mange of the legs, base of the beak, vent area, and back of parakeets and canaries, respectively. Lesions respond well to daily applications of mineral oil to all areas where mites are likely to be found, including the vent area. The oil tends to loosen crusts, which should be carefully removed.

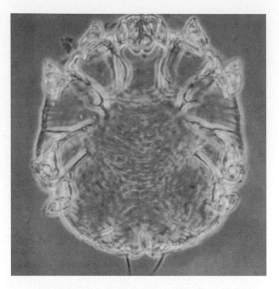

FIGURE 1-87 *Knemidokoptes* female (×200).

Rotenone-orthophenylphenol (Goodwinol ointment) or ivermectin mixed with a few drops of dimethyl sulfoxide (DMSO) and applied to lesions with a cotton swab are suitable topical treatments. Ivermectin administered orally or intramuscularly at 0.2 mg/kg presents several advantages over topical acaricides: only one (or in particularly serious cases two) treatment is necessary. It does not mat down feathers or get in the birds' eyes and is apparently well tolerated (Ryan, 1986).

Knemidokoptes gallinae, the depluming mite of chickens, pigeons, pheasants, and geese, is found at the base of the feathers on the back, on top of the wing, and on the vent, breast, and thighs. It causes intense pruritus, leading in turn to feather pulling.

Family Psoroptidae

Psoroptes

The legs are long, and the pretarsi have long, three-segmented pedicels (Figure 1-88). *Psoroptes ovis* causes a very **serious and reportable form of a mange** (scabies or "scab") in cattle, sheep, and horses. Psoroptic mange is prevalent among cattle herds in the southwestern United States but relatively rare elsewhere in North America. *Psoroptes cuniculi* is very common and causes ear canker in rabbits and a less severe form of otic acariasis in goats and horses.

P. ovis does not burrow in the epidermis but remains at the base of the hairs and pierces the skin with its styletlike chelicerae. This manner of feeding results in exudation of serum, which hardens to form a scab. The mites are best demonstrated under the edges of these scabs, so it is inefficient to submit

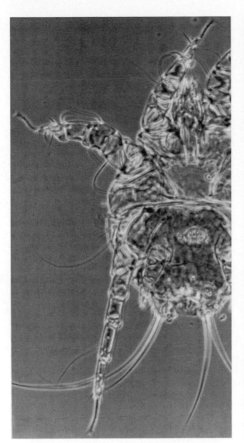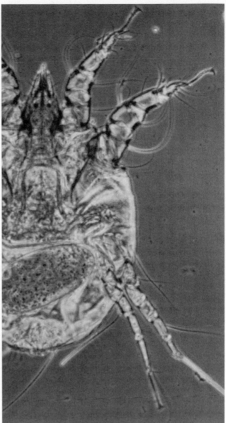

FIGURE 1-88 *Psoroptes* male (*left*, ×110) and female (*right*, ×110).

great wads of wool to the laboratory, especially if the scabs are not included in the shipment. Psoroptic scab is particularly devastating in sheep, especially those maintained principally for the production of high-quality wool. Pruritus is usually intense. At first, tags of wool are observed projecting from the fleece and clinging to fence posts, door jambs, trees, and other convenient objects against which an itchy sheep might obtain some measure of relief. Progressively more and more wool is shed or rubbed away by the frantic sheep, and pustules appear on the denuded, hardened, thickened, and excoriated skin. As the pustules become confluent and overlain by a scab of coagulated serum and foreign material, the area ceases to be suitable for the mites, and they move on to fresh territory. In this way, the lesions tend to spread over the surface of the body. The sheep become greatly debilitated by psoroptic scab and may even die of it. *P. ovis* may survive off the host for several days or weeks. Therefore effective control requires both acaricidal treatment of all infested livestock and either disinfection or 2- to 4-week vacating of contaminated enclosures and vehicles (Wilson, Blachut, and Roberts, 1977).

P. cuniculi is a ubiquitous parasite of the external ear canal and can frequently be demonstrated in apparently normal rabbits. When infested rabbits are placed under stress, as for example when a doe kindles, the population of mites tends to explode and the ear canal is laid waste as a result. A full-blown case of **ear canker** without secondary bacterial infection will respond amazingly well and heal in a dramatic fashion after the subcutaneous administration of ivermectin. Prevention is possible by weekly instillation of a few drops of mineral oil into the ear canal of each rabbit in the colony. *P. cuniculi* produces a less severe form of otic acariasis in goats and horses.

Chorioptes bovis

Pretarsi of *Chorioptes bovis* have short, unsegmented pedicels on the first, second, and fourth pairs of legs of the female and on all legs of the male; the male has two turretlike lobes on the posterior margin of the body (Figures 1-89 and 1-90). *C. bovis* is a cosmopolitan, superficially dwelling parasite, displaying a distinct preference for the tail, escutcheon, and legs of cattle, where it feeds on epithelial debris.

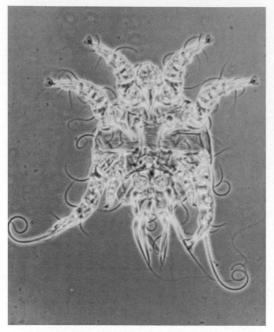
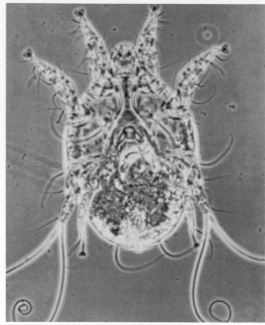

FIGURE 1-89 *Chorioptes* male (*left*, ×120) and female (*right*, ×140). The female has pretarsi on the first, second, and fourth pairs of legs; the male has pretarsi on all four pairs.

Although cattle are the principal hosts, *C. bovis* also may be found on the tail and legs of horses, sheep, and goats and in the ear canal of rabbits. Asymptomatic infestation is far more common than obvious dermatitis.

Chorioptic mange in cattle usually appears during late winter as a superficial, mildly pruritic, flaky dermatitis involving the tail, escutcheon, and hind legs. Whereas stanchioned animals are made miserable because they are unable to take appropriate action to relieve the itching, for unconfined cattle, chorioptic mange is probably not much more serious a burden than a crop of chewing lice and, like a suit of woolen underwear, may help keep them warm by encouraging physical activity. Chorioptic mange tends to disappear soon after the cattle are turned out to pasture in spring. *C. bovis,* like the pinworm *Oxyuris equi,* is an identifiable cause of tail rubbing in horses.

C. bovis causes exudative dermatitis on the lower legs and scrota of rams. In extreme cases the crusts may be 5 cm thick. Deterioration of semen quality was associated with chorioptic mange lesions covering more than one third of the scrotum and was apparently related to elevation of testicular temperature (Rhodes, 1975).

Otodectes cynotis

Pretarsi of *Otodectes cynotis* have short, unsegmented pedicels on the first and second pairs of legs of the female and on all legs of the male; the body of the male is only weakly bilobed posteriorly (Figure

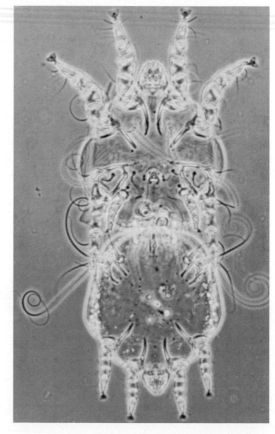

FIGURE 1-90 *Chorioptes* male and deutonymph (×140). The deutonymph has pretarsi on the first and second pairs of legs.

1-91). *O. cynotis* infests the external ear canal and adjacent skin of dogs, cats, foxes, and ferrets, causing intense irritation. Copious production of dark cerumen is characteristic of otodectic otitis. Aural pruritus sometimes causes the animal to rub and scratch its ears and shake its head violently enough to produce hematoma of the aural pinna. The mites may be demonstrated by swabbing the ear canal with a cotton applicator and then placing the applicator on a dark background under a lamp or on a sunny windowsill. The heat will drive the mites out of the debris, and they will be seen as tiny white specks moving against the dark background. The number of mites present in the cat's ear can be quite remarkable. Preisler (1985) reported more than 8500 mites in the ear canal of a cat. When large numbers of mites are present in the canal, the cat's ear tends to contain a dry, waxy, light-colored, parchmentlike material in sheets, with large numbers of mites present in each layer.

Other Astigmatid Mites

Hair-clasping mites of the superfamily Listrophoroidea have one or more pairs of legs variously flattened, bowed, or otherwise modified for clasping a hair. Examples include *Chirodiscoides caviae,* a parasite of guinea pigs (Figure 1-92) and *Myocoptes musculinus*, a parasite of rodents (Figure 1-93). *Lynxacarus radovskyi* is a hair-clasping mite of domestic cats in Florida, Puerto Rico, Hawaii, Australia, and Fiji (Figure 1-94); hordes of these tiny mites clinging to the hairs impart a scruffy appearance (Greve and Gerrish, 1981). Not all hair-clasping mites belong to the superfamily Listrophoroidea or even to the suborder Astigmata. For examples of exceptions, see *Myobia* and *Radfordia* later.

Feather mites occur in variety and abundance. Most are members of several superfamilies of Astigmata. Feather mites are usually external, but some live within the quills. Others, such as members of the family Epidermoptidae, burrow in the skin and may cause a mangelike condition. Astigmatid feather mites may be distinguished from prostigmatid feather mites such as *Syringophilus* by their sarcoptiform pretarsi.

Two families of Astigmata have evolved as internal parasites of birds: *Laminosioptes* (Laminosioptidae) occur in subcutaneous nodules in chickens, and several genera of the family Cytoditidae are parasites of the air sacs and respiratory passages of chickens, canaries, and other birds.

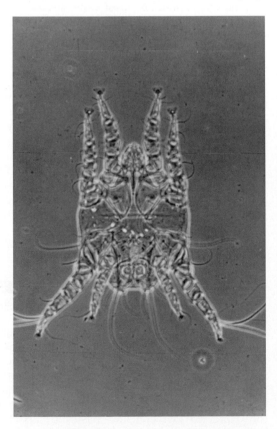
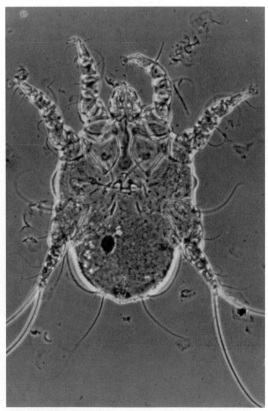

FIGURE 1-91 *Otodectes* male (*left*, ×110) and female (*right*, ×120). The female has pretarsi on the first and second pairs of legs; the male has pretarsi on all four pairs.

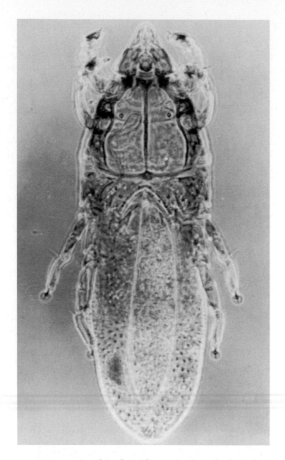

FIGURE 1-92 *Chirodiscoides caviae* female (×220).

Members of the families Acaridae and Glyci-phagidae are free-living mites that feed on organic matter. They may be found in grain, cheeses, dried fruit, and other stored food products. Contact with these mites and their detritus may cause urticaria and dermatitis in human beings. "Grain mites" are frequently found as pseudoparasites in fecal smears. They may be distinguished from parasitic astigmatids by the shape of the female genital opening, which is a transverse or U-shaped slit in the parasites but a more or less longitudinal slit in grain mites.

Suborder Cryptostigmata, Oribatid Mites

The Cryptostigmata, or oribatid mites, are free-living inhabitants of humus, some of which serve as intermediate hosts to tapeworms of the family Anoplocephalidae. When ingested by an oribatid mite, the larva in the egg of the tapeworm *Moniezia* develops into a cysticercoid, the larval stage of which is infective for the ruminant definitive host.

Suborder Prostigmata, Prostigmatid Mites

The Prostigmata is a polyphyletic amalgamation including both free-living species and such diverse obligate parasites as pilosebaceous mites *(Demodex)*, hair-clasping mites *(Myobia)*, and "chiggers" (Trombiculidae).

Family Demodicidae

Demodex

These tiny, wormlike mites with short, stubby legs (Figure 1-95) live in the hair follicles and sebaceous glands of mammals. Several distinct species of *Demodex* often parasitize the same host animal, but each species tends to be restricted to a particular habitat. For example, two species, *Demodex folliculorum* and *Demodex brevis*, live in the skin of almost every human face, *D. folliculorum* in the hair follicles, and *D. brevis* in the sebaceous glands (Desch and Nutting, 1972), where they eat the epithelial cells. Some important pest species are as follows.

Demodex canis is present in small numbers in the skin of most normal dogs (see Figure 1-95). Pups acquire *D. canis* infection from their dams during the nursing period, and most cases of demodectic mange occur between 3 and 6 months of age. Affected dogs harbor much larger than normal populations of *D. canis*, apparently as a result of immunodeficiency, and display circumscribed areas of erythema and alopecia around the eyes and mouth and over bony projections on the extremities. There is no evidence of pruritus. If the lesions remain thus localized, the prognosis for clinical recovery is excellent; the majority of such cases are mild and the animals recover spontaneously with the attainment of sexual maturity. However, a few cases persist, and these tend to become generalized and intractable and may prove fatal. In generalized demodicosis, the hair becomes sparse over wider expanses and the skin becomes coarse, dry, and erythematous ("red mange"). Concomitant staphylo-coccal pyoderma is the rule in generalized cases; pustules develop, break open, and ooze. Severe cases are associated with a disagreeable odor. Generalized canine demodicosis is difficult to ameliorate and probably impossible to cure.

Demodex bovis mites are part of the normal fauna of bovine skin, but sometimes pinhead- to egg-sized nodules appear, usually on the neck and forequarters. Occasionally, only the eyelids, vulva, or scrotum are involved. If a fresh nodule is nicked with a sharp scalpel, a thick, toothpastelike pus can sometimes be expressed that contains masses of *D. bovis* mites, but older lesions consist only of scar tissue and are devoid of mites. Bovine demodectic mange

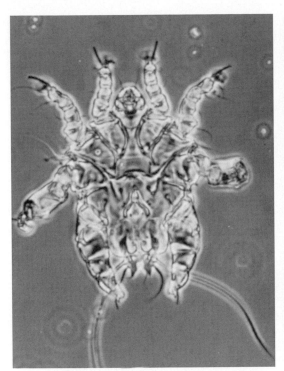
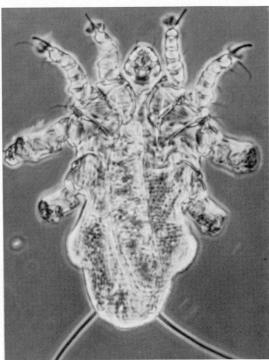

FIGURE 1-93 *Myocoptes musculinus* male (*left*, ×230) and female (*right*, ×230), an astigmatid hair-clasping parasite of laboratory rodents. Notice how the third pair of legs of the male and third and fourth pairs of legs of the female are modified for hair clasping. The first two pairs of legs have sarcoptiform pretarsi.

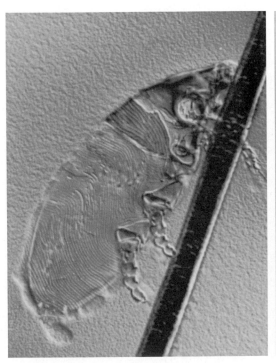
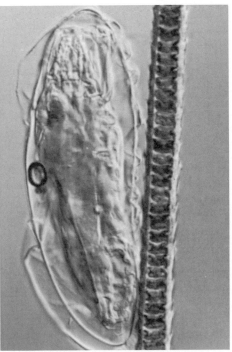

FIGURE 1-94 *Lynxacarus radovskyi* (Listrophoroidea), a hair-clasping mite of the cat. *Left*, Adult mite (×168); *right*, egg with larva (×425).
(Specimens courtesy Dr. Robert Foley.)

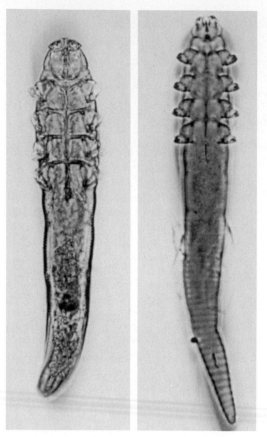

FIGURE 1-95 *Demodex canis (left)* and *D. cati (right)* (×390).

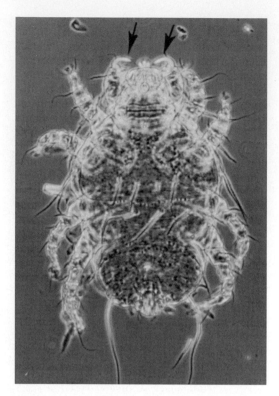

FIGURE 1-96 *Cheyletiella yasguri* (×130). Notice the formidable palpal claws *(arrows)*.

is practically incurable, even though individual lesions typically regress, because new nodules form to take their place. However, an unusual case of bilateral lower palpebral demodicosis in a dairy cow, characterized by chronic eosinophilic granulomatous cellulitis but without appreciable pus formation, resolved spontaneously within 3 months (Gearhart, Crissman, and Georgi, 1981).

Demodex ovis is rarely noticed but probably rather common; mites infest the meibomian glands and the hair follicles and sebaceous glands of primary hairs of the general body skin but are most numerous on the neck, flanks, and shoulders. A second species parasitizing sheep, *Demodex aries,* appear to be confined to areas with very large sebaceous glands such as the vulva, prepuce, and nostrils (Desch, 1986).

Demodex caprae causes a nodular dermatitis in milk goats.

Demodex caballi is a harmless parasite of the meibomian glands of horses. The horse is also host to a second species, *Demodex equi,* that is about half as long (190 to 232 m) as *D. caballi* (Desch and Nutting, 1978).

Demodex cati is rarely noticed (see Figure 1-94). Dermatitis associated with *D. cati* is usually localized on the head and in the ear canals.

Demodex cuniculi is a relatively rare parasite of the rabbit.

Demodex phylloides is found in nodules around the eyes and on the snouts of pigs. These lesions later spread over the underside of the body.

Family Cheyletiellidae

Cheyletiella spp. are easily recognized by their big palpal claws, M-shaped gnathosomal peritremes, and comblike tarsal appendages (Figure 1-96). *Cheyletiella yasguri* occurs on dogs, *Cheyletiella blakei* on cats, and *Cheyletiella parasitivorax* on rabbits. Humans may serve as an accidental or transitory host. Pups infested with *C. yasguri* develop "walking dandruff" on their backs, a dermatitis with branlike exfoliative debris that stirs with the movements of these rather large mites. The Georgi's observed a caged cat that passed *C. blakei* in its feces for several weeks. Presumably this cat was ingesting these mites while grooming itself, but there was no macroscopically visible skin lesion and they could find no mites in the fur. Other genera of the family Cheyletiellidae are parasites of birds. *Cheyletiella* spp. survive longer off the host than other mange mites, and the premises may remain a source of reinfestation after treatment of affected animals.

Family Psorergatidae

Psorobia ovis, the sheep itch mite, sporadically causes pruritus and fleece derangement in sheep by rubbing and through chewing by the infested host. The course is very chronic. Lambs younger than 6 months appear unaffected, and generalization may require 3 or 4 years. The mite is minute, almost discoidal, and has radially arranged legs. *Psorobia bos* is a nonpathogenic mite of cattle. *Psorergates simplex,* the subcutaneous mite of mice, may cause a mangelike condition. To demonstrate mites, skin an infested mouse and look for pockets of mites on the underside of the dermis.

Family Myobiidae

Myobiid mites cause dermatitis in stocks of laboratory rodents. In myobiids, the first pair of legs is modified for clasping hair (Figure 1-97), whereas in *Myocoptes* spp., the third pair of legs of the male and third and fourth pairs of the female are so modified (see Figure 1-93). *Myobia musculi* attacks laboratory mice, and *Radfordia ensifera* attacks laboratory rats. Alopecia and erythema of the dorsal neck region are typical; severe cases are characterized by self-inflicted excoriations. Stress of overcrowding is frequently responsible for converting an asymptomatic infestation of hair-clasping mites into an outbreak of serious skin disease.

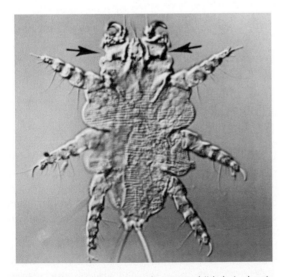

FIGURE 1-97 *Myobia musculi,* a myobiid hair-clasping parasite of laboratory rodents. The first pair of legs *(arrows)* is modified for hair clasping (×170).

Family Harpyrhynchidae

Harpyrhynchids are rounded mites, resembling psorergatids, that cause mangelike conditions in birds. Several genera include species that burrow in feather follicles or form large crusted cysts in the skin.

Family Syringophilidae

Syringophilids are nonpathogenic inhabitants of the lumen of feather quills.

Family Trombiculidae

Larvae (**chiggers**) of the family Trombiculidae are parasitic, but the nymphs and adults are free-living. These bright red or orange, six-legged larvae are likely to be found on the skin or in the ears of cats or dogs, on the faces or pasterns of sheep and other ungulates, and under the wings or around the vents of chickens and other birds. Infestation is usually acquired in wild or semiwild landscapes; the distribution of these nuisances is remarkably spotty, but wherever they are found, chiggers are infamous. Microscopically, the scutum is useful for recognizing a chigger as such and for generic and species identification with the help of keys. Focus on the dorsal surface (the surface opposite the one with the coxae) to see the scutum (Figures 1-98 and 1-99). Chiggers remain on the skin for several days unless dislodged by the scratching host, and their saliva, injected into the skin, disintegrates host cells and the resulting material is taken into the mite as food. The surrounding skin hardens and a tube called a **stylostome** is formed in which the mouthparts remain until the chigger is replete or dislodged. The fully developed stylostome extends from the surface of the epidermis into the dermis and is lined by necrotic cells of the stratum germinativum. Pruritus is intense and may be protracted for many days after the chigger has been removed. Twenty-four hours after infestation with more than 2000 larvae of *Neotrombicula autumnalis*, two male Yorkshire Terriers developed paresis involving first the hind legs, then the forelegs. The nervous signs disappeared within 3 days after repeated acaricidal (propoxur) and symptomatic therapy (Prosl, Rabitsch, and Brabenetz, 1985).

Recently, a new syndrome, straelensiosis, was reported to be affecting dogs in Europe. This is due to a trombiculid mite. Some 22 dogs over a period of 5 years in the south of France were found to be suffering from a chronic, painful, extensive-to-generalized dermatitis that was associated with papular crusts and suppurations (Bourdeau et al, 2001). The mite was described as *Straelensia cynotis* by Fain and Le Net (2001). This larval

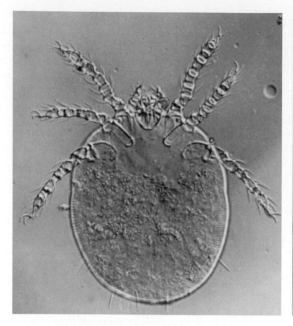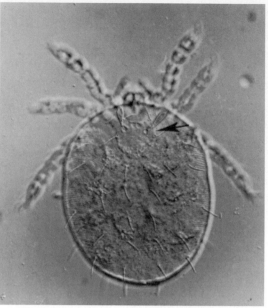

FIGURE 1-98 *Walchia americana*, a trombiculid mite (chigger). *Left*, The ventral surface is in focus; *right*, the dorsal surface. The scutum *(arrow)* with its two sensillae (large plumose setae) and four or five setae is helpful in identifying chiggers; it is on the dorsal surface near the anterior end of the body (×170).

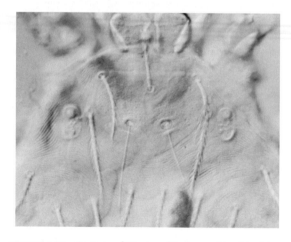

FIGURE 1-99 Scutum of *Neotrombicula* sp. (Trombiculidae: Prostigmata; ×425).

trombiculid enters the hair follicle, where it stays for an extensive period with its stylostome directed into the dermis.

Family Pyemotidae

Pyemotes

"Hay itch mites" of the genus *Pyemotes* are parasites of various insect larvae that are grain-destroying pests. *Pyemotes tritici* is a tiny elongate mite that becomes enormously distended when gravid; males and females are sexually mature at birth.

People and domestic animals that come into contact with infested grains, straw, hay, and the like may be attacked by these mites and develop an erythematous and intensely pruritic papular and vesicular rash. An outbreak of dermatitis in 12 horses and many persons in Florida was attributed to *P. tritici* received in a shipment of alfalfa hay (Kunkle and Greiner, 1982).

Family Tarsonemidae

Acarapis woodi is the tracheal mite of honey bees. These mites entered the United States through Texas and Florida in 1984, coming from Mexico and Europe. These mites, along with *Varroa* and the beetle, *Aethina,* have been responsible for the remarkable reduction of honey bee populations in the United States. These small mites live within the trachea of the honey bee. Females move from bee to bee, entering the adult bee through the first thoracic spiracle. Large numbers can build up in the tracheal tubes. The mites within the tubes cause problems with thermoregulation of hives in winter and cause bees to die outside of hives because they cannot elevate their metabolic rate high enough to stay warm when they fly on cool days. Treatment has been performed using the addition of menthol chips or oil of wintergreen to hives (Williams, 2000). Though this seems to afford some protection, it may be that most susceptible hives have already disappeared.

Treatment of Mite Infestations

Dogs and Cats

Sarcoptes

Selamectin is probably the treatment of choice for sarcoptic mange in dogs and is labeled for this application (Shanks et al, 2000). Subcutaneous ivermectin is also routinely used to treat sarcoptic mange. Other effective acaricides include amitraz, benzyl benzoate, lime sulfur, phosmet, and rotenone. In most cases, with these other compounds, treatment must be repeated several times over a period of weeks.

S. scabiei and other sarcoptiform parasites may temporarily infest people who come into intimate contact with mangy dogs and cats. In this case, acaricidal treatment of the pet is the key to lasting success in curing the people. On the other hand, proper scabies contracted from another human being causes very persistent dermatitis and misery unless effectively treated and, of course, has little or nothing to do with dogs and cats.

Notoedres

Selamectin topically applied to cats will probably treat notoedric mange. Ivermectin (0.3 mg/kg) has been successfully used to treat numerous cats with notoedric mange (Foley, 1991a). The standard treatment previously for N. cati infestations in cats was lime sulfur. With lime sulfur, the cat is first bathed and then dipped or washed with a 1:40 solution of lime sulfur in warm water. This treatment is applied weekly for at least 6 weeks.

Otodectes

Ivermectin 0.01% in an otic suspension (ACAREXX) has been approved for cats and dogs where 0.5 ml of the suspension is applied to each ear canal. This treatment will also prevent the development of the eggs of this mite (Bowman et al, 2001). Subcutaneous ivermectin (0.2 to 0.225 mg/kg) injected on one or two occasions with a 3-week interval between injections has proven highly successful in treating ear mites in cats (Foley, 1991b). Otodectes ear infestations also respond to pyrethrin- and rotenone-containing compounds. With these products, the ear canal should be thoroughly cleaned before instillation of the acaricidal solution. The application of 1 to 2 ml of mineral oil to the ear canal followed by 30 seconds of massage repeated every 2 or 3 days will often cure dogs and cats of their ear mite infestations (Bourma et al, 2001).

Demodex

D. canis is susceptible to benzyl benzoate, rotenone, ronnel, and cythioate (Manson and Malynicz, 1969). The localized form of demodectic mange may be controlled by applying rotenone ointment or benzyl benzoate lotion. These drugs have very little residual activity and therefore must be applied daily. The treatment of generalized demodectic mange is a challenge and frequently proves to be a frustrating experience for the clinician and client alike. A 1% alcoholic solution of rotenone is applied to one third of the body every day until skin scrapings are negative for D. canis. Amitraz is approved for the control of generalized demodicosis in dogs. Amitraz is applied topically as an aqueous suspension (10.6 ml concentrate per 2 gal or 7.6 L of water) at 2-week intervals for a total of three to six applications (Folz et al, 1983). It is recommended that treatment be continued until no viable mites can be found in skin scrapings at two successive treatments. A brood bitch with asymptomatic D. canis infection may be bred, but a bitch with demodectic mange or a history of demodectic mange should be spayed. A dog with amitraz-resistant demodicosis was successfully treated by the daily oral treatment with ivermectin (0.6 mg/kg); the dog took 4 months to become clinically normal (Paradis and Laperriere, 1992). Of 30 dogs placed on daily oral milbemycin oxime (0.52 to 3.8 mg/kg) for 12 months, 16 dogs were cured, 9 cleared but relapsed, and 5 dogs never cleared their mite infestations (Miller et al, 1993).

Cheyletiella

C. yasguri in dogs responds well to the application of topical 65% permethrin, and all mites were gone within 1 week of treatment (Endris et al, 2000). Milbemycin oxime has also been used to treat dogs with naturally occurring cheyletiellosis (White, Rosychuk, and Fieseler, 2001). Canine cheyletiellosis has also been successfully treated using fipronil (Chadwick, 1997). Cheyletiella is also susceptible to amitraz. The premises should be sprayed with a residual organophosphate insecticide such as diazinon to destroy these rather hardy mites.

C. yasguri of dogs and C. blakei of cats also attack people, especially those who share their beds with their pets. Curiously, C. blakei rarely produces obvious lesions on cats, but the owner may be aware of frequent bites. If C. blakei infestation is suspected, one can attempt to collect mites from the fur with a bit of Scotch tape. However, the diagnosis is more often reached fortuitously when the mites or their eggs are found in a routine fecal flotation. Because cats so meticulously groom themselves, a fecal flotation often affords a better sample of what is on the cat's exterior than direct examination does.

Ruminants

Chorioptes

Chorioptic mange usually responds to standard louse treatments. Crotoxyphos, coumaphos, or lime sulfur suspension as spray or dip controls chorioptic mange mites on lactating dairy cows. Eprinomectin can be applied to lactating dairy cattle without withholding of milk and is approved for the treatment of chorioptic mange.

Sarcoptes

Sarcoptic mange should be reported to state disease control authorities and treatment carried out under their supervision. Lactating dairy cows can now be treated with eprinomectin, which is labeled for *Sarcoptes* infestations of cattle. Sarcoptic mange of beef cattle and nonlactating dairy cattle is treated with avermectins, ivermectin, moxidectin, doramectin, or eprinomectin. It also can be treated with sprays or dips containing lime sulfur, phosmet, and tetrachlorvinphos.

Psoroptes

Psoroptic scabies in cattle or sheep should be reported to state disease control authorities and treatment carried out under their supervision. Coumaphos, phosmet, and hot lime sulfur are approved by APHIS as official dips for psoroptic scabies in cattle, and injectable ivermectin is approved as a systemic acaricide (Wright, 1986). Most of the macrocyclic lactones are labeled for treating psoroptic mange in cattle. Cattle treated with ivermectin must be isolated from untreated cattle for 2 weeks after treatment and withheld from slaughter for the required period. There is no ivermectin approved for the treatment of chorioptic mange in sheep in the United States. Holding facilities vacated by sheep or cattle with psoroptic mange should be left vacant for at least 2 weeks to give the mites time to die off before housing new stock (Wilson, Blachut, and Roberts, 1977).

Horses

Severe irritation caused by mange mites may lead to serious self-mutilation by affected horses. Treatment with macrocyclic lactones should prove efficacious. Mange is contagious and sometimes communicable. Isolate mangy horses and sterilize all water buckets, brushes, curry combs, and the like. Stalls should be thoroughly disinfected or left vacant for 2 to 3 weeks.

Swine

Ivermectin is highly effective in treating sarcoptic mange in swine. Sarcoptic mange in swine also responds to malathion sprays applied twice at an interval of 2 weeks.

Rodents and Lagomorphs

Notoedric mange *(Notoedres douglasi)* affecting two fox squirrels *(Sciurus niger)* responded dramatically to a single subcutaneous injection of ivermectin at 0.5 mg/kg body weight (Evans, 1984).

Myocoptes musculinus and *M. musculi* infestations were eliminated from laboratory mice by subcutaneous injection of ivermectin 0.2 mg/kg body weight (Wing, Courtney, and Young, 1985). Application of 0.5 mg active permethrin per mouse as 0.25% dust mixed with the bedding was convenient and eliminated *M. musculi* infestations in experimental mice (Bean-Knudsen, Wagner, and Hall, 1986).

Guinea pigs infected with *T. caviae* have been shown to respond well to treatment with ivermectin (McKellar et al, 1992). The guinea pigs were first treated with ivermectin 0.5 mg/kg orally, subcutaneously, or percutaneously, and then treated 1 week later with a subcutaneous dose of ivermectin 0.5 mg/kg.

Ear canker in rabbits *(P. cuniculi)* responds to two subcutaneous injections of ivermectin at 0.2 mg/kg administered 14 days apart (Bowman, Fogelson, and Carbone, 1992).

■ CLASS PENTASTOMIDA

Pentastomids, or "tongueworms," are highly specialized arthropods, as unlikely as that may seem. The adult parasites live in the respiratory passages of predacious reptiles, birds, and mammals. Eggs containing four- or six-legged larvae are discharged with the nasal secretions. If ingested by an appropriate intermediate host, usually a member of some species likely to fall prey to the predator in question, these larvae invade the tissues, develop, and encyst in the viscera as nymphs that resemble the adults in all particulars except for mature reproductive organs. The body is annulated, and the anterior, subterminal stoma is flanked by two pairs of retractable hollow fangs or hooks (Figure 1-100).

Linguatula serrata occurs in the nasal and paranasal sinuses of dogs and cats, where it causes bleeding, catarrhal inflammation, and some impediment to respiration. Cattle, sheep, rabbits, and other animals serve as intermediate hosts; fully developed nymphs, the form infective for carnivorans, are found encysted in the lymph nodes and serous membranes.

Kazacos et al (2000) reported on a Basenji-cross dog that had been born and spent time in Cameroon, Africa. It seems that the dog must have ingested some quantity of python feces containing the eggs of pentastomes of the genus *Armillifer*. The dog had been ill for several years, and when it became acutely ill 2 years after first admission, it was unresponsive to treatment and euthanatized. It was found to have a massive visceral infection with the nymphs of this pentastomid (Figures 1-101 and 1-102).

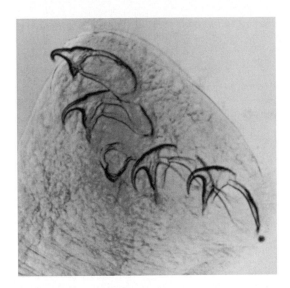

FIGURE 1-100 Stoma and hooks of a pentastomid nymph from a South American otter (×35).

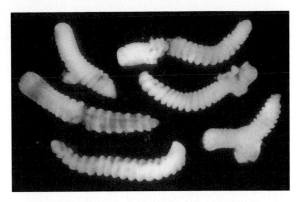

FIGURE 1-102 *Armillifer armillatus.* Nymphs of this pentastomid teased from the tissues of the dog in Figure 1-101. Several of the nymphs have been damaged during the teasing process. (Courtesy Dr. Kevin R. Kazaco, School of Veterinary Medicine, Purdue University, West Lafayette, Indiana.)

■ CLASS CRUSTACEA
Copepods

Copepods are crustaceans of importance to veterinary medicine because they serve as intermediate hosts of both cestodes and nematodes. There are three major groups of copepods, the calanoids, cyclopoids, and harpacticoids; the cyclopoids compose the group that typically has been found to be important intermediate hosts of the parasites of domestic animals. Copepods have shrimp-shaped bodies and five pairs of swimming legs (Figure 1-103). The antenna on each side of the head usually branches into two stalks. There may or may not be a single simple eye. Copepods reproduce sexually, and the males often have a

modified antenna that is used in copulation. The females typically carry egg sacks that contain developing eggs. Most copepods are grazers of phytoplankton, but some can be carnivorous, and a few are parasites in their own right. There are 11 molts that occur, separating 12 larval stages. The first five molts produce six larval forms of the naupliar type, the next five molts produce the developmental stages called copepodites (typically a new body segment is added with each molt), and the final molt produces the adult male or female. While grazing, the copepods will ingest either the coracidia of tapeworms or the hatched larvae of nematodes. They will then serve as either transport

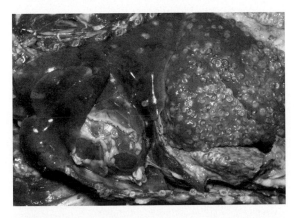

FIGURE 1-101 *Armillifer armillatus.* Viscera of a dog showing the liver, lungs, and heart containing large numbers of the very large coiled nymphs of this pentastomid parasite whose adults are found in pythonid snakes.

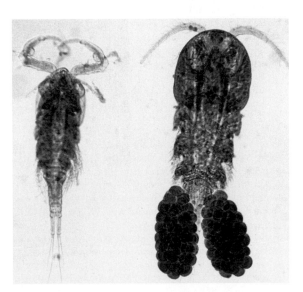

FIGURE 1-103 Copepods, male and female. The female bears the two large egg sacks that are typical of many of these free-living crustaceans.

hosts or as required intermediate hosts. Important parasites that utilize copepods include *Spirometra*, *Diphyllobothrium*, and *Dracunculus* species.

■ REFERENCES

Abbitt B, Abbitt LG: Fatal exsanguination of cattle attributed to an attack of salt marsh mosquitoes *(Aedes sollicitans), J Am Vet Med Assoc* 179:1397–1400, 1981.

Agarwal GP, Chandra S, Saxena AK: Feeding habits of dog louse *Heterodoxus spiniger* (End.) (Mallophaga, Amblycera), *Z. Angewandte Entomol* 94:134–137, 1982.

Andress ER, Campbell JB: Inundative release of pteromalid parasitoids (Hymenoptera: Pteromalidae) for the control of stable flies, *Stomoxys calcitrans* (L.) (Diptera: Muscidae) at confined cattle installations in west central Nebraska, *J Econ Entomol* 87:714–722, 1994.

Anziani OS, Guglielmone AA, Signorini AR, et al: *Haematobia irritans* in Argentina, *Vet Rec* 132:588, 1993.

Anziani OS, Loreficce C: Prevention of cutaneous myiasis caused by screw worm larvae *(Cochliomyia hominivorax)* using ivermectin, *J Vet Med B Infect Dis Vet Public Health* 40:287–290, 1993.

Arendt WJ: *Philornis* ectoparasitism of pearly-eyed thrashers. I. Impact on growth and development of nestlings, *Auk* 102:281–292, 1985.

Arrioja-Dechert A: *Compendium of veterinary products*, Port Huron, Mich, 1997, North American Compendiums.

Atwell RB, Campbell FE, Evans EA: Prospective survey of tick paralysis in dogs, *Aust Vet J* 79:412–418, 2001.

Baird CR: Development of *Cuterebra jellisoni* (Diptera: Cuterebridae) in six species of rabbits and rodents, *J Med Entomol* 8:615–622, 1971.

Baird CR: Development of *Cuterebra ruficrus* (Diptera: Cuterebridae) in six species of rabbits and rodents with a comparison of *C. ruficrus* and *C. jellisoni* third instars, *J Med Entomol* 9:81–85, 1972.

Baird CR, Podgore JK, Sabrosky CW: *Cuterebra* myiasis in humans: six new case reports from the United States with a summary of known cases (Diptera: Cuterebridae), *J Med Entomol* 19:263–267, 1982.

Baker NF, Farver TB: Failure of brewer's yeast as a repellent to fleas on dogs, *J Am Vet Med Assoc* 183:212–214, 1983.

Bean-Knudsen DE, Wagner JE, Hall RD: Evaluation of the control of *Myobia musculi* infestations on laboratory mice with permethrin, *Lab Anim Sci* 36:268–270, 1986.

Beasley VR, Wolf GA, Fischer DC, et al: Cantharidin toxicosis in horses, *J Am Vet Med Assoc* 182:283–284, 1983.

Bequaert J: A monograph of the Melophaginae, or ked-flies, of sheep, goats, deer, and antelopes (Diptera: Hippoboscidae), *Entomol Am* 22:1–220, 1942.

Blagburn BL, Vaughan JL, Lindsay DS, et al: Efficacy dosage titration of lufenuron against developmental stages of fleas *(Ctenocephlides felis felis)* in cats, *Am J Vet Res* 55:98–101, 1994.

Bourdeau P, Degorce F, Poujade A, et al: *Straelensiosis* (Straelensia cynotis), *a new and severe parasitosis in dogs*, Proceedings of the eighteenth conference of the World Association for the Advancement of Veterinary Parasitology, Stressa, Italy, 2001.

Bowman DD, Fogelson ML, Carbone LG: Effect of ivermectin on the control of ear mites *(Psoroptes cuniculi)* in naturally infested rabbits, *J Am Vet Med Assoc* 53:105–109, 1992.

Bowman DD, Giovengo SL: Identification of adult and nymphal ticks, *Vet Tech* 12:505–509, 1991.

Bowman DD, Katz S, Fogarty EA: Effects of an ivermectin otic suspension on egg hatching of the cat ear mite, *Otodectes cynotis*, in vitro, *Vet Therapeut* 2:311–316, 2001.

Burgdorfer W, Barbour AD, Hayes SF, et al: Lyme disease: a tick-borne spirochetosis? *Science* 216:1317–1319, 1982.

Burghardt HF, Whitlock JH, McEnerney PJ: Dermatitis due to *Simulium* (black flies), *Cornell Vet* 41(3):311–313, 1951.

Chadwick AJ: Use of a 0.25% fipronil pump spray formulation to treat canine cheyletiellosis, *J Small Anim Pract* 38:261–262, 1997.

Chandler AC, Read CP: *Introduction to parasitology*, ed 10, New York, 1961, John Wiley & Sons.

Chitwood MB, Stoffolano JG: First report of *Thelazia* sp. (Nematoda) in the face fly, *Musca autumnalis*, in North America, *J Parasitol* 57:1363–1364, 1971.

Cilek JE, Schreiber ET: Diel host-seeking activity of *Chrysops celatus* (Diptera: Tabanidae) in northwest Florida, *Florida Entomol* 79:520–525, 1996.

Clare AC, Medleau L: Case management workshop (mosquito bite hypersensitivity in a cat), *Vet Med* 92:728–733, 1997.

Coe M: Unforeseen effects of control, *Nature* 327:367, 1987.

Cogley TP, Anderson JR, Cogley LJ: Migration of *gasterophilus intestinalis* larvae (Diptera: Gasterophilidae) in the equine oral cavity, *Int J Parasitol* 12:473–480, 1982.

Cogley TP: Key to the eggs of the equid stomach bot flies *Gasterophilus* Leach, 1817 (Diptera: Gasterophilidae) utilizing scanning electron microscopy, *Systematic Entomol* 16:125–133, 1991.

Craig T: *The prevalence of bovine parasites in various environments within the lowland tropical country of Guyana*, doctoral dissertation, College Station, 1976, Texas A&M University.

Craig T: Horse parasites and their control, *Southern Class* 12–15, 1984.

DeMarmels J: *Cistudinomyia* (Diptera: Sarcophagidae) causing myiasis in a Venezuelan gecko (Sauria, Geckonidae), *Entomol Mont Mag* 130:222–225, 1994.

Desch CE: *Demodex aries* sp. nov., a sebaceous gland inhabitant of the sheep, *Ovis aries*, and a redescription of *Demodex ovis* Hirst, 1919, *N Z J Zool* 13:367–375, 1986.

Desch C, Nutting WB: *Demodex folliculorum* (Simon) and *D. brevis* Akbulatova of man: redescription and reevaluation, *J Parasitol* 58:169–177, 1972.

Desch CE, Nutting WB: Redescription of Demodex caballi (=D. folliculorum var. equi Railliet, 1895) from the horse, *Equus caballus, Acarologia* 20:235–240, 1978.

Dobson P, Tinembart O, Fisch RD, et al: Efficacy of nitenpyram as a systemic flea adulticide in dogs and cats, *Vet Rec* 147:709–713, 2000.

Doebler SA: The rise and fall of the honeybee: mite infestations challenge the bee and the beekeeping industry, *BioScience* 50:738–742, 2000.

Dougherty CT, Knapp FW, Burrus PB, et al: Face flies (*Musca autumnalis* De Geer) and the behavior of grazing beef cattle, *Appl Anim Behav Sci* 35:313–326, 1993.

Dougherty CT, Knapp FW, Burrus PB, et al: Behavior of grazing cattle exposed to small populations of stable flies *(Stomoxys calcitrans* L.), *Appl Anim Behav Sci* 42:231–248, 1994.

Dryden MW, Bruce AB: Development of a trap for collecting newly emerged *Ctenocephalides felis* (Siphonaptera: Pulicidae) in homes, *J Med Entomol* 30:901–906, 1993.

Dryden MW, Long GR, Gaafar SM: Effects of ultrasonic collars on *Ctenocephalides felis* on cats, *J Am Vet Med Assoc* 195:1717–1718, 1989.

Eagleson JS, Thompson DR, Scott PG, et al: (1993): Field trials to confirm the efficacy of ivermectin jetting fluid for control of blow fly strike in sheep, *Vet Parasitol* 51:107–112, 1993.

Edwards FW, Oldroyd H, Smart J: *British blood-sucking flies,* London, 1939, British Museum (Natural History).

Elzen PJ, Baxter JR, Westervelt D, et al: Field control and biology studies of a new pest species, *Aethina tumida* Murray (Coleoptera, Nitidulidae), attacking European honey bees in the Western Hemisphere, *Apidologie* 30:361–366, 1999.

Endris RG, Reuter VE, Nelson JD, et al: Efficacy of 65% permethrin applied as a topical spot-on against walking dandruff caused by the mite, *Cheyletiella yasguri*, in dogs, *Vet Therapeut* 1:273–279, 2000.

Evans RH: Ivermectin treatment of notoedric mange in two fox squirrels, *J Am Vet Med Assoc* 185:1437–1438, 1984.

Eyre P, Boulard C, Deline T: Local and systemic reactions in cattle to *Hypoderma lineatum* larval toxin: protection by phenylbutazone, *Am J Vet Res* 42:25–28, 1981.

Fain A, Le Net JL: A new larval mite of the genus *Straelensia* Vercammen-Granjean and Kolebinova, 1968 (Acari: Leeuwenhoekiidae) causing nodular dermatitis of dogs in France, *Int J Acarol* 26:339–345, 2001.

Farkas R, Hall MJR, Daniel M, et al: Efficacy of ivermectin and moxidectin injection against larvae of *Wohlfartia magnifica* (Diptera: Sarcophagidae) in sheep, *Parasitol Res* 82:82–86, 1996.

Fehrenbach P: Where have all the flea dollars gone? *Pest Control Technol* 24:23, 36, 40, 1996.

Foil LD, Hogsette JA: Biology and control of tabanids, stable flies, and horn flies, *Rev Sci Tech* 13:1125–1158, 1994.

Foil LD, DeRoven SM, Morrison DG: Economic benefits of horn fly control for beef production: fall-calving cows and stocker cattle, *Louisiana Agric* 39:12–13, 1996.

Foley RH: A notoedric mange epizootic in an island's cat population, *Feline Pract* 19:8–10, 1991a.

Foley RH: Parasitic mites of dogs and cats, *Compen Contin Ed Pract Vet* 13:783–800, 1991b.

Folz SD, Kratzer DD, Conklin RD, et al: Chemotherapeutic treatment of naturally acquired generalized demodicosis, *Vet Parasitol* 13:85–93, 1983.

Gearhart MS, Crissman JW, Georgi ME: Bilateral lower palpebral demodicosis in a dairy cow, *Cornell Vet* 71:305–310, 1981.

Geden CJ, Rutz DA, Bishop DR: Cattle lice (Anoplura, Mallophaga) in New York: seasonal population changes, effects of housing type on infestations of calves, and sampling efficiency, *J Econ Entomol* 83:1435–1438, 1990.

Geden CJ, Rutz DA, Miller RW, et al: Suppression of house flies (Diptera: Muscidae) on New York and Maryland dairies using releases of *Muscidifurax raptor* (Hymenoptera: Pteromalidae) in an integrated management system, *Environ Entomol* 21:1419–1426, 1992.

Gerhardt RR, Allen JW, Green WH, et al: The role of face flies in an episode of infectious bovine keratoconjunctivitis, *J Am Vet Med Assoc* 180:156–159, 1982.

Gherardi SG, Sutherland SS, Monzu N, et al: Field observations on body strike in sheep affected with dermatophilosis and fleece-rot, *Aust Vet J* 60:27–28, 1983.

Greve JH, Gerrish BS: Fur mites *(Lynxacarus)* from cats in Florida, *Feline Pract* 11:28–30, 1981.

Hall RD, Doisy KE, Teasley CH: *Walk-through trap to control horn flies on cattle*, Agricultural Guide G1195, Columbia, 1987, University of Missouri-Columbia Extension Division.

Harman A: Honey bees: more than just honey, *FDA Veterinarian Newsletter* 12(2):1998.

Haufe WO: Growth of range cattle protected from horn flies *(Haematobia irritans)* by ear tags impregnated with fenvalerate, *Can J Anim Sci* 62:567–573, 1982.

Hawkins JA, Adams WV, Cook L, et al: Role of horse fly *(Tabanus fuscicostatus* Hine) and stable fly *(Stomoxys calcitrans* L.) in transmission of equine infectious anemia to ponies in Louisiana, *Am J Vet Res* 34:1583–1586, 1973.

Hayes RO, Doane OW, Sakolsky G, et al: Evaluation of attractants in traps for greenhead fly (Diptera: Tabanidae) collections on a Cape Cod, Massachusetts, salt marsh, *J Am Mosq Control Assoc* 9:436–440, 1993.

Heffner RS, Heffner HE: Effect of cattle ear mite infestation on hearing in a cow, *J Am Vet Med Assoc* 182:612–614, 1983.

Hibler CP, Adcock JL: Elaeophorosis. In Davis JW, Anderson RC, editors: *Parasitic diseases of wild mammals*, Ames, 1971, Iowa State University Press.

Hink WF, Fee BJ: Toxicity of D-limonene, the major component of citrus peel oil, to all life stages of the cat flea, *Ctenocephalides felis* (Siphonaptera: Pulicidae), *J Med Entomol* 23:400–404, 1986.

Hinkle NC, Koehler PG, Patterson RS: Larvicidal effects of boric acid and disodium octaborate tetrahydrate to cat fleas (Siphonaptera: Pulicidae), *J Med Entomol* 32:424–427, 1995.

Hinrichsen VL, Whitworth UG, Breitschwerdt EB, et al: Assessing the association between the geographic distribution of deer ticks and seropositivity rates to various tick-transmitted disease organisms in dogs, *J Am Vet Med Assoc* 218:1092–1097, 2001.

Jagger T, Banks I, Walker A: Traveling ticks, *Vet Rec* 139:476, 1996.

James MT: *The flies that cause myiasis in man*, Misc Pub No 631, Washington, DC, 1948, U.S. Department of Agriculture.

Jubb TF, Vasallo RL, Wroth RH: Suppurative otitis in cattle associated with ear mites *(Raillietina auris), Aust Vet J* 70:354–355, 1993.

Karesh WB, Robinson PT: Ivermectin treatment of lice infestations in two elephant species, *J Am Vet Med Assoc* 187:1235–1236, 1985.

Kazacos KR, Kapke EJ, Widmer WR, et al: *"Out of Africa": massive visceral pentastomiasis in a dog*, Proceedings of the forty-fifth annual meeting of the American Association of Veterinary Parasitologists, Salt Lake City, Utah, 2000, Abstract 8.

King JM: *Pneumonyssus caninum*, *Vet Med* 83:1216, 1988.

Kitselman CH, Grundman AW: Equine encephalomyelitis virus isolated from naturally infected *Triatoma sanguisuga* Le Conte, Tech Bull 50, Manhattan, Kan, 1940, Kansas State College Agricultural Experiment Station.

Kleynhans KPN: *Musca nevilli* sp. Nov. (Diptera: Muscidae), a dung-breeding fly from South Africa, *Onderstepoort J Vet Res* 54:115–118, 1987.

Knipling EF, Wells RW: Factors stimulating hatching of eggs of *Gasterophilus intestinalis* de Geer and the application of warm water as a practical method of destroying these eggs on the host, *J Econ Entomol* 28:1065–1072, 1935.

Konstantinov SA: Quantitative evaluation of the principal phases of horse-fly (Tabanidae) attack on cattle in natural conditions, *Parazitologicheskii Sbornik* 37:73–100, 1992 (abstracted in CAB Abstracts AN# 950507013).

Konstantinov SA: The range of attack, distance, and character of daily flying of horse-flies of the genus *Hybomitra* (Diptera: Tabanidae), *Parazitologiia* 27:419–426, 1993 (in Russian).

Kraus SJ, Glassman LH: The crab louse: review of physiology and study of anatomy as seen by the scanning electron microscope, *J Am Venereal Dis Assoc* 2:12–18, 1976.

Krinsky WL: Animal disease agents transmitted by horse flies and deer flies (Diptera: Tabanidae), *J Med Entomol* 13:225–275, 1976 (review).

Kummel BA, Estes SA, Arlian LG: *Trixacarus caviae* infestation of guinea pigs, *J Am Vet Med Assoc* 177:903–908, 1980.

Kummerfeld N, Hinz KH: Diagnose und Terapie der durch die Luftsackmilbe *(Sternostoma tracheacolum)* bei Finken (Fringillidae) und Prachtfinken (Estrilididae) verursachten Acariasis, *Kleintierpraxis* 27:95–104, 1982.

Kunkle GA, Greiner EC: Dermatitis in horses and man caused by the straw itch mite, *J Am Vet Med Assoc* 181:467–469, 1982.

Kutzer E: Ektoparasitenbekampfung mit ivermectin (Ivomec) bei Schalenwild (Rothirsch, Reh, Widschwein), *Mitteil Dtsch Gschft Allg Angwndt Entomol* 6:217–222, 1988.

Kwochka KW, Gram D, Kunkle GA, et al: Clinical efficacy of selamectin for the control of fleas on dogs and cats, *Vet Therapeut* 1:252–260, 2000.

Lane RS, Burgdorfer W: Transovarial and transstadial passage of *Borrelia burgdorferi* in the western black-legged tick, *Ixodes pacificus* (Acari: Ixodidae), *Am J Trop Med Hyg* 37:188–192, 1987.

Levot GW, Sales N: Effectiveness of a mixture of cyromazine and diazinon for controlling flystrike on sheep, *Aust Vet J* 76:343–344, 1998.

Linquist DA, Abusowa M, Hall MJR: The new world screwworm fly in Libya: a review of its introduction and eradication, *Med Vet Entomol* 6:2–8, 1992.

Lissman BA, Bosler EM, Camay H, et al: Spirochete-associated arthritis (Lyme disease) in a dog, *J Am Vet Med Assoc* 185:219–220, 1984.

Madigan JE, Pusterla N, Johnson E, et al: Transmission of *Ehrlichia risticii*, the agent of Potomac horse fever, using naturally infected aquatic insects and helminth vectors: preliminary report, *Equine Vet J* 32:275–279, 2000.

Mally M, Kutzer E: Zur Tabanidenfauna Österreichs und Betrachtungen zu ihrer medizinischen Bedeutung, *Mitt Österr Ges Tropenmed Parasitol* 6:97–193, 1984.

Mandigers PJJ, van der Hage MH, Dorrstein GM: Eee veldoderzoek naar de effectiviteit van ivermectine in proyleenglycol bij de behandeling van schurft bij cavias, *Tijdschr Diergeneesk* 118:42–46, 1993.

Manson ER, Malynicz GL: The use of cythioate in the treatment of demodectic mange in the dog, *Aust Vet J* 45:533–534, 1969.

Marchionado AA: Biology, economic effect, and control of the horn fly, *Anim Health Nutr* May/June:6–10, 1987.

Mather TN, Ribiero JMC, Spielman A: Lyme disease and babesiosis: acaricide focused on potentially infected ticks, *Am J Trop Med Hyg* 36:609–614, 1987.

Matushka FR, Spielman A: The emergence of Lyme disease in a changing environment in North America and Central Europe, *Exptl Appl Acarology* 2:337–353, 1986.

McKellar QA, Midgley DM, Galbraith EA, et al: Clinical and pharmacological properties of ivermectin in rabbits and guinea pigs, *Vet Rec* 130:71–73, 1992.

McLaughlin RF, Addison EM: Tick *(Dermacentor albipictus)*-induced winter hair loss in captive moose *(Alces alces)*, *J Wildlife Dis* 22:502–510, 1986.

McMahon MJ, Gaugler R: Effect of salt marsh drainage on the distribution of *Tabanus nigrovittatus* (Diptera: Tabanidae), *J Med Entomol* 30:474–475, 1993.

Meleney WP, Kim KC: A comparative study of cattle-infesting *Haematopinus* with redescription of *H. quadripertusus* Fahrenholz, 1916 (Anoplura: Haematopinidae), *J Parasitol* 60:507–522, 1974.

Michener GR: Lethal myiasis of Richardson's ground squirrels by the sarcophagid fly *Neobillieria citellovora*, *J Mammol* 74:148–155, 1993.

Miller WH, Scott DW, Wellington JR, et al: Clinical efficacy of milbemycin oxime in the treatment of generalized demodicosis in adult dogs, *J Am Vet Med Assoc* 204:1426–1429, 1993.

Molina CG, Euzeby J: Activite de l'ivermectine sur *Melophagus ovinus*, *Sci Vet Med Comp* 84:133–134, 1982.

Moorhouse DE: *On the morphogenesis of the attachment cement of some ixodid ticks*, Proceedings of the third International Congress of Acarology, Prague, Czechoslovakia, 1973, pp 527–529.

Moorhouse DE, Tatchell RJ: The feeding processes of the cattle tick *Boophilus microplus* (Canestrini): a study in host-parasite relations. Part I. Attachment to the host, *Parasitology* 56:623–632, 1966.

Mundell AC, Ihrke PJ: Ivermectin in the treatment of *Pneumonyssoides caninum*: a case report, *J Am Anim Hosp Assoc* 26:393–396, 1990.

Muniz RA, Coronado A, Anziani OS, et al: Efficacy of injectable doramectin in the protection of castrated cattle against field infestations of *Cochliomyia hominivorax*, *Vet Parasitol* 58:327–333, 1995.

Nevill EM: Preliminary report on the transmission of *Parafilaria bovicola* in South Africa, *Onderstepoort J Vet Res* 41:41–48, 1975.

Nevill EM: The epidemiology of *Parafilaria bovicola* in the Transvaal Bushveld of South Africa, *Onderstepoort J Vet Res* 52:261–267, 1985.

Olander HJ: The migration of *Hypoderma lineatum* in the brain of a horse: a case report and review, *Pathol Vet* 4:477–483, 1967.

Paradis M, Laperriere E: Efficacy of daily ivermectin treatment in a dog with amitraz-resistant generalized demodicosis, *Vet Dermatol* 3:85–88, 1992.

Peterson HO, Roberts IH, Becklund WW, et al: Anemia in cattle caused by heavy infestation of the bloodsucking louse *Haematopinus eurysternus*, *J Am Vet Med Assoc* 122:373–376, 1953.

Piesman J: Field studies on Lyme disease in North America, *Can J Infect Dis* 2:55–57, 1991.

Pobst D, Richards C: *The caddisfly handbook: an Orvis guide*, New York, 1999, The Lyons Press.

Pound JM, Miller JA, George JE, et al: Systemic treatment of white-tail deer with ivermectin-medicated bait to control free-living populations of lone star ticks (Acari: Ixodidae), *J Med Entomol* 33:385–394, 1996.

Preisler J: Incidence of ear mites, *Otodectes cynotis*, on some carnivores in the territory of CSR, *Folia Parasitol (Praha)* 32:82, 1985.

Price RE, Stromberg PC: Seasonal occurrence and distribution of *Gasterophilus intestinalis* and *Gasterophilus nasalis* in the stomachs of equids in Texas, *Am J Vet Res* 48:1225–1232, 1987.

Principato M: Classification of the main macroscopic lesions produced by larvae of *Gasterophilus* spp. (Diptera: Gasterophilidae) in free-ranging horses in Umbria, *Cornell Vet* 78:43–52, 1988.

Prosl H, Rabitsch A, Brabenetz J: Zur Bedeutung der Herbstmilbe—*Neotrombicula autumnalis* (Shaw 1790)—in der Veterinärmedizin: Nervale Symptome bei Hunden nach massiver Infestation, *Tierärztl Prax* 13:57–64, 1985.

Pruett JH, Kunz SE: Warble stage development of third instars of *Hypoderma lineatum* (Diptera: Oestridae), *J Med Entomol* 33:220–223, 1996.

Pusterla N, Johnson E, Chae JS, et al: Infection rate of *Ehrlichia risticii*, the agent of Potomac horse fever, in freshwater stream snails *(Juga yrekaensis)* from northern California, *Vet Parasitol* 92:151–156, 2000.

Rainey JW: Equine mortality due to *Gasterophilus* larvae (stomach bots), *Aust Vet J* 24:116–119, 1948.

Ramsay GW, Mason PC: Chicken mite *(D. gallinae)* infesting a dog, *N Z Vet J* 62:701, 1975.

Rhodes AP: Seminal degeneration associated with chorioptic mange of the scrotum of rams, *Aust Vet J* 51:428–432, 1975.

Riek RF: Studies on allergic dermatitis (Queensland itch) of the horse. I. Description, distribution, symptoms, and pathology, *Aust Vet J* 29:177–184, 1953a.

Riek RF: Studies on allergic dermatitis of the horse. II. Treatment and control, *Aust Vet J* 29:185–187, 1953b.

Roberts FHS: *Insects affecting livestock,* Sydney, 1952, Angus and Robertson Ltd.

Roncalli RA: Efficacy of ivermectin against *Oestrus ovis* in sheep, *Vet Med Small Anim Clin* 79:1095–1097, 1984.

Rooney JR: Gastric ulceration in foals, *Pathol Vet* 1:497–503, 1964.

Rosenstein M: Paralysis in chickens caused by larvae of the poultry tick *Argas persicus, Avian Dis* 20:407–409, 1976.

Rothschild M, Schlein Y, Parker K, et al: The flying leap of the flea, *Sci Am* 229:92–100, 1973.

Ryan T: Cnemidocoptic mite infestation in cage birds, *Mod Vet Pract* 67:525–526, 1986.

Sabrosky CW, Bennett GF, Whitworth TL: *Bird blow flies (Protocalliphora) in North America (Diptera: Calliphoridae) with notes on the palearctic species*, Washington DC, 1989, Smithsonian Institute Press.

Schoeb TR, Panciera RJ: Blister beetle poisoning in horses, *J Am Vet Med Assoc* 173:75–77, 1978.

Schoeb TR, Panciera RJ: Pathology of blister beetle poisoning in horses, *Vet Pathol* 16:18–31, 1979.

Scholl PJ, Barrett CC: Technique to extract *Hypoderma* sp. (Diptera: Oestridae) larvae from the backs of cattle, *J Econ Entomol* 79:1125–1126, 1986.

Schroeder HO: Habits of the larvae of *Gasterophilus nasalis* (L.) in the mouth of the horse, *J Econ Entomol* 33(2):382–384, 1940.

Shanks DJ, McTier TL, Behan S, et al: The efficacy of selamectin in the treatment of naturally acquired infestations of *Sarcoptes scabiei* on dogs, *Vet Parasitol* 91:269–281, 2000.

Shoop WL, Egerton JR, Eary CH, et al: Eprinomectin: a novel avermectin for use as a topical endectocide for cattle, *Int J Parasitol* 26:1237–1242, 1996.

Silverman J, Rust MK, Reierson DA: Influence of temperature and humidity on survival and development of the cat flea, *Ctenocephalides felis* (Siphonaptera: Pulicidae), *J Med Entomol* 18:78–83, 1981.

Sinclair J: The reappearance of warble fly in Britain, 1993–1994, *State Vet J* 5:9–10, 1995.

Smiley RL, O'Connor BM: Mange in *Macaca arctoides* (Primates: Cercopithecidae) caused by *Cosarcoptes scanloni* (Acari: Sarcoptidae) with possible human involvement and descriptions of the adult male and immature stages, *Int J Acarol* 6:283–290, 1980.

Smith PH, Dallwitz R, Wardhaugh KG, et al: Timing of larval exodus from sheep and carrion in the sheep blow fly, *Lucilia cuprina, Entomol Exptl Aplicata* 30:157–162, 1981.

Spielman A: Human babesiosis in Nantucket Island: transmission by nymphal *Ixodes* ticks, *Am J Trop Med Hyg* 25:784–787, 1976.

Stanchi ND, Grisolia CS: Uso de ivermectina en el tratamiento de le acariasis (*Ophionyssus* sp.) de ofidios, *Vet Argent* 3:578–581, 1986.

Steve PC, Lilly JH: Investigations on transmissibility of *Moraxella bovis* by the face fly, *J Econ Entomol* 58:444–446, 1965.

Strickler JD, Walker ED: Seasonal abundance and species diversity of adult Tabanidae (Diptera) at Lake Lansing Park—North Michigan, *Great Lakes Entomol* 26:107–112, 1993.

Theiler A: Diseases, ticks, and their eradication, *Agr J S Afr* 1:491–508, 1911.

Thomas GD, Hall RD, Berry IL: Diapause of the horn fly (Diptera: Muscidae) in the field, *Environ Entomol* 60:1092–1097, 1987.

Timm RM, Lee RE Jr: Do bot flies, *Cuterebra* (Diptera: Cuterebridae), emasculate their hosts? *J Med Entomol* 18(4):333–336, 1981.

Torres S: Infectious gastroenteritis in wild cats, *N Am Vet* May:297–299, 1941.

Underwood PC, Dikmans G: Gastralgia in a horse due to bot infestation, *Vet Med* 38:12–13, 1943.

Waddell AH: The pathogenicity of *Gasterophilus intestinalis* in the stomach of the horse, *Aust Vet J* 48:332–335, 1972.

Wall R, Strong L: Environmental consequences of treating cattle with the antiparasitic drug ivermectin, *Nature* 327:418–421, 1987.

Warburg A, Saraiva E, Lanzaro GC, et al: Saliva of *Lutzomyia longipalpis* sibling species differs in its composition and capacity to enhance leishmaniasis, *Philos Trans R Soc Lond B Biol Sci* 345:223–230, 1994.

Washburn RH, Klebsadel LJ, Palmer JS, et al: The warble fly problem in Alaska reindeer, *Agroborealis* 12:23–28, 1980.

Wells RW, Knipling EF: A report of some recent studies on species of *Gasterophilus* occurring in horses in the United States, *Iowa State Coll J Sci* 12:181–203, 1938.

White SD, Rosychuk RAW, Fieseler KV: Clinicopathologic findings, sensitivity to house dust mites and efficacy of milbemycin oxime treatment of dogs with *Cheyletiella* sp. infestation, *Vet Dermatol* 12:13–18, 2001.

Willadsen P, Bird P, Cobon GS, et al: Commercialization of a recombinant vaccine against *Boophilus microplus, Parasitology* 110:543–550, 1995.

Williams DF: A veterinary approach to the European honey bee *(Apis mellifera), Vet J* 160:61–73, 2000.

Williams KJ, Summers BA, de Lahunta A: Cerebrospinal cuterebriasis in cats and its association with feline ischemic encephalopathy, *Vet Pathol* 35:330–343, 1998.

Wilson GWC: Control of warble fly in Great Britain and the European Community, *Vet Rec* 118:653–656, 1986.

Wilson GI, Blachut K, Roberts IH: The infectivity of scabies (mange) mites, *Psoroptes ovis* (Acarina: Psoroptidae), to sheep in naturally contaminated enclosures, *Res Vet Sci* 22:292–297, 1977.

Wilson ML, Telford SR, Piesman J, et al: Reduced abundance of immature *Ixodes dammini* (Acari: Ixodidae) following elimination of deer, *J Med Entomol*, 25:224–228, 1988.

Wing SR, Courtney CH, Young MD: Effect of ivermectin on murine mites, *J Am Vet Med Assoc* 187:1191–1192, 1985.

Wright FC: Control of psoroptic scabies of cattle with fenvalerate, *Vet Parasitol* 21:37–42, 1986.

CHAPTER 2

PROTOZOANS

Most protozoans are free-living organisms, and of those that live as parasites in the bodies of mammals, only a small proportion is associated with disease. Even then, their etiological significance is sometimes unclear. For example, certain intestinal flagellates multiply when the host has diarrhea. In such cases, the presence of large numbers of flagellates in the fecal smear is the result rather than the cause of the diarrhea. On the other hand, there are protozoans that indeed behave as primary pathogens, and these are responsible for some of the most important diseases of humans and domestic animals. These diseases are the malarias, piroplasmoses, and coccidioses caused by apicomplexans and the trypanosomiases caused by sarcomastigophoran hemoflagellates.

■ SUBPHYLUM SARCOMASTIGOPHORA
Flagellates

Flagellates bear one or more long, slender **flagella** (sing., **flagellum**) for locomotion. The flagellum is also called an **undulipodium** by those engaged in protozoology to accentuate its structural differences with the flagellum of bacteria. Flagellates multiply asexually by binary fission, and certain species form resistant cysts. The parasitic flagellates can be divided into two main groups according to their location in the host's body and type of life history. The **hemoflagellates** (e.g., *Trypanosoma* and *Leishmania*) live in the blood, lymph, and tissue spaces and are typically transmitted from host to host by bloodsucking insects. There is no collective term for the others, so we will call them **mucosoflagellates.** These live in the alimentary or genital tract, usually in intimate association with the mucous membrane, and are transmitted from host to host in the feces or genital effluvia. Certain mucosoflagellates are transmitted as trophozoites (e.g., *Trichomonas*), others as cysts (e.g., *Giardia*).

Hemoflagellates
Trypanosoma and Leishmania

A trypanosome is an elongated, spindle-shaped cell with a single nucleus lying near the middle of its length and a single **flagellum** that arises near a large mitochondrion with copious DNA called a **kinetoplast** and passes out of the anterior end of the cell (Figure 2-1). During development in both mammalian and arthropod hosts, trypanosomes can undergo considerable morphological change. Four morphological forms are distinguished in the case of *Trypanosoma cruzi*. The **amastigote** lacks a flagellum, whereas the other three forms all have a flagellum but differ with respect to the location of the kinetoplast. The kinetoplast lies posterior to the nucleus in the **trypomastigote,** immediately anterior to the nucleus in the **epimastigote,** and near the anterior end of the cell in the **promastigote.** The flagellum lies in the edge of an **undulating membrane** as it courses from kinetoplast to the

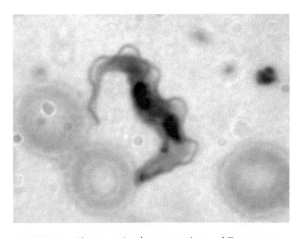

FIGURE 2-1 Giemsa-stained trypomastigote of *Trypanosoma brucei.* With the tsetse-transmitted trypanosomes, dividing forms, like the one in this image, can be observed in blood smears (×4000).

anterior end of the cell body of the trypomastigote. Infection of the arthropod host occurs when it ingests the blood of an infected mammal. Infection of the mammalian host occurs by one of two mechanisms, depending on the species of trypanosome involved: either through the bite of the infected arthropod or by contamination of the host's mucous membranes or abraded skin by its feces. The former are called **salivarian,** and the latter **stercorarian** trypanosomes. Most salivarians are pathogenic and most stercorarians are nonpathogenic, but the pathogenic stercorarian *Trypanosoma cruzi* is an important exception to this generalization.

Tsetse-transmitted trypanosomes are of major significance in sub-Saharan Africa (see Figure 2-1). *Trypanosoma brucei* and *Trypanosoma congolense* cause fatal **nagana disease** in domestic ruminants but are only mildly pathogenic in the indigenous wild ruminants. The wild ruminants thus serve as reservoirs of *T. brucei* and *T. congolense,* which are conveyed through the bites of tsetses (*Glossina* spp.) to domestic livestock. These trypanosomes and tsetses defend vast areas of African grazing lands against invasion by domestic livestock. Humans have been striving to introduce their domestic animals into these areas for a long time without remarkable success, and where they have succeeded, they have often destroyed the grasslands by overgrazing and turned them into deserts.

T. brucei multiplies by longitudinal binary fission in the blood, lymph, and cerebrospinal fluid of the mammalian host. The trypomastigotes, the only stage in the mammalian host, that are ingested by the tsetse when it feeds on the blood of an infected mammal multiply in the insect's midgut, undergo metamorphosis, and migrate to the salivary glands, where they reach the infective **metacyclic** trypomastigote stage and are then ready to be injected into the mammalian host at the next feeding. *Trypanosoma gambiense* and *Trypanosoma rhodesiense,* the etiological agents of African **sleeping sickness** in human, are closely related to *T. brucei.*

Trypanosoma vivax is a form of considereable importance to livestock in West Africa. The reservoir hosts are wild ungulates. The living trypanosome is active in fresh blood films, hence the name "vivax." In cattle the infection may be without signs, or there may be acute or chronic disease. In peracute disease, there may be a high parasitemia associated with extensive hemorrhages throughout the mucosal and serosal surfaces of the body. In the chronic disease, cattle will become anemic and emaciated, with signs of severe wasting. Similar disease has been reported in goats and sheep. *T vivax* has been exported from Africa to South America where the reservoir appears to be deer. Outside of Africa, the disease is transmitted mechanically by biting flies.

Trypanosoma evansi occurs in Asia, tropical America, and Africa north of the Sahara and causes **surra** of all species of domestic animals. Flies of the family Tabanidae and vampire bats serve as vectors. In South American horses, *Tryponosoma equinum* causes a disease called **mal de Caderas,** which is similar to surra.

Trypanosoma equiperdum is unique among trypanosomes in not requiring an intermediate host. Transmission among hosts occurs through direct sexual contact and results in the equine venereal disease called **dourine.** The acute stage is characterized by swelling of the genitalia and a mucoid discharge in which *T. equiperdum* can usually be demonstrated. As the acute signs subside, circular, flattened, "silver dollar" plaques appear in the skin and then disappear within several hours or days to be replaced by others. The chronic stage of dourine is marked by emaciation, paresis, intermittent fever, and finally death. Dourine was eradicated from the United States in 1920 and again in 1949 but has since reappeared at least once. The eradication of *T. equiperdum* from North America was made possible to a great extent by the work of a Canadian veterinarian, Edward Watson, who worked on the disease for some 15 years, was the first to identify the trypanosome in horses in North America, and developed a complement fixation test that could be used to identify infected horses in the field. Identified horses were then destroyed. Thus, within 16 years the disease had been identified and eradicated from the Canadian provinces (Derbyshir and Nielsen, 1997).

Not all trypanosomes transmitted by the bites of arthropod vectors are exotic and tropical, but most of them are nonpathogenic. *Trypanosoma cervi* was identified in 29 of 45 Alaskan reindeer *(Rangifer tarandus)* examined over a 2-year period and in 98% of white-tailed deer *(Odocoileus virginianus)* in southern Florida examined over a 5-year period (Telford et al, 1991). *T. cervi* also infects elk and mule deer in the United States and is apparently without pathogenic effect (Kingston et al, 1982). *Trypanosoma theileri* (pronounced "tyler-eye") is a harmless parasite of cattle transmitted by tabanid flies, and *Trypsanoma melophagium* is an equally harmless parasite of sheep transmitted by *Melophagus ovinus;* both are distributed worldwide. Occasionally, *T. theileri* contaminates culture media that have been enriched with "sterile" bovine serum, much to the surprise and confusion of the microbiologist. It is interesting that *M. ovinus,* which is first cousin to a tsetse, is almost universally infected with a trypanosome, albeit fortunately a harmless one.

T. cruzi (Figure 2-2), the etiological agent of American trypanosomiasis **(Chagas' disease)** of human and dog, is transmitted by triatomin bugs of the genera *Triatoma, Rhodnius,* and *Panstrongylus* in South and Central America and in Texas, Arizona, New Mexico, California, and Oklahoma (Fox et al, 1986). *T. cruzi* was also observed in hunting dogs in central Virginia that had lymphadenopathy but did not yet have clinical signs of cardiomyopathy (Barr et al, 1995). Five of 400 raccoons *(Procyon lotor)* examined in Maryland were infected (Walton et al, 1958). Opossums, armadillos, rats, guinea pigs, cats, raccoons, and monkeys serve as reservoirs of infection in the wild. *T. cruzi* amastigotes multiply by binary fission in mammalian cells, including reticuloendothelial, neural, and glial cells, but most important, in cardiac and smooth muscle cells. Amastigotes released by rupture of the host cell change into trypomastigotes, which then appear in the circulating blood to invade other cells or to be ingested by the bug as it feeds. Trypomastigotes of *T. cruzi* are rarely, if ever, seen dividing in blood smears prepared from circulating blood. The trypanosomes multiply and undergo metamorphosis in the bug's hindgut and are eventually passed in the feces that the bug almost invariably passes while feeding on its sleeping victim. Trypanosomes enter the body by going through the oral, nasal, and conjunctival mucosae or by infectious bug feces being rubbed into abrasions in the skin. Infection can also occur through the placenta or by blood transfusion, and accidental self-injection presents a potential hazard of infection to persons handling blood samples from infected animals, even those specimens in which trypomastigotes cannot be demonstrated in blood films. Trypomastigotes are difficult to demonstrate in the blood of long-term carriers, and one must turn to serology, culture, or **xenodiagnosis** for recourse. In xenodiagnosis, uninfected bugs are allowed to feed on the suspected individual, and their hindguts are later examined for trypanosomes, a cumbersome and inefficient procedure at best. In dogs, acute disease is characterized by lymphadenopathy and clinical signs associated with acute myocarditis: pale mucous membranes, lethargy, ascites, hepatomegaly, splenomegaly, and tachyrhythmia (Barr, 1991). The signs during the chronic stage of the disease are related to congestive myocardial failure. Megaesophagus and other mega-syndromes described in humans with chronic Chagas' disease have not been reported in dogs.

Leishmania donovani causes several clinical forms of **visceral leishmaniasis (kala-azar),** and *Leishmania tropica* causes several clinical forms of **cutaneous** and **mucocutaneous leishmaniasis** in humans, dogs, rodents, and wild mammals. These

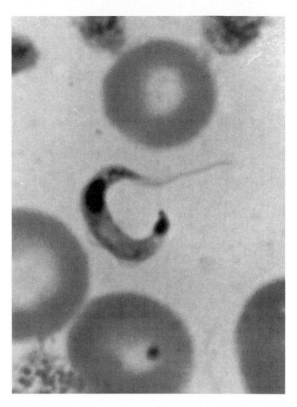

FIGURE 2-2 *Trypanosoma cruzi* in a Wright's stained buffy coat preparation from a naturally infected dog (×4000). (Specimen provided by Dr. Stephen C. Barr.)

diseases are mostly confined to the tropics, where they are transmitted by psychodids of the genera *Phlebotomus* in the Eastern Hemisphere and *Lutzomyia* in the Western Hemisphere. A case of dermal leishmaniasis involving the ears of a domestic cat was reported from south-central Texas. Radical pinnectomy was performed before the cat was returned to its owners to prevent it from serving as a source of infection to sand flies (Craig et al, 1986). Visceral leishmaniasis has also been reported in a colony of American foxhounds in Oklahoma (Anderson et al, 1982) and in a colony of English foxhounds in Ohio (Swenson et al, 1988). The Ohio outbreak involved one case of chronic illness and death, and positive serum titers in eight of 25 other colony dogs. Because the dead dog had been born and raised in the research colony and because more than a third of the other dogs in the colony carried titers to *L. donovani,* the authors concluded that transmission of the disease must have occurred in Ohio, most likely through the agency of an insect vector. In 1999 additional infections were reported from a group of working foxhounds kenneled at a hunt club in New York State. The initial presentation involved signs including bleeding, wasting, seizures, hair loss, and kidney failure. A number of the dogs died, and Dr. Breitschwerdt and colleagues at North Carolina State University recovered *Leishmania* organisms from synovial fluid. Further testing of foxhounds from around the United States revealed that of 11,000 foxhounds in U.S. and Canadian hunt packs, some 12% had antibodies to *Leishmania* organisms, although most were without signs (Enserink, 2000). Infected dogs were found in 21 states in the United States and southern Canada, with most cases in the eastern portion of North America. It is unclear at this time how the infection is being spread between dogs, although it is being guessed that transmission is by means of sand flies when the dogs are taken to southern states for hunts.

Visceral leishmaniasis in dogs (Figure 2-3) often is seen with cutaneous manifestations. Dogs are considered major reservoirs for human infections with this parasite and have been the targets of eradication programs in a manner similar to rabies control programs (Oliveira-dos-Santos et al, 1993). The need to develop a means of preventing canine

infections on a large scale has resulted in attempts to develop vaccines that will prevent canine infections (Mayrink et al, 1996). Horses will also sometimes have cutaneous lesions, and horses in Puerto Rico have been found infected with this parasite (Ramos Vara et al, 1996).

Mucosoflagellates

Trichomonads

Trichomonads are characteristically pear-shaped and have a rodlike axostyle that protrudes from the more pointed posterior end. There are three to five anterior flagella and an undulating membrane with a trailing flagellum running along its free edge. Special techniques are required for the differentiation of trichomonad genera on purely morphological grounds. Therefore, practical diagnosis is based on host and site specificity and on the number of anterior and trailing flagella.

Tritrichomonas foetus (Figure 2-4) is found in the vagina, uterus, macerated fetus, prepuce, penis, epididymis, and vas deferens. The organism displays

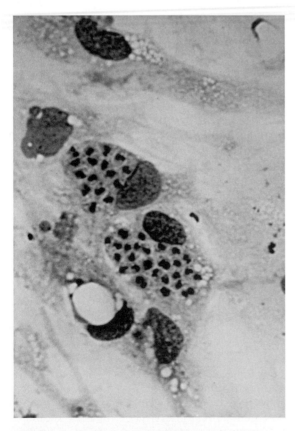

FIGURE 2-3 *Leishmania donovani* in dog spleen smear stained with Giemsa stain. Note two macrophages containing amastigotes, each with a nucleus and kinetoplast (×1100).

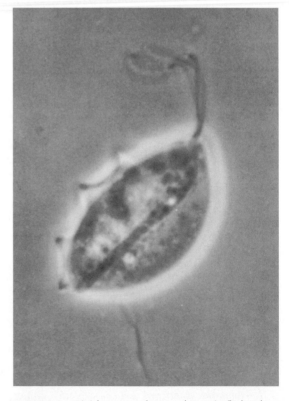

FIGURE 2-4 *Tritrichomonas foetus*, electronic flash, phase contrast photomicrograph of living organism from a culture provided by Dr. S.J. Shin (×5500). The three anterior flagella, undulating membrane, trailing flagellum, and axostyle are clearly visible.

considerable pleomorphism, varies from 10 to 25 μm in length, and has three anterior flagella and a long, trailing flagellum that extends beyond the undulating membrane. In collecting samples to isolate *T. foetus,* it is important to avoid fecal contamination and consequent potential confusion with intestinal flagellates.

Bovine genital trichomoniasis is a venereal disease manifested in cows and heifers by infertility, abortion up to 5 months after breeding, pyometra, and occasional fetal mummification. Infection in beef cattle remains relatively common in some parts of the United States; 16% of 57 herds sampled in California had at least one infected bull (BonDurant et al, 1990). Although infection is inapparent in bulls, *T. foetus* trophozoites can be demonstrated by direct microscopic examination or by culture of preputial swabs or washings. The infected bull is usually responsible for spreading trichomoniasis in the herd, and artificial insemination is recommended as a control measure when feasible. The *T. foetus* trophozoites are transferred from the penis to the vagina during copulation. However, semen is usually not infectious unless contaminated with preputial fluid during artificial collection. Semen contaminated in this way will remain infectious despite the addition of diluents, antibiotics, and freezing (Fitzgerald, 1986). Infected bulls should be culled, and in those situations in which artificial insemination is impractical, they should be replaced with younger, uninfected bulls. However, failure on the part of the artificial insemination technician to observe effective hygienic precautions in conducting vaginal examinations for the detection of estrus may totally negate the benefits of artificial insemination as a control measure (Goodger and Skirrow, 1986). *T. foetus* can usually be demonstrated in the vaginal secretions or washings of virgin heifers 14 to 20 days after service by an infected bull. Infected cows should be given at least 4 months of sexual rest, during which time *T. foetus* trophozoites usually disappear from the reproductive tract. Whether inseminated naturally or artificially, cows and heifers must first be given sexual rest so their reproductive tracts will be cleared of *T. foetus* before gestation begins; otherwise the infection will be perpetuated in the developing embryo (Fitzgerald, 1986). Metronidazole administered intravenously at 75 mg/kg three times at 12-hour intervals is indicated for the treatment and control of *T. foetus* infections in cows.

Trichomonas spp. occur as oral parasites on various hosts and tend to multiply in the presence of pyorrhea, much as their intestinal counterparts multiply in the presence of diarrhea. One species, *Trichomonas vaginalis,* causes vaginitis in women;

it is transmitted by sexual intercourse, with men playing the role of asymptomatic carriers. *Trichomonas gallinae* causes necrotic ulcerations in the esophagus, crop, and proventriculus of pigeons, turkeys, and chickens.

Nonpathogenic species of *Tritrichomonas, Trichomitus, Tetratrichomonas,* and *Pentatrichomonas* occur in the cecum and colon of various domestic animals. These organisms tend to multiply in fluid feces, and many cases of diarrhea are mistakenly attributed to them for this reason. Their abundance in fluid feces is often the effect of and not the cause of the diarrhea. However, it is hard to ascertain whether they cause disease. Romatowski (2000) described pentatrichomoniasis with diarrhea in four kittens. Gookin et al (1999) examined the effect of pentatrichomoniasis in a large number of cases and found most infections in cats younger than 1 year with the feces being pasty to semiformed.

Treatment

Trichomonas infections in puppies may be controlled with metronidazole administered orally at 66 mg/kg once daily for 5 consecutive days (Buckner and Ewing, 1977). Romatowski (2000) treated cats with both metronidazole and enroflaxcin and suggested that the long-term daily administration of enrofloxacin stopped the soft stools. Gookin et al (1999) tried paromomycin, fenbendazole, and furazolidone, and in all cases had mixed success.

Monocercomonas spp. resemble *Trichomonas* but lack an undulating membrane. *Monocercomonas* spp. are nonpathogenic; *Monocercomonas ruminantium* is found in the rumen of cattle.

Histomonas meleagridis is a cosmopolitan parasite of the cecum and liver of turkeys, chickens, pheasants, guinea fowl, and the like. The cecal nematode *Heterakis gallinarum* serves as paratenic host for *Histomonas meleagridis.* When a bird ingests an infective *H. gallinarum* egg, it acquires a nonpathogenic nematode and a pathogenic protozoan parasite at one stroke. The protozoan, released from the nematode larva, spends about a week as a flagellate resident of the cecal lumen before it loses its flagella and invades the subepithelial tissues of the wall as an ameboid organism. Inflammation and necrosis of the cecal wall and the liver are particularly severe and cause a high mortality in turkeys. *H. meleagridis* trophozoites discharged in bird droppings perish within hours, but they remain infective for years within the larvated eggs of *H. gallinarum* in soil. Earthworms serve as paratenic hosts for *H. gallinarum* larvae, and because birds like to eat them, they actually facilitate infection with both this nematode and its protozoan guest.

The trichomonads discussed thus far do not form cysts; *Giardia* does.

Giardia

The number of species of *Giardia* that exist is open to question. On the basis of differences in the shape of the **median bodies,** there appear to be at least three: *Giardia lamblia (Giardia duodenalis)* in mammals, *Giardia muris* in mice, and *Giardia ranae* in frogs, but there may be many more. About 7% of the world's human population harbors *Giardia* in their small intestines, but little is known about the epidemiology of this organism, especially with regard to the possible role of other mammals as sources of human infection. *Giardia* cysts are commonly found in the feces of dogs, cats, cattle, sheep, goats, llamas, and other domestic and wild mammals, and although cross-transmission between hosts can occur, we actually know little about how often it happens. It has been suggested that dairy calves and other hoofed livestock are mainly hosts to what has been termed *Assemblage B* (O'Handley et al, 2000; Thompson et al, 2000). On the other hand, humans tend to be infected mainly with genotypes of organisms called *Assemblage A*. It appears that most cattle shed the "B" type unless they have somehow been around humans and picked up the "A" type. People are probably capable of being infected with both types, but for the most part, people get infected with *Giardia* from other people, at least with the type that is considered the predominantly human type.

Giardia trophozoites are adapted for attachment to the mucous epithelial cells of the small intestine. The *Giardia* **trophozoite** cell is shaped like a teardrop, with one side pushed in to form a sucking disc. Within the cell are two nuclei, each with a large endosome (Feulgen-negative nucleolus) that makes the organism look like a tennis racket with eyes when viewed bottom side up under the compound microscope. Other subcellular structures include two slender axonemes, four pairs of flagella, and a pair of median bodies. All of the other intestinal flagellates are found in the cecum and colon but *Giardia* parasitizes the small intestine, in which the trophozoites attach to the mucosal cells by their sucking discs. Trophozoites usually form infective cysts before passing out with the feces. The mature **cyst** containing two potential trophozoites is the form usually found in the feces of infected hosts. Although trophozoites may also be passed, especially with diarrheal stools, they are incapable of causing infection and soon die.

Giardia infection in humans may be inapparent or cause severe enteritis. Diagnosis is usually based on finding the distinctive cysts in the feces. Sometimes, however, no evidence of infection can be found in the feces of patients with severe giardial enteritis. *Giardia* is generally considered capable of causing enteritis and diarrhea in dogs,

yet we have observed *Giardia* cysts in scores of well-formed canine fecal samples. The question of transmission of *Giardia* from animals to humans has not been settled; feces-contaminated water supplies appear to figure in the epidemiology of human infection.

Diagnosis

Trophozoites may be demonstrated in direct smears of diarrheal feces (Figure 2-5). Cysts (Figure 2-6) may be concentrated by fecal flotation in zinc sulfate of specific gravity 1.18 but tend to shrink and become distorted beyond recognition in sucrose and other flotation media. Phase contrast microscopy is helpful in identifying *Giardia* trophozoites and cysts. If phase contrast microscopy is unavailable, a drop of Lugol's solution of iodine at the edge of the coverslip will stain the trophozoites and cysts and make them easier to identify. *Giardia* cysts are frequently found in the normal stools of asymptomatic hosts, but in occasional cases of clinical giardiosis neither cysts nor trophozoites can be found in the feces. A comparison of the zinc sulfate flotation method with an ELISA (enzyme-linked immunosorbent assay) that was developed to diagnose giardiasis in humans found that the flotation method was slightly more sensitive in the examination of feces containing cysts (Barr et al, 1992).

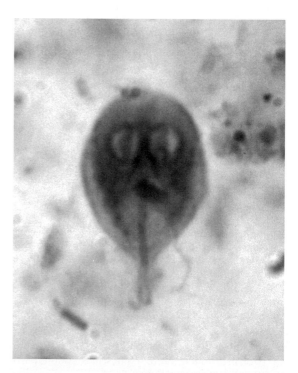

FIGURE 2-5 *Giardia lamblia,* iron hematoxylin-stained trophozoite from human feces (×3000).

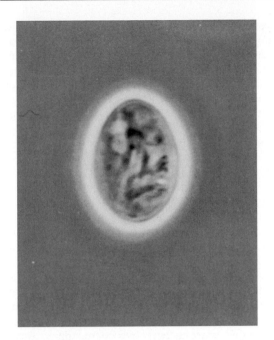

FIGURE 2-6 Cyst of *Giardia* from the feces of a cat. The four nuclei are visible at the upper pole of the cyst (×2280).

In dogs, diarrhea may begin as early as 5 days after exposure to infection (Abbitt et al, 1986); cysts first appear in the feces after about a week or two. In cats, *Giardia* trophozoites are found in the jejunum and ileum instead of the duodenum. The principal clinical sign is persistent diarrhea resulting from intestinal malabsorption; the feces of infected cats are often mucoid, pale, soft, and more than usually malodorous (Kirkpatrick, 1986). In calves, *Giardia* was associated with chronic diarrhea marked by high morbidity, negligible mortality, absence of response to electrolytes and antibiotics, and clinical and parasitological response to dimetridazole within 48 hours (St. Jean et al, 1987). In lambs, the careful examination of production parameters in bottle-reared and experimentally infected animals showed that neonatal giardiasis caused extended times for lambs to reach slaughter weight and decreased carcass weight (Olson et al, 1995). The enumeration of cysts in the feces of ewes around lambing time revealed that there was a periparturient increase in cyst production by ewes that peaked between the time of lambing and 4 weeks afterward (Xiao et al, 1994).

Treatment

Dogs may be treated for giardiasis with fenbendazole at the same dosage used for helminthes (Barr et al, 1994; Zajac et al, 1998). Treatment with albendazole ([Valbazen] 25 g/kg every 12 hours for a total of four doses) has been shown to stop the shedding of *Giardia* cysts by infected dogs (Barr

et al, 1993). Albendazole therapy has the potential of inducing bone marrow toxicosis in dogs and cats; therefore, veterinarians should observe caution in using this drug for treating giardiasis (Stokol et al, 1997). Other treatments that have also been used for canine giardiasis include quinacrine (6.6 mg/kg twice a day for 5 days), metronidazole (22 mg/kg orally twice a day for 5 days), and tinidazole (44 mg/kg once daily for three days) (Zimmer and Burrington, 1986).

Giardia infections in cats may be treated safely and effectively with the same dosage schedule of metronidazole (Zimmer, 1987). Cats probably can also be successfully treated for giardiasis with febantel, albendazole, or fenbendazole, but only febantel has been approved for use in cats as an anthelmintic.

Fenbendazole and albendazole administered to calves at varying doses for different periods have both been proved efficacious against *Giardia* (O'Handley et al, 1997; Xiao et al, 1996). For fenbendazole, all treatments with a single dose of 10 mg, with 10 or 20 mg administered daily for 3 days, or with 0.833 mg administered daily for 6 days were effective. For albendazole, a dose of 20 mg administered daily for 3 days was effective.

Dimetridazole was administered orally to infected calves in 250 ml of water at a dosage of 50 mg/kg for 5 days. The calves cleared their feces of cysts and stopped their diarrhea within 48 hours (St. Jean et al, 1987).

For treatment of giardiasis in parakeets, three doses of dimetridazole at 1.5 mg/30 g of body weight at 12-hour intervals by stomach tube were more effective than supplying drinking water containing 200 ppm of this chemical to the birds for 5 days. Metronidazole therapy was not effective (Scholtens et al, 1982).

Control of *Giardia* infection involves prevention of fecal contamination of feed and water supplies and sanitation and disinfection of the environment with Lysol (2% to 5%), Sterinol (1%), or chlorine bleach (sodium hypochlorite, 1%) (Kirkpatrick, 1986).

Amebas
Intestinal Amebas

Entamoeba histolytica is principally a parasite of the large intestine and causes **amebic dysentery** in humans, an endemic disease of the tropics that occurs sporadically in the temperate regions. Amebic abscess of the liver is a serious, frequently life-threatening sequela. Humans also host a few nonpathogenic amebas *(Entamoeba dispar, Entamoeba hartmanni, Entamoeba coli, Iodamoeba butschlii* and *Endolimax nana),* some of which are shared with domestic animals. *E histolytica* and other amebas appear to cause little if any harm to domestic animals. Amebic trophozoites and cysts frequently appear in fresh fecal smears of perfectly healthy cattle, sheep, goats, horses, and swine but are usually overlooked. These have been described in the past as separate species (e.g., *Entamoeba bovis* and *Entamoeba ovis*) but have received almost no attention in recent years.

However, special cases exist in which amebas are of clinical importance, notably in primates. For example, a case of gastric amebiasis characterized by anorexia, diarrhea, and weight loss was reported in the silvered leaf monkey (*Presbytis cristatus*, Palmieri et al, 1984). The normal high pH level (5.0 to 6.7) of the stomach of leaf monkeys and the stress of capture, shipment, and confinement were considered to have contributed to the extensive gastric involvement observed. *Entamoeba invadens* causes severe disease and death in captive reptiles. For example, 200 of 500 red-footed tortoises *(Geochelone carbonaria)* imported into southern Florida died over a period of 2 months, showing signs of anorexia, listlessness, and diarrhea. Necropsy examination revealed necrosis of the duodenal mucosa and multifocal hepatic necrosis. Amebas were found in both duodenal and hepatic lesions histologically (Jacobson et al, 1983).

The parasitic amebas reproduce asexually, usually by binary fission. Actively parasitic forms, called **trophozoites**, display ameboid motion when recovered from fresh feces and kept at body temperature. Most species form cysts, which in certain cases are multinuclear. Trophozoites are more likely to be found in fluid feces and cysts in formed feces.

Treatment of *Entamoeba histolytica* Infections

Little is known about the treatment of canine amebiasis. In humans, metronidazole is the drug of choice in the treatment of intestinal and hepatic amebiasis and is therefore a logical choice for treating canine amebiasis. Roberson (1977) suggests oral administration of 50 mg of metronidazole per kilogram body weight daily for 5 days.

Facultative Amebiasis

Facultative amebas are free-living most of the time, but can cause serious disease if they enter human hosts. These pathogens are best known for causing disease in humans (e.g., fulminate primary amebic meningoencephalitis [*Naegleria fowleri*, mainly], chronic amebic encephalitis [*Acanthamoeba culbertsoni* and other spp.], and acanthamoeba keratitis) (Barnett et al, 1996; Schaumberg et al, 1996; Sell et al, 1997). However, cases of amebic encephalitis

have been reported from other animals, including dogs, gibbons, sheep, cattle, beavers, and tapirs (Lozano Alarcon et al, 1997). More recently a new ameba, *Balamuthia mandrillis,* was found to cause disease in a mandrill from the San Diego Zoo (Visvesvara et al, 1993). This parasite has also killed gorillas, an orangutan, and a horse (Canfield et al, 1997; Kinde et al, 1998; Rideout et al, 1997). Human cases have also been reported (Deol et al, 2000).

■ SUBPHYLUM CILIOPHORA (CILIATES)
Balantidium coli

Balantidium coli, a normal element of the intestinal fauna of the pig and rat, is very large as single cells go, measuring up to 150 µm in length (Figure 2-7). The cell surface is covered with **cilia** (singular, **cilium**) arranged in rows with a tuft of longer ones surrounding the peristome, or "cell mouth." Prominent organelles include a large macronucleus, a smaller micronucleus, two contractile vacuoles, and a number of food vacuoles in the cytoplasm. *B. coli* reproduces by transverse fission and forms cysts up to 60 µm in diameter.

Although harmless to the pig and usually harmless to humans, *B. coli* occasionally causes ulceration of the human large intestine, manifested clinically as diarrhea and occasionally as **dysentery** (diarrhea with abdominal pain, straining, and blood and mucus in the stools). Diagnosis of *B. coli* infection is based on the demonstration of motile trophozoites in direct smears of diarrheal feces or cysts in flotation preparations of formed feces. Acute enteritis characterized by watery diarrhea and lethargy involving four gorillas in the Los Angeles Zoo was attributed to *B. coli* infection (Teare and Loomis, 1982). Lowland gorillas affected with balantidiasis did not accept metronidazole well and were treated with intramuscular injections of dehydroemetine dihydrochloride (Gual-Sill and Pulido-Reyes, 1994).

Symbiotic Ciliates

The forestomachs of ruminants and the cecums and colons of horses abound with large, somewhat bizarre ciliates that are neither pathogenic nor indispensable to their hosts (Figure 2-8). Sometimes they are found in the lungs of ruminants at necropsy, the result of agonal inspiration of ruminal contents and nothing more.

■ SUBPHYLUM APICOMPLEXA

The Apicomplexa (Sporozoa) of interest to us are all obligate intracellular parasites that cause disease

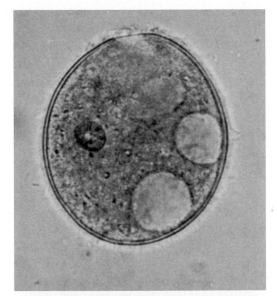

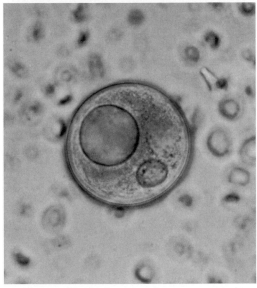

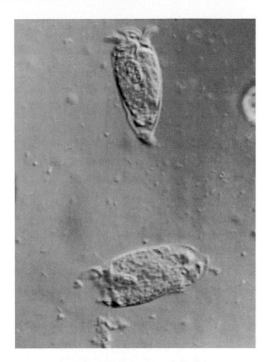

FIGURE 2-8 Ciliates of the large intestine of the horse (×425).

FIGURE 2-7 *Balantidium coli.* **A,** Trophozoite (electronic flash photomicrograph) of motile ciliate (×700). **B,** Cyst (×425). Trophozoites abound in the large intestine of normal swine, and cysts are passed in their feces. *Balantidium coli* has been incriminated in human colonic disease ranging from mild colitis to an ailment resembling amebic dysentery.

by destroying those cells. The most important members are the **coccidians,** many of which develop in epithelial cells of the alimentary canal and cause a form of enteritis called **coccidiosis,** and the **hemosporidians,** which develop in erythrocytes and cause hemolytic anemia. Coccidians are transmitted mainly by fecal contamination and reproduce by rigid sequences of asexual and sexual phases of multiplication and development that, in an important minority of cases, require an alternation of hosts. Hemosporidians are transmitted by bloodsucking

arthropods and include the **piroplasms,** which are transmitted by ixodid ticks, and the **plasmodia,** which are transmitted by dipterans, in which they complete the sexual phases of their life histories.

Coccidians

The functional unit of coccidian ontogeny is the **zoite,** a motile, banana- or cigar-shaped cell, rounded at one end and pointed at the other (apical) end (Figure 2-9). It is the zoite that migrates in the host and invades cells, and it is the zoite that represents the beginning and end point of every coccidian life process. Relationship to a particular portion of the life history is denoted by a prefix. Thus, **sporozoites** are infective forms found in sporulated **oocysts** (pronounced "oh'oh-sists"). Sporozoites invade host cells, in which they form many **merozoites** by a kind of multiple internal fission called **schizogony** (pronounced "ski-zog o-ne"; synonym, **merogony**); **tachyzoites** divide rapidly, **bradyzoites** divide slowly, and soon. The genera *Eimeria, Isospora, Hammondia, Sarcocystis,* and *Toxoplasma* present an orderly sequence of increasing biological complexity and therefore are taken up in that order.

Eimeria

The general form of coccidian life history is represented by the genus *Eimeria,* species of which

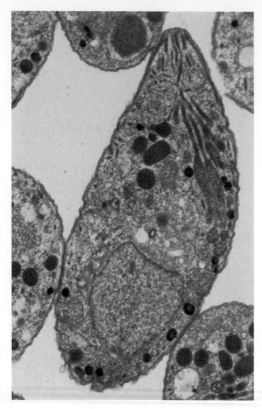

FIGURE 2-9   Tachyzoite of *Toxoplasma gondii* from a mouse (×22,500).
(TEM courtesy Dr. John F. Cummings.)

are gastrointestinal parasites of a wide range of vertebrate hosts. This life history includes both asexual multiplication and sexual multiplication. Sexual multiplication culminates in the formation of oocysts, which are discharged with the feces, and in the development, within each of these oocysts, of eight infective organisms, sporozoites. The life history of *Eimeria* should be learned by heart because it serves as a basis for all of the other coccidians. The illustrated diagram of Figure 2-10 may prove helpful in mastering the following details.

Schizogony (Merogony)

If the infective, sporulated oocyst is ingested by a suitable host, the sporozoites emerge, and each may enter an epithelial or lamina propria cell, round up as a **trophozoite**, grow larger, and become a first-generation **schizont** (pronounced "skiz ont," [**meront**]). The trophozoite, schizont, and all other intracellular stages of *Eimeria* are surrounded by a membrane-lined **parasitophorous vacuole** in the host cell cytoplasm or, in some cases, nucleoplasm. This schizont produces **first-generation merozoites** that burst the cell and invade fresh cells to become **second-generation schizonts.** There may be several

more schizogonic generations, but two or three are the limit for many of the important species of *Eimeria*. The number of asexual generations, the type and location of the host cells parasitized, and the number of merozoites formed at each generation depend on the species of coccidium in question. The salient attributes of schizogony are (1) an exponential increase in the number of zoites arising from a single sporozoite, (2) destruction of host cells in proportion to the degree of infection, and (3) automatic suspension of the asexual process after a fixed number of repetitions.

Gametogony

A merozoite produced by the final schizogony (i.e., a **telomerozoite**) enters a fresh host cell and develops into either a male or female gametocyte or developing sex cell. The female gametocyte (**macrogametocyte** or **macrogamont**) enlarges, stores food materials, and induces hypertrophy of both cytoplasm and nucleus of its host cell. When mature, it is called a **macrogamete** or female sex cell. The male gametocyte (**microgametocyte** or **microgamont**) undergoes repeated nuclear division and becomes multinucleate. Each nucleus is finally incorporated into a biflagellate **microgamete** or male sex cell. Of the many microgametes formed by the microgametocyte, only a small fraction finds and fertilizes macrogametes to form **zygotes.** A wall forms around the zygote by the coalescence of hyaline granules at its periphery to form an **oocyst**. The oocyst is released by rupture of the host cell and passes out with the feces to undergo **sporulation**. Within a day or two, if provided with adequate moisture, moderate temperatures, and sufficient oxygen, the single cell (**sporont**) in the oocyst divides into four **sporoblasts.** Each sporoblast develops into a **sporocyst,** which contains two haploid **sporozoites,** thus becoming an infective, **sporulated oocyst** and completing the cycle (Figure 2-11). The life history of *Eimeria* is presented again in schematic form in Figure 2-12.

Isospora

The genus *Isospora* (I-sos por-rah) once included species now assigned to the genera *Hammondia, Toxoplasma, Besnoitia,* and *Sarcocystis* because the sporulated oocysts of all of these genera contain two sporocysts, each of which contains four sporozoites (Figure 2-13). The life history of *Isospora felis* resembles that of *Eimeria* except that its sporozoites may encyst (singly) in the tissues of a mouse. As Figure 2-14 indicates, a cat may become infected with *I. felis* by ingesting either sporulated oocysts or sporozoite-infected mice. The mouse thus serves as a facultative paratenic host for *I. felis*.

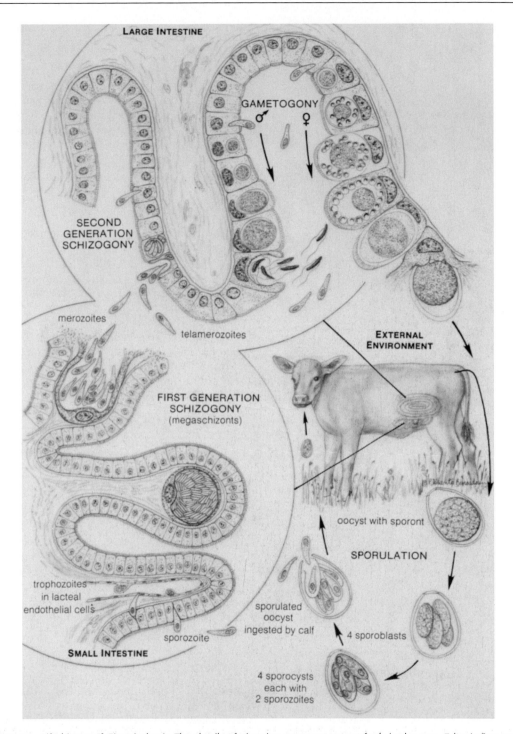

FIGURE 2-10 Life history of *Eimeria bovis*. The details of eimerian ontogeny are set forth in the text. *E bovis* first-generation schizonts are megaschizonts and develop in central lacteal cells of the small intestine. Second-generation schizogony and gametogony occur in epithelial cells of the large intestine. Clinical signs are associated with the large intestinal phase of infection.

Enteric Coccidiosis

A particular species of *Eimeria* or *Isospora* tends to be restricted to a narrow range of hosts, but each host species may be parasitized by a number of different species of coccidians simultaneously. Antemortem diagnosis of coccidian infection (i.e., **coccidiosis**) is based on identification of oocysts in the host's feces. Host specificity and the form of

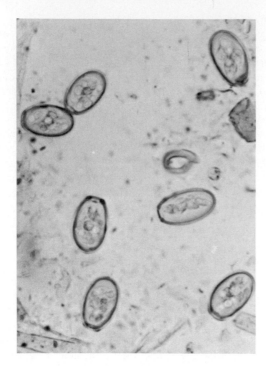

FIGURE 2-11 *Eimeria magna* oocysts, sporulated, from the feces of a domestic rabbit (×425).

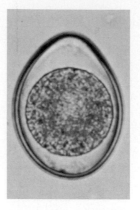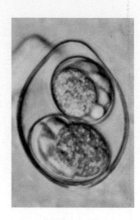

FIGURE 2-13 *Isospora felis* unsporulated oocyst *(left)* and sporulated oocyst *(right)* (×1074).

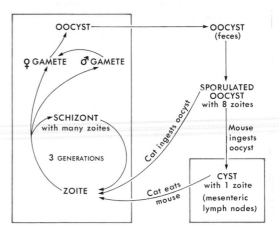

FIGURE 2-14 Life history of *Isospora felis*.

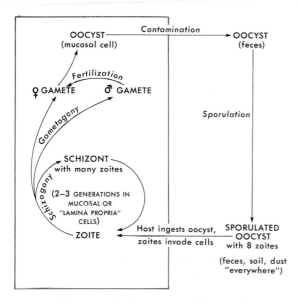

FIGURE 2-12 Life history of a typical *Eimeria* sp.

the oocyst usually suffice for identification to the species level, but micrometry and sporulation of the oocysts must occasionally be resorted to in order to distinguish between certain species (see Chapter 5). Postmortem diagnosis is based on gross and microscopic lesions, which vary considerably with the host and parasite species involved, and on

the demonstration of the sexual or asexual stages of the parasites. Schizonts, gamonts, oocysts, and intermediate stages lie surrounded by their parasitophorous vacuoles in the cytoplasm (or nucleus, in a few cases) of enterocytes, lamina propria cells, or endothelial cells of the central lacteal of the villus. Although these are most elegantly displayed by histological techniques, direct smears or squash preparations are just as dependable as hematoxylin and eosin (H&E) slides and are quicker and less expensive. Oocysts and merozoites can often be demonstrated in smears or concentrates of the intestinal contents. Contrast microscopy or staining with Wright's or Giemsa stain is helpful in demonstrating sporozoites.

It is important to understand that the mere identification of coccidian oocysts in the feces of a host does not justify a diagnosis of the disease coccidiosis unless the history and clinical signs are in accord. Large numbers of oocysts may be counted in the feces of perfectly healthy hosts, and surveys reveal prevalence rates on the order of 30% to 50% in a wide range of host species. On the other hand, severe and even fatal coccidiosis sometimes occurs during the early asexual stages of infection before oocysts have had time to develop. In such cases, disease is manifest, but oocysts have not yet appeared in the feces. Chronic diarrhea is the cardinal sign of coccidiosis and results from the destruction of intestinal epithelium by hordes of multiplying organisms. Diarrhea has many causes, only one of which is coccidian infection, so the diagnosis of coccidiosis is always uncertain in individual cases. In other words, diarrhea plus oocyst shedding does not infallibly equal coccidiosis. However, as regularly recurring episodes of illness characterized by diarrhea in successive populations of young puppies, kittens, calves, lambs, kids, piglets, chicks, ducklings, poults, or other domestic or wild animals, outbreaks of coccidiosis become predictable events and leave the diagnostician in little doubt as to the etiology. Given a closed breeding colony with reasonably steady environmental conditions, clinical coccidiosis will regularly appear in each new wave of young mammals or birds unless effective prophylactic measures have been exercised.

It is often repeated that coccidian infection is "self-limiting," implying that the population of infecting organisms grows to a maximum and then more or less abruptly fades away to extinction or to a low level as the host develops immunity. Small numbers of oocysts may be shed in the feces for several weeks or even months, but infection remains otherwise inapparent. Should the now relatively immune host be exposed to a different species of coccidian, the same pattern will be repeated. Thus immunity to coccidian infection tends to be highly specific and reasonably protective but incomplete. Some animals shed oocysts while remaining healthy for months or years. Such animals have sufficient protective immunity to limit but not exclude infection in the presence of continued exposure.

The disease *coccidiosis* results from either overwhelming infection or the interaction of moderate levels of infection and stress. The level of environmental contamination with oocysts is best affected by removing all manure and getting all surfaces as clean as it is feasible to do. There is no reliable and practical disinfectant. Drying and direct sunlight are most effective in destroying oocysts when these agents happen to be available. Administration of anticoccidian drugs (coccidiostats) during exposure of young susceptible animals permits infection to occur and immunity to develop but limits infection sufficiently to abort disease. Such drugs are virtually indispensable to intensive systems of poultry, goat, cattle, sheep, dog, and cat production.

Dogs and Cats

True infection of dogs and cats with species of *Isospora* must be distinguished from pseudoparasitism arising from the various gustatory habits of these hosts. A dog with a history of recurrent diarrhea and oocyst shedding seems like an "open and shut case" until the oocysts turn out to belong to a parasite of the squirrel *Sciurus carolinensis*. It would then seem that dietary indiscretion and not protozoan infection is probably to blame for the diarrhea. In fact, almost all puppies and kittens experience infection with *Isospora* at some time during the early months of their lives. More than once I have observed *Isospora* oocysts in the feces of puppies and kittens raised in elaborately controlled gnotobiotic colonies, and infection always occurs in well-managed colonies in which less stringent levels of sanitation are practiced.

Isospora canis, Isospra ohioensis, and *Isospra burrowsi* in dogs and *I. felis* and *Isospora rivolta* in cats are the species most commonly involved in coccidian infection and disease in these hosts. Clinical signs may precede oocyst shedding in particularly acute infections. Diarrhea is copious and watery, and may persist for several weeks. Response to treatment is seldom dramatic.

Cattle

All calves experience infection with one or more species of *Eimeria* during their first year of life, so finding a few oocysts in the diarrheal feces of a sick calf does not itself justify a diagnosis of coccidiosis. However, authentic outbreaks of coccidiosis do occur, especially in cattle up to 2 years of age, and these outbreaks are most often attributed to either *Eimeria zuernii* or *Eimeria bovis*. Both of these species undergo two asexual cycles; the first culminates in the formation of schizonts in the lamina propria cells *(E. zuernii)* or endothelial cells of the lacteals *(E. bovis)* of the villi of the lower ileum. The megaschizonts of *E. bovis* are macroscopically visible (about 250 µm) and contain more than 100,000 merozoites. The schizonts of *E. zuernii* are unobtrusive because of their small size and deeper location. The second-generation schizonts are microscopic and occur in the epithelial cells of the cecum and colon, which is also the site of gametogony. The onset of clinical signs coincides with the beginning of gametogony and results from the mechanical disruption of mucosal cells by the sexual stages. In severe cases, so few epithelial cells remain that serum and blood are lost from the capillaries of the denuded lamina propria. The prepatent period for *E. bovis* is 16 to 21 days; the prepatent period for *E. zuernii* is 12 to 14 days.

Winter coccidiosis in calves characterized by bloody diarrhea and tenesmus is a distinctive clinical entity. Severe cold weather and other stresses may precipitate clinical disease at infection levels that might otherwise not produce symptoms.

Nervous coccidiosis may affect as many as one third of the cattle in some herd outbreaks of coccidiosis, especially in beef cattle in the northwestern United States and western Canada. In addition to acute diarrhea, affected animals display muscular tremors, convulsions, opisthotonus, nystagmus, blindness, and a mortality rate of about 50%. The pathogenesis of nervous coccidiosis is unknown, but more than 90% of the cases occur during the coldest months of the year, from January to March. Canadian workers have reported the presence of a heat-labile toxin in the serum of calves with nervous coccidiosis that can transfer neurologic signs to inoculated mice (Isler et al, 1987). *Eimeria alabamensis* and *Eimeria auburnensis* are occasionally incriminated in outbreaks of clinical coccidiosis (Radostits and Stockdale, 1980).

Sheep and Goats

At one time, sheep and goats were thought to share the same species of *Eimeria*; however, gradually two complete sets of species names are emerging to reflect the predominant opinion that sheep and goats harbor similar but distinct sets of coccidian species. Specific diagnosis is based on morphological identification of oocysts in sugar flotation concentrates of feces. Micrometry and sporulation of oocysts in 1% of potassium dichromate solution may be resorted to if necessary for differentiating similar species.

In sheep, clinical coccidiosis is especially likely to occur after shipping and is probably precipitated by the associated stress. In lambs experimentally infected with *Eimeria ovinoidalis*, oocysts appear in the feces about 14 days after infection, and if the infections are severe, deaths will occur beginning about 3 weeks after infection. Goats appear to be much more susceptible, and coccidiosis is a serious problem in raising kids in many goat herds. Clinical signs typically follow weaning by 2 to 3 weeks, but coccidiosis should be suspected whenever diarrhea is observed in kids older than 2 weeks. Weaker, heavily infected kids are likely to die; the stronger and less heavily infected survive but fail to grow normally. Pasty to watery diarrhea and dehydration are typical. Bloody stools and tenesmus, frequently observed in calves with coccidiosis, are not typical of the disease in sheep and goats. Diarrhea may precede oocyst shedding by several days. In such cases of suspected prepatent coccidiosis, examine direct fecal smears for merozoites. Necropsy examination reveals many 3- to 6-mm irregular, whitish, raised lesions. Smears or squash preparations made from these lesions reveal *Eimeria* in various stages of development.

Horses

Eimeria leuckarti is the only species of enteric coccidian reported from North American horses. A survey of naturally acquired *E. leuckarti* infection conducted on 13 Kentucky breeding farms revealed *E. leuckarti* in 67 (41%) of the foals on 11 of those farms. Oocysts, demonstrated by flotation in concentrated sucrose (S.G. 1.275), were first shed in the feces when the foals were 15 to 123 days old and continued to be shed sporadically for as long as 4 months (Lyons et al, 1988).

Oral administration of 50 thousand to 2 million oocysts to yearling ponies led to patent infections in 33 to 37 days, and oocyst shedding continued for as long as 12 days. Schizonts were not observed; gametocytes developed in lamina propria cells of the villi in the small intestine. No clinical signs of disease were observed in these artificially infected ponies (Barker and Remmler, 1972). *E. leuckarti* infection thus appears to be prevalent, at least in foals in Kentucky, but relatively harmless.

Swine

Pigs are host to eight species of *Eimeria* and one of *Isospora,* of which only the latter appears to be of significant clinical importance (Vetterling, 1965). *Isospora suis* causes neonatal coccidiosis in 1- to 2-week-old pigs. Clinical signs include diarrhea, dehydration, and weight loss; morbidity tends to be high and mortality low or moderate. Susceptibility to infection falls rapidly with age. Although 400,000 oocysts of *I. suis* may kill a 1-day-old pig, only mild and transient diarrhea ensues if infection is postponed until the pig reaches 2 weeks of age. The prepatent period is 5 days, and oocyst shedding lasts 1 to 3 weeks. Pigs surviving infection with *I. suis* are solidly immune to reinfection with this species. Porcine neonatal coccidiosis is to be differentiated from enteritides associated with *Strongyloides ransomi,* toxigenic *Escherichia coli,* transmissible gastroenteritis virus, rotavirus, and *Clostridium perfringens* type C. *I. suis* infection is rarely observed in adult swine, and the epidemiology of porcine neonatal coccidiosis remains problematical (Stuart et al, 1980; Lindsay et al, 1992).

Birds

The subject of coccidiosis in domestic poultry forms too large and complex a body of information to be accommodated on these pages. The reader is referred to standard texts on avian diseases.

Treatment and Control

Treatment of isolated cases of fully developed coccidiosis is a matter of supportive therapy because by the time oocysts are detected in the feces, no available drug will have much effect on the population of coccidians infecting that particular host. Controlling coccidiosis in populations of susceptible animals is a challenging proposition, and heavy reliance is placed on chemicals administered prophylactically. The objective of anticoccidian prophylaxis is to afford sufficient protection to the exposed animal to allow it to develop immunity without getting sick in the process. The chemicals reduce the magnitude of challenge and thereby prevent coccidiosis; they do not prevent the infection. However, do not expect the chemical to perform miracles. Too much contamination of the environment with oocysts and, even more important, too much stress placed on the hosts are conditions that cannot be overcome by the best of chemicals.

Dogs and Cats

Coccidiosis outbreaks in dogs and cats involving *Isospora* spp. can be controlled with sulfonamide drugs. Sulfadimethoxine is administered to dogs for the treatment of coccidian enteritis according to the following schedule: 55 mg/kg for the first day and 27.5 mg/kg for the next 4 days or until the dog is symptom free for at least 2 days.

Ruminants

Whatever chemical agent is chosen, efficient control of coccidiosis requires that exposure of ruminants to oocysts and stressful conditions be minimized. Adequate stall space, clean mangers, plenty of clean air, and dry footing are as essential as they are rare. Never mix calves, sheep, or goats of different ages or sizes in the same pen. As a matter of regular routine, all animals should be observed attentively for several minutes a day at a time that neither the stockman nor his stock has other urgent business. If any sick animals are observed, they should be removed to a separate pen for supportive treatment. This measure is doubly beneficial; it reduces exposure of the sick to unnecessary stress and of the healthy to extra oocysts. As soon as coccidiosis has been diagnosed in one or a few of the animals, all of the other young ruminants on the premises should be treated prophylactically with an anticoccidian agent. Coccidian infection (coccidiasis) is inevitable. Coccidian disease (coccidiosis) can be prevented or at least ameliorated by sound husbandry and appropriate medication.

Cattle

Clinical coccidiosis in calves caused by *E. bovis* and *E. zuernii* may be treated with amprolium (thiamin antagonist), monensin (an ionophore), or sulfa drugs (e.g., sulfamethazine, sulfadimethoxine, and sulfquinoxaline). Actually, once oocysts have appeared in the feces, it is too late in the course of infection for specific chemotherapy to benefit the animal appreciably. Chemotherapy is certainly outweighed in importance by supportive therapy, especially that directed toward maintenance of fluid balance. Amprolium may be administered for 5 days in the drinking water at a concentration intended to deliver a dose of 10 mg/kg body weight per day. Usually, it is better to administer medication individually to clinically ill animals because the sickest and neediest animals are the least likely to receive their share with mass treatment methods. Sulfamethazine is administered orally at a dosage rate of 140 mg/kg body weight daily for 3 days (Radostits and Stockdale, 1980).

For prophylaxis, amprolium is administered to calves in the feed or drinking water for 21 days during natural exposure to oocysts at a concentration intended to deliver 5 mg/kg per day. Decoquinate is recommended as an aid in the prevention of coccidiosis caused by *E. bovis* and *E. zuernii* in ruminating calves and older cattle. Decoquinate is fed at a dosage level of 0.5 mg/kg for at least 28 days during periods when there is risk of exposure to oocysts; it is ineffective in the treatment of already established infections. Lasalocid is sold as a feed additive and administered at 1 mg/kg daily. Horses must not be allowed to ingest feed that contains lasalocid. Monensin is sold as a feed additive for improved feed efficiency and the control of coccidiosis and is fed at the rate of 100 to 360 mg per head per day. Horses must never be allowed access to feed containing monensin because the toxic dose for this species is only about one tenth of that for cattle (Langston et al, 1985). There are also several sulfa-based products available for coccidiosis control.

Sheep

Decoquinate, lasalocid, and sulfaquinoxaline are approved for coccidiosis control in sheep. Sulfaquinoxaline is to be administered in the water for 3 to 5 days. Decoquinate is administered as for cattle at 0.5 mg/kg for at least 28 days. Lasalocid is administered to sheep in feed so that they get between 15 and 70 mg per head per day. Again, do not let horses get at feed containing lasalocid.

Goats

Decoquinate and monensin are approved for preventing coccidiosis in nonlactating goats. For prophylaxis, herd conditions may require that kids be medicated continuously from 2 weeks until they are several months of age. Decoquinate may be mixed with the feed to supply 0.5 mg/kg per day or mixed with salt (4 lb of 6% decoquinate premix with 100 lb of salt). Monensin is fed at the rate of 20 g of monensin sodium per ton on a 90% dry matter basis. This is offered as the sole ration. Do not let horses get into feed containing monensin. Amprolium is not approved for goat kids in the United States. Experimentally, amprolium may be administered to goat kids with coccidiosis at a considerably higher dose rate than is recommended for calves (25 to 50 mg/kg of body weight). Overdose with amprolium may lead to fatal polioencephalomalacia from thiamin deficiency. Sulfa drugs may be used for treating coccidiosis only in sufficiently hydrated kids because sulfa drugs damage the kidneys if insufficient water is available to keep them in solution.

Older goats, while remaining free of clinical signs, may shed oocysts for extended periods and serve as the ultimate source of infection for kids. In problem herds, it may prove necessary to isolate kids at birth from their dams, feed them artificially, and include a coccidiostat in the starter ration for several months. In more favorable situations, it may suffice to provide a clean, disinfected stall and wash the does' udders carefully before kids are allowed to nurse. Stress or exposure to a previously unencountered species of *Eimeria* may lead to temporary bouts of diarrhea in adult goats. Much of the information and perspectives on goat coccidiosis presented here are those of Smith and Sherman, 1994.

Horses
E. leuckarti appears to be nonpathogenic, which is fine because no treatment is available for this infection.

Swine
Medication of piglets suffering from neonatal coccidiosis appears to be futile. Rigorous sanitation probably represents the most effective investment. "The following sanitation program has been recommended: steam clean farrowing crates; wet down the crates with an ammonia- orphenol-containing disinfectant and let them stand overnight; and steam clean the following day" (Stuart and Lindsay, 1986).

Cryptosporidium

Cryptosporidium spp. are tiny (oocytes are 4 to 8 μm in diameter, depending on species and stage) coccidians that undergo schizogony, gametogony, and sporogony in parasitophorous vacuoles usually in the microvillous borders of enteric epithelial cells but also in the gallbladder and the respiratory and renal epithelium, especially in immune-compromised hosts. A wide range of vertebrates serves as hosts, and cross-infection among host species occurs. Currently, the species *Cryptosporidium parvum* is undergoing a division by molecular taxonomists. Recognized species of *C. parvum*–like parasites in mammals now include *C. parvum*, *Cryptosporidium wrairi* (guinea pigs), *Cryptosporidium felis*, *Cryptosporidium canis*, and probably soon to be described new species from pigs and marsupials. Most humans are infected with a type of *C. parvum* that is called *Genotype 1 (C. hominus),* whereas cattle are usually infected with *Genotype 2* (Sulaiman et al, 1998; Widmer et al, 2000). People can be infected with Genotype 2 (as veterinarians well know from the reports of veterinary students who have been infected [Anderson et al, 1982]), but Genotype 1 does not infect cattle or other animals. Typically, however, it seems that with *Cryptosporidium*, as with *Giardia*, most people get their infections from people most of the time; occasionally, people get infected with the animal form of the disease, usually in rural settings (Ong et al, 1999). The large species in cattle that had been called *Cryptosporidium muris* is now recognized as a distinct species, *Cryptosporidium andersoni* (Lindsay et al, 2000). *C. parvum* occurs usually in calves younger than 3 weeks, and *C. andersoni* typically in older calves. In immune-deficient individuals, such as AIDS patients, *C. parvum* is autoinfective and capable of generating life-threatening infections (Current, 1985).

Life History
Infective oocysts containing four sporozoites are discharged in the feces and serve to disseminate the infection (Figure 2-15). The oocysts remain viable for months unless exposed to extremes of temperature (below 0° C, above 65° C), desiccation, or impracticably concentrated disinfectants (5% ammonia, 10% formalin). When ingested by a suitable host, the oocyst opens along a preexisting suture line to release the four sporozoites that invade the microvillous border of the gastric glands (*C. muris*, Tyzzer, 1907, 1910) or lower half of the small intestine (*C. parvum*, Tyzzer, 1912). In parasitophorous vacuoles in the microvillous border, the cryptosporidians undergo schizogony, gametogony, fertilization, and sporogony. Some oocysts go through excystation internally, providing the mechanism for autoinfection that accounts for the chronicity of certain cases in immune-sufficient hosts and lethal hyperinfection in immune-deficient hosts.

Clinical Signs
Inapparent infection is common in many mammalian, avian, reptilian, and piscine hosts. For example, *Cryptosporidium* was found in the microvillous borders of enterocytes of 5% (184 of 3491) of 1- to 30-week-old pigs submitted for diagnostic necropsy, but according to Sanford, "Only 26 per cent of the cryptosporidia-infected

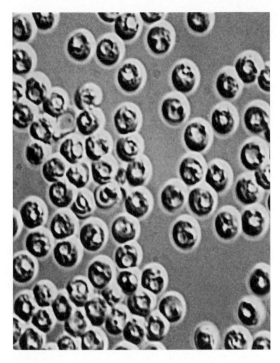

FIGURE 2-15 Purified oocysts of *Cryptosporidium parvum* in water (×1400).

pigs had diarrhea and most of those had other primary diarrheagenic agents or lesions capable of causing their diarrhea" (Sanford, 1987). On the other hand, debilitating diarrhea may be associated with infection, (e.g., in calves within the first 3 weeks of life). Although *C. parvum* is usually the culprit in clinical cryptosporidiosis in mammals, *C. andersoni* may cause mild diarrhea in cattle of all ages, especially young adults. Immunocompromised hosts may develop a life-threatening hyperinfective form of cryptosporidiosis, as is the case with many human AIDS patients (Ma and Soave, 1983). Severe cryptosporidiosis has been reported to be associated with immunocompromise induced by feline leukemia virus (FeLV) in a cat (Monticello et al, 1987) and in Arabian foals with inherited combined immunodeficiency. In the latter case, however, it was not possible to separate the effects of *Cryptosporidium* and concurrent adenoviral infection (Snyder et al, 1987).

Diagnosis

Cryptosporidium oocysts are difficult to see on fecal slides because they are colorless, transparent, and small; *C. parvum* is 5.0 by 4.5 μm and *C.*

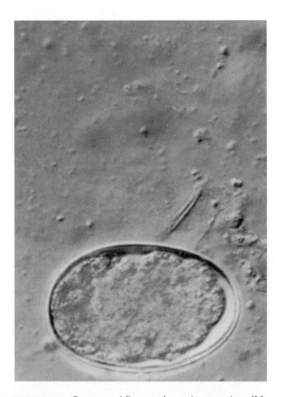

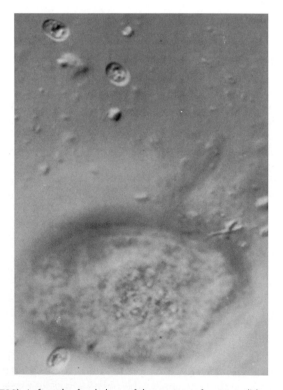

FIGURE 2-16 *Cryptosporidium andersoni* oocysts in calf feces (×780). *Left*, at the focal plane of the contour of a strongylid egg, no *Cryptosporidium* oocysts are visible. *Right*, At the focal plane of the uppermost surface of the strongylid egg (i.e., immediately under the coverslip), three *Cryptosporidium andersoni* oocysts are now visible. All competent microscopists constantly adjust the fine focus as they view and scan. Sorry, but *Cryptosporidium parvum* is even smaller.

andersoni is 7.4 by 5.6 μm (Upton and Current, 1985). Concentrated sucrose solution (specific gravity 1.33) is the flotation medium of choice for concentrating oocysts of *Cryptosporidium*. Use the coverslip variant of the flotation concentration technique, which is described in Chapter 5 in the section on "Qualitative Fecal Examination," can be used. The oocysts appear as tiny subspherical objects that may be dented by osmotic extraction of water by the hypertonic medium. They tend to lie immediately below the coverslip, so focus on the top of an air bubble to find the best focal plane for *Cryptosporidium* oocysts (Figure 2-16). The oocyst walls may have a pinkish hue that helps in finding them; the pinkish hue is due to chromatic aberration and is best developed by objective lenses of modest quality. The cyst walls are clear and colorless under a highly corrected objective lens. Questionable objects may be examined under the highest magnification to demonstrate the sporozoites. Phase contrast microscopy is helpful, and a number of staining procedures (e.g., methylene blue, Giemsa stain, iodine wet mount, modified Kinyoun acid-fast smear) have been recommended to increase the optical contrast and stain-confusing yeasts differentially. However, the most serious obstacle to the correct microscopic diagnosis of cryptosporidiosis is inexperience and insecurity on the part of the microscopist. The best procedure is to keep examining feces from 1- to 3-week-old calves with the 40× objective and suitably stopped brightfield illumination until you see *Cryptosporidium* oocysts. If in doubt, check for sporozoites under higher power. Once you have seen the oocysts, you will have acquired the most essential ingredient of accurate diagnosis. Exacting microscopic technique pays dividends, especially as one nears the resolution limits of the light microscope. Köhler illumination, described in all microscope manuals, is indispensable. Several assays designed for in-office use are approved for the detection of the *C. parvum* antigen in human feces, and the test, although expensive, appears to work well on bovine samples.

Treatment

There is no effective specific treatment for *Cryptosporidium* infection.

Toxoplasma

Life History

Toxoplasma gondii is an enteric coccidian of the domestic cat *(Felis catus)* and other members of the family Felidae. Cats are the only known definitive hosts, and therefore only infected cats shed oocysts of this parasite in their feces. The oocyst is small (11 to 13 μm; Figure 2-17), contains a single

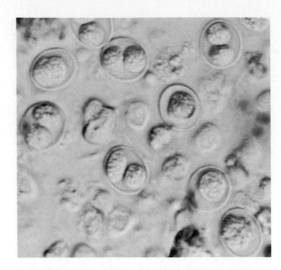

FIGURE 2-17 *Toxoplasma gondii* oocysts in cat feces (×1030). Sporulation has already begun, and half of the cysts are already in the two-sporoblast stage.

sporont, and is noninfective when passed in the feces. Sporulation is completed in 1 to 5 days and results in formation of two sporocysts, each of which contains four sporozoites. Fully sporulated oocysts are infective on ingestion to essentially all warm-blooded animals including cats (Figure 2-18). Therefore, almost any warm-blooded animal may serve as a paratenic host of *T. gondii* (Dubey, 1986a, 1986b). A **paratenic host** is a host in which a parasite may grow or multiply, but the growth or development is not required by the parasite to complete its life cycle.

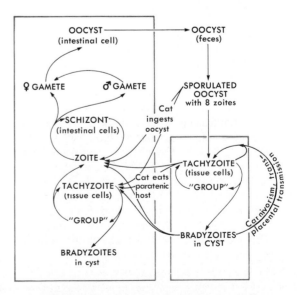

FIGURE 2-18 Life history of *Toxoplasma gondii.*

On ingestion, sporulated oocysts rupture in the intestine and release the sporozoites. These enter and multiply in cells of the intestine and associated lymph nodes to form rapidly multiplying stages, **tachyzoites,** which spread to all other tissues of the body; there they invade cells and continue to multiply. Eventually, tissue cysts containing slowly dividing forms, **bradyzoites,** are formed in the brain, striated muscles, and liver and remain viable for the life of the host. Bradyzoites are infective on ingestion to essentially all warm-blooded animals and behave in the manner similar to that just described for sporozoites. Thus, paratenic hosts become infected with *T. gondii* by ingesting sporulated oocysts from cat feces or bradyzoites in the tissues of other paratenic hosts. Transplacental transmission of tachyzoites from dam to fetus in utero also occurs but varies in importance from species to species of host (Dubey, 1986a, 1986b).

When a member of the cat family ingests tissue cysts of *T. gondii* (Figure 2-19), the bradyzoites penetrate the epithelial cells of the small intestine, undergo a series of asexual cycles, and finally undergo the sexual cycle, which culminates in the shedding of oocysts. Cats shed *Toxoplasma* oocysts in their feces 3 to 10 days after eating mice infected with encysted bradyzoites but not until 19 to 48 days after ingesting sporulated oocysts (Dubey and Frenkel, 1976). Apparently, the asexual reproduction preceding formation of bradyzoites in the paratenic host satisfies a major portion of the developmental requirements preceding sexual reproduction. Cats may also serve as paratenic hosts inasmuch as multiplication of tachyzoites and cyst formation occur in their extraintestinal tissues (Dubey, 1986b); cats are also capable of developing systemic disease (Meier et al, 1957).

Importance

Like other coccidians, *T. gondii* destroys cells, and the explosive multiplication of tachyzoites of this organism is potentially devastating to the intermediate host. On first exposure to *T. gondii* infection, adult humans with intact immune systems suffer a brief if unpleasant illness marked by variable combinations of fever, myalgia, lymphadenopathy, anorexia, and sore throat that is probably rarely diagnosed as to exact etiology. The situation is far more grave for hosts with deficient immune responses such as fetuses, neonates, older adults, and those with congenital or acquired immune deficiency diseases. The greatest concern attaches to exposure of human fetuses to the hazard of death, congenital malformation, or mental retardation that may result from exposure of the nonimmune mother to *T. gondii* infection during pregnancy. Although women with circulating antibody to *T. gondii* need

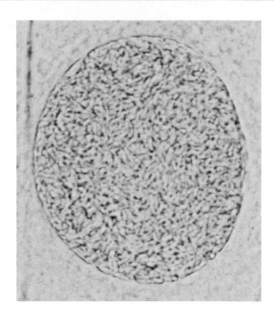

FIGURE 2-19 *Toxoplasma gondii* cyst in a mouse's brain (×4600). This is a fresh, temporary mount prepared by simply squashing the brain tissue between the coverslip and slide.

not worry about exposing their unborn babies to congenital toxoplasmosis, such women account for only about 30% of the population at risk. The other 70% must be careful to avoid cat feces and uncooked meat during pregnancy (Dubey, 1986a, 1986b).

Adult cattle appear to be resistant to toxoplasmosis, whereas sheep and goats are susceptible, usually manifesting toxoplasmosis as abortion due to focal placentitis (Dubey, 1986d, 1987). Aborting ewes and does need not be culled because they probably will not repeat the performance. *T. gondii* infection is highly prevalent in pigs, and uncooked pork may be an important source of human infection (Dubey, 1986a, 1986c).

Treatment

Humans may contract toxoplasmosis either by ingesting sporulated oocysts from the feces of an infected cat or by eating uncooked meat of animals containing *T. gondii* cysts. "Pregnant women should eat only adequately cooked meat and either leave the cleaning of cat litter pans to someone else or wear disposable gloves" (Frenkel and Dubey, 1972). They are also well advised to wash lettuce and other fresh vegetables carefully; avoid contact with newborn lambs, kids, and fetal membranes; and shun unpasteurized goat's milk.

A cat shedding oocysts of *T. gondii* should be hospitalized to prevent exposure of its owner until it stops shedding oocysts, usually in less than 2 weeks. Reinfection, if it occurs, results in low-grade shedding of oocysts of short duration. Intercurrent *Isospora* infection may also trigger a brief output of *T. gondii* oocysts. However, in general, having once passed through a patent *T. gondii* infection, the particular cat remains a relatively minor source of infection. Thus, the cat that has a history of shedding *T. gondii* oocysts and/or is serologically positive is probably a safer pet than the cat that has never been exposed to this organism (Dubey, 1986b).

According to Dr. S.C. Barr, cats clinically ill with toxoplasmosis can be treated with clindamycin hydrochloride. The drug should be given orally with food. Start at 25 mg/kg twice daily and work up to 50 mg/kg twice daily. If the cat goes off its feed, withhold the drug for 24 hours and then start the clindamycin again at the level of 25 mg/kg. Cats should be treated for a minimum of 2 weeks. Cats can also be treated with clindamycin phosphate intramuscularly at 12.5 to 25 mg/kg twice daily, pyrimethamine orally at 0.25 to 0.5 mg/kg with 30 mg/kg sulfonamide given twice daily, or trimethoprim and sulfadiazine orally at 15 mg/kg twice daily, all for 4 weeks (Lindsay et al, 1997). Pyrimethamine causes megaloblastic anemia or leukopenia, and therapy should be discontinued if there is no response in 30 days.

Neospora

Neospora caninum was originally described as a parasite of the domestic dog (Dubey et al, 1988). It was initially identified in litter mates dying of signs related to polyradiculitis (Core et al, 1983; Bjerkås

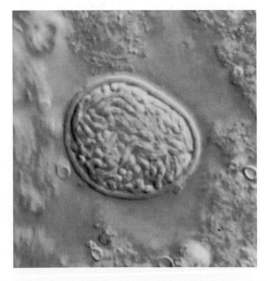

FIGURE 2-20 *Neospora caninum* cyst from dog brain homogenate (×1000).

et al, 1984). The cysts seen in neural tissues (Figure 2-20) were characterized by the possession of a cyst wall thicker than that of *T. gondii,* which is the apicomplexan it is thought to most closely resemble. In transplacentally infected puppies, the typical presentation is a flaccid hindlimb paresis. In cases where there is adult onset of the disease, presentation includes neurological signs, nodular dermatitis, pneumonia, urine and fecal incontinence, hepatitis, myocarditis, and myositis. More recently, *N. caninum* was recognized as a major cause of bovine abortion among dairy cows around the world (Anderson et al, 1991; Barr et al, 1997). Abortions due to this parasite are common, and between 10% and 20% of abortions in dairy cows probably are due to this parasite. *Neospora* abortions tend to peak at midgestation, and calves infected in utero after this time tend to survive. Abortions may occur in subsequent pregnancies, but more typically, future births produce calves that are congenitally infected. It seems that serologically positive calves will ultimately give birth to calves that are infective and seropositive. It has been suggested that seropositive cows produce less milk than seronegative cows and are more likely to be culled earlier (Thurmond and Hietala, 1996, 1997, 1999).

In 1998, the *N. caninum* of cattle was shown to use dogs as definitive hosts (McAllister et al, 1998). The oocyst shed in the feces of dogs is indistinguishable from those of *T. gondii* and *Hammondia* spp. Oocyst shedding by dogs was confirmed (Lindsay et al, 1999), but it has been hard to get dogs to produce large numbers of oocysts on a regular basis. This has made it difficult to study means of prevention or to more fully understand the importance of dogs relative to environmental contamination. Several diagnostic assays, immunologic and molecular, are now available for the detection of *N. caninum* infections. It appears that cattle do not typically serve as hosts of *T. gondii*, and there have been no cases of neosporosis reported from humans. Thus, at this time, it would appear that the ingestion of rare beef does not pose a threat of human infection with either of these parasites. Treatment of lactating dairy cows is especially problematic, and no drug therapy is currently available. Intervet offers a vaccine that aids in the prevention of infection with bovine neosporosis.

Neospora hughesi was described in 1998 from material collected from a horse (Marsh et al, 1998). The differentiation was based on molecular differences among the equine, bovine, and canine isolates. The differences between *N. hughesi* and the bovine and canine isolates were later confirmed with material collected from a horse in Oregon (Dubey et al, 2001).

Hammondia

Hammondia hammondi, a rather rare parasite of the cat, goes beyond *I. felis* by multiplying in the tissues of an intermediate host, pigs, rats, mice, goats, hamsters, and dogs. *Hammondia heydorni* is a similar parasite that uses dogs, foxes, and coyotes as the final host and cattle, sheep, goats, camels, water buffalo, guinea pigs, and dogs as intermediate hosts. The zoites first multiply rapidly (tachyzoites); they then form cysts in which they multiply slowly (bradyzoites). The net result is the multiplication and storage of zoites in cysts in the tissues of an animal that is likely to fall prey to a cat or dog final host. As indicated in Figure 2-21 for *H. hammondi,* only sporulated oocysts from cat feces are infectious for mice, and only bradyzoites from mouse tissues are infectious for cats. Thus, *H. hammondi* has an obligatory two-host life history. Tachyzoites are neither infectious to cats nor transmittable to the progeny of pregnant female mice via the placenta, as is true of *T. gondii.* The oocysts of these species are morphologically indistinguishable from those of *T. gondii, N. caninum,* or each other.

An argument has been made (Mehlhorn and Heydorn, 2000) that *H. heydorni* is the same as *N. caninum* and that *H. hammondi* is the same as *T. gondii.* These authors argue five major points:

1. *T. gondii* comprise pathogenic and nonpathogenic strains with clinical signs also being dependent on the host infected with the final host being infected with either tissue cysts or oocysts.

2. *H. hammondi* is indistinguishable from *T. gondii* and should be considered solely a less virulent strain with the belief that cats could perhaps be infected with oocysts.
3. *H. heydorni* is a parasite of the dog where the dog does not become infected by ingesting oocysts.
4. *N. caninum* should be considered a virulent form of *H. heydorni.*
5. *N. hughesi* is the same as *N. caninum.*

This work has engendered significant debate among those working on these parasites with arguments and data appearing on both sides (Frenkel and Dubey, 2000; Heydorn and Mehlhorn, 2001; Hill et al, 2001; McAllister, 2000; Mugridge et al, 1999; Riahi et al, 2000).

Sarcocystis

Species of *Sarcocystis,* like *H. hammondi,* have an obligatory two-host life history but differ in that only sexual reproduction occurs in the definitive host and that sporogony is completed there. Fully sporulated oocysts and sporocysts are discharged in the host's feces, and no development occurs in the external environment. Asexual reproduction, including schizogony and sarcocyst formation, occurs only in the intermediate host. The brady-zoites in **sarcocysts** differ from those in *Hammondia* cysts in that they develop into gametocytes instead of schizonts when ingested by the definitive host. Bradyzoites represent a state of arrested development, or **hypobiosis.** Like sporozoites in a sporulated oocyst, bradyzoites in a sarcocyst must enter a definitive host to develop further. The life history of *Sarcocystis* is portrayed diagrammatically in Figure 2-22.

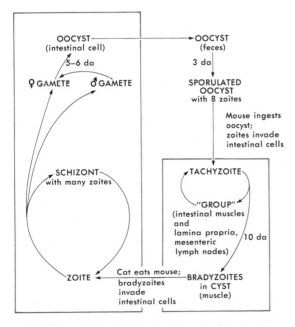

FIGURE 2-21 Life history of *Hammondia hammondi.*

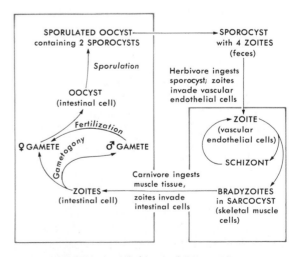

FIGURE 2-22 Life history of *Sarcocystis* sp.

TABLE 2-1 ■ **Host Relationships of Some Species of *Sarcocystis***

Intermediate Hosts	Definitive Hosts		
	Dog	Cat	Human
Cattle	S. cruzi	S. hirsuta	S. hominis
Sheep	S. tenella	S. arieticanis S. gigantea	S. medusiformis
Goat	S. capracanis	—	—
Swine	S. miescheriana	S. porcifelis?	S. suihominis
Horses	S. bertrami	S. fayeri	S. equicanis
Cottontail rabbit	S. leporum	—	—
Mouse	—	S. muris	—
Mule deer	S. hemionilatrantis	—	—

The host relationships of several species of *Sarcocystis* are summarized in Table 2-1. Normally, the carnivorous host becomes infected by eating the infected flesh of the herbivorous host, and the herbivorous host becomes infected by ingesting sporocytes from the feces of the carnivorous host. Schizogony and encystment occur exclusively in the herbivorous host, and gametogony, fertilization, and sporulation occur exclusively in the carnivorous host. *Sarcocystis* usually causes no illness in the carnivore, but schizogony in the endothelium of the herbivore may result in serious or fatal disease.

Cattle become infected with *Sarcocystis cruzi* when they ingest its sporocysts discharged in dog feces. Two schizogonic generations occur in the vascular endothelium, the first generation principally in the endothelium of the mesenteric arteries and the second in the endothelium of capillaries throughout the body. At least one more schizogonic generation occurs in circulating mononuclear cells. Merozoites released from second- or later-generation schizonts enter striated muscle cells and, in certain cases, nerve cells to form sarcocysts. Sarcocyst formation is a slow process requiring several months. The dog becomes infected when it consumes uncooked beef containing sarcocysts of *S. cruzi*. Thus the cycle of infection can be interrupted either by cooking beef scraps to be fed to dogs or by preventing canine fecal contamination of cattle feedstuffs. The economic importance of subclinical bovine sarcocystosis remains to be assessed, but clinical disease and death losses have occurred in cases in which 10,000 or more sporocytes were ingested over a short time interval (Frelier et al, 1977, Dubey and Fayer, 1983). Clinical signs in cattle are associated with release of the second wave of merozoites about 4 to 6 weeks after infection

and consist of protracted fever, anemia, lymphadenopathy, anorexia, diarrhea, hypersalivation, weakness, and hair loss about the eyes, neck, and perhaps most noticeably, the tail switch.

Infection of sheep with 10 thousand to 50 million *Sarcocystis tenella* sporocytes was studied experimentally. A total of 25 to 50 million sporocysts led to death in 16 to 19 days from occlusion of the mesenteric arteries by first-generation schizonts. Sheep infected with 10 million and fewer sporocysts had anemia, hepatitis, and myocarditis related to the second schizogonic generation. Neurological signs and lesions of encephalomyelitis were also observed in these artificial *S. tenella* infections in sheep (Dubey, 1988).

Equine Protozoal Myeloencephalitis Organism

This organism causes severe neurological disease in horses of both sexes and all ages. Clinical signs include stumbling, paresis, lameness, ataxia, recumbency, constipation, urinary incontinence, diaphoresis, muscle atrophy, and other manifestations of neural degeneration depending on the location of the lesions (Mayhew and Greiner, 1986). The equine protozoal myeloencephalitis (EPM) organism has been identified as a species of *Sarcocystis* and was named *Sarcocystis neurona* (described by Dubey et al, 1992). It was suggested that the parasite in the horse was synonymous with *Sarcocystis falcatula*, originally described from cysts in the muscles of the rose-breasted grosbeak with an opossum final host (Dame et al, 1995; Fenger et al, 1995). Thus, it was put forth that horses were infected by the ingestion of feed or forage contaminated with sporocysts shed in opossum feces (Figure 2-23). When grown in

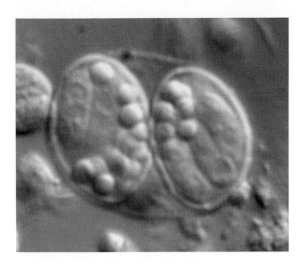

FIGURE 2-23 Sporocysts of *Sarcocystis neurona* passed in the feces of a opossum fed infected muscle from an experimentally infected cat (×4100).
(Specimen courtesy Dr. J.P. Dubey, USDA, Beltsville, Maryland.)

culture, the stages of *S. falcatula* from birds infected with sporocysts from opossum feces produced schizonts similar to those of the EPM organisms (Figure 2-24). The experimental infection of horses, however, failed to produce disease on almost all occasions (Fenger et al, 1997; MacKay, 1997). Work has since suggested that the organisms differ biologically with respect to pathology in the avian hosts and also molecularly, and they are no longer considered synonymous (Marsh et al, 1997).

Opossums are still considered the host that is shedding sporocysts into the environment. Recent work has shown that opossums shed sporocysts of *S. neurona* and four other distinct sporocyts in their feces as determined morphologically and molecularly (Cheadle et al, 2001). It is also now known that cats, striped-skunks, and nine-banded armadillos can be infected with muscle stages of *S. neurona* (Cheadle et al, 2001; Tanheuser et al, 2001). It has also been discovered that raccoons are capable of having myocarditis and encephalitis that are due to *S. neurona* infections (Hamir and Dubey, 2001).

Diagnosis

An antemortem diagnosis is based solely on clinical signs of neurological disease, and none of these is pathognomonic. Three providers (Equine Biodiagnostics Inc. [EBI] and Neogen Corporation, both in Lexington, Kentucky, and The Diagnostic Laboratory of Michigan State University) perform diagnostic tests consisting of Western blot analysis of serum or cerebrospinal fluid. EBI also performs a polymerase chain reaction with cerebrospinal fluid. A positive diagnosis is based on histopathological demonstration of the EPM organisms in association with lesions in the central nervous system (Figure 2-25).

Treatment

A 4- to 12-week course of pyrimethamine at 0.1 to 0.25 mg/kg given orally once daily after an initial dose of 0.5 mg/kg, plus trimethoprim/sulfadiazine at 7.5 to 10 mg/kg given orally twice daily for a total daily dose of 15 to 20 mg forms a basis for

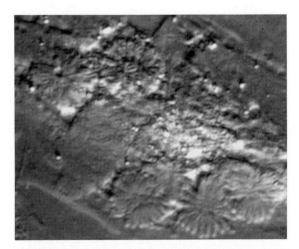

FIGURE 2-24 Schizonts of *Sarcocystis neurona* in a culture of bovine turbinate cells (illuminated with Hoffmann modulation optics). Culture was initiated with merozoites from the nervous tissue of a naturally infected horse (×400).

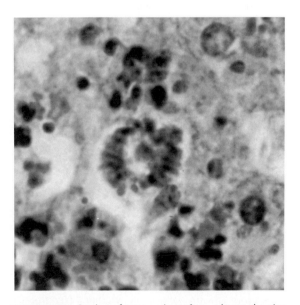

FIGURE 2-25 Section of nervous tissue from a horse showing the characteristic rosette of organisms that is not uncommonly seen in infections with *Sarcocystis neurona*, the causative agent of equine protozoal myeloencephalitis (EPM) (×1800).

EPM therapy. "Certainly, hundreds of horses suspected of having EPM have been treated as discussed, and not all have died. With survival, however, no definitive diagnosis is possible; therefore, cure rates cannot be given" (Mayhew and Greiner, 1986).

Protozoal Encephalomyelitis Organism

Sheep

Apicomplexan encephalomyelitis of adult sheep may be caused by *S. tenella* and other *Sarcocystis* species (Dubey, 1988).

Cattle

Dubey et al (1987) described a case of encephalitis in an 18-month-old steer apparently caused by a *Sarcocystis*-like organism.

Besnotia

Large cysts (0.5 mm) containing bradyzoites occur in the skin of cattle, where they cause scleroderma, and in various tissues of other animals. Oocysts resembling those of *Toxoplasma* are shed in the feces of cats.

Klossiella

Klossiella equi is a parasite of the renal epithelium of the horse, and *Klossiella muris* is a parasite of the renal epithelium of the mouse (see Fig. 5-165). The life histories of these parasites have yet to be worked out in detail; neither species appears to be pathogenic under ordinary circumstances. However, Anderson et al (1988) reported tubular necrosis and nonsuppurative interstitial nephritis in an older, immune-compromised pony. Reinmeyer et al (1983) were first to demonstrate the sporocysts of *K. equi* in the urine of a 2-year-old Standardbred gelding with immune deficiency. These transmission stages are rarely observed; they, like the pathological changes reported by Anderson et al (1988), were observed in immune-deficient horses.

Hepatozoon

The *Hepatozoon* species commonly causing disease in dogs in the United States has now been assigned the name *Hepatozoon americanum* (Macintire et al, 1997; Panciera et al, 1997, Vincent-Johnson et al, 1998). Throughout the rest of the world, the disease seems to be caused by a different species, *Hepatozoon canis* (Smith, 1996). The vector of *Hepatozoon americanum* is now known to be *Amblyomma maculatum* (Mathew et al, 1998 and 1999). In the case of *H. canis*, dogs acquire their infections by ingesting an infected tick, *Rhipicephalus sanguineus*. Ticks become infected by ingesting a blood meal that contains neutrophils and monocytes that harbor the gamonts of the parasite. Sexual replication in the gut of the tick results in the production of oocysts containing infective sporozoites. After dogs become infected by ingesting the tick, there are schizonts that occur in various tissues, and finally, the gamonts are found that occur in white blood cells. *H. canis* typically seems to cause subclinical infections, and the diagnosis is typically made by finding gamonts in the peripheral blood. In the case of infection with *H. americanum*, there is typically severe disease, with dogs having marked neutrophilic leukocytosis. Dogs with *H. americanum* often have significant joint pain associated with myositis and periosteal bone proliferation, which can be revealed in radiographs. Lesions occur primarily on the diaphysis of the more proximal long bones of the limbs; however, flat and irregular bones are frequently involved (Panciera et al, 2000). Lesions involving metacarpals, metatarsals, and digits are infrequent. The earliest observed periosteal lesions in experimentally infected dogs were observed 32 days after exposure to sporulated oocysts of *H. americanum* with hypertrophy and hyperplasia of osteoprogenitor cells, and osteoblasts appearing in the cellular zone of the periosteum. The osseous lesions are similar to those of hypertrophic osteopathy in domestic dogs and other mammalian species. Diagnosis of *H. americanum* typically requires the examination of muscle tissue collected at biopsy or during necropsy to reveal the schizonts. With *H. americanum* infection, there is a large cystic form of the organism that occurs in skeletal muscles that has not been observed in other parts of the world. Also, the meronts typically seen in multiple organs of the body with the occurrence of *H. canis* infection in dogs from other parts of the world are not seen in dogs infected in the United States. In a report of two cases of infection in the United States, treatment with toltrazuril failed to prevent relapse in most of the 11 treated dogs; treatment of three dogs with a combination of trimethoprim sulfate, pyrimethamine, and clindamycin also failed to prevent relapse (Macintire et al, 1997). Macintire et al (1997) suggested that primaquine phosphate has proven efficacious in treating dogs infected with *H. canis* in Africa. Of the 22 dogs reported in the study by Macintire et al (1997), 7 were humanely killed because of chronic wasting, 6 died of the disease, 3 were lost to follow-up, and 6 were alive at the time of the report. Three of the living dogs were free of clinical signs, whereas the other three dogs had chronic wasting disease with intermittent periods of remission and relapse.

Hemosporidians

Piroplasmoses
Babesia

Babesia spp. are apicomplexan parasites of the erythrocytes (Figure 2-26). *Babesia bigemina* causes bovine piroplasmosis ("Texas fever"), a disease characterized in the acute phase by pyrexia (up to 42° C), hemoglobinuria, anemia, icterus, and splenomegaly. The apple-seedlike piroplasms are found in pairs in the erythrocytes, which they destroy, releasing hemoglobin in the process and giving rise to the characteristic clinical manifestations. Transmission of infection among cattle occurs through the bite of the one-host ticks *Boophilus annulatus* and *Boophilus microplus;* the piroplasms multiply in the ovary of the female tick and thereby infect the larvae that hatch from her eggs. In the United Kingdom, piroplasmosis is transmitted by *Ixodes ricinus* and can be transmitted experimentally by parenteral injection of infected erythrocytes. Calves are much less susceptible than older cattle. The greater susceptibility of older hosts holds for all species of *Babesia* and is greatly increased by splenectomy.

Texas fever was once endemic south of the thirty-fifth parallel in the United States, but a cattle-dipping campaign launched in 1906 to eradicate *B. annulatus* virtually eliminated the disease by 1940. This prodigious effort was successful mainly because of the high degree of specificity displayed by *B. annulatus* for its bovine host. Other mammals can serve as hosts, but most

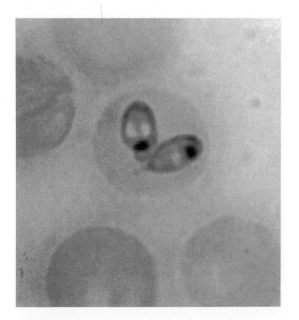

FIGURE 2-26 *Babesia canis* in Giemsa-stained blood film from a dog (×4000).

B. annulatus ticks are found on cattle. Therefore, when the cattle were rounded up for dipping, most of the feeding tick population was rounded up with them. *B. microplus,* on the other hand, infests a broad range of hosts. When *B. microplus* is involved, eradication of bovine piroplasmosis is virtually impossible with contemporary methods.

Babesia bovis, *Babesia divergens*, and *Babesia argentina* cause bovine piroplasmosis in various parts of the world. Each uses one or more different species of tick vectors. Other species of *Babesia* infect sheep *(Babesia ovis),* horses *(Babesia caballi, Babesia equi),* swine *(Babesia trautmanni),* and dogs *(Babesia canis, Babesia gibsoni).*

Canine piroplasmosis is cosmopolitan in distribution (Lobetti et al, 1998). Dogs are infected with two species of these parasites, *B. canis* and *B. gibsoni. B. canis* is the larger form with pear-shaped trophozoites, 4 to 5 μm long, typically being found in pairs in the erythrocytes. *B. gibsoni* is smaller, 3 μm long, and usually round to oval in shape. *B. gibsoni* is transmitted by *R. sanguineus, Haemaphysalis bispinosa,* and *Haemaphysalis longicornis.* The species *B. canis* has been divided into three subspecies: *Babesia canis canis* of Europe transmitted by *Dermacentor reticulatus, Babesia canis vogeli* of northern Africa and North America transmitted by *R. sanguineus,* and *Babesia canis rossi* of southern Africa transmitted by *Haemapophysalis leachi.* Fortunately, the subspecies in North America and Europe do not produce the fulminate form of disease seen in southern Africa. A survey of greyhounds in Florida has shown that large numbers (46% of 383 greyhounds) have antibodies to *B. canis* (Taboada et al, 1992), but most do not have clinical signs. Clinical signs when present include depression, anorexia, ancmia, and splenomegaly. The strain of *Babesia* in Florida appears mainly to cause disease in puppies for which the major diagnostic feature is anemia. Diagnosis is based on demonstrating trophozoites of the parasites in the erythrocytes in Giemsa-stained blood films or serology.

Theileria

Theileria parva, the etiological agent of East Coast fever of African cattle, occurs in the erythrocytes, lymphocytes, and endothelial cells and is transmitted interstadially by *Rhipicephalus* and *Hyalomma* spp. East Coast fever is characterized by dyspnea, emaciation, weakness, tarry feces, and exceptionally heavy mortality.

Cytauxzoon

CYTAUXZOON FELIS. Cytauxzoonosis is a sporadic but rapidly and usually fatal disease of domestic cats occurring predominantly in the south central

United States (Blouin et al, 1984). Clinical signs consist of pyrexia, anemia, icterus, and dehydration; death occurs within a few days. Wright's- or Giemsa-stained blood smears reveal 1- to 2-μm organisms with light blue cytoplasm and dark red nucleus in the erythrocytes (Figure 2-27). Late in the course of cytauxzoonosis, enormous reticuloendothelial cells packed with schizonts appear in the peripheral blood. Histologically, parasitized reticuloendothelial cells nearly occlude the lumens of small- and medium-sized veins in the lungs, spleen, and lymph nodes (Wightman et al, 1977). The bobcat *Lynx rufus* has a parasitemia but no clinical signs of disease and may be the natural reservoir host of *C. felis* (Kier et al, 1982, Glenn et al, 1982). Curiously, blood from parasitemic bobcats injected intraperitoneally into domestic cats led to a persistent erythroparasitemia but no clinical signs of disease. However, when *Dermacentor variabilis* nymphs were fed on a splenectomized parasitemic bobcat, allowed to molt to the adult stage, and then fed on two splenectomized domestic cats, the latter died in 13 and 17 days with typical lesions of cytauxzoonosis (Blouin et al, 1984). Thus, experimentally at least, *D. variabilis* serves as a transstadial vector of *C. felis* from the reservoir host *L. rufus* to the highly susceptible accidental host *F. catus* and leads to lethal infection with the schizogonic stages of this piroplasm. Iatrogenic cytauxzoonosis has been induced in a specific pathogen-free cat by the inoculation of mononuclear cells from a Florida panther *(Felis concolor coryi),* in an attempt to determine whether the panther was infected with feline immunodeficiency virus (Butt et al, 1991). The cat died 12 days after inoculation with typical schizonts of *C. felis* occluding the pulmonary veins (see Figure 2-27).

Treatment of Piroplasmoses

DOGS AND CATS. *Babesia canis* infection usually responds to a single intramuscular injection of 3.5 mg diminazene (Berenil) per kilogram or to subcutaneous injections of 15 mg phenamidine (Ganaseg) per kilogram (Lewis and Huxsoll, 1977; Roberson, 1977). *B. gibsoni* infections are not as readily curable with these drugs as is *B. canis* (Ruff et al, 1973). In Okinawa, diminazine aceturate (3 mg/kg injected intramuscularly on two consecutive days) and pentamidine isethionate (16.5 mg/kg injected intramuscularly on two consecutive days) appeared to cure *B. canis* infection and effected satisfactory clinical response in *B. gibsoni*–infected dogs but did not clear their blood of parasites (Farwell et al, 1982). None of these drugs are available for routine clinical use in the United States. Trypan blue and acridine derivatives (e.g., acriflavin) also have been used in the treatment of babesiosis.

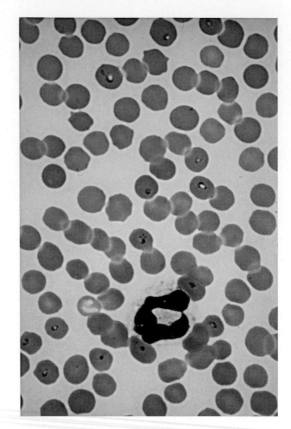

FIGURE 2-27 Giemsa-stained blood film from a cat showing the appearance of the *Cytauxzoon felis* organisms within the red blood cells (×1200). (Courtesy Dr. Tracy W. French.)

For cytauxzoonosis, attempts to treat experimentally infected cats with parvaquone and buparvaquone, two drugs used to treat bovine theileriosis, failed to prevent the death of the infected cats (Motzel and Wagner, 1990). A cat that had a 2-day history of lethargy and anorexia rapidly progressed to become seriously icteric with dark-brown urine and began a 10-day course of enrofloxacin followed by a 5-day course of tetracycline (Walker and Cowell, 1995). *C. felis* organisms were present in the blood of the cat after the 10-day course of enrofloxacin, but were not present in blood samples collected 6 and 15 weeks after discharge. Greene et al (1999) successfully treated six of seven cats with two intramuscular injections (2 mg/kg body weight) of diminazene (five cats) or imidocarb (one cat); one cat died after the first injection of diminazene. More recently, cats have been identified surviving natural infections with *C. felis* (Meinkoth et al, 2000). Eighteen cats from northwestern Arkansas and northeastern Oklahoma were initially identified through piroplasms in blood smears. Clinical signs in most cats were similar to those described for cytaux-zoonosis, but four did not have symptoms. The parasitemia was generally persistent throughout follow-up (i.e., for up to 154 days). Only one cat was treated with imidocarb, and all cats survived. The authors postulate that they may be dealing with a less virulent strain of this parasite.

HORSES. *Babesia caballi* and *B. equi* are susceptible to many antiprotozoal drugs, but in the United States, none are approved for use in horses. Imidocarb dipropionate is administered subcutaneously at 2 mg/kg repeated once after 24 hours for the treatment of *B. caballi*, and at 4 mg/kg repeated at 72-hour intervals for *B. equi*.

Malarias
Plasmodium

Plasmodium spp. are the etiological agents of malarias of humans, nonhuman primates, rodents, birds, and reptiles (mainly lizards). Mammalian malarias are transmitted by anopheline mosquitoes and avian malarias by culicine mosquitoes; the vectors of reptilian malarias are largely unknown.

LIFE HISTORY. Sporozoites injected into the host by the infected mosquito during feeding enter cells such as hepatocytes, become trophozoites, and undergo schizogony. This first multiplication of *plasmodia* in hepatocytes is termed **preerythrocytic schizogony.** Merozoites released when the hepatocyte ruptures invade erythrocytes or reticulocytes of the circulating blood, pass through a trophozoite phase, and then undergo schizogony. In certain species of *Plasmodium*, some of these merozoites reinvade hepatocytes to continue **exoerythrocytic schizogony,** which is held accountable by some authorities for relapses after therapeutic elimination of erythrocytic infection by chloroquine, quinine, and the like. Merozoites released when the infected erythrocytes rupture reinvade other erythrocytes and again undergo schizogony. Each generation of erythrocytic merozoites occupies approximately 24, 48, or 72 hours, depending on the species of *Plasmodium* involved. Synchronization of schizogony and consequent erythrocyte destruction leading to cyclic bouts of chills and fever is typical of certain malarias, particularly those of humans. The terms *quotidian, tertian,* and *quartan* refer to recurrence of fever daily, on the third day (i.e., at 48 hours), and on the fourth day (i.e., at 72 hours), the anomaly in nomenclature arising from inconsistency in the inclusion of zero in the system of natural numbers as applied to the reckoning of time. Eventually, some merozoites develop into either microgametocytes or macrogametocytes, which are the stages infective for the mosquito. When a suitable species of mosquito feeds on a malarious host, the microgametocytes and macrogametocytes in the blood meal mature, and the microgametes fertilize the macrogametes to form zygotes. The zygotes then elongate to form motile **ookinetes,** which migrate to the hemocoel side of the mosquito's midgut, where each develops into an oocyst. Thousands of sporozoites develop within each oocyst by a budding process similar to schizogony and are released into the hemocoel when the oocyst ruptures. Those sporozoites that reach the salivary glands are ready to infect another host next time the mosquito takes a blood meal and thus complete the rather involved life history of *Plasmodium*. In humans, the symptoms of malaria are extremely variable, and diagnosis depends on the demonstration of plasmodia in fixed, stained blood smears. Fatality can usually be attributed to cerebral involvement, renal failure, or pulmonary hemorrhage.

IDENTIFICATION. Differentiation of species of *Plasmodia* is based on study of Giemsa-stained thin blood smears and recognition of rather subtle morphological features of the early trophozoite ("ring form"), ameboid late trophozoite, schizont, and male and female gametocytes. The color and distribution of hematin in the cytoplasm of the parasite, as well as cytoplasmic stippling and other morphological alterations of the infected erythrocyte, are also taken into account. The diagnosis of malaria is clearly a job for an expert.

SIMIAN MALARIA. About 20 species of *Plasmodium* have been described from nonhuman primates, some of which (e.g., *P. knowlsi, P. cynomolgi*) are transmissible to humans through the bites of infected anopheline mosquitoes. The diagnosis of simian malaria is of particular interest to laboratories where imported primates are experimental animals (Coatney et al, 1971). Old World monkeys may also be infected with *Hepatocystis*.

AVIAN MALARIA. Avian malaria is a complex of diseases caused by many species of *Plasmodium* (Figure 2-28). *Haemoproteus* and *Leucocytozoon,* considered later, also cause malaria-like infections in birds.

Haemoproteus

Haemoproteus spp. are parasites of birds, turtles, and lizards. Schizogony occurs in vascular endothelial cells of various organs, and only gametocytes appear in circulating erythrocytes. In blood films fixed with methanol and stained with Giemsa, the gametocytes appear as elongate, sometimes horseshoe-shaped cells embracing the erythrocyte nucleus; the cytoplasm of the gametocyte contains pigment granules accumulating as a result of the incomplete digestion of hemoglobin. Various species of *Haemoproteus* are transmitted by *Culicoides,* Hippoboscidae, or *Chrysops,* which

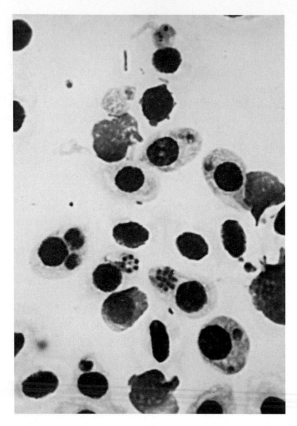

FIGURE 2-28 *Plasmodium* sp. in a blood smear from a bald eagle (*Haliaetus leucocephalus*). There are several schizonts apparent in this photomicrograph of a blood film (×1400).

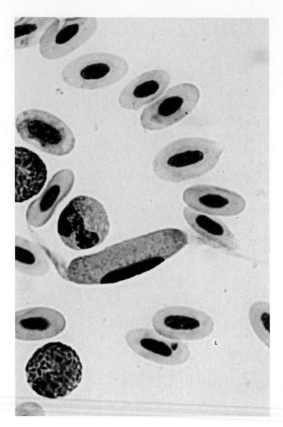

FIGURE 2-29 *Leucocytozoon* sp. in the blood smear from a red-tailed hawk (×1400).

become infected when they ingest erythrocytes containing gametocytes. Fertilization, development of oocysts, and salivarian transmission of sporozoites to the vertebrate host resemble the corresponding events in the life history of *Plasmodium*. *Haemoproteus* is essentially nonpathogenic.

Leucocytozoon

Leucocytozoon spp. are parasites of domestic and wild birds; *L. simondi* causes acute, fatal disease of ducks and geese, as does *L. caulleryi* in chickens, and *L. smithi* in turkeys. Schizogony occurs in hepatocytes and vascular endothelial cells of various tissues, producing merozoites that invade erythroblasts, erythrocytes, lymphocytes, and monocytes, and there develop into gametocytes. *Leucocytozoon* gametocytes differ from those of *Plasmodium* and *Haemoproteus* in not containing pigment granules and in greatly distorting the host cell (Figure 2-29). Some gametocytes are round and push the host cell nucleus to one side so that it forms a cap on the parasite. Others are oval or elliptical in cells that become elongated and bizarre in appearance as the parasite grows. *Simulium* spp. serve as intermediate hosts.

Hepatocystitis

Hepatocystis spp. are parasites of the lower monkeys, fruit bats, and squirrels of the Old World. Schizogony occurs in hepatocytes, requires 2 months, and results in large schizonts called **merocysts.** Merozoites released from merocysts invade erythrocytes and develop into gametocytes. *Culicoides* spp. are the probable vectors.

■ REFERENCES

Abbitt B, Huey RL, Eugster AK, et al: Treatment of giardiasis in adult greyhounds, using ipronidazole-medicated water, *J Am Vet Med Assoc* 188:67–69, 1986.

Anderson BC, Donndelinger T, Wilkins RM, et al: Cryptosporidiosis in a veterinary student, *J Am Vet Med Assoc* 180:408–409, 1982.

Anderson DC, Buckner RG, Glenn BL, et al: Endemic canine leishmaniasis, *Vet Pathol* 17:94–96, 1982.

Anderson ML, Blanchard PC, Barr BC, et al: *Neospora*-like protozoan infection as a major cause of abortion in California dairy cattle, *J Am Vet Med Assoc* 198:241–244, 1991.

Anderson WI, Picut CA, Georgi ME: *Klossiella equi*-induced tubular nephrosis and interstitial nephritis in a pony, *J Comp Pathol* 98, 363–366, 1988.

Barker IK, Remmler O: The endogenous development of *Eimeria leuckarti* in ponies, *J Parasitol* 58, 112:122, 1972.

Barr BC, Bjerkas I, Buxton D, et al: Neosporosis: report of an International *Neospora* workshop, *Comp Cont Ed Pract Vet* 19(suppl):S120–S126, 1997.

Barr SC: American trypanosomiasis in dogs, *Comp Cont Educ Pract Vet* 13:745–755, 1991.

Barr SC, van Beek O, Carlisle-Nowak MS, et al: *Trypanosoma cruzi* infection in Walker Hounds from Virginia, *Am J Vet Res* 56:1037–1044, 1995.

Barr SC, Bowman DD, Erb HN: Evaluation of two test procedures for diagnosis of giardiasis in dogs, *Am J Vet Res* 53:2028–2031, 1992.

Barr SC, Bowman DD, Heller RL: Efficacy of fenbendazole against giardiasis in dogs, *Am J Vet Res* 55:988–990, 1994.

Barr SC, Bowman DD, Heller RL, et al: Efficacy of albendazole against giardiasis in dogs, *Am J Vet Res* 54:926–928, 1993.

Bjerkås I, Mohn SF, Presthus J: Unidentified cyst-forming sporozoon causing encephalomyelitis and myositis in dogs, *Z Parasitenkd* 70:271–274, 1984.

Blouin EF, Kocan AA, Glenn BL, et al: Transmission of *Cytauxzoon felis* Kier, 1979 from bobcats, *Felis rufus* (Schreber), to domestic cats by *Dermacentor variabilis* (Say), *J Wildlife Diseases* 20:241–242, 1984.

BonDurant RH, Anderson ML, Blanchard P, et al: Prevalence of trichomoniasis among California beef herds, *J Am Vet Med Assoc* 196:1590–1593, 1990.

Buckner RG, Ewing SA: Trichomoniasis. In *Current Veterinary Therapy VI*, Philadelphia, WB Saunders Co, p. 970.

Butt MT, Bowman DD, Barr MC, et al: Iatrogenic transmission of *Cytauxzoon felis* from a Florida panther *(Felis concolor coryi)* to a domestic cat, *J Wildl Dis* 27:342–347, 1991.

Canfield PJ, Vogelnest L, Cunningham ML, et al: Amoebic meningoencephalitis caused by *Balamuthia mandrillaris* in an orangutan, *Aust Vet J* 75:97–100, 1997.

Cheadle MA, Dame JB, Greiner EC: Sporocyst size of isolates of *Sarcocystis* shed by the Virginia opossum *(Didelphis virginiana)*, *Vet Parasitol* 95:305–311, 2001.

Cheadle MA, Tanhauser SM, Dame JB, et al: The nine-banded armadillo *(Dasypus novemcinctus)* is an intermediate host for *Sarcocystis neurona: Int J Parasitol* 31:330–335, 2001.

Cheadle MA, Yowell CA, Sellon DC, et al: The striped skunk *(Mephitis mephitis)* is an intermediate host for *Sarcocystis neurona: Int J Parasitol* 31:843–849, 2001.

Coatney GR, Collins WE, Warren McW, et al: The Primate Malarias, Washington, DC, 1971, US Government Printing Office.

Core DM, Hoff EJ, Milton JL: Hindlimb hyperextension as a result of *Toxoplasma gondii* polyradiculitis, *J Am Hosp Assoc* 19:713–716, 1983.

Craig TM, Barton CL, Mercer SH, et al: Dermal leishmaniasis in a Texas cat, *Am J Trop Med Hyg* 35:1100–1102, 1986.

Current WL: Cryptosporidiosis, *J Am Vet Med Assoc* 187:1334–1338, 1985.

Dame JB, MaKay RJ, Yowell CA, et al: *Sarcocystis falcatula* from passerine and psittacine birds: Synonymy with *Sarcocystis neurona*, agent of equine protozoal myeloencephalitis, *J Parasitol* 81:930–935, 1995.

Deol I, Robledo L, Meza A, et al: Encephalitis due to a free-living amoeba *(Balamuthia mandrillaris)*: case report with literature review, *Surg Neurol* 54:611–616, 2000.

Dubey JP: Toxoplasmosis, *J Am Vet Med Assoc* 189:166–170, 1986a.

Dubey JP: Toxoplasmosis in cats, *Feline Practice* 16:12–26, 1986b.

Dubey JP: A review of toxoplasmosis in pigs, *Vet Parasitol* 19:181–233, 1986c.

Dubey JP: A review of toxoplasmosis in cattle, *Vet Parasitol* 22:177–202, 1986d.

Dubey J: Toxoplasmosis in goats, *Agri-Practice* 8:43–52, 1987.

Dubey JP: Lesions in sheep inoculated with *Sarcocystis tenella* sporocysts from canine feces, *Vet Parasitol* 26:237–252, 1988.

Dubey JP, Carpenter JL, Speer CA, et al: Newly recognized fatal protozoan disease of dogs, *J Am Vet Med Assoc* 192:1269–1285, 1988.

Dubey JP, Davis SW, Speer CA, et al: *Sarcocystis neurona* n. sp. (Protozoa: Apicomplexa), the etiologic agent of equine protozoal myeloencephalitis, *J Parasitol* 77:212–218, 1992.

Dubey JP, Fayer R: Sarcocystosis, *Br Vet J* 139:371–377, 1983.

Dubey JP, Frenkel JK: Feline toxoplasmosis from acutely infected mice and the development of *Toxoplasma* cysts, *J Protozool* 23:537–546, 1976.

Dubey JP, Liddell S, Mattson D, et al: Characterization of the Oregon isolate of *Neospora hughesi* from a horse, *J Parasitol* 87:345–353, 2001.

Dubey JP, Perry A, Kennedy MJ: Encephalitis caused by a *Sarcocystis*-like organism in a steer, *J Am Vet Med Assoc* 191:231–232, 1987.

Enserink M: Has leishmaniasis become endemic in the U.S.? *Science* 290:1881,1883, 2000.

Farwell GE, LeGrand EK, Cobb CC: Clinical observations on *Babesia gibsoni* and *Babesia canis* infections in dogs, *J Am Vet Med Assoc* 180:507–511, 1982.

Fayer R, Dubey JP: Comparative epidemiology of coccidia: clues to the etiology of equine protozoal myeloencephalitis, *Int J Parasitol* 17:615–620, 1987.

Fenger CK, Granstrom DE, Gajadhar AA, et al: Experimental induction of equine protozoal myeloencephalitis in horses using *Sarcocystis* sp. sporocysts from the opossum *(Didelphis virginiana)*, *Vet Parasitol* 68:199–213, 1997.

Fenger CK, Granstrom DE, Langemeir JL, et al: Identification of opossums *(Didelphis virginiana)* as the putative definitive hosts of *Sarcocystis neurona*, *J Parasitol* 81:911–916, 1995.

Fitzgerald PR: Bovine trichomoniasis, *Vet Clin N Am Food Animal Practice* 2(2):277–282, 1986.

Fox JC, Ewing SA, Buckner RG, et al: *Trypanosoma cruzi* infection in a dog from Oklahoma, *J Am Vet Med Assoc* 189:1583-1585, 1986.

Frelier P, Mayhew IG, Fayer R, et al: Sarcocystosis: a clinical outbreak in dairy calves, *Science* 195:1341–1342, 1977.

Frenkel JK, Dubey JP: Toxoplasmosis and its prevention in cats and man, *J Infect Dis* 12:664–673, 1972.

Frenkel JK, Dubey JP: The taxonomic importance of obligate heteroxeny: distinction of *Hammondia hammondi* from *Toxoplasma gondii*—another opinion, *Parasitol Res* 86:783–786, 2000.

Glenn BT, Rolley RE, Kocan AA: *Cytauxzoon*-like piroplasms in erythrocytes of wild-trapped bobcats in Oklahoma, *J Am Vet Med Assoc* 181(11):1251–1253, 1982.

Goodger WJ, Skirrow SZ: Epidemiologic and economic analyses of an unusually long epizootic of trichomoniasis in a large California dairy herd, *J Am Vet Med Assoc* 189:772–776, 1986.

Gookin JL, Breitschwerdt EB, Levy MG, et al: Diarrhea associated with trichomonosis in cats, *J Am Vet Med Assoc* 215:1450–1454, 1999.

Greene CE, Latimer K, Hopper E, et al: Administration of diminazene aceturate or imidocarb dipropionate for treatment of cytauxzoonosis in cats, *J Am Vet Med Assoc* 215:497–500, 1999.

Gual-Sill F, Pulido-Reyes J: Tratamento de la balantidiasis en gorilas de tierras bajas en el Zoologica de Chupultepec, Ciudad de Mexico, *Vet Mexico* 25:73–75, 1994.

Hamir AN, Dubey JP: Myocarditis and encephalitis associated with *Sarcocystis neurona* infection in raccoons (Procyon lotor), *Vet Parasitol* 95:335–340, 2001.

Heydorn AO, Mehlhorn H: Further remarks on *Hammondia hammondi* and the taxonomic importance of obligate heteroxeny, *Parasitol Res* 87:573–577, 2001.

Hill DE, Liddell S, Jenkins MC, et al: Specific detection of *Neospora caninum* oocysts in fecal samples from experimentally-infected dogs using the polymerase chain reaction, *J Parasitol* 87:395–398, 2001.

Homan W, van Gorkom T, Kan YY, et al: Characterization of Cryptosporidium parvum in human and animal feces by single-tube nested polymerase chain reaction and restriction analysis, *Parasitol Res* 85:707–712, 1999.

Isler CM, Bellamy JEC, Wobeser GA: Labile neurotoxin in serum of calves with "nervous" coccidiosis, *Canad J Vet Res* 51:253–260, 1987.

Jacobson E, Clubb S, Greiner E: Amebiasis in red-footed tortoises, *J Am Vet Med Assoc* 183:1192–1194, 1983.

Kier AB, Wagner JE, Morehouse LG: Experimental transmission of *Cytauxzoon felis* from bobcats *(Lynx rufus)* to domestic cats *(Felis domesticus)*, *Am J Vet Res* 43:97–101, 1982.

Kinde H, Visvesvara GS, Barr BC, et al: Amebic meningoencephalitis caused by *Balamuthia mandrillaris* (leptomyxid ameba) in a horse, *J Vet Diag Invest* 10:378–381, 1998.

Kingston N, Morton JK, Dietrich R: *Trypanosoma cervi* from Alaskan reindeer *Rangifer tarandus, J Protozool* 29(4):588–591, 1982.

Kirkpatrick CE: Feline giardiasis: a review, *J Sm Anim Pract* 27:69–80, 1986.

Langston VC, Galey F, Lovell R, et al: Toxicity and therapeutics of monensin: a review, *Food Animal Pract* 80:75–84, 1985.

Lewis GE, Huxsoll DL: Canine babesiosis. In Kirk RW, editor: *Current Veterinary Therapy VI*, Philadelphia, WB Saunders Co, p. 1330.

Lindsay DS, Blagburn BL, Dubey JP: Feline toxoplasmosis and the importance of the *Toxoplasma gondii* oocyst, *Comp Cont Ed Pract Vet* 19:448–506, 1992.

Lindsay DS, Blagburn BL, Powe TA: Enteric coccidial infections and coccidiosis in swine, *Comp Cont Educ Pract Vet* 14:698–702, 1992.

Lindsay DS, Current WL, Taylor JR: Effects of experimentally induced *Isospora suis* infection on morbidity, mortality, and weight gains in nursing pigs, *Am J Vet Res* 46:1511–1512, 1985.

Lindsay DS, Dubey JP, Duncan RB: Confirmation that the dogs is a definitive host for *Neospora caninum*, *Vet Parasitol* 82:327-333, 1999.

Lindsay DS, Upton SJ, Owens DS, et al: *Cryptosporidium andersoni* n. sp. (Apicomplexa: Cryptosporiidae) from cattle, *Bos Taurus, J Euk Microbiol* 47:91–95, 2000.

Lobetti RG: Canine babesiosis, *Comp Cont Ed Pract Vet* 20:418–431, 1998.

Lyons ET, Drudge JH, Tolliver SC: Natural infection with *Eimeria leuckarti:* prevalence of oocysts in feces of horse foals on several farms in Kentucky during 1986, *Am J Vet Res* 49:96–98, 1988.

Ma P, Soave R: Three-step stool examination for cryptosporidiosis in 10 homosexual men with protracted watery diarrhea, *J Infect Dis* 147:824–828, 1983.

Macintire DK, Vincent-Johnson N, et al: Hepatozoonosis in dogs: 22 cases (1989–1994), *J Am Vet Med Assoc* 210:916–922, 1997.

MacKay RJ: Equine protozoal myeloencephalitis, *Vet Clin N Am Eq Pract* 13:79–96, 1997.

Marsh AE, Barr BC, Packham AE, et al: Description of a new *Neospora* species (Protozoa: Apicomplexa: Sarcocystidae), *J Parasitol* 84:983–991, 1998.

Marsh A, Barr BC, Tell LA, et al: *In vitro* cultivation and experimental inoculation of *Sarcocystis falcatula* and *S. neurona* merozoites into budgerigars, Abstract 121, 42nd Annual Meeting of the Am Assoc. Vet. Parasitol, Reno, Nev.

Mathew JS, Ewing SA, Panciera RJ, et al: Sporogonic development of *Hepatozoon americanum* (Apicomplexa) in its definitive host, *Amblyomma maculatum* (Acarina), *J Parasitol* 85:1023–1031, 1999.

Mathew JS, Ewing SA, Panciera RJ, et al: Experimental transmission of *Hepatozoon americanum* Vincent-Johnson et al, 1997 to dogs by the Gulf Coast tick, *Amblyomma maculatum* Koch, *Vet Parasitol* 80:1–14, 1998.

Mayhew IG, Greiner EC: Protozoal diseases, *Vet Clin N Am, Equine Pract Parasitol* 2(2):439–445, 1986.

Mayrink W, Genaro O, Silva JCF, et al: Phase I and II open clinical trials of a vaccine against *Leishmania chagasi* infections in dogs, *Mem Inst Oswaldo Cruz* 91:695–697, 1996.

McAllister MM: *Neospora caninum*: its oocysts and its identity: an opinion, *Parasitol Res* 86:860, 2000.

McAllister MM, Dubey JP, Lindsay DS, et al: Dogs are definitive hosts of *Neospora caninum, Int J Parastiol* 28:1473--1478, 1998.

Mehlhorn H, Heydorn AO: *Neospora caninum*: is it really different from *Hammondia heydorni* or is it a strain of *Toxoplasma gondii?* An opinion, *Parasitol Res* 86:169–178, 2000.

Meier H, Holzworth J, Griffiths RC: Toxoplasmosis in the cat— fourteen cases, *J Am Vet Med Assoc* 131:395–414, 1957.

Meinkoth J, Kocan AA, Whitworth L, et al: Cats surviving natural infection with *Cytauxzoon felis:* 18 cases (1997-1998), *J Vet Intern Med* 14:521–525, 2000.

Monticello TM, Levy MG, Bunch SE, et al: Cryptosporidiosis in a feline leukemia virus-positive cat, *J Am Vet Med Assoc* 191:705–706, 1987.

Motzel SL, Wagner JE: Treatment of experimentally induced cytauxzoonosis in cats with parvaquone and buparvaquone, *Vet Parasitol* 35:131–138, 1990.

Mugridge NB, Morrison DA, Heckeroth AR, et al: Phylogenetic analysis based on full-length large subunit ribosomal RNA gene sequence comparison reveals that *Neospora caninum* is more closely related to *Hammondia heydorni* than to *Toxoplasma gondii, Int J Parasitol* 29:1545–1556, 1999.

O'Handley RMO, Olson ME, Fraser D, et al: Prevalence and genotypic characterisation of *Giardia* in dairy calves from Western Australia and Western Canada, *Vet Parasitol* 90:193–200, 2000.

O'Handley RM, Olson ME, McAllister TA, et al: Efficacy of fenbendazole for treatment of giardiasis in calves, *Am J Vet Res* 58:384–388, 1997.

Oliveira-dos-Santos AJ, Nascimento EG, Silva MP, et al: Report on a visceral and cutaneous leishmaniasis focus in the town of Jequie, State of Bahia, Brazil, *Rev Inst Med Trop Sao Paulo* 35:583–584, 1993.

Olson ME, McAllister TA, Deselliers L, et al: Effects of giardiasis on production in a domestic ruminant (lamb) model, *Am J Vet Res* 56:1470–1474, 1995.

Ong CSL, Eisler DL, Goh SH, et al: Molecular epidemiology of cryptosporidiosis outbreaks and transmission in British Columbia, Canada, *Am J Trop Med Hyg* 61:63–69, 1999.

Palmieri JR, Dalgard DW, Connor DH: Gastric amebiasis in a silvered leaf monkey, *J Am Vet Med Assoc* 185:1374–1375, 1984.

Panciera RJ, Gatto NT, Crystal MA, Helman RG, Elly RW: Canine hepatozoonosis in Oklahoma, *J Am Anim Hosp Assoc* 33:221–225, 1997.

Panciera RJ, MathewJS, Ewing SA, Cummings CA, Drost WT, Kocan AA: Skeletal lesions of canine hepatozoonosis caused by *Hepatozoon americanum, Vet Pathol* 37: 225–230, 2000.

Radostits OM, Stockdale PHG: A brief review of bovine coccidiosis in western Canada, *Can Vet J* 21:227–230, 1980.

Ramos Vara JA, Ortiz Santiago B, Segales J, Dunstan RW: Cutaneous leishmaniasis in twochorses, *Vet Pathol* 33: 731–734, 1996.

Reinmeyer CR, Jacobs RM, Spurlock GN: A coccidial oocyst in equine urine, *J Am Vet Med Assoc* 182:1250–1251, 1983.

Riahi H, Leboutet MJ, Labrousse F, Bouteille B, Darde ML: Monoclonal antibodies to *Hammondia hammondi* allowing an immunological differentiation from *Toxoplasma gondii, J Parasitol* 86:1362–1366, 2000.

Rideout BA, Gardiner CH, Stalis IH, Zuba JR, Hadfield T, Visvesvara GS: Fatal infections with *Balamuthia mandrillaris* (a free-living amoeba) in gorillas and other old world primates, *Vet Pathol* 34:15–22, 1997.

Roberson E: Antiprotozoal drugs. In Jones LM, Booth NH, McDonald LE, editors: *Veterinary pharmacology and therapeutics*, Ames, The Iowa State University Press, p. 1095.

Romatowski J: *Pentatrichomonas hominis* infection in four kittens, *J Am Vet Med Assoc* 216:1270–1272, 2000.

Ruff MD, Fowler JL, Fernau RC, et al: Action of certain antiprotozoal compounds against *Babesia gibsoni* in dogs, *Am J Vet Res* 34:641–645, 1973.

Sanford SE: Enteric cryptosporidial infection in pigs: 184 cases (1981–1985), *J Am Vet Med Assoc* 190:695–698, 1987.

Scholtens RG, New JC, Johnson S: The nature and treatment of giardiasis in parakeets, *J Am Vet Med Assoc* 180:170–173, 1982.

Smith MC, Sherman DM: *Goat medicine,* Philadelphia, Lea & Febiger.

Smith TG: The genus *Hepatozoon* (Apicomplexa: Adeleina), *J Parasitol* 82:565–585, 1996.

Snyder SP, England JJ, McChesney AE: Cryptosporidiosis in immunodeficient Arabian foals, *Vet Pathol* 15:2–17, 1987.

St Jean G, Couture Y, Dubreuil P, et al: Diagnosis of *Giardia* infection in 14 calves, *J Am Vet Med Assoc* 191:831–832, 1987.

Stokol T, Randolph JF, Nachbar S, et al: Development of bone marrow toxicosis after albendazole administration in a dog and cat, *J Am Vet Med Assoc* 210:753–1756, 1997.

Stuart BP, Lindsay DS: Coccidiosis in swine, *Vet Clin N Am, Food Anim Pract* 2(2):455–468, 1980.

Stuart BP, Lindsay DS, Ernst JV, et al: *Isospora suis enteritis* in pigs, *Vet Pathol* 17:84–93, 1980.

Sulaiman IM, XiaoLH, Yang CF, et al: Differentiating human from animal isolates of *Cryptosporidium parvum, Emerg Infect Dis* 4:681–685, 1998.

Swenson CL, Silverman J, Stromberg PC, et al: Visceral leishmaniasis in an English foxhound from an Ohio research colony, *J Am Vet Med Assoc* 193:1089–1092, 1988.

Taboada J, Harvey JW, Levy MG, et al: Seroprevalence of babesiosis in greyhounds in Florida, *J Am Vet Med Assoc* 200:47–50, 1992.

Tanhauser SM, Cheadle MA, Massey ET, et al: The nine-banded armadillo *(Dasypus novemcinctus)* is naturally infected with *Sarcocystis neurona, Int J Parasitol* 31:325–329, 2001.

Teare JA, Loomis MR: Epizootic of balantidiasis in lowland gorillas, *J Am Vet Med Assoc* 181(11):1345–1347, 1982.

Telford SR, Forrester DJ, Wright SD, et al: The identity and prevalence of trypanosomes in white-tailed deer *(Odocoileus virginiana)* in southern Florida, *J Helm Soc Wash* 58:19–23, 1991.

Thompson RCA, Hopkins RM, Homan WL: Nomenclature and genetic groupings of Giardia infecting mammals, *Parasitol Today* 16:210–213, 2000.

Thurmond MC, Hietala SK: Culling associated with *Neospora caninum* infection in dairy cows. *Am J Vet Res* 57:1559–1562, 1996.

Thurmond MC, Hietala SK: Effect of *Neosporum caninum* infection on milk production in first-lactation dairy cows, *J Am Vet Med Assoc* 210:672–674, 1997.

Thurmond MC, Hietala SK: Culling associated with *Neospora caninum* infection in dairy cows. *Am J Vet Res* 57:1559–1562, 1999.

Tyzzer EE: A sporozoan found in the peptic glands of the common mouse, *Proc Soc Exptl Biol Med* 5:12–13, 1907.

Tyzzer EE: An extracellular coccidium, *Cryptosporidium muris* (gen. et sp. nov.), of the common mouse, *J Med Res* 18:487–509, 1910.

Tyzzer EE: *Cryptosporidium parvum* (sp. nov.), a coccidium found in the small intestine of the common mouse, *Arch Protistenk* 26:394–412, 1912.

Upton SJ, Current WL: The species of *Cryptosporidium* (Apicomplexa: Cryptosporidiidae) infecting mammals, *J Parasitol* 71:625–629, 1985.

Vetterling JM: Coccidia (Protozoa: Eimeriidae) of swine, *J Parasitol* 51:897–912, 1965.

Vincent-Johnson NA, Macintire DK, Lindsay DS, Lenz SD, Baneth G, Shkap V, Blagburn BL: A new *Hepatozoon* species from dogs: description of the causative agent of canine hepatozoonosis in North America, *J Parasitol* 83:1165–1172, 1998.

Visvesvara GS, Schuster FL, Martinez AJ: *Balamuthia mandrillaris,* n. g., n. sp., agent of amebic meningoencephalitis in humans and other animals, *J Euk Microbiol* 40:504–514, 1993.

Walker DB, Cowell RL: Survival of a domestic cat with naturally acquired cytauxzoonosis, *J Am Vet Med Assoc* 206:1363–1365, 1995.

Walton BC, Bauman PM, Diamond LS, et al: Isolation and identification of *Trypanosoma cruzi* from raccoons in Maryland, *Am J Trop Med Hyg* 7:603–610, 1958.

Widmer G, Akiyoshi D, Buckholt MA, et al: Animal propagation and genomic survey of a genotype 1 isolate of *Cryptosporidium parvum, Mol Biochem Parasitol* 108;187–197, 2000.

Wightman SR, Kier AB, Wagner JE: Feline cytauxzoonosis: clinical features of a newly described blood parasite disease, *Feline Practice* 7(3):23–26, 1977.

Xiao L, Herd RP, McClure KE: Periparturient rise in the excretion of *Giardia* sp. cysts and Cryptosporidium parvum oocysts as a source of infection for lambs, *J Parasitol* 80:55–59, 1994.

Xiao L, Saeed K, Herd RP: Efficacy of albendazole and fenbendazole against *Giardia* infection in cattle, *Vet Parasitol* 61:165–170, 1996.

Zajac AM, LaBranche TP, Donoghue AR, et al: Efficacy of fenbendazole in the treatment of experimental *Giardia* infection in dogs, *Am J Vet Res* 59:61–63, 1998.

Zimmer JF: Treatment of feline giardiasis with metronidazole, *Cornell Vet* 77:383–388, 1987.

Zimmer JF, Burrington DB: Comparison of four protocols for the treatment of canine giardiasis, *J Am Anim Hosp Assoc* 22:168–172, 1986.

CHAPTER 3

HELMINTHS

The parasitic worms belong to the phyla Platyhelminthes ("flat worms," "flukes," and "tapeworms"), Nemathelminthes or Nematoda ("roundworms"), Acanthocephala ("thorny-headed worms"), and Annelida ("segmented worms," "night-crawlers"). "Tongueworms" of the parasitic class Pentastomida are also wormlike in appearance, but being of the phylum Arthropoda, are discussed in Chapter 1. This list of helminth taxa does not exhaust Nature's bounty of "small, elongate, and slender, creeping or crawling animals, usually soft-bodied, naked, and limbless or nearly so; any animal having a real or fancied resemblance to an angleworm or earthworm" (*Webster's New International Dictionary*, ed 2, Springfield, Mass, 1935, G & C Merriam Co). However, it does include all of the worms in which veterinarians are particularly interested. The phylum Platyhelminthes contains three classes: Turbellaria, Trematoda, and Cestoda. All are typically soft-bodied, flattened dorsoventrally, and hermaphroditic. The Turbellaria (planarians) are mostly free-living, carnivorous flatworms. Aquarists finding planarians in fish tanks may mistake them for parasites, but otherwise they are of only passing interest to veterinarians. The trematodes (flukes) of importance to veterinary medicine may be found as adults in the intestine, bile ducts, lungs, blood vessels, or other organs of their vertebrate final hosts. Adult cestodes (tapeworms) are parasites of the intestine of vertebrates, and their larvae are parasites of different vertebrates or of invertebrates. The class Cestoda includes many important parasites of domestic animals and is the subject of the second portion of this section.

■ CLASS TREMATODA

The class Trematoda contains three orders: Monogenea, Aspidogastrea, and Digenea. Monogeneans and most Aspidogastreans undergo direct development and are parasites of aquatic and amphibious animals. *Gyrodactylus* and *Dactylogyrus,* for example, are common and pathogenic monogenean parasites of the skin and gills of aquarium fishes. These two orders of parasites are of interest to few veterinarians. The trematodes of importance to most veterinarians are the digenetic trematodes.

Order Digenea
Life History

The order Digenea is so called because its members undergo indirect development with sexual and asexual generations parasitizing alternate hosts. All flukes infecting dogs, cats, ruminants, horses, and swine are digeneans. The life history of *Fasciola hepatica,* depicted in Figure 3-1, is typical of the order.

Adult *F. hepatica* flukes (Figure 3-2) live in the bile ducts of ruminant and other mammalian hosts. Their eggs are carried first to the bowel lumen with the bile and then to the exterior with the feces. When deposited, each of these eggs consists of a fertilized ovum and a cluster of vitelline cells enclosed in an operculated capsule (Figure 3-3). Only if the egg falls into water will a ciliated larva called a **miracidium** develop inside it (Figure 3-4). The miracidium is completely covered with cilia and has a conical papilla at its anterior end for boring into the snail intermediate host, a pair of eye spots, a brain, a rudimentary excretory system, and a cluster of germinal cells, the progenitors of the next generation of larvae (Figure 3-5). The miracidium, which is fully developed and ready to hatch after 2 to 4 weeks at summer temperatures, escapes from the egg capsule by pushing aside the operculum and swims about in search of a suitable species of snail (e.g., *Lymnaea truncatula*). If it fails to find such a snail within 24 hours, the miracidium exhausts its energy stores and dies.

If the miracidium is more fortunate, it bores into the snail's body, loses its ciliated covering, migrates to the gonad or digestive gland (often referred to as the *liver*), and forms a **sporocyst.** Each germinal

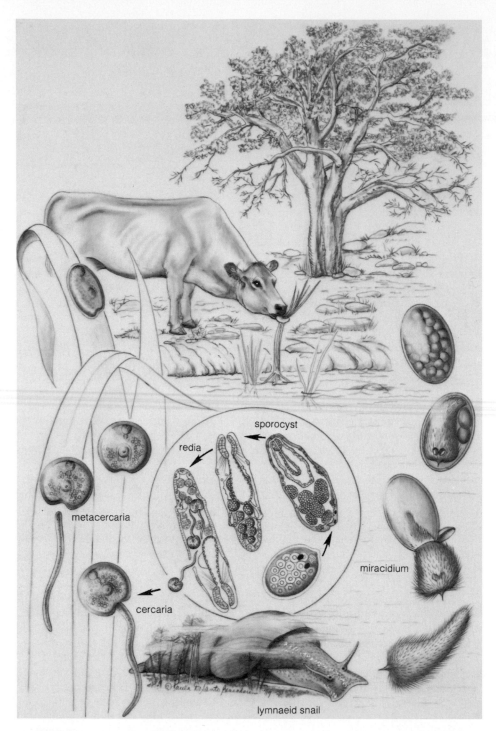

FIGURE 3-1 Life history of *Fasciola hepatica*. The adult liver flukes produce fertile eggs that leave the host by way of the common bile duct and intestinal tract. If these eggs are carried to water, a ciliated miracidium develops within them over a period of several weeks or months, depending on the temperature of the water. On hatching, the miracidia seek certain species of Lymnaeid snails in which they develop and multiply through one generation of sporocysts and two of rediae. The second generation of rediae produce free-swimming cercariae that leave the snail and encyst as metacercariae on various submerged objects, including aquatic vegetation. Ruminants and other animals become infected with *F. hepatica* when they ingest aquatic plants contaminated with metacercariae.

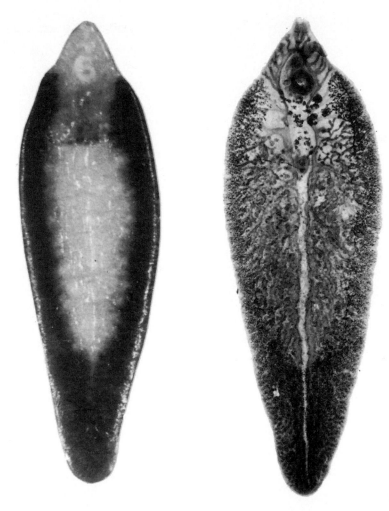

FIGURE 3-2 Adult *Fasciola hepatica* liver fluke. *Left,* An uncleared specimen; *right,* a cleared, stained specimen (×6.5).

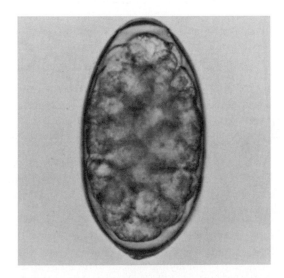

FIGURE 3-3 Egg of *Fasciola hepatica* from a sheep's bile duct (×380).

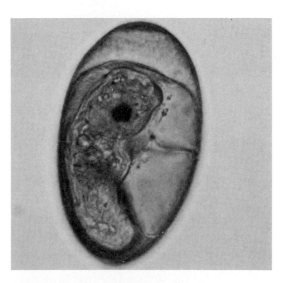

FIGURE 3-4 Egg of *Fasciola hepatica* containing a fully developed miracidium (×380).

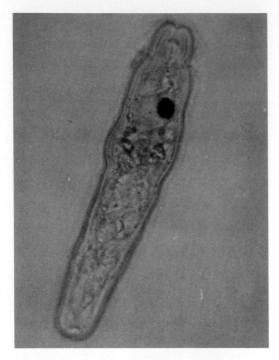

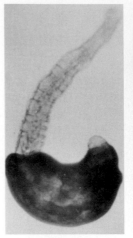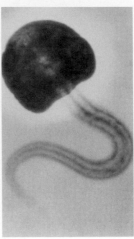

FIGURE 3-7   Cercariae of *Fasciola hepatica*. (Electronic flash photomicrograph, approx. ×125.)

FIGURE 3-5   Miracidium of *Fasciola hepatica* swimming; electronic flash photomicrograph (approx. ×400).

cell, by growth and repeated divisions, becomes a **germinal ball,** and each germinal ball develops into a **redia** (Figure 3-6).

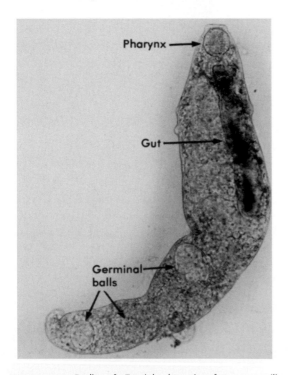

FIGURE 3-6   Redia of *Fasciola hepatica* from a snail's digestive gland (×90).

The rediae grow until they burst the sporocyst wall and are thus liberated into the tissues of the snail. The redia has a mouth and digestive organs and eats its way through the snail's tissues. Like the sporocyst, the redia is packed with germinal balls, these being the progenitors of a second generation of rediae. Each germinal ball of second-generation rediae develops into yet a third kind of larva, the **cercaria** (Figure 3-7).

The cercaria is a tadpolelike larva with a discoidal body and a long tail for swimming. The cercaria displays certain adult organs (e.g., oral and ventral suckers, mouth, pharynx, forked intestine, and excretory canals with flame cells) and primordia of the reproductive organs. Special secretory cells alongside the pharynx are purely larval structures; they secrete a cyst wall within which the final larval stage will lie in wait for a grazing ruminant. When fully developed in a month or two of summer temperatures, the cercaria leaves the redia through a birth pore and makes its way out through the snail's tissues and into the surrounding water. After a brief swim, the cercaria migrates a short distance above the water level on the surface of some plant and encysts, losing its tail in the process to become a **metacercaria,** the stage that is infective to sheep and other grazing mammals (Figure 3-8).

When ingested, the metacercarial cyst is digested in the host's small intestine. The young fluke, now called a **marita,** penetrates the wall of the intestine and crosses the peritoneal space to the liver, which it penetrates. After several weeks of boring about in the hepatic parenchyma, the maritas enter the bile ducts, mature into adult flukes, and begin laying eggs at about a month and a half after infection. The complete life cycle of *F. hepatica* thus encompasses 3 or 4 months under

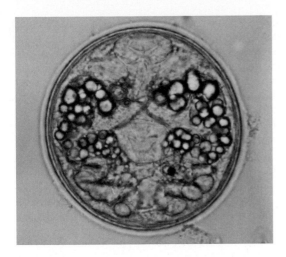

FIGURE 3-8   Metacercaria of *Fasciola hepatica* (×250).

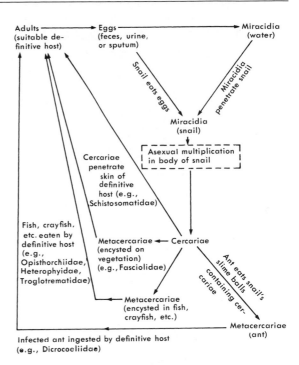

FIGURE 3-9   Some life history variations followed by trematode parasites of domestic animals.

favorable conditions. Therefore exposure to this parasite and patent infection tend to be rather more widely separated in time than is the case of most ruminant parasitisms.

Digenean trematodes are very discriminating in their choice of snail hosts, and the geographical distribution of trematode species is therefore largely dictated by the geographic distribution of suitable species of snails. Adult trematodes, on the other hand, seem to be able to make do with a rather broad range of definitive host species.

The metacercarial stage determines what food the host must eat to obtain an infection with an adult fluke. The strategies used by different trematodes vary (Figure 3-9). The metacercariae of asciolids and paramphistomatids encyst on vegetation and have a strategic advantage when it comes to getting into grazing ruminants. For the troglotrematids, heterophyids, and opisthorchiids, the metacercariae encyst in intermediate hosts such as fish, crayfish, and crabs, and fish-eating mammals tend to serve as the final hosts. The diplostomatids are found within amphibia or other vertebrate paratenic hosts, whereas the dicrocoeliids encyst in arthropods. The schistosomatids differ from other trematodes in that there is no metacercarial stage; rather, the cercariae penetrate the skin of the final host. Sometimes humans eat foodstuffs that put them in contact with possible trematode infections (e.g., *F. hepatica* has found its way into humans by way of watercress, and *Dicrocoelium dendriticum* has entered humans through the ingestion of ants containing metacercariae).

Identification

An adult trematode is typically little more than a bag of reproductive organs with both sexes represented. Typically, there are two testes and one ovary, the anatomical positions of which provide diagnostic criteria. The genital pore may be identified by the convergence of male and female reproductive ducts. Usually the presence of a cirrus, or intromittent organ, helps to identify the male duct and a procession of well-tanned eggs the female duct. The oral sucker surrounds the mouth, which is connected by way of the esophagus to a pair of blind ceca. The ceca are simple tubular sacs in most species but are intricately branched in the family Fasciolidae. The ventral sucker or acetabulum is often but not always near the genital pore. In the family Heterophyidae, both the ventral sucker and the genital pore are enclosed in an invagination, the ventrogenital sac, and an extra genital sucker or gonotyl surrounds the genital opening. The anatomical structures most used as taxonomic characters are labeled in Figure 3-10. Diagnostic criteria sufficient for identification of these families are presented in the following discussion. In general, identification of trematodes to family level combined with the host and organ listings provided in Chapter 5 will result in sufficiently precise diagnosis to serve practical needs. An excellent guide to the identification of families and genera of trematodes of North America north of Mexico is S.C. Schell's *Handbook of Trematodes of North America North of Mexico* (Moscow, Idaho, 1985, University Press of Idaho). Because only a limited

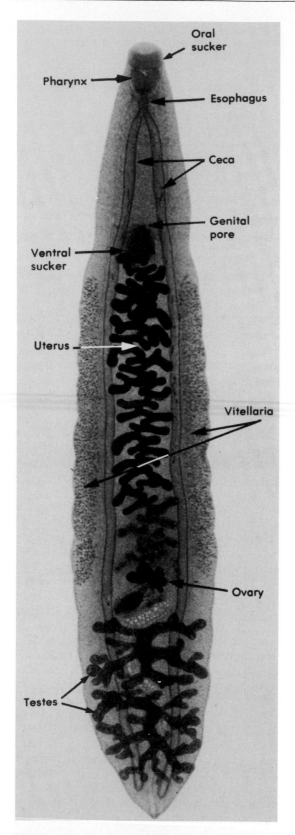

FIGURE 3-10 *Clonorchis sinensis* (Opisthorchiidae; ×30).

set of trematode species is likely to be found in domestic animals in any particular locality, knowledge of the endemic species is valuable. Sometimes the only way to acquire this information is to submit collections for expert identification. The specimens should be relaxed by overnight storage at 5° C and fixed in formaldehyde and acetic acid in alcohol (FAA) or shipped fresh and packed in plenty of ice in a well-insulated container.

A Few Representative Families of Trematodes

Trematodes Acquired by Eating Metacercariae Encysted on Vegetation

Family Fasciolidae

IDENTIFICATION. The body is large and leaflike with suckers close together at the anterior end; the ceca have numerous diverticula; and the ovary and testes are dendritic (see Figures 3-2 and 3-11). *F. hepatica, Fasciola gigantica,* and *Fascioloides magna* are parasites of the liver and bile ducts of herbivorous mammals and man. *Fasciolopsis buski* is a parasite of the small intestine of pigs and humans in Asia; the ceca of this species do not have diverticula. Antemortem diagnosis of chronic fascioliasis is by demonstration of the large operculate eggs (see Figure 3-3) in the feces. Saturated sucrose floats but distorts the eggs, which nevertheless remain recognizable. Sedimentation techniques are preferred, however.

LIFE HISTORY. The life history of *F. hepatica,* as presented in the preceding section, is typical of the family. The geographic distribution of *F. hepatica* is worldwide but discontinuous. In North America, *F. hepatica* is found in the Gulf Coast States, Pacific Northwest, the Caribbean, and eastern Canada. The lymnaeid snails that serve as intermediate hosts require neutral soils that remain reasonably moist throughout the year and tend to flourish where winters are not so cold as to destroy the eggs and juvenile stages, thus permitting the parasite population to survive its season of hardship in both definitive host and environment. Because soil characteristics may vary dramatically within very short distances, it is not uncommon for one "fluky pasture" to contain all of the *F. hepatica* snails and metacercariae, whereas the rest of the farm may afford safe grazing. Small streams, ponds, and marshy areas are obvious snail-breeding areas, but any depression (e.g., rut, dead furrow) that can hold a bit of water for a while can serve as a source of infection during periods of adequate rainfall.

Transmission of fascioliasis occurs between February and July in Louisiana (Malone et al, 1984), but in the northwestern states transmission

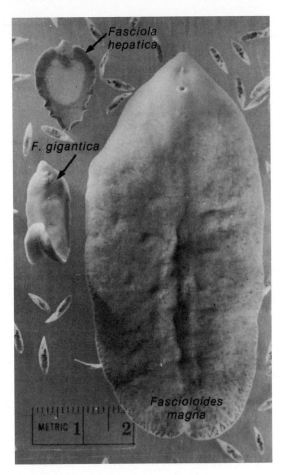

FIGURE 3-11 Liver flukes of ruminants. *Fasciola hepatica*, *Fascioloa gigantica*, and *Fascioloides magna* belong to the family Fasciolidae. The small flukes scattered about are *Dicrocoelium dendriticum* of the family Dicrocoeliidae.

F. magna, one of the largest known trematodes, is widely scattered over North America. Adult *F. magna* are found in cysts that communicate with the bile ducts of its normal definitive host, the white-tailed deer *(Odocoileus virginianus).* In cattle, these cysts usually do not communicate with the bile ducts, and in sheep and goats *F. magna* maritas fail to mature and the juvenile flukes wander aimlessly and destructively in the liver tissue. Therefore *F. magna* infection is nonpatent in cattle, sheep, and goats and cannot be diagnosed by fecal examination in these hosts. Aimlessly migrating *F. magna* maritas are likewise very destructive in llamas, dama deer, sika deer, and other cervids in game farms and "petting zoos" where white-tailed deer probably serve as the source of infection.

IMPORTANCE. Several clinical syndromes may be associated with liver fluke infection, depending on the numbers and stage of development of the parasite and on the presence or absence of *Clostridium novyi.* **Acute fluke disease** occurs during invasion of the liver by recently ingested metacercariae. In heavy invasions, the trauma inflicted by the maritas tunneling about in the liver and consequent inflammatory reaction result in highly fatal clinical illness characterized by abdominal pain with a disinclination to move. Postmortem examination reveals an abdominal cavity containing blood-stained exudate and an enlarged, friable liver covered with fibrin tags; large numbers of maritas can be recovered from the cut surfaces. Heavy invasions of the sort associated with acute fluke disease may occur when lambs are turned into pastures containing marshy areas that were heavily contaminated the previous season.

In certain cases, all that is needed to precipitate rapidly fatal disease is a minor trauma that provides clostridial organisms with some damaged and poorly oxygenated tissue in which to multiply and secrete their deadly toxins. Even the minor trauma associated with the migrations of a few *F. hepatica* (or *Taenia hydatigena* larvae) is enough to provide an appropriate environment for *C. novyi.* As is typical of clostridial infections, sheep die so fast that they hardly have time to be sick. Necropsy reveals focal liver necrosis and extensive subcutaneous hemorrhage; the latter is possibly responsible for the colloquial name "black disease." *C. novyi* also causes a lethal condition called *big head* in young rams, but here the precipitating trauma results from contests of physical prowess instead of parasite migrations.

Chronic fluke disease is associated with the presence of adult trematodes in the bile ducts and characterized by the classical clinical signs of liver fluke infection. There is gradual loss of condition,

gradually builds through the pasture season and reaches a peak during November (Hoover et al, 1984). Summer drought tends to interrupt the cycle on the Gulf Coast, whereas winter cold tends to do the same in the Northwest. However, special circumstances may produce unexpected results. For example, outbreaks of fascioliasis during periods of drought form an apparent paradox that can be explained as follows. When drought has laid waste to the rest of the pasture, green vegetation is still to be found at the water hole, and livestock may be forced to graze on aquatic plants, which they ordinarily eschew as unpalatable. Such plants are likely to be heavily contaminated with the resistant metacercariae of *F. hepatica,* and concentrated grazing on them may result in serious levels of infection. Because metacercariae are extremely resistant to drying, infection may follow feeding of hay grown on infested meadows far removed from the scene of an outbreak.

progressive weakness, anemia, and hypoproteinemia with development of edematous subcutaneous swellings, especially in the intermandibular space and over the abdomen. Necropsy reveals distended, thickened bile ducts packed with adult trematodes. In cattle, the fibrotic ducts later calcify to produce what looks like a branching system of clay pipes. Isseroff, Sawma, and Reino (1977) demonstrated that the bile duct hyperplasia of fascioliasis is related to the excretion of large amounts of the amino acid proline by *F. hepatica*. Isseroff et al (1979) have adduced evidence to the effect that proline synthesis and excretion by *F. hepatica* may account, at least in part, for the anemia that often accompanies infection with this fluke.

The presence of one fluke leads to condemnation of the liver in slaughtering establishments inspected by the U.S. Department of Agriculture (USDA). Tindall (1985) reported that almost one third of livers from cattle raised in Puerto Rico were condemned during the year ending in October 1984. Following Puerto Rico, in order of percentage of livers condemned, were Florida, Nevada, Oregon, Idaho, Utah, Washington, and California. Probably, liver condemnations far outweigh losses caused by clinical fascioliasis in economic importance.

F. magna causes considerable economic loss by producing wasted cattle livers condemned as unfit for human consumption, and its destructive migrations in the livers of sheep and goats virtually preclude small ruminant production in endemic areas.

TREATMENT AND CONTROL. Clorsulon (Curatrem) is administered to cattle orally as 8.5% suspension at a dosage rate of 7 mg/kg for treatment of immature and adult *F. hepatica* infections (Malone, Ramsey, and Loyacano, 1984; Courtney et al, 1985; Yazwinski et al, 1985). The dose of clorsulon (2 mg/kg) administered with ivermectin as Ivomec Plus is only efficacious against the adults of *F. hepatica*. Clorsulon is not licensed for use in dairy cattle of breeding age, and cattle must not be treated within 8 days of slaughter.

Albendazole is indicated for the removal of liver fluke from cattle at a dosage rate of 10 mg/kg of body weight and from sheep at 7.5 mg/kg. Albendazole is not licensed for use in dairy cattle of breeding ages, and cattle must not be treated within 27 days of slaughter. Albendazole (15 mg/kg) was effective in eliminating adult *F. hepatica* and in reducing the death rate among naturally infected goats in Montana (Leathers et al, 1982).

Other effective flukicides (diamphenethide, nitroxynil, oxyclozanide, rafoxanide, triclabendazole) are not available in the United States.

F. magna presents a more difficult problem in domestic ruminants. Both clorsulon (24 mg/kg) and albendazole (26 mg/kg) were reasonably effective against immature and adult *F. magna* in its natural host, the white-tailed deer (Foreyt and Drawe, 1985). However, a drug must kill essentially all immature *F. magna* to benefit infected sheep and goats because survival of only a few maritas is potentially lethal in these hosts. In sheep, a single treatment with clorsulon (15 mg/kg) 8 weeks after inoculation with metacercariae of *F. magna* was not sufficiently effective to be of practical value (Conboy et al, 1988), whereas closantel (15 mg/kg orally or 7.5 mg/kg intramuscularly) was considered to "meet the need" (Stromberg et al, 1985). Unfortunately, closantel is unavailable to veterinarians in the United States.

Theoretically, aquatic snails can be controlled by draining swamps or by broadcasting molluscicides on the snail-infested waters. However, the continued existence of flukes where they have always been indicates that snail control measures are impracticable in many cases. Areas connected by streams with other snail-infested regions are generally not amenable to snail control measures. Periodic anthelmintic medication may help to reduce contamination of pastures with fluke eggs. When periods of drought or cold destroy *F. hepatica* eggs and snails weakened by infection with this parasite, control measures based on anthelmintic medication alone may produce satisfactory results. On the other hand, when large populations of eggs and infected snails are able to survive the year around, these must be attacked directly as well.

Family Paramphistomadtidae

IDENTIFICATION. The ventral sucker is at the posterior end of the body; the ventral sucker of other trematodes is either on the ventral surface of the body or absent (Figure 3-12). Genera include *Paramphistomum, Calicophoron,* and *Cotylophoron* (rumen flukes), *Gastrodiscoides hominis* (a parasite of the intestine of humans, monkeys, and apes), and *Megalodiscus* spp. (parasites of the colon and cloaca of frogs).

LIFE HISTORIES. Eggs of *Paramphistomum cervi* are undeveloped when passed in the feces of cattle, sheep, and goats. Miracidia develop in eggs deposited in water and hatch to invade snails of the genera *Physa, Bulinus, Galba,* and *Pseudosuccinea,* in which cercariae develop through one sporocyst and two redial stages. On emergence from the snail, the cercaria swims away to encyst on aquatic vegetation. Thus the extramammalian portion of the life history of *Paramphistomum* genus is very much like that of Fasciola. Metacercariae of *Paramphistomum* species excyst in the upper small intestine and migrate through the abomasum back to the rumen. In heavy infections, migration to the rumen tends to be prolonged, and disease of several

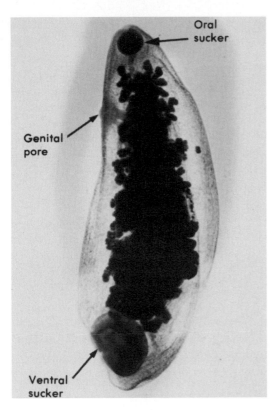

FIGURE 3-12 A "rumen fluke" of the family Paramphistomatidae (×16).

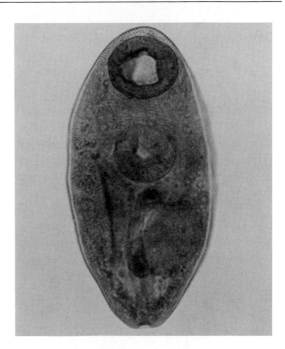

FIGURE 3-13 *Nanophyetus salmincola* (Troglotrematidae; ×108).

months' duration may result. Once arrived in the rumen and reticulum, the adult paramphistomes are relatively harmless (Rolfe and Boray, 1987).

Instead of encysting on aquatic vegetation as do other paramphistomatids, *Megalodiscus* cercariae encyst on the skin of frogs and tadpoles. The frogs become infected when they eat pieces of molted epidermis or tadpoles bearing metacercariae.

TREATMENT. Clorsulon at 2 mg/kg in combination with ivermectin at 0.2 mg/kg was ineffective in treating immature rumen flukes (Rolfe and Boray, 1993). Hexachlorophene in a single dose of 20 mg/kg and oxyclozanide in two doses of 19 mg/kg 3 days apart were both highly efficient against juvenile and adult paramphistome flukes, predominantly *Calicophoron calicophorum*, in cattle (Rolfe and Boray, 1987). Unfortunately, neither of these chemicals is available for use in domestic ruminants in the United States.

Trematodes Acquired by Eating Fish, Crayfish, Crabs, and Other Intermediate Hosts

Family Troglotrematidae

IDENTIFICATION. The genital pore is immediately posterior to the ventral sucker; the genital pore of other trematodes is located elsewhere. The location of the genital pore and the fact that the testes lie opposite one another are the only characteristics that unite the diverse assemblage of genera thrown together in the family Troglotrematidae. Troglotrematids of veterinary importance are parasites of the intestines (*Nanophyetus* sp., Figure 3-13) or lungs (*Paragonimus* sp., Figures 3-14 and 3-15).

LIFE HISTORIES. *Nanophyetus salmincola* adults parasitize the small intestine of piscivorous carnivorans of the Pacific Northwest. Eggs are undeveloped when passed in the host's feces. Miracidia require about 3 months to develop in eggs laid in water and hatch spontaneously still later. The miracidia penetrate the freshwater snail *Oxytrema silicula* in which cercariae develop in rediae. After emergence from the snail, these cercariae penetrate the skin of salmonid fishes and

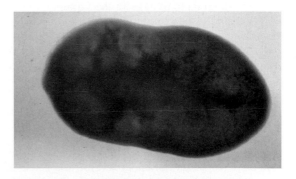

FIGURE 3-14 *Paragonimus kellicotti*, living adult worm recovered at necropsy from a cyst in the lung of a cat (Troglotrematidae; ×9).

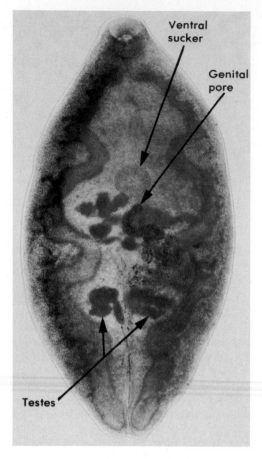

FIGURE 3-15 *Paragonimus kellicotti* (Troglotrematidae; ×13).

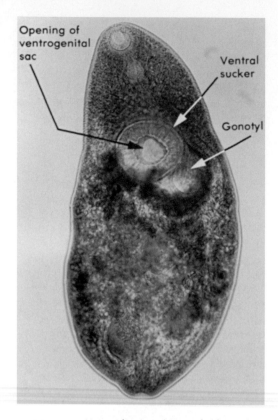

FIGURE 3-16 *Heterophyes* sp. (Heterophyidae; ×8). (Courtesy Dr. John Pearson, University of Queensland.)

encyst in various tissues. Eating salmon or trout infected with metacercariae of this trematode infects the dog, cat, coyote, fox, bear, raccoon, or mink. *N. salmincola* is host in turn to a rickettsial agent, *Neorickettsia helminthoeca*, the etiological agent of "salmon poisoning" in dogs. Salmon poisoning, characterized by hemorrhagic enteritis and lymph node enlargement, is diagnosed by the presence of trematode eggs in the patient's feces, and is usually fatal unless treated with broad-spectrum antibiotics.

Paragonimus kellicotti occurs, usually in pairs, in pulmonary cysts. Cats, dogs, and many species of wild mammals in North America may become infected by eating crayfish containing the encysted cercariae or by eating animals that have recently fed on crayfish. The large, vase-shaped eggs (see Figure 5-20) are swept up the tracheobronchial tree, swallowed, and passed out with the feces. If the eggs arrive in water, miracidia develop and hatch in about 2 weeks and enter an operculate snail, *Pomatiopsis lapidaria,* in which cercariae develop through one sporocyst and two redial stages. The cercariae leave the snail and encyst as metacercariae in crayfish. Radiographically demonstrable cysts develop in the lungs of cats at 28 days, and eggs are first shed in the feces about a month after infection. Signs of respiratory disease may be associated with *P. kellicotti* infection.

TREATMENT. Praziquantel, 23 mg/kg 3 times a day for 3 days, has been shown to be highly efficacious in removing *P. kellicotti* from the lungs of cats and dogs (Bowman et al, 1991). Fenbendazole, 50 mg/kg for 10 to 14 days, is also highly effective against these lung flukes (Dubey et al, 1979), as is albendazole, at a dosage rate of 25 mg/kg twice daily for 14 days. Praziquantel, 7 mg to 38 mg administered subcutaneously or intramuscularly, has also been shown to be highly effective in the removal of *N. salmincola* from dogs and coyotes (Foreyt and Gorham, 1988).

Family Heterophyidae

IDENTIFICATION. The ventral sucker and genital pore are withdrawn in a ventrogenital sac; one or more **gonotyls** (muscular suckers surrounding the genital pore) may be present (Figure 3-16). *Metagonimus yokagawi* and *Heterophyes heterophyes* are parasites of cats, dogs, pigs, and humans in East

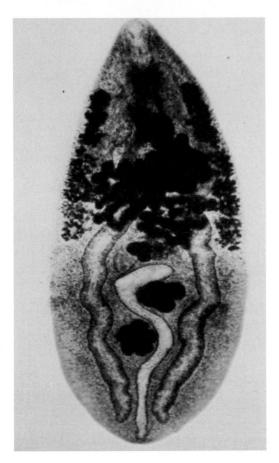

FIGURE 3-17 *Parametorchis* sp. (Opisthorchiidae; ×50).

Asia; infection is acquired by eating insufficiently cooked fish in which metacercariae have encysted. *Cryptocotyle lingua*, a parasite of gulls and terns, produces severe enteritis in dogs, foxes, and minks a few days after they have eaten a small North Atlantic fish, the cunner, in which metacercariae are found in the subcutaneous tissues surrounded by black host capsules. The appearance of infected fish leads to the colloquial name "black spot disease." A black host capsule is also observed surrounding various other species of trematode metacercariae and is not peculiar to *C. lingua*. Cercariae of *C. lingua* develop in the periwinkle *Littorina littorea*, a marine snail.

Family Opisthorchiidae

IDENTIFICATION. The uterus and ovary are anterior to the testes. There is no cirrus sac, and the genital pore is immediately anterior to the ventral sucker of these flat, translucent, fusiform, or oval parasites of the bile and pancreatic ducts of mammals, birds, and reptiles (see Figures 3-10 and 3-17). Opisthorchiids might be confused with dicrocoeliids because they are similar in size, shape, and location

in the host, but in dicrocoeliids, the ovary is posterior to the testes. Species include *Opisthorchis tenuicollis, Opisthorchis felineus, Metorchis conjunctus, Metorchis albidus, Parametorchis complexus, Clonorchis sinensis,* and others.

LIFE HISTORY OF OPISTHORCHIS TENUICOLLIS. The adult trematodes are parasites of the bile and pancreatic ducts and small intestine of dogs, cats, foxes, pigs, and humans. When deposited in the host's feces, eggs containing miracidia are eaten by a snail *Bithynia tentaculata*, in which cercariae develop in rediae. The cercariae encyst as metacercariae in carp, bream, and roach. The definitive host becomes infected by eating these freshwater fish.

IMPORTANCE. Opisthorchids display a rather low order of host specificity, and each species is capable of infecting many species of fish-eating mammals. Uncomplicated infection with moderate numbers of opisthorchiids is usually asymptomatic, but chronic infection with heavy worm burdens may lead to severe hepatic insufficiency.

TREATMENT. Lienert (1962) used hexachlorophene in a single oral dose of 20 mg/kg for the treatment of opisthorchiasis in dogs and cats. Praziquantel at 100 mg/kg should be efficacious.

Trematodes Acquired by Eating Arthropods or Vertebrate Paratenic Hosts

Family Dicrocoeliidae

IDENTIFICATION. The body is translucent. The ovary is posterior to the testes of these parasites of the gallbladder and bile and pancreatic ducts of mammals, birds, and reptiles (Figures 3-18 and 3-19).

LIFE HISTORY OF *DICROCOELIUM DENDRITICUM*. Whereas most trematode life histories involve water, this species is adapted to a sequence of hosts that frequent dry habitats. Adult *D. dendriticum* are parasites of the bile ducts of sheep, cattle, pigs, deer, woodchucks, and cottontail rabbits. Embryonated eggs deposited in the host's droppings are ingested by the terrestrial snail *Cionella lubrica* in which long-tailed cercariae develop in daughter sporocysts. As the cercariae leave the sporocysts, the snail secretes mucus around masses of them to form so-called slime balls in which they are expelled from the snail. The slime balls are apparently esteemed as food by the ant *Formica fusca*, in which the cercariae encyst as metacercariae. The definitive host becomes infected by inadvertently ingesting infected ants while grazing; the metacercariae excyst in the small intestine and migrate up the common bile duct into the finer ramifications of the biliary tree.

IMPORTANCE. *D. dendriticum* causes no clinical illness in cattle, lambs, or yearling sheep, but these trematodes are long-lived and the pathological

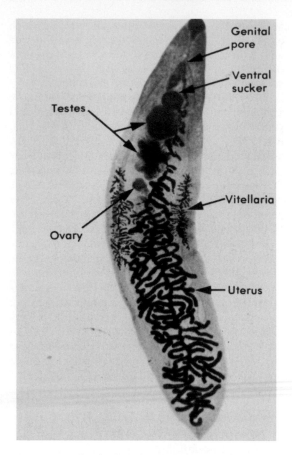

FIGURE 3-18 *Dicrocoelium dendriticum* (Dicrocoeliidae; ×25).

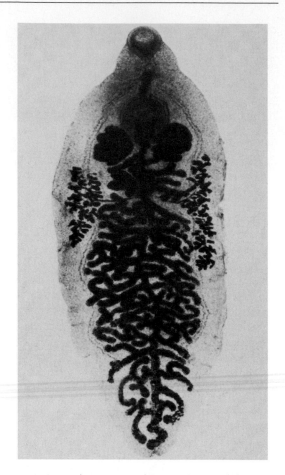

FIGURE 3-19 *Platynosomum fastosum* (Dicrocoeliidae; ×24).

changes in the liver increase in severity and extent with the duration of the infection. Therefore in older sheep, *D. dendriticum* infection causes progressive hepatic cirrhosis manifested clinically as cachexia, lowered wool production, decreased lactation, and premature aging. In short, *D. dendriticum* makes sheep husbandry unprofitable by curtailing the reproductive life of the ewe flock.

TREATMENT. Albendazole administered orally to sheep at 15 to 20 mg/kg is highly effective against adult *D. dentriticum* (Theodorides et al, 1982).

PLATYNOSOMUM FASTOSUM. This parasite of the bile and pancreatic ducts of cats occurs in the southeastern United States and the Caribbean (see Figure 3-19). Infection is acquired by eating lizards, toads, geckos, and skinks containing metacercariae (Chung et al, 1977; Eckerlin and Leigh, 1962).

TREATMENT. Nitroscanate, 100 mg/kg, and praziquantel, 20 mg/kg, markedly reduced the number of *Platynosomum* eggs passed in the feces of cats (Evans and Green, 1978). On the suggestion to a practitioner in Florida that it might be possible to treat platynosomiasis with elevated doses of praziquantel, the reply was that the last infected cat

presenting with hepatic dysfunction died when so treated. Thus it was thought that surgical removal of the flukes was the best course of therapy. Albendazole is another logical choice.

EURYTREMA PROCYONIS. This common parasite of the pancreatic duct of the raccoon was reported from a New York State domestic cat with a 2-year history of weight loss and vomiting probably resulting from pancreatic fibrosis and atrophy (Anderson et al, 1987). A cat infected with *E. procyonis* stopped shedding eggs in its feces after a 6-day course of 30 mg/kg of fenbendazole (Roudebush and Schmidt, 1982).

Trematodes Acquired by Eating Amphibia or Vertebrate Paratenic Hosts
Family Diplostomatidae

IDENTIFICATION. The body of these intestinal parasites of birds and mammals is divided into a flattened or spoon-shaped forebody containing oral and ventral suckers and a bulbous tribocytic organ, and a cylindrical hindbody containing the reproductive organs (Figure 3-20). The forebody will

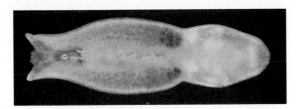

FIGURE 3-20 *Alaria canis* (Diplostomatidae, living specimen detached from mucosal epithelium showing the forebody and hindbody, with the forebody having a ventral groove for wrapping around a bit of host mucosa (×8).

wrap around the mucosa of the intestinal tract, forming a firm attachment between the fluke and the host's intestinal epithelium (Figure 3-21). Diplostomatids are most likely to be confused with members of the families Strigeidae, which have cup-shaped forebodies and leaflike tribocytic organs, and Cyathocotylidae, which have bulbous tribocytic organs but undivided bodies.

LIFE HISTORY OF *ALARIA* (FIGURE 3-22). The large, unembryonated egg (see Figure 5-20, *A*) is passed in the feces of the infected canid. If the egg is deposited in water, a miracidium develops and hatches in about 2 weeks to penetrate a snail of the genus *Helisoma* in which cercariae develop in daughter sporocysts. Each cercaria that succeeds in penetrating the skin of a tadpole transforms into a

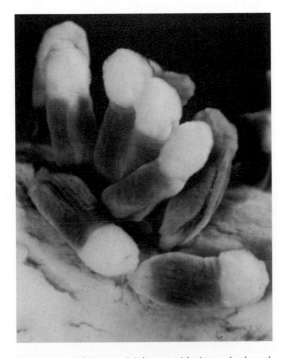

FIGURE 3-21 *Alaria* sp. (Diplostomatidae) attached to the mucosa of a dog's small intestine (×6.5).

special larval stage called a **mesocercaria,** which is limited to *Alaria* spp. and a few closely related genera. If the tadpole is eaten by a frog, snake, or mouse, the mesocercariae take up residence and wait for their new host to fall prey to a dog or other suitable definitive host. The frog, snake, or mouse that harbors these mesocercariae is called a **paratenic host** or **collector host,** which, by definition, is a host in which immature stages may survive indefinitely but undergo no essential development. The paratenic host helps to distribute the parasite in space and time and often bridges the gap of food preferences or overcomes some other obstacle to the union of parasite and definitive host. When a dog eats a paratenic host, the mesocercaria migrates directly through the diaphragm to the lungs, where it transforms into a metacercaria. In a few weeks, the metacercaria migrates up the trachea, is swallowed, and matures in the intestine. Eggs appear about 3 to 5 weeks after ingestion of mesocercariae (see Figure 3-22).

Mice infected with mesocercariae transmit *Alaria marcianae* to their sucklings through the milk and, when mature, these offspring can transmit the infection in the same fashion. If a female cat becomes infected with *A. marcianae* during lactation, the mesocercariae will not develop into metacercariae in her lungs but instead will migrate to her mammary glands to infect her kittens. The kittens then behave as definitive hosts and develop patent infections (Shoop and Corkum, 1984).

IMPORTANCE. Adult *Alaria* spp. are attached to the mucous membrane of the small intestine but apparently do their host little harm. However, because the mesocercariae migrate through the lungs and sometimes wander into other tissues, they may at times cause clinical illness. For example, a case of human infection with mesocercariae of *Alaria americana* terminated fatally as a result of extensive pulmonary hemorrhage. The circumstances suggested that the person had eaten inadequately cooked frogs' legs while hiking (Freeman et al, 1976).

TREATMENT. Infections with the adult trematode within the intestinal tract of dogs and cats can be treated with praziquantel and probably epsiprantel. The typical cestocidal dosage will be efficacious in most cases.

Families Allocreadiidae, Hemiuridae, and Lecithodendriidae

In the case of Potomac horse fever caused by *Erhlichia risticii,* it is thought that horses are becoming infected by the ingestion of caddis flies or mayflies containing the metacercariae of various trematodes (Madigan et al, 2000); one of six horses fed pools of aquatic insects became infected with *E. risticii* after being fed pools of mature caddis

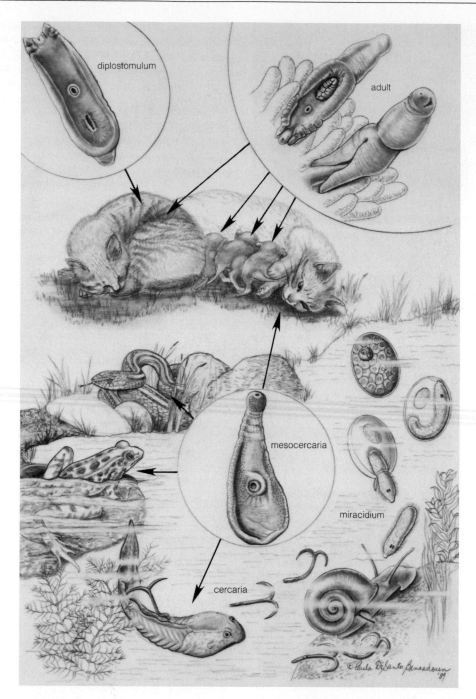

FIGURE 3-22 Life history of *Alaria marcianae* (Diplostomatidae). Miracidia develop in eggs deposited in water, hatch, and enter planorbid snails of the genus *Helisoma* where they develop into forked-tailed cercariae. Cercariae penetrate the skin and enter the tissues of tadpoles of the leopard frog *Rana pipiens* where, undergoing only minor changes, they remain as mesocercariae. If the tadpole is eaten by a frog, snake, bird, or mammal, the mesocercariae invade the tissues of these paratenic hosts but again remain mesocercariae. However, when mesocercariae in tadpoles or any of the paratenic hosts are ingested by a male or nonlactating female cat, they penetrate the diaphragm and develop into metacercariae of the diplostomulum type in the lungs. Finally, diplostomula pass up the trachea and down the esophagus to mature and reproduce in the small intestine. If mesocercariae are ingested by a lactating queen, they migrate to the mammary glands and are shed in the milk to develop into adult worms in the kittens. Some mesocercariae remain in the tissues of the queen to infect future litters.
(Diagram and notes modified from Pearson [1956] and Shoop and Corkum [1984a, 1984b].)

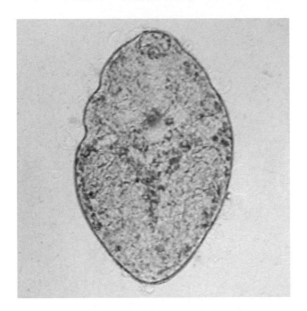

FIGURE 3-23 Lecithodendriid metacercaria recovered from a caddis fly in California incriminated as a vector of Potomac horse fever.
(Courtesy Dr. John E. Madigan, School of Veterinary Medicine, University of California, Davis, California.)

flies *(Discosmoecus gilvipes).* Operculate snails, *Elimia livescens* of the family Pleuroceridae, that were shedding virgulate cercariae (typically cercariae of the Lecithodendriidae) were dissected and the trematode cercariae and sporocysts were examined in pools for the presence of *E. risticii* DNA by amplification using the polymerase chain reaction (PCR). Of 209 pools of trematodes so examined, 50 were found to be positive for *E. risticii* DNA with PCR (Kanter et al, 2000). Trematodes of the family Lecithodendriidae are typically found in bats, so it is suspected that the cercariae from the snails go on to form metacercariae (Figure 3-23) in the aquatic larvae of various flies (e.g., caddis flies and mayflies) that are infectious to the bats after they become flying adults. Horses become infected when the adult flies fall into and are consumed with feed or water.

Another bit of the puzzle showed that an *Ehrlichia* sp. very closely related to *E. risticii* could be isolated from both the tissues and trematodes recovered from rainbow trout *(Oncorhynchus mykiss)* from a creek in northern California (Pusterla et al, 2000). The trematodes in this case were members of the genera *Deropegus* (family Hemiruidae) and *Crepidostomum* and *Creptotrema* (family Allocreadiidae). These trematodes live in the intestine and gall bladder of the trout as adults. The metacercarial stage is probably found in the larval stages of various aquatic flies (e.g., caddis flies and mayflies), although members of the family

Hemiuridae are thought to have larval stages mainly in crustacea. If this agent infects horses, it is thought that as with the trematodes of bats, the horses are infected by the ingestion of adult flies harboring the metacercarial stages of this parasite.

Trematodes Acquired by Skin Penetration
Family Schistosomatidae
Schistosomiasis caused by *Schistosoma mansoni, Schistosoma haematobium,* and *Schistosoma japonicum* is second only to malaria as a scourge of mankind, especially in the Caribbean area, South America, Africa, and Eastern Asia. Domestic animals in various tropical areas may be affected with *Schistosoma bovis* (cattle and sheep), *Schistosoma indicum* (horses, cattle, goats, and, in India, buffalo), *Schistosoma nasale* (cattle in India), *Schistosoma suis* (swine and dogs in India), and *Schistosoma matheei* (sheep, southern Africa). In Japan and the Philippines, *S. japonicum* is a serious parasite of human and animal alike. In North America, schistosomes present only two small problems: *Heterobilharzia americana,* a parasite of raccoon, nutria, bobcat, rabbit, and dog in the area extending from Florida along the Gulf Coast into Texas and north at least as far as Kansas, and "swimmer's itch," a dermatitis caused by cercariae of wild waterfowl schistosomes *(Trichobilharzia, Austrobilharzia,* and *Bilharziella* spp.) penetrating and abortively migrating in human skin. Of course, many cases of human schistosomiasis exist in North America among immigrants from endemic localities, but human schistosomiasis is unlikely to become endemic in the United States because the snail intermediate hosts *(Biomphalaria, Tropicorbis, Oncomelania,* and *Bulinus* spp.) do not occur here.

IDENTIFICATION. Sexes are separate, with the slender female lying in the gynecophoric canal of the somewhat stouter male (Figure 3-24). Adult schistosomes are parasites of veins of the digestive and urinary tracts of birds and mammals. Other trematodes are hermaphroditic and parasitize tissues other than blood vessels. Eggs lack an operculum and contain a fully developed miracidium when discharged in the feces (e.g., *S. mansoni, S. japonicum)* or urine (e.g., *S. haematobium);* eggs of some species are armed with a spine. Other trematode eggs have a polar operculum and lack a spine. Schistosome eggs hatch on exposure to water, so feces must be suspended in 0.85% sodium chloride (NaCl) solution when sedimenting eggs of these parasites. A miracidium hatching technique (Goff and Ronald, 1980) increases the probability of detecting patent *H. americana* infection in dogs. The eggs of *H. americana* are rather spherical and possess only a slight bump on

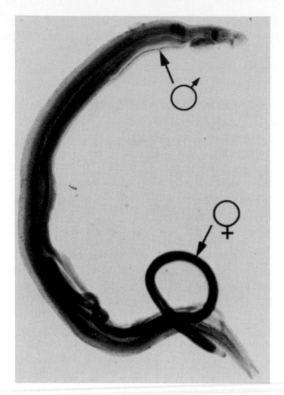

FIGURE 3-24 *Schistosoma* spp. (Schistosomatidae; ×24). The body of the slender female can be seen protruding from the gynecophoric groove of the stouter male.

one side rather than a spine as seen in *S. mansoni* and *S. haematobium*.

LIFE HISTORY OF *HETEROBILHARZIA AMERICANA*. The miracidium hatches soon after the egg comes in contact with water and then enters a freshwater snail, *Lymnaea cubensis,* in which cercariae develop in daughter sporocysts. On emergence from the snail, the cercariae penetrate the skin of a raccoon, nutria, bobcat, rabbit, or dog and migrate by way of the lungs to the liver. After a period of development in the liver, mature males and females make their way to the mesenteric veins and mate, the more or less cylindrical female lying in the gynecophoric groove of the male. The eggs, laid in the terminal branches of the mesenteric veins, passively work through the bowel wall to the lumen and escape with the feces. The eggs evoke a granulomatous reaction that eventually prevents their egress and favors their carriage to other organs, with the consequent production of widely disseminated granulomas. The life histories of other schistosomes differ only in detail from that of *H. americana*.

TREATMENT OF *HETEROBILHARZIA AMERICANA* INFECTION. Fenbendazole administered orally at 40 mg/kg for 10 days completely removed *H. americana* from one artificially infected dog, whereas an untreated control dog remained infected

(Ronald and Craig, 1983). Praziquantel and epsiprantel are also logical choices for treating *H. americana* infection.

Information on some trematodes of veterinary importance can be found in Table 3-1.

■ CLASS CESTODA

Tapeworms belong to the class Cestoda of the phylum Platyhelminthes and resemble trematodes in having acoelomate parenchymatous bodies and in having both sexes represented in the same individual. An adult tapeworm is essentially a chain (**strobila**) of independent, progressively maturing reproductive units, one end of which is capable of attachment to the wall of the host's intestine by a holdfast organ or **scolex.** In a fully developed adult tapeworm, all stages of development are displayed in a linear array starting at the scolex and terminating at the distal end. Although from a reproductive viewpoint a tapeworm appears to be a colony instead of an individual, all segments are served by common osmoregulatory and nervous systems, and the animal moves in a rhythmic and coordinated manner by means of the concerted activity of two zones of muscle fibers found in each segment. There are no organs of prehension or digestion; all nutrients are absorbed through the tapeworm's specialized integument. The body of an adult tapeworm is so flattened that for the purposes of argument it can be said to have two surfaces and two edges. This shape affords maximum surface area per unit volume, a distinct asset for an animal that absorbs all of its nourishment through its skin. Some tapeworms grow to considerable size. The strobila of *Taenia saginata,* for example, may contain as many as 2000 segments and reach a length of 3.6 m (30 feet) in the human small intestine (Arundel, 1972).

Two orders of the class Cestoda are of greatest interest to veterinarians: Pseudophyllidea and Cyclophyllidea. The order Pseudophyllidea is represented by only two genera of importance to most veterinarians: *Diphyllobothrium* and *Spirometra*. Both use copepods as the first intermediate host in which the **oncosphere** develops into a second-stage larva called a **procercoid.** The second intermediate host may be a fish, amphibian, or reptile and supports development of the procercoid into a third-stage larva called a **plerocercoid.** The definitive host becomes infected when it ingests a second intermediate host containing **plerocercoids.** Pseudophyllideans are associated with aquatic food chains. The order Cyclophyllidea contains five families of veterinary importance: Taeniidae, Mesocestoididae, Anoplocephalidae, Dipylidiidae, and Hymenolepididae. Most cyclophyllideans require only one

TABLE 3-1 ■ Information on Some Trematodes of Veterinary Importance

Family	Genera and species	Geographic distribution	Hosts	Location in host	Disease	Length of adult	Length of egg	Second intermediate host	Prepatent period
Fasciolidae	*Fasciola hepatica*	Tropics and U.S.	Herbivorus mammals and humans	Bile ducts	Hepatic fibrosis	3 cm	120 μm	Metacercariae on vegetation	60 days
	Fasciola gigantica	Africa	humans	Bile ducts	Hepatic fibrosis	5 cm	120 μm	Metacercariae on vegetation	60 days
	Fasciolopsis buskii	Asia	Pigs and humans	Intestine	Intestinal upset	8 cm	120 μm	Metacercariae on vegetation	90 days
	Fascioloides magna	U.S. and Europe	White-tailed deer	Liver (cysts)	Kills other ceruids, sheep, nonpatent cysts in cattle	10 cm	120 μm	Metacercariae on vegetation	270 days
Paramphistomidae	*Paramphistomum* and *Cotylophoron*	Worldwide	Ruminants	Rumen	Intestinal damage by immature flukes	10 mm	120 μm	Metacercariae on aquatic vegetation	80 days
Troglotrematidae	*Nanophyetus salmincola*	North Pacific rim	Dogs and cats	Intestine	Transmits *Neorickettsia helminthoeca*	1 mm	80 μm	Fish	7 days
	Paragonimus kellicotti	Eastern U.S.	Minks, dogs, cats	Lungs	Cysts in lungs	6 mm	90 μm	Crayfish	30 days
Heterophyidae	*Cryptocotyle*	U.S.: East coast	Birds	Intestine	Enteritis	2 mm	30 μm	Fish	14 days
	Heterophyes	Middle East	Dogs and cats	Intestine	Enteritis	2 mm	30 μm	Fish	14 days
Opisthorchidae	*Opisthorchis*	Asia and Europe	Dogs and cats	Bile ducts	Very little	6 mm	30 μm	Fish	30 days
	Metorchis	U.S.	Foxes, pigs	Bile ducts	Very little	6 mm	30 μm	Fish	17 days
	Clonorchis	Asia	Dogs and cat	Bile ducts	Very little	6 mm	30 μm	Fish	60 days
Dicrocoelidae	*Dicrocoelium dendriticum*	New York, Quebec, British Columbia, Europe	Sheep, cattle, pigs, deer, woodchucks	Bile ducts	Fibrosis with chronic disease	10 mm	40 μm	Ants	80 days

Continued

TABLE 3-1 ■ Information on Some Trematodes of Veterinary Importance—cont'd.

Family	Genera and species	Geographic distribution	Hosts	Location in host	Disease	Length of adult	Length of egg	Second intermediate host	Prepatent period
	Platynosum fastosum	Caribbean and southern U.S.	Cats	Bile ducts and gall bladder	Fibrosis, vomiting, jaundice, diarrhea	7 mm	45 µm	Lizards	30 days
Diplostomidae	*Alaria canis*	Northern U.S. and Canada	Dogs and foxes	Intestine	Very little	4 mm	100 µm	Frogs, paratenic hosts	35 days
	Alaria marcianae *Fibricola texensis*	Southern U.S.	Raccoons and opossums						
Schistosomatidae	*Schistosoma mansoni*	Worldwide	Humans	Mesenteric veins	Hepatic fibrosis	10–20 mm; sexes separate	55–145 µm; lateral spine	None, penetrate skin	60 days
	Schistosoma haematobium	Africa	Humans	Veins of urinary bladder	Erosion of bladder wall	10 mm; sexes separate	60 × 140 µm; terminal spine	None, penetrate skin	70–84 days
	Schistosoma japonicum	Asia	Humans, cats, mammals	Mesenteric veins	Hepatic fibrosis	10 mm; sexes separate	58 × 85 µm; no spine	None, penetrate skin	35–42 days
	Schistosoma bovis	Africa	Cattle	Mesenteric veins	Hepatic fibrosis	10 mm; sexes separate	62 × 207 µm; terminal spine	None, penetrate skin	42 days
	Schistosoma margrebowiei	Africa	Horses, ruminants	Mesenteric veins	Hepatic fibrosis	10 mm; sexes separate	60 × 80 µm; no spine	None, penetrate skin	38 days
	Bivitellobilharzia loxodontae	Africa	Elephants	Mesenteric veins	Hepatic fibrosis	10 mm; sexes separate	71 × 87 µm; no spine	None, penetrate skin	???
	Heterobilharzia americana	U.S.	Raccoons, dogs, opossums	Mesenteric veins	Hepatic fibrosis	10 mm; sexes separate	70 × 87 µm; no spine	None, penetrate skin	60 days
	Bird genera	Worldwide	Birds	Skin	Nonpatent dermatitis	10 mm; sexes separate		None, penetrate skin	Does not become patent

intermediate host. Depending on the family of tapeworm, the intermediate host may be a mammal (Taeniidae) or an arthropod (Anoplocephalidae, Dipylidiidae, Hymenolepididae). Members of the Mesocestoididae are thought to require two intermediate hosts, the second of which may be a mammal, bird, or reptile, but so far, the hypothesized second-stage larvae and first intermediate host have not been identified. Cyclophyllideans produce oncospheres with a protective capsule of embryonic membrane origin and are associated with terrestrial food chains.

Almost all tapeworms require at least two and some require three hosts to complete their life histories. *Vampirolepis* (=*Hymenolepis*; =*Rodentolepis*) *nana*, a cyclophyllidean parasite of mice and sometimes of humans, is exceptional in being able to complete its life history within the confines of a single individual.

Cestodes produce eggs that when fully developed contain a first-stage larva called an **oncosphere.** Oncospheres develop into second-stage larvae in the body cavities or tissues of an intermediate host. Usually, the second-stage larva is infective for the definitive host on ingestion. However, in certain prominent cases, the second-stage larva must first develop into a third-stage larva in a second intermediate host before it is ready to infect the definitive host. The **oncosphere** is the first-stage larva and is infective for the first (or only) intermediate host. The oncosphere consists of a **hexacanth** embryo surrounded by two embryonic membranes. The first-stage larva, or hexacanth embryo, is infective to the first intermediate host and develops in this host into a second-stage larva. In most cyclophyllideans of interest to us, there is only one intermediate host, and the second-stage larva is the stage infective to the definitive host in which it matures. In the Mesocestoididae (in which the second-stage larva is still hypothetical) and in the Pseudophyllidea, the second-stage larvae are infective to the second intermediate host in which it develops into a third-stage larva. The third-stage larvae of mesocestoidids and pseudophyllideans are the form infective for the definitive host. The second and third larval stages of these various tapeworms have their own names that are presented later in the discussion of their respective life histories.

In a teleological sense, the objective of larval development is to form a scolex in a kind of intermediate host that is likely, for one reason or another, to be ingested by a suitable definitive host. Because this objective has been reached in such diverse hosts as mites and cattle, there is considerably more variation in size and form among larval cestodes than among adults. It is at this point that uniformity of structure and function gives way to diversity. Therefore details of larval development are discussed in connection with life histories in the following characterization of cestode families.

When an infective tapeworm larva first arrives in the intestine of its definitive host, most of the infective larva's body is digested away, leaving only the scolex and a bit of undifferentiated tissue called the **neck.** The scolex attaches to the intestinal wall, and the neck begins to bud off segments. These segments remain attached to one another to form the chain mentioned previously. At first the segments remain undifferentiated, but ovaries, testes, vitellaria, and other reproductive organs gradually begin to take shape in the segments some distance removed from the neck. These reproductive organs gradually mature, eggs and sperm are formed, and fertilization occurs. Depending on the kind of tapeworm, the fertilized eggs either are discharged through a uterine pore or accumulate in the segment. Therefore the terminal segments of a mature tapeworm are found to be empty in the former case and packed full of eggs like ripe seedpods in the latter.

The anatomical details and nomenclature of the genitalia are important in detailed taxonomic work but need not be emphasized here because a reliable identification usually can be made on the basis of host identity and somewhat more accessible morphological features as outlined later. However, differences do exist between cyclophyllideans and pseudophyllideans that are important in diagnosis and in understanding their particular life histories.

Pseudophyllidean Tapeworms

The **holdfast** of pseudophyllideans has only two shallow, longitudinally grooved **bothria** for locomotion and attachment (Figure 3-25). The two most important genera, *Diphyllobothrium* and *Spirometra,* have no hooks to assist the weak grip of the bothria. The considerable area of contact between the long chain of broad segments and the intestinal mucosa apparently affords sufficient traction to maintain the tapeworm in place.

Pseudophyllidean segments have a uterine pore that permits the escape of eggs (Figure 3-26). Segments over a considerable length of the strobila discharge their eggs until their supply is exhausted. The terminal segments of pseudophyllidean tapeworms become senile rather than gravid and are usually detached in short chains rather than individually. Thus the diagnosis of pseudophyllidean infection depends on distinguishing the operculate eggs in fecal sediments from those of trematodes, which sometimes is not an easy matter.

The pseudophyllidean oncosphere and its two membranes are surrounded in turn by an operculate

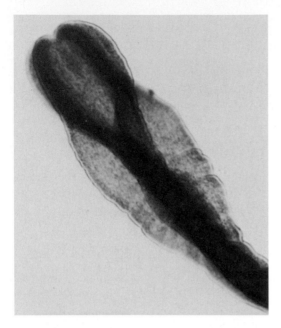

FIGURE 3-25 *Diphyllobothrium latum* (Diphyllobothriidae), scolex of stained, permanent mount (×50).

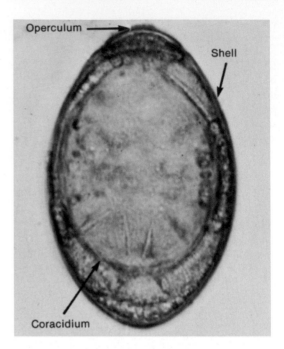

FIGURE 3-27 Egg of *Spirometra mansonoides* (Diphyllobothriidae) (×1300). The capsule of diphyllobothriid eggs is operculate; this one contains a fully developed coracidium.

shell (Figure 3-27). The outermost membrane remains behind in the shell when the oncosphere, now surrounded only by its ciliated inner membrane or **embryophore,** pops open the operculum of the shell and swims away (Figure 3-28). The ciliated pseudophyllidean oncosphere is called a **coracidium.**

Family Diphyllobothriidae

IDENTIFICATION. The scolex of *Diphyllobothrium latum* and *Spirometra mansonoides* has two slitlike grooves (see Figure 3-25). Mature segments are broader than long (see Figures 3-26 and 3-29). The uterus consists of a spiral tube with four to eight loops on each side and opens to the outside through

a midventral uterine pore behind the genital pore. The reproductive organs are concentrated at the centers of the segments (see Figure 3-29). Operculated eggs are discharged through the uterine pore.

LIFE HISTORY. Whereas cyclophyllidean development involves only one intermediate host, pseudophyllideans require at least two, of which the first

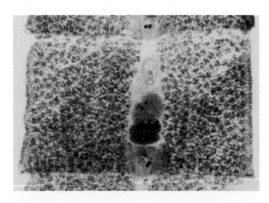

FIGURE 3-26 Mature segment of *Diphyllobothrium latum* (×60).

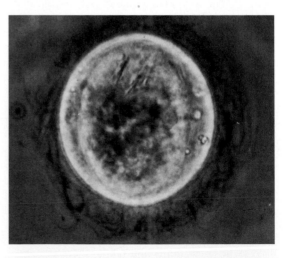

FIGURE 3-28 Coracidium of *Spirometra mansonoides*, phase contrast electronic flash photomicrograph of the free-swimming organism (×1200).
(Culture courtesy Dr. Justus Mueller [deceased].)

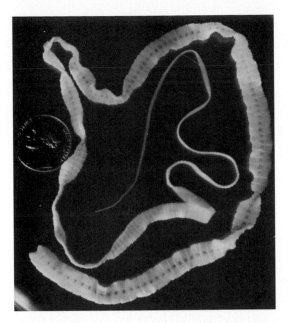

FIGURE 3-29 *Spirometra mansonoides* (Diphyllobothriidae), entire specimen from a cat. Notice how small the scolex is relative to the mature segments and also the central location of the genitalia throughout the length of the tapeworm.

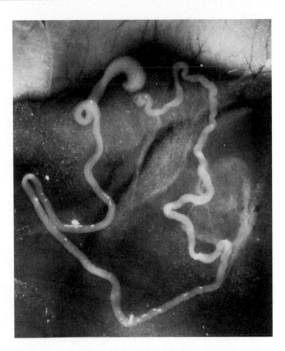

FIGURE 3-31 *Spirometra mansonoides* plerocercoid larva in the subcutaneous tissues of a white mouse. (Photograph courtesy Dr. Robert Smith [about twice natural size]; culture courtesy Dr. Justus Mueller [deceased].)

is a copepod and the second is a vertebrate. When ingested by a copepod, the **coracidium** (oncosphere with ciliated embryophore) develops into a solid wormlike **procercoid** within the body cavity (Figure 3-30). When the infected copepod is ingested by a second intermediate host, the procercoid enters its musculature or connective tissues and develops into a **plerocercoid** (Figure 3-31). The plerocercoid is notable for its ability to parasitize a series of predatory **paratenic hosts** until a suitable definitive host is found. Thus when a pike eats a minnow infected with the plerocercoids of *D. latum,* these merely invade the flesh of the pike and remain plerocercoids. However, when a human, a

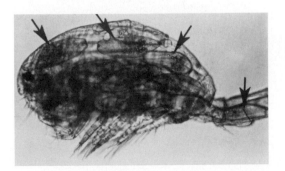

FIGURE 3-30 Copepod *(Cyclops vernalis)* with body cavity filled with procercoids of *Spirometra mansonoides*; electronic flash photomicrograph of living organisms (×70).

dog, or a cat eats either the minnow or the pike, the plerocercoid matures into an adult tapeworm with the **prepatent period** (i.e., the time between infection and the appearance of detectable stages, which in this case, are found in the feces) being about 5 or 6 weeks. *D. latum* procercoids develop in copepods of the genus *Diaptomus*, and its plerocercoids develop in fish. Definitive hosts of *D. latum* include humans, dogs, mongooses, walruses, seals, sea lions, bears, foxes, and minks (Wardle and McLeod, 1952). S. mansonoides procercoids develop in copepods of the genus *Cyclops*. Its plerocercoids develop in "any class of vertebrates except fishes"; even kittens fed procercoids support development of plerocercoids, which appear in the flat muscles of the body wall and subcutaneous fascia (Mueller, 1974). The natural intermediate host is probably the water snake *Natrix,* and the natural definitive host is probably the bobcat *Lynx rufus.* Other definitive hosts of *S. mansonoides* include the domestic cat and dog and the raccoon (Mueller, 1974). The life history is illustrated in Figure 3-32; animals can begin shedding eggs in the feces as soon as 10 days after the ingestion of the larval plerocercoid stage.

An Eastern Asian species, *Spirometra mansoni,* does use frogs, rabbits, and birds for development of the plerocercoid. Once upon a time not so very

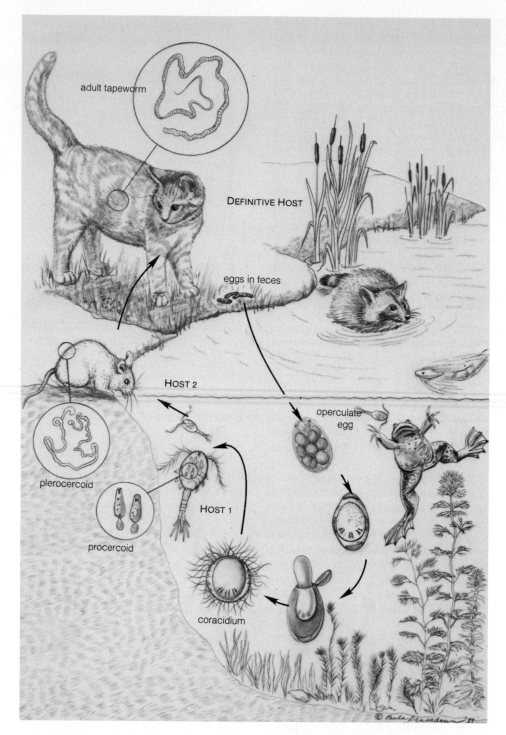

FIGURE 3-32 Life history of *Spirometra mansonoides*, a pseudophyllidean tapeworm. Coracidia develop and hatch from eggs deposited in water and swim about until they are ingested by copepods of the genus *Cyclops*. Shedding its ciliated coat, the hexacanth embryo develops into a procercoid larva in the body cavity of the copepod. If an infected copepod is swallowed by any vertebrate except a fish, the procercoids develop into plerocercoids, which tend to locate in the subcutaneous tissues and flat muscles of the body wall. Plerocercoids survive predation of their hosts and remain plerocercoids in their new hosts unless the new host happens to be a cat. Plerocercoids develop into adult *S. mansonoides* tapeworms in the small intestine of the domestic cat and bobcat.

long ago, it was the custom in parts of the Eastern Asia to apply the incised body of a freshly caught frog as a poultice to wounds, sore eyes, and the like. (This behavior is not so unlike the once common application of a raw steak to "reduce the bruising" associated with a black eye.) The plerocercoids of *S. mansoni*, if present in the tissues of the frog, would then transfer to the human host and migrate about in the subcutaneous connective tissues, a condition dubbed **sparganosis** in the human medical literature. The plerocercoids (**spargana**) of *S. mansonoides* are also capable of causing human sparganosis, as Mueller and Coulston (1941) demonstrated by experiments on themselves where they inserted spargana into the tissues of their arms.

D. *latum* and *S. mansonoides* are less obtrusive than other tapeworm parasites of dogs and cats because they do not detach segments but release their eggs more or less continuously through the uterine pores of their mature segments. Therefore the client usually is unaware of *Diphyllobothrium* and *Spirometra* infection unless a whole tapeworm or a long chain of senile segments is discharged at once. *Diphyllobothrium* infection is acquired by eating uncooked predatory freshwater fish. *S. mansonoides* can be passed experimentally from the copepod through such diverse second intermediate hosts as frogs and mice. In the type locality (Syracuse, New York), *Natrix*, a water snake, is frequently found infected with *S. mansonoides* plerocercoids.

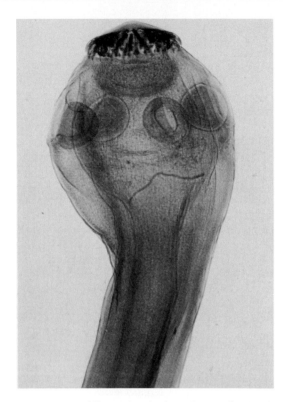

FIGURE 3-33 Holdfast and neck of *Taenia* spp., showing four suckers and nonretractable rostellum with hooks (×40).

Families of Cyclophyllidean Cestodes

Compared with the rest of the mature worm, which may be several meters long in the larger species, the **scolex** is minute, frequently measuring less than a millimeter. The cyclophyllidean scolex has four radially disposed muscular suckers that serve for attachment and locomotion (Figure 3-33). These suckers and the tissue immediately surrounding them are quite mobile. Dr. Georgi watched a severed scolex of *Taenia pisiformis* "walk" with remarkable agility across the bottom of a Petri dish. Each sucker in turn was advanced on a stalk of tissue and fixed to the bottom of the dish. Then the scolex was drawn toward the point of fixation by contraction of the stalk of tissue, another sucker advanced, and so on. At the apex of most cyclophyllidean scolices there is a dome-shaped projection, the **rostellum,** which is sometimes retractable into the scolex and may be armed with small hooks. In the family Taeniidae, a nonretractable rostellum is armed with two concentric rows of hooks. Strong muscles operate these hooks in a concerted and rhythmic clawing motion. The points are projected in a manner similar to a cat baring its claws, but in a centrifugal direction. This clawing motion ceases once the scolex has found safe anchorage in the intestinal wall. Cyclophyllidean families that lack rostellar hooks (e.g., Anoplocephalidae, Mesocestoididae) tend to have more strongly developed suckers to make up for it.

Segments of cyclophyllidean strobila have genital pores for fertilization but no opening to allow the eggs to escape from the uterus. Thus the eggs accumulate until the segment becomes packed full like a ripe seedpod. As they reach the end of the chain, these gravid segments are detached and pass out with the feces or crawl out the anus onto the perianal skin. Therefore cyclophyllidean infections are usually diagnosed by identifying gravid segments on the host or in its environment.

Cyclophyllidean oncospheres are fully developed when passed in the feces of the definitive host and are immediately infective for the intermediate host. These oncospheres lack a true shell and technically should not be called eggs, but most authors call them this and so shall we. The outer membrane of the cyclophyllidean oncosphere serves as a protective capsule in some species. However, the outer membrane of taeniid oncospheres is delicate and usually has been lost by the time they appear in a host's feces. The inner embryonic membrane

(embryophore) serves as a protective coat for the taeniid oncosphere. In anoplocephalids, the embryophore is a distinctive pear-shaped body **(pyriform apparatus),** and in taeniids it consists of a rather thick layer of prismatic blocks. The eggs of *Dipylidium caninum* are clustered in packets formed by outpocketings of the uterine wall.

Teratological development of cestode larvae is not at all uncommon, and occasionally cases are observed in which larval tapeworm tissue behaves much like a malignant neoplasm. For example, Williams et al (1985a) reported a fatal case of peritoneal cestodiasis in a dog from which parasites actually passed out through a poorly healing laparotomy incision, and 500 ml of parasite tissue was recovered from the peritoneal cavity at necropsy. The parasites were too abnormal both grossly and histologically to identify, even by careful comparison with specimens of the most likely candidates, *Mesocestoides corti, Taenia crassiceps,* and *Taenia multiceps.*

Family Taeniidae
Taenia

IDENTIFICATION. Adult tapeworms of the genus *Taenia* measure from tens to hundreds of centimeters in length, depending on the species in question and degree of maturity of the specimen. The scolex has four suckers and a nonretractable rostellum

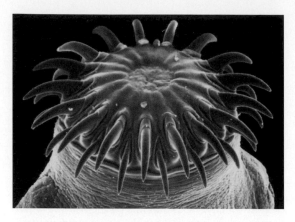

FIGURE 3-34 *Taenia taeniaeformis* (Taeniidae), scanning electron micrograph by Dr. Ronald Minor (×90). The rostellum of taeniid tapeworms is nonretractable and is armed with a row of long hooks and a concentric row of short hooks.

armed with two rows of hooks (see Figures 3-33 and 3-34). The segments are more or less rectangular with unilateral genital pores alternating irregularly from one side to the other along the strobila (Figure 3-35). The eggs in gravid segments are typical of the family (Figure 3-36). Differentiation of genera and species is based on number and sizes of rostellar hooks and on morphology of mature segments and may require the services of an expert (Verster, 1969).

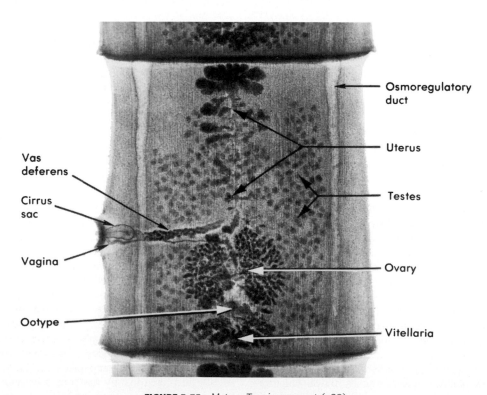

FIGURE 3-35 Mature *Taenia* segment (×22).

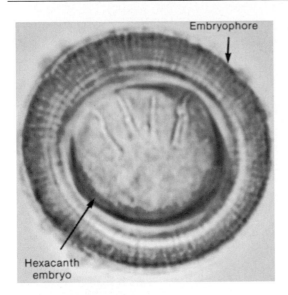

Embryophore

Hexacanth embryo

FIGURE 3-36 Egg of *Taenia taeniaeformis* (Taeniidae) of the cat (×2000). The capsule of taeniid eggs is fragile; eggs in fecal smears have usually lost their capsules.

LIFE HISTORY. Gravid taeniid segments (Figure 3-37) are shed and exit from the carnivorous definitive host through the anus. The segments crawl about on the pelage of the host or surface of the fecal mass, emptying themselves of their eggs (oncospheres) in the process. Therefore any segment collected after it has been out for more than a few minutes may contain few if any eggs. If ingested by a suitable vertebrate intermediate host (usually a species normally taken as prey by the definitive host), the egg hatches and the hexacanth embryo enters the wall of the intestine and migrates to its organ of predilection, usually the liver and peritoneal membranes or the skeletal and cardiac muscles. Here the hexacanth embryo grows, cavitates, and differentiates to form the second-stage larva, which is infective to the definitive host. The fully developed second-stage larva of the family Taeniidae consists of a fluid-filled bladder with one or more scolices (often called a **bladderworm**) and is surrounded by a connective tissue capsule formed by the vertebrate intermediate host.

Until the middle of the nineteenth century, the relationship of bladderworms to tapeworms was not recognized. Therefore different stages of the same species were described and named as distinct species belonging to separate phyla. For example, *Cysticercus cellulosae* was placed in the now defunct phylum Cystica, whereas its parent, *Taenia solium*, was referred to the defunct phylum Vermes. The older names of the larval stages are still occasionally used to identify the morphologically different larval stages of tapeworms. Such usage is

helpful in describing pathological specimens because it eliminates the need of writing "the cysticercus of *Taenia* such-and-such." However, because the specific names of the adult and larval stages often differ, these additional names can add to the confusion that sometimes surrounds the events in the development of different species of tapeworm. Thus their use has been minimized herein as much as possible.

When a second-stage larva is ingested by a suitable definitive host, the bladder is digested away, the scolex embeds itself in the mucosa of the small intestine, and the neck begins to bud off segments to form the strobila. Eggs of taeniid tapeworms first appear in the feces in 6 to 9 weeks after ingestion of the larva. Williams and Shearer (1982) observed a prepatent period of 34 to 80 days for *Taenia taeniaeformis* in cats, and the infections remained patent for 7 to 34 months.

There are four basic kinds of taeniid second-stage larvae: the **cysticercus, strobilocercus, coenurus,** and **hydatid.** Members of the genus *Taenia* typically form cysticerci, strobilocerci, and coenuri, depending on the species in question. A **cysticercus** (Figures 3-38 and 3-39) consists of a single bladder with one scolex. A **strobilocercus** (Figure 3-40) is a cysticercus that has already begun to elongate and segment while still in the intermediate host, and a **coenurus** (Figure 3-41) consists of a single bladder with many scolices, each with the potential of developing into a mature tapeworm. **Hydatids** are formed by members of the genus *Echinococcus* and are of two kinds, **unilocular hydatid cysts** and **alveolar hydatids,** both of which often contain thousands of scolices. Usually, one *Taenia* oncosphere develops into only one bladderworm. However, in the case of *T. crassiceps*, asexual multiplication (budding) results in many cysticeri surrounded by a single host-tissue capsule. Such a structure may easily be mistaken for a hydatid cyst by the unwary observer. Many coenuri branch and ramify extensively to form very complex structures (Figure 3-42), and teratological malformations may result in diverse and complex structures.

CYSTICERCOSIS. The cysticercus of the canine taeniid tapeworm *T. hydatigena* migrates through the liver tissue and encysts on the peritoneal membranes of cattle, sheep, swine, and certain wild ungulates. Massive invasions, such as when entire tapeworm segments are ingested, result in acute traumatic hepatitis, and even small numbers of migrating *T. hydatigena* larvae are capable of precipitating "black disease" in the presence of *C. novyi*. However, frank disease is rarely caused by this larval tapeworm, and the principal economic loss results from condemnation of infected livers by meat inspection authorities.

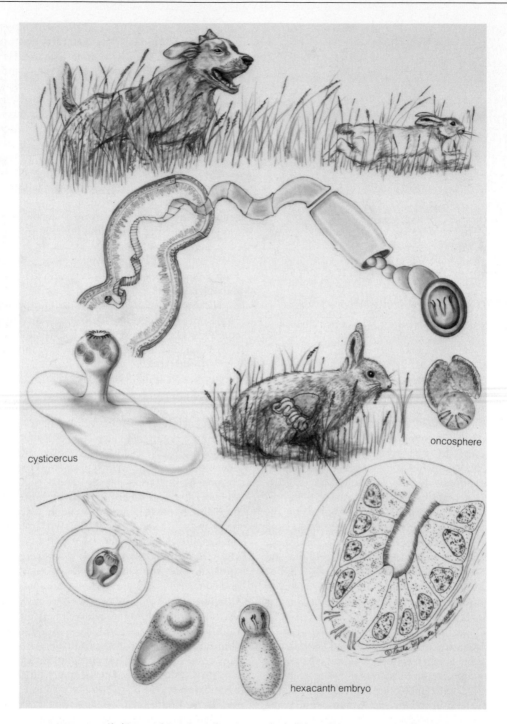

FIGURE 3-37 Life history of *Taenia pisiformis*, a cyclophyllidean tapeworm. Oncospheres (eggs) of *T. pisiformis* are shed in the feces of dogs. If ingested by a cottontail rabbit, *Sylvilagus floridanus*, the hexacanth embryo hatches, invades the mucosa of the small intestine, and makes its way to the liver. Tunneling through the liver, the hexacanth grows, cavitates to form a bladder, and develops a holdfast organ complete with two rows of hooks and four suckers. Fully developed cysticerci may remain in the liver, but they are more often found encapsulated on the peritoneal surfaces of the mesentery. When a dog eats an infected rabbit, the bladder is digested, leaving only the holdfast and adjacent neck. The holdfast attaches to the wall of the small intestine, and segments begin to form at the neck.

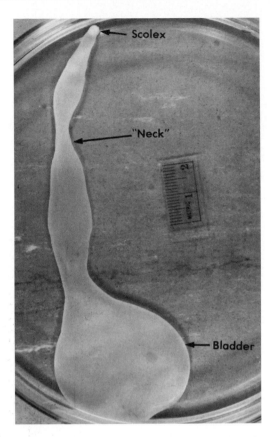

FIGURE 3-38 Cysticercus of *Taenia hydatigena* (Taeniidae). The bladder of this particular species has an attenuated "neck" region; hence the old larval name *Cysticercus tenuicollis*.

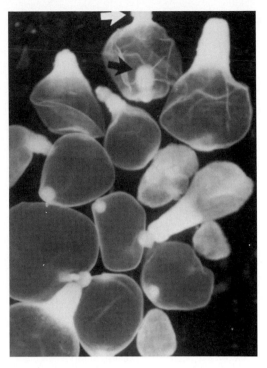

FIGURE 3-39 Cysticerci from a mole rat. Notice the cyst with two scolices (×6.5). The distinction between cysticercus and coenurus is sometimes finely drawn.

The cysticercus of a second canine taeniid tapeworm, *Taenia ovis*, infects the cardiac and skeletal muscles of sheep and represents the most important pathological lesion found by United States inspectors in imported Australian mutton. In one instance $1,540,000 worth of boneless mutton (12.5% of the total shipment) had to be sold as pet food or shipped back to Australia (Arundel, 1972).

The cysticercus of a third canine taeniid tapeworm, *Taenia pisiformis,* is found in the liver and peritoneal cavity of rabbits. This tapeworm is the most common taeniid tapeworm of dogs in the United States. It also indicates how well the process works because every dog that is so infected must have eaten a rabbit or parts of a rabbit and this means that many rabbits are infected by grazing near where *Taenia pisiformis* segments have been shed.

The cysticercus of the "unarmed" human tapeworm *T. saginata* encysts in the striated muscles of cattle, especially the heart and muscles of mastication. The cystericus has an **unarmed scolex,** so-called because both the larval and adult forms of this tapeworm lack the hooks typical of other *Taenia* spp. Taeniid eggs survive the rigors of the septic

tank, as well as many contemporary municipal sewage treatment processes, and because defecating out-of-doors is unavoidable when hunting or camping out (and because the segments can leave the host by crawling out through the anal opening), it is easy to see how cattle pastures become contaminated with *T. saginata* eggs. The cysticerci that develop when these eggs are ingested by cattle are relatively inconspicuous and easily overlooked by the lover of rare or raw ("cannibal sandwich") beef. Consequently, *T. saginata* is a common parasite in the United States and would be far more common but for the vigilance of our meat inspectors. Condemnation of carcass meats for the presence of *T. saginata* cysticerci results in great economic loss. Sometimes this loss is concentrated in a particular lot of cattle and borne by a single producer. Under such circumstances, the economic loss caused by *T. saginata* ceases to be an abstract figure and becomes of immediate concern, not only to the unlucky producer, but to his veterinarian, too. The problem is that some person, most likely a farm or feedlot employee, has a tapeworm and has defecated or shed segments in or near the cattle feed. People are generally uncooperative under such circumstances, and the culprit is rarely identified.

In southeast Asia (e.g., Thailand, Indonesia, Korea, Taiwan, and the Philippines), there is a

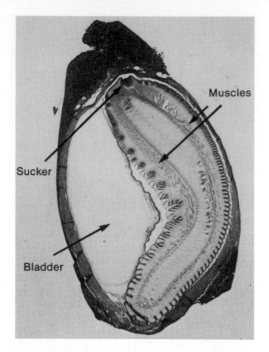

FIGURE 3-40   Strobilocercus of *Taenia taeniaeformis* in the liver of a muskrat (*Ondatra zibethica*) (×10). The plane of the section includes two of the suckers at the anterior end, a section of the body, and the bladder at the posterior end of the larva. Notice the two zones of muscle fibers in the body parenchyma, typical of adult tapeworm segments. This larva is a very common parasite of meadow voles *(Microtus pennsylvaticus).* Meadow voles are relished by cats, which serve as definitive hosts of *T. taeniaeformis.*

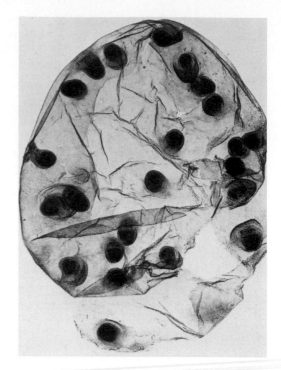

FIGURE 3-41   A coenurus (×2). Notice the many scolices attached to a rather thin-walled bladder.

cysticercus with hooks that is found in the liver of pigs (occasionally cattle) and does not occur in muscle. When this form develops to the adult stage in humans, the hooks are lost, and the tapeworm appears morphologically and molecularly very similar to *T. saginata*. This form has caused significant economic losses in pigs in the area where it occurs and is thought to be maintained by the habit of humans eating raw liver. This form has been designated a separate subspecies with the name *Taenia saginata asiatica* (Fan et al, 1995; Hoberg et al, 2001).

The cysticercus of the human tapeworm *T. solium* represents a significant hazard to human health. People become infected with *T. solium* by ingesting the cysticerci in undercooked pork. After the tapeworm matures, the person's feces contain a steady supply of eggs, which may be conveyed to the mouth at any time by a lapse in personal hygiene. When the eggs reach the stomach, the oncospheres hatch out, enter the gut wall, and wander far and wide in the body, slowly developing into cysticerci. Apparently the *milieu intérieur* of humans resembles that of swine closely enough to satisfy the development requirements of the

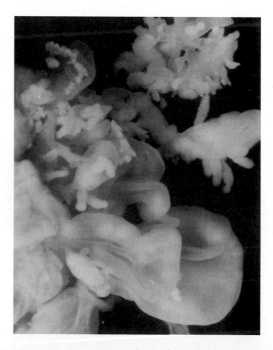

FIGURE 3-42   A coenurus from the subcutaneous and intermuscular connective tissues of a cottontail rabbit (*Sylvilagus floridanus*) (×2). This bladder displays marked budding and ramification in growth.

cysticercus. In humans, the signs depend on where the cysticerci localize, and sites may include the eye, brain, or spinal cord. Rare cases of human cysticercosis and coenurosis are also caused by larvae of canine taeniids.

STROBILOCERCUS. The larva of the cat tapeworm *T. taeniaformis* is a strobilocercus (see Figure 3-40). This larval stage is not of any significant zoonotic potential.

COENUROSIS. The coenurus of the canine taeniid tapeworm *T. multiceps* invades the cranial cavity of sheep, goats, and sometimes cattle. As the cyst grows over a period of 6 or 8 months, neurological signs of progressive space occupation slowly develop. There may be blindness, incoordination, walking in circles, and pressing the head against walls, tree trunks, and the like. Finally, the animal lies down and dies. The most common diseases that might be confused with cerebral coenurosis are bacterial encephalitis (listeriosis) and parelaphostrongylosis. Intracranial surgery is the only cure for cerebral coenurosis but lies beyond economic reality for sheep unless the shepherd is very skillful with his jackknife. The location of the larva within the skull makes some people wonder how the scolices ever reach a dog's stomach, but they must not realize that a good stout dog can crush a sheep's skull with one bite. As in the case of *T. hydatigena* and *T. ovis,* control can be based only on excluding dogs and other canids from sheep pastures. Unfortunately, this is often next to impossible.

Cerebral coenurosis in cats appears in isolated cases (Georgi et al, 1969; Hayes and Creighton, 1978; Kingston et al, 1984; Smith et al, 1988). Marked by severe neurological disturbances, it is invariably fatal. The responsible species is probably *T. multiceps* or *Taenia serialis.*

Echinococcus

IDENTIFICATION. The genus *Echinococcus* contains two species of special importance to veterinary medicine, *Echinococcus granulosus* and *Echinococcus multilocularis,* which are very small (2 to 8 mm long) adult tapeworms having only four or five segments of which only the terminal segment is gravid (Figure 3-43). In *E. granulosus,* 45 to 65 testes are generally distributed, and the genital pore is located at or posterior to the middle of the segment. In *E. multilocularis,* 17 to 26 testes are found posterior to the genital pore, which is located anterior to the middle of the segment. **Caution:** Human hydatid infection may be acquired by ingesting the eggs of *Echinococcus* spp.; wear gloves and wash carefully when handling the feces of potentially infected carnivores.

E. granulosus is a parasite of the dog, coyote, wolf, and dingo. Its larva is a hydatid cyst in sheep,

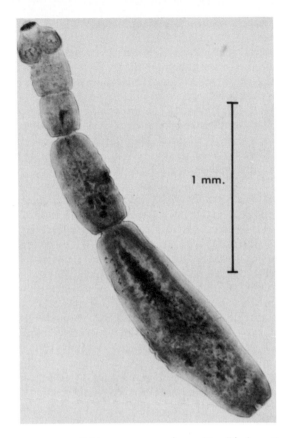

FIGURE 3-43 *Echinococcus granulosus* (Taeniidae), entire worm (×44).

swine, cattle, humans, moose, caribou, kangaroos, and others. Species vary in their suitability as intermediate hosts. Hydatid cysts found in sheep are usually fertile, whereas those in cattle tend to be sterile. Subspecies of *E. granulosus* differ in their preferences for intermediate hosts. For example, *Echinococcus granulosus granulosus* hydatids belong to the subspecies adapted to sheep and humans, whereas *Echinococcus granulosus equinus* is the subspecies found in horses, asses, and mules. The hydatid membrane may bud off daughter cysts either internally or externally. The whole structure occupies progressively more space as it grows, but hydatid cysts do not infiltrate, in contrast to alveolar hydatids. Pathogenic effects of hydatid cysts include pressure atrophy of surrounding organs and allergic reactions to hydatid fluid leaks. Rupture of a fertile hydatid cyst may scatter bits of germinative membrane, scolices, and brood capsules throughout the pleural or peritoneal cavity and result in multiple hydatidosis. Pulmonary hydatid cysts may rupture into a bronchus, the contents coughed up, and the lesion healed. Hydatid cysts that remain intact eventually die and degenerate, but the course is protracted.

E. granulosus is endemic in North and South America, England, Africa, the Middle East, Australia, and New Zealand. *E. multilocularis* is endemic in north-central Europe, Alaska, Canada, and central United States as far south as Illinois and Nebraska (Ballard and Vande Vusse, 1983).

HYDATID DISEASE. The **unilocular hydatid cyst** is the second-stage larva of *E. granulosus* and is infective to dogs and other canids that serve as definitive hosts (Figure 3-44). Starting as an oncosphere less than 30 μm in diameter, the larva grows very slowly and infrequently exceeds more than a few centimeters in diameter in slaughtered sheep and cattle. Because humans live longer, a fertile hydatid infecting man may grow very large and interfere with the function of neighboring organs by pressing against them. The hydatid membrane is surrounded by, but usually not attached to, an inflammatory connective tissue capsule. The space between the host and the parasite generally contains a small volume of clear, colorless, or light-yellow liquid. Brood capsules, each containing many scolices, develop from the germinal epithelium lining the laminated hydatid membrane (Figure 3-45). Some of these rupture, releasing scolices to form a sediment of so-called hydatid sand in the hydatid fluid (Figure 3-46). Endogenous daughter cysts may be found free in the fluid-filled cyst cavity or attached to the germinal epithelium. Exogenous daughter cysts are

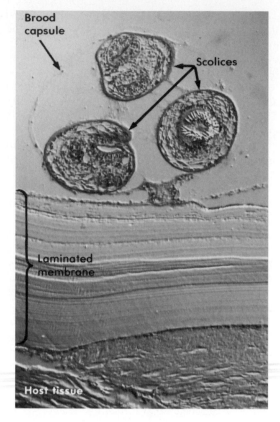

FIGURE 3-45 *Echinococcus granulosus* hydatid cyst with brood capsule containing three scolices (×202).

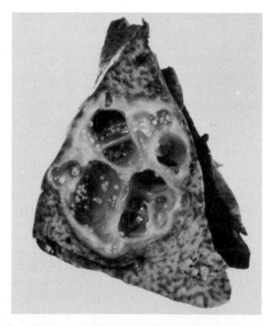

FIGURE 3-44 A hydatid cyst *(Echinococcus granulosus)* in the liver of a horse (about natural size). This horse displayed no clinical signs of hepatic involvement despite the presence of 20 to 30 cysts like the one illustrated.

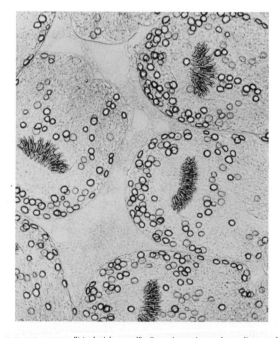

FIGURE 3-46 "Hydatid sand" (i.e., invaginated scolices of *Echinococcus granulosus*) found free in the hydatid fluid (×130). This material was recovered from the hydatid cyst of Figure 3-42.

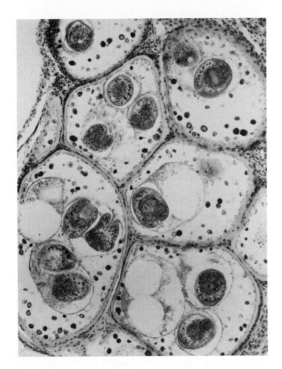

FIGURE 3-47 *Echinococcus multilocularis* alveolar hydatid (×108).

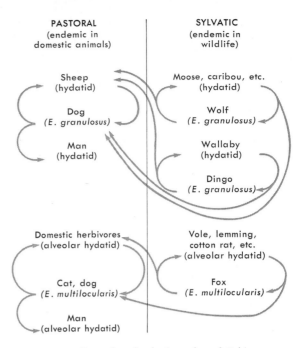

FIGURE 3-48 Pastoral and sylvatic cycles of *Echinococcus granulosus* and *Echinococcus multilocularis*.

relatively unusual; they may be found in the pericystic space between the hydatid membrane and the host connective tissue capsule. Sterile hydatids lack brood capsules, scolices, and daughter cysts; their identification in cattle and swine is necessarily somewhat presumptive.

Alveolar hydatid cysts are second-stage larvae of *E. multilocularis* and are infective to dogs, foxes, and cats, which serve as definitive hosts (Figure 3-47). Alveolar hydatids develop in voles, lemmings, cattle, horses, swine, and humans. They are characterized by exogenous budding that does not remain contained within the reactive connective tissue capsule but continuously proliferates and infiltrates surrounding tissue like a malignant neoplasm. Alveolar hydatid infection proves invariably fatal in a few years.

Both *E. granulosus* and *E. multilocularis* tend to establish sylvatic cycles when suitable predator-prey relationships exist in the wildlife population of a region. Therefore *E. granulosus* cycles are maintained among wild ruminants and wolves in the Canadian north woods and among wallabies and dingoes in Australia. Natural nidi of *E. multilocularis* are maintained in various rodents and foxes. The sylvatic cycle reaches humans through their domesticated animals. Dogs that scavenge the entrails of wild game infected with *Echinococcus* spp. become direct sources of hydatid infection to humans and their domestic

animals. Contamination of pastures with the feces of infected wild carnivorans also results in hydatid infection of domestic ruminants and swine. The establishment of a pastoral cycle may then result from the feeding of uncooked offal from these domestic animals to dogs and, in the case of *E. multilocularis*, to cats (Figure 3-48).

The direct source of human infection is, in most instances, the domestic dog or cat, and scrupulous hygiene is the first line of defense. Periodic anthelmintic medication of dogs or cats, depending on the species of tapeworm involved, carries the threat one step further away. In the case of a well-established sylvatic cycle, this is about as far as it is practical to go. *Echinococcus* infection may be reduced to insignificant incidence in cases in which it is limited to a pastoral cycle and thus accessible to manipulation by humans. Destruction of all stray dogs, regimented anthelmintic medication of the rest, and prohibition against feeding uncooked offal to dogs and cats are mandatory.

A campaign against hydatid disease has been in effect in Iceland since 1864. At the outset, about one of six or seven people and virtually all ages of slaughter sheep and cattle harbored hydatid cysts, and about one fourth of the dogs were infected with the adult worm. By 1900 the human infection rate had fallen dramatically and has almost reached the point of nonexistence. The campaign, devised by Dr. Harald Krabbe of the Royal Veterinary and Agricultural University of Copenhagen, consisted of alerting the public to the need to observe strict hygiene in dealing with dogs, destroying all cysts and infected offal, and administering mandatory anthelmintic medication to all dogs (Palsson, 1976). Thus salutary results in *Echinococcus* control can be achieved in a century or so, provided there is no sylvatic cycle to complicate the issue. In Australia, for example, a sylvatic cycle involving kangaroos and *Canis dingo* would have to be considered in any eradication attempt. "Obviously the denial of sheep offal to domestic dogs will not eliminate infection if dogs have access to macropods in dingo-infested areas" (Herd and Coman, 1975). In the United States, *E. granulosus* appears to be most prevalent in sheep-raising areas of Utah (Loveless et al, 1978) and California. In California, the spread of echinococcosis appears to be related to a quaint transhumant form of husbandry in which bands of sheep migrate from place to place under the control of contract Basque shepherds from Spain and France. These shepherds, for the most part, are ignorant of the epidemiology of hydatid disease and feed their dogs mostly on dead sheep (Araujo et al, 1975).

Other Cyclophyllidean Tapeworms

The second-stage larvae of all of the following cyclophyllidean families are **cysticercoids** of one kind or another. A cysticercoid may be thought of as a cysticercus small enough to fit into the body of an arthropod. It is small and solid rather than cavitated but has an inverted (or at least introverted) scolex. The cysticercoids of *Mesocestoides* spp. have yet to be identified, remarkable as that may seem in this enlightened age. However, the specialists nevertheless seem certain that a cysticercoid stage of *Mesocestoides* spp. must precede the well-known **tetrathyridium** found in a wide range of mammals, birds, and reptiles.

Family Anoplocephalidae

IDENTIFICATION. *Moniezia* spp. have unarmed scolices with four large suckers and very wide segments with bilateral genitalia. They are found in the small intestine of cattle, sheep, and goats (*Moniezia benedeni, Moniezia expansa,* and *Moniezia caprae*). Interproglottidal glands at the posterior margin of each segment extend the full width of *M. expansa* but occupy only the midzone of the *M. benedeni* segment (Figure 3-49). The egg of *Moniezia* sp. found in cattle feces is one of the few eggs that appears square, and internally the pear-shaped (pyriform apparatus) characteristic of anoplocephalid eggs can be seen (Figure 3-50).

Thysanosoma actinioides, the "fringed tapeworm," is found in the common bile duct and duodenum of

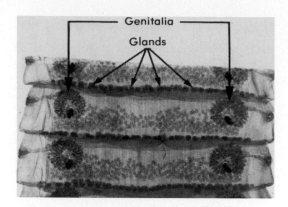

FIGURE 3-49 Mature segments of *Moniezia expansa* (Anoplocephalidae) (×5).

virtually all ruminant species except cattle. Ligature of the bile duct within 5 minutes of slaughter has revealed that these worms are probably found almost exclusively in the intestine of the living animal (Boisvenue and Hendrix, 1987). The endemic areas of *T. actinioides* are the western parts of North and South America, especially mountainous areas. *Wyominia tetoni* is found in the bile ducts and duodenum of mountain sheep *(Ovis canadensis). T. actinioides* has wide segments with bilateral genitalia and a *fringe* of outgrowths at the posterior border of each segment. *W. tetoni* resembles *T. actinioides,* but its segments are not fringed. *Thysaniezia, Stilesia,* and *Avitellina* spp. are exotic anoplocephalids of ruminants.

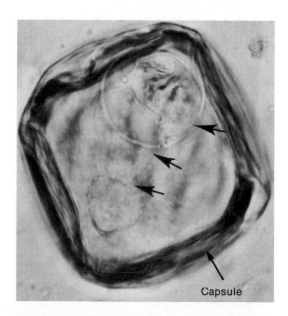

FIGURE 3-50 Egg of *Moniezia* sp. (Anoplocephalidae) of ruminants (×1100). The pear-shaped embryophore *(arrows)* is typical of anoplocephalid eggs.

Anoplocephala magna and *Paranoplocephala mammilana* (Figure 3-51) are relatively harmless parasites in the small intestine of horses. *Anoplocephala perfoliata* (Figure 3-52) is found mainly in the cecum but also tends to cluster in the ileum near the ileocecal valve, where it is associated with ulceration and reactive inflammation of the ileal wall. This clustering results in ulceration of the mucous membrane and inflammation with thickening and induration of the deeper layers of the intestinal wall. These pathological changes probably account for some cases of persistent diarrhea and may predispose to intussusception of the ileum into the cecum or rupture of the bowel wall in the vicinity of the ileocecal valve (Barclay et al, 1982; Beroza et al, 1983). Proudman and Edwards (1993) published work showing an association between infection with *A. perfoliata* and ileocecal colic in horses. Diagnosis of *A. perfoliata* infection is based on distinguishing the eggs from those of *A. magna* and *P. mammilana*. *A. perfoliata* eggs and segments frequently cannot be demonstrated, either by flotation or sedimentation techniques, in the feces of horses known to be heavily infected with this parasite, a paradox for which we are unable to offer a satisfactory explanation. For this reason, an enzyme-linked immunosorbent assay (ELISA) has been used to examine the immunoglobulin G (IgG) of horses to determine infection with this parasite. In a case-control study with this means of detection, horses with tapeworms had a 26 times greater risk of developing spasmodic colic (Proudman et al, 1993). What is important is that horses be treated occasionally with something other than ivermectin (i.e., something that will kill tapeworms).

The tapeworms of cattle, sheep, and goats all belong to the family Anoplocephalidae. The life histories of only a few anoplocephalids have been documented, but those that have involve an arthropod intermediate host in which the infective cysticercoid develops. Infection purportedly results from the incidental ingestion of these infected arthropods by the grazing animal. Pasture renovation is recommended to destroy the surface layer of

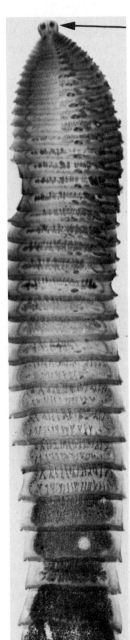

Scolex

Genitalia maturing

Uterus beginning to fill with eggs

Segments gravid

Segments about to detach

FIGURE 3-51 *Paranoplocephala mamillana* (Anoplocephalidae), entire tapeworm (×3).

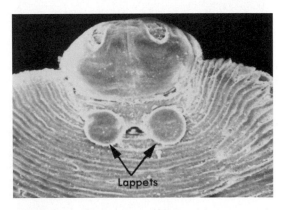

Lappets

FIGURE 3-52 *Anoplocephala perfoliata* (Anoplocephalidae), scanning electron micrograph (×18). The scolex of *A. perfoliata* is about 2 mm in diameter and has four large suckers and four projections called *lappets*.

humus and thus the habitat of oribatid mites, which are the intermediate host of at least some of these cestodes. However, there seems to be little experimental basis to support this recommendation. Fortunately, adult tapeworms are relatively nonpathogenic. Those species that invade the bile ducts cause condemnation of the liver at slaughter and in this way lead to considerable economic loss. However, the most common reason for a veterinarian's wish for a drug to remove adult tapeworms from ruminants seems related to the difficulty of persuading the average client that those big white worms are relatively harmless. It is easier to worm the stock than to convince the stockman.

LIFE HISTORY. Free-living oribatid mites serve as hosts for cysticercoids of *Moniezia* spp. of sheep and cattle, *Bertiella* spp. of primates, and *Cittotaenia* spp. of the European wild rabbit. *Thysanosoma actinoides* is apparently transmitted by "booklice" or "barklice" of the family Psocidae, order Psocoptera. Psocopterans resemble mallophagan lice but are entirely free living and have no other known relationship to parasite life histories.

Family Dipylidiidae

IDENTIFICATION. In *D. caninum*, *Diplopylidium* spp., and *Joyeuxiella* spp., the scolex has four suckers and a retractable rostellum armed with several circles of thornlike hooks (Figure 3-53).

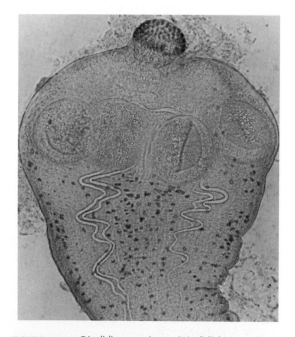

FIGURE 3-53 *Dipylidium caninum* (Dipylidiidae), scolex of fresh mount (×108). The scolex of *D. caninum* is less than 0.5 mm in diameter; the rostellum is retractable and armed with small thornlike hooks.

Segments are shaped like cucumber seeds and have bilateral genital pores. The genital apertures of *D. caninum* lie slightly behind the middle of the segment (i.e., away from the scolex), and each egg capsule may contain from 5 to 30 eggs. The genital apertures of the Middle Eastern, African, and Australasian parasites *Diplopylidium* and *Joyeuxiella* lie before the middle of the segment (i.e., toward the scolex), and each capsule contains a single egg.

LIFE HISTORY. Cysticercoids of *D. caninum* develop in fleas (*Ctenocephalides* spp.) and biting lice *(Trichodectes canis),* and the dog acquires this tapeworm while nipping its insects (Figure 3-54). Children also may become infected in this way. Cysticercoids of *Diplopylidium* and *Joyeuxiella* develop in coprophagous beetles; reptiles and small mammals serve as second intermediate hosts.

D. caninum requires only 2 to 3 weeks to develop from a cysticercoid into a segment-shedding tapeworm. Thus the benefits of anthelmintic therapy are particularly short-lived unless fleas and biting lice also are brought under control. It has been shown that the developing cysticercoids require a day or so in a flea that has found a mammalian host to be warm enough to finish their ultimate development to the infective stage (Pugh, 1987).

Family Hymenolepididae

The family Hymenolepididae contains many species that occur in birds and two mammalian parasites. *Hymenolepis diminuta* is a parasite of the small intestine principally of rodents but occasionally also of dogs and even humans (Ehrenford, 1977). The eggs of this tapeworm can be found in the feces (Figure 3-55). The cysticercoid of *H. diminuta* develops in fleas, flour beetles, and a rather wide range of other insects (Figure 3-56). *Vampirolepis* (=*Hymenolepis*; =*Rodentolepis*) *nana* is also a parasite of rodents and humans, and its second-stage larva is a cysticercoid in fleas and flour beetles or in the intestinal mucosa of its definitive host. *V. nana* can complete its life history within the intestinal tract of a mouse or a human. Some of the eggs hatch within the intestine, and the hexacanth embryos burrow into the mucous membrane to form cysticercoids that later reenter the lumen to complete their development as mature tapeworms. The rest of the eggs pass out with the feces to await ingestion by flour beetles or fleas, in which the cysticercoids develop. Thus *H. diminuta* requires fleas, flour beetles, or other insects as intermediate hosts, whereas *V. nana* may or may not. Because the eggs discharged in feces are infective to humans, *V. nana* infection in laboratory rodent stocks constitutes something of a health hazard to personnel. Because *H. diminuta* infection requires ingestion of an infected insect, human infection with this tapeworm

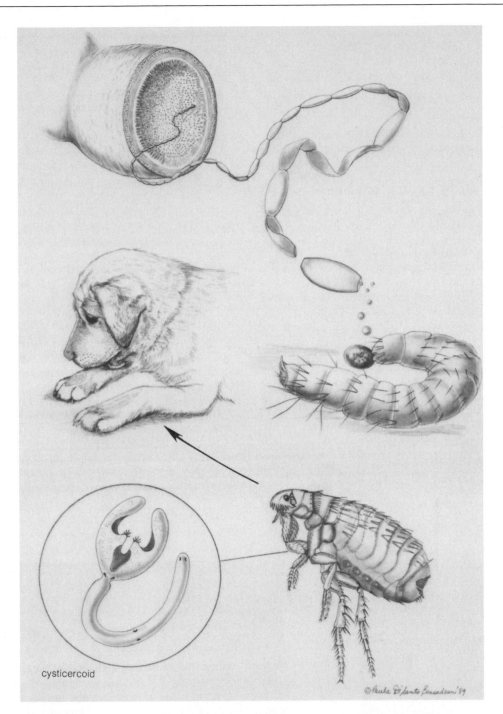

cysticercoid

FIGURE 3-54 Life history of *Dipylidium caninum*. Gravid segments discharge their egg packets as they move about. Larvae of *Ctenocephalides* chew their way into egg packets and ingest the oncospheres of the tapeworm. The hexacanth embryo enters the body cavity of the flea larva and remains there through its metamorphosis. After the adult flea emerges from the cocoon, the hexacanth develops into a cysticercoid in 2 or 3 days. If such a flea is ingested by the definitive host as during self-grooming, the cysticercoids develop into adult tapeworms in the small intestine.

is less probable but does occur. Hymenolepids have three testes and a single ovary; *V. nana* has a single circle of hooks on its scolex, whereas *H. diminuta* has no hooks.

Family Mesocestoididae

IDENTIFICATION. The scolex of *Mesocestoides* spp. has four suckers but no hooks. Mature segments have a mediodorsal genital pore, and eggs accumulate in

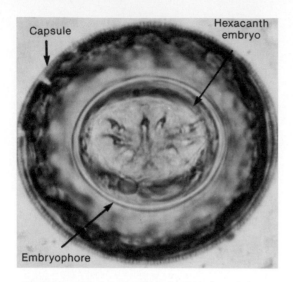

FIGURE 3-55 Egg of *Hymenolepis diminuta* (Hymenolepidae), a common parasite of rodents (×900).

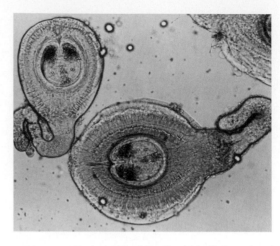

FIGURE 3-56 Cysticercoids of *Hymenolepis diminuta* (×90).

a special, thick-walled parauterine organ as the segments mature (Figure 3-57). Gravid segments detach from the strobila and carry their relatively small burden of oncospheres to the outside world.

LIFE HISTORY. The complete life history of the genus *Mesocestoides* has yet to be worked out. The larval form infective for the definitive host is a third-stage larva called a **tetrathyridium** and is found in the peritoneal cavity of mammals and reptiles and in the lungs of birds. A cysticercoid larval stage is hypothesized to precede the tetrathyridium, possibly developing from the oncosphere in a coprophilic insect (Loos-Frank, 1991).

Mesocestoides infection of dogs and cats results from predation on snakes, birds, and small mammals. Some clients find it difficult to accept that their civilized pets are using their long, sharp teeth in an atavistic way, especially sportsmen with expensive bird dogs and vegetarians with cats. However, the carnivoran must be denied prey if *Mesocestoides* infection is to be prevented. Most taeniids have about a 2-month prepatent period, but *Mesocestoides* spp. may start discharging segments

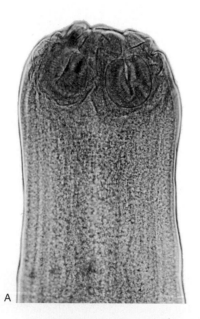
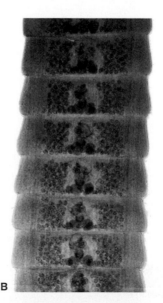
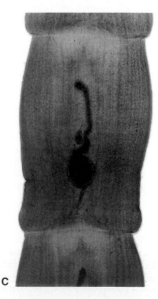

FIGURE 3-57 *Mesocestoides* sp. **A,** Scolex (×108). **B,** Mature segments (×16). **C,** Gravid segments (×16).

TABLE 3-2 ■ Information on Some Tapeworms of Veterinary Importance

Cestode family genus species	Final hosts	Geographical distribution	Egg	Intermediate hosts	Larval stage infective to final host	Prepatent period	Scolex	Segment
Diphyllobothriidae diphyllobothrium	Dogs, cats, humans, bears, pigs, seals	Cold climate, freshwater	Operculate 66 × 44 μm	Copepod,* fish†	Plerocercoid	40 days	Slitlike, no hooks	Square, medial uterine pore
Spirometra	Dogs, cats, lynx, raccoons	U.S., Australia, Far East	Operculate 66 × 44 μm	Copepod*; tadpoles, snakes, rodents†	Plerocercoid "sparganum"	15–30 days	Slitlike, no hooks	Square, medial uterine pore
Mesocestoididae mesocestoides	Raccoons, dogs, cats	Worldwide	Eggs confined to parauterine organ	Reptiles and mammals†; first host still unknown	Tetrathyridium	20–30 days	Muscular, 4 suckers, no hooks	Small, sesame seed–like, with contained parauterine organ
Taeniidae Taenia pisiformis	Dogs	Worldwide	Taeniid egg, 30 μm	Cottontail rabbits	Cysticercus	56 days	Muscular, 4 suckers, claw-hammer–shaped hooks	Square, single lateral pore
Taenia hydatigena	Dogs	Worldwide	Taeniid egg, 30 μm	Mainly sheep	Cystecercus	51 days	Muscular, 4 suckers, claw-hammer–shaped hooks	Square, single lateral pore
Taenia ovis	Dogs	Worldwide	Taeniid egg, 30 μm	Mainly sheep	Cysticercus		Muscular, 4 suckers, claw-hammer–shaped hooks	Square, single lateral pore
Taenia taeniaeformis	Cats	Worldwide	Taeniid egg, 30 μm	Mice and rats	Strobilocercus	40 days	Muscular, 4 suckers, claw-hammer–shaped hooks	Square, single lateral pore
Taenia serialis	Dogs	Worldwide	Taeniid egg, 30 μm	Cottontail rabbits	Coenurus		Muscular, 4 suckers, claw-hammer–shaped hooks	Square, single lateral pore
Taenia multiceps	Dogs	Worldwide	Taeniid egg, 30 μm	Mainly sheep	Coenurus	30 days	Muscular, 4 suckers, claw-hammer–shaped hooks	Square, single lateral pore

Continued

TABLE 3-2 ■ Information on Some Tapeworms of Veterinary Importance—cont'd.

Cestode family genus species	Final hosts	Geographical distribution	Egg	Intermediate hosts	Larval stage infective to final host	Prepatent period	Scolex	Segment
Echinococcus granulosus	Dogs, other canids	Sheep areas	Taeniid egg, 30 μm	Mainly sheep	Unilocular hydatid cyst	45–60 days	Muscular, 4 suckers, claw-hammer–shaped hooks	Very small, usually not seen
Echinococcus multilocularis	Foxes, dogs	Holarctic	Taeniid egg, 30 μm	Voles, mice and rats	Multilocular hydatid cyst	28 days	Muscular, 4 suckers, claw-hammer–shaped hooks	Very small, usually not seen
Dipylidiidae Dipylidium caninum	Dogs, cats, other felids and canids	Worldwide	Eggs passed in egg packets	Fleas	Cysticercoid	21 days	Four suckers, retractable rostellum, thorn-shaped hooks	Pumpkin seed-shaped with pores on both sides
Anoplocephalidae moniezia benedeni	Cattle	Worldwide	Square	Oribatid mites	Cysticercoid	40 days	Unarmed	Much wider than long
Moniezia expansa	Sheep	Worldwide	Squarish to round	Oribatid mites	Cysticercoid	25–45 days	Unarmed	Much wider than long
Moniezia capra	Goats	Worldwide	Squarish to round	Oribatid mites	Cysticercoid	???	Unarmed	Much wider than long
Thysanosoma actinoides	Ruminants, not cattle	Mountains of North and South America	Elongate, small	Book lice (Psocidae)	Cysticercoid	???	Unarmed	Fringed
Anoplocephala magna	Equids	Worldwide	Round	Oribatid mites	Cysticercoid	4–6 wk	Unarmed	Much wider than long
Anoplocephala perfoliata	Equids	Worldwide	Round	Oribatic mites	Cysticercoid	4–6 wk	Unarmed with lappets	Usually see whole worm
Paranoploceph-ala mammilana	Equids	Worldwide	Round	Oribatid mites	Cysticercoid	4–6 wk	Unarmed	Much wider than long

*First intermediate host.
†Second intermediate host.

in hardly more than 2 weeks after infection, thereby imparting the impression that the anthelmintic has not worked at all. To make matters worse, *M. corti* tapeworms multiply asexually in the intestines of dogs. If this species is not totally eliminated by anthelmintic medication, it will repopulate the intestine even without further exposure (Eckert et al, 1969).

Information of some tapeworms of veterinary importance may be found in Table 3-2.

Treatment of Adult Tapeworm Infections
Dogs and Cats

Adult tapeworm infections cause little harm or inconvenience to dogs and cats. It is true that infected dogs frequently sit down and drag their bottoms, but so do uninfected dogs. No doubt a tapeworm segment wandering about the perineum tickles. Although this phenomenon must certainly be included in the list of etiologies for **pruritus ani,** distended anal sacs are more frequently to blame. The veterinarian who treats pruritus ani by expressing anal sacs will obtain better results than another who prescribes anthelmintics for this condition.

A tapeworm segment crawling about on their pet's tail or freshly passed feces offends most clients, and the civilized world makes quite a business of poisoning tapeworms. For lasting results to be obtained, the source of infection must also be dealt with, or the segments will reappear and the client may not.

There are many drugs with proven efficacy against the tapeworms affecting dogs and cats. Dichlorophene, nitroscanate, praziquantel, and epsiprantel all show activity against one or more tapeworm genera, but almost all fail against one or another genus.

The cestocidal drug, praziquantel, in a single 5 mg/kg oral or subcutaneous dose, eliminates 100% of both immature and adult *T. hydatigena, T. pisiformis, T. ovis, T. taeniaeformis, E. granulosus, E. multilocularis, M. corti,* and *D. caninum* from dogs and cats (Dey-Hazra, 1976; Rommel et al, 1976; Anderson et al, 1978; and Thomas and Gönnert, 1978). Praziquantel at a dosage of 7.5 mg/kg for 2 consecutive days eliminated 100% of *Diphyllobothrium erinacei,* and a single dose of 35 mg/kg eliminated all *D. latum* from infected cats (Sakamoto, 1977). Praziquantel in combination with pyrantel pamoate and febantel also has been shown efficacious in removing infections from *E. granulosus* and *E. multilocularis.* Epsiprantel at 2.75 mg/kg in cats and 5.5 mg/kg in dogs is efficacious against *D. caninum, T. pisiformis,* and *T. taeniaeformis.* Doses of 7.5 mg/kg were required to clear all dogs of infections from adult *E. multilocularis* (Arru et al, 1990).

Nitroscanate is active against adult *E. granulosus* (Boray et al, 1979). Fenbendazole administered for 3 days at 50 mg/kg is effective against *T. pisiformis.*

Ruminants

For *Moniezia* infection in the United States, fenbendazole has been approved as a cattle anthelmintic at 5 mg/kg. Overseas, fenbendazole is marketed for *Moniezia* control at a higher dose of 7.5 mg/kg. Albendazole also can be used in cattle in the United States for treatment of *Moniezia* infection at the approved dose of 10 mg/kg. Oxfendazole is also approved for treating *Moniezia* infection in cattle at a dose of 4.5 mg/kg.

Albendazole is effective against *Thysanosoma* infection in sheep at 7.5 mg/kg. Fenbendazole at 10 mg/kg also appears to be effective (Bergstrom et al, 1988), as also is praziquantel at 40 mg/kg (Martinez, 1984). *T. actinoides* infections were treated experimentally with 10 g of dichlorophene per animal (Ryff et al, 1950).

Stilesia (exotic) infections are difficult to treat. Praziquantel at a dose of 2.5 mg/kg was extremely effective against *Moniezia* infection in sheep, but doses of 8 to 15 mg/kg were required for the treatment of *Avitellina centripunctata, Stilesia globipunctata,* and *Stilesia hepatica* (Bankov, 1975, 1976; Thomas and Gönnert, 1978). Dichlorophene at a rate of 250 mg/kg (Guilhon and Graber, 1960) was completely effective against *S. globipunctata* but was inactive against *S. hepatica* in sheep.

Horses

A. perfoliata was reported by Kelly and Bain (1975) as very susceptible to 15 mg/kg micronized mebendazole, but Slocombe found this drug to be without effect at dose levels below 35 mg/kg. Slocombe (1979) found pyrantel at 13.2 to 19.8 mg base/kg highly effective. The daily feeding of pyrantel tartrate (2.64 mg/kg) to horses significantly reduces tapeworms in both adult horses and yearlings, with most treated animals becoming free of this parasite (Greiner and Lane, 1994; Lyons et al, 1997b). Lyons et al (1992) found praziquantel at 1 mg/kg to be highly effective in the removal of *A. perfoliata* from horses.

■ PHYLUM NEMATODA

Body form is remarkably constant among nematodes, a fact that may simplify the anatomy lesson but that somewhat aggravates the difficulties of identification and taxonomic classification. It is helpful in understanding nematode anatomy and physiology to appreciate the significance of their unique high-turgor pressure method of maintaining sufficient corporeal rigidity to permit rapid locomotion by sinusoidal undulation. Crofton (1966) brilliantly expounded these relationships in his book *Nematodes,* and the following discussion represents a summary of his exposition.

Nematodes have a relatively large body cavity **(pseudocoelom)** containing fluid under pressure that varies up to one half atmosphere above that of the surrounding medium. The body cuticle contains inelastic fibers so arranged that an increase in internal pressure causes an increase in length but minimal change in diameter. This anisometric cuticle and high internal pressure thus maintain a relatively constant body diameter. Nematodes do not have a circular muscle layer. Rather, all of the somatic musculature is oriented longitudinally and divided into dorsal and ventral fields by lateral expansions of the hypodermis, the **lateral chords.** A muscle cell of either field is connected by a cytoplasmic process to its respective (dorsal or ventral) median nerve. Thus dorsal and ventral flexion of the body are made possible by independent contraction of the corresponding muscle field, and longitudinal waves of contraction result in the sinusoidal pattern characteristic of nematode locomotion.

The high internal pressure also exerts its influence on the structure and organization of the internal organs. For the lumen of the intestine to be filled with food, some sort of pump is essential to overcome the tendency of the pseudocoelomic fluid pressure to collapse it, and most nematodes have a well-developed muscular esophagus for this purpose. Defecation, on the other hand, is accomplished by the contraction of a *dilator ani* muscle (there is no sphincter) that opens the end of the digestive tube and allows it to empty.

The basic **excretory system** consists of paired unicellular glands with a common midventral excretory pore in the neck region and ducts that, in some forms, run nearly the full length of the body in the substance of the lateral chords.

Male nematodes are smaller than the females of their species. Their caudal ends may terminate in a cuticular expansion supported by muscular rays. This so-called **copulatory bursa** reaches its highest development among the strongylids and is used to grasp the female (Figure 3-58). The **copulatory spicules,** used to dilate the vulva of the female, are cuticular structures that develop by sclerotization of folds of the dorsal wall of the cloaca. Spicules are often paired, but some species have only one (e.g., *Trichuris* sp.) or none (e.g., *Trichinella* sp); they vary greatly in size and shape among species and are often used as diagnostic characters. In many species, accessory sclerotizations of the cloacal wall serve as guides for the spicules. A spicule guide in

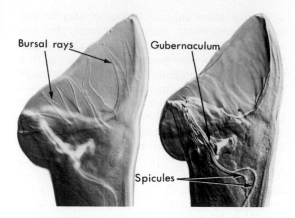

FIGURE 3-58 Surficial *(left)* and sagittal *(right)* aspects of the copulatory bursa of *Cyathostomum labiatum,* a typical member of the order Strongylida, superfamily Strongyloidea (×64).

the dorsal wall is called a **gubernaculum,** and one located in the ventral wall is called a **telamon.** The primary male reproductive organs consist of a single convoluted tube with regions structurally and functionally differentiated as testis, seminal vesicle, and vas deferens. The terminal portion of the vas deferens with its strong muscular coat is called the **ejaculatory duct,** which empties into the cloaca. Some male nematodes have two reproductive ducts, but none of these are animal parasites.

The female reproductive system is also tubular and usually has two branches (i.e., didelphic) but may be monodelphic or even multidelphic. Regions structurally and functionally differentiated as ovary, oviduct, uterus, and vagina communicate through the vulva with the exterior. The vulva is

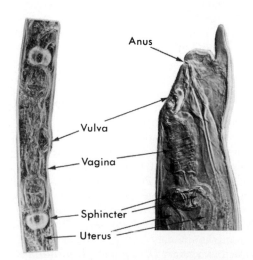

FIGURE 3-59 Ovijectors of a representative of the superfamily Trichostrongyloidea *(left)* and of the superfamily Strongyloidea *(right)* (×64).

ventral in position and may be located near the oral end (opisthodelphic), caudal end (prodelphic), or near the middle of the body (amphidelphic). The location and special anatomical features of the vulva are useful in identification (Figure 3-59). In female strongylids, a muscular ovijector regulates the discharge of eggs from the uterus. The eggs contained in the terminal portion of the uterus are valuable aids in identifying nematodes. See Chapter 5 for illustrations of nematode eggs.

All rational control efforts are based on an understanding of the life history and behavior of both host and parasite. A general outline of the ontogenetic development of a nematode is shown in Figure 3-60. What appears to be a rich and confusing diversity of life histories among various orders of nematodes can all be related and rationalized according to this basic pattern. Embryonic development is, of course, a continuous process with change accompanying every cell division. The "one-cell," "morula," and "vermiform embryo" stages are arbitrarily chosen from this continuum because they are the stages of egg development most frequently encountered in diagnostic procedures. The difference between a vermiform embryo and a first-stage larva is that the former contains only cell clusters as organ primordia, whereas the latter displays clearly recognizable organs such as esophagus, intestine, and excretory glands. A microfilaria is an example of a vermiform embryo, developing into a larva only after it has been ingested by a mosquito. Each larval stage is separated from the next by a **molt** marked by metamorphosis of the larva and **ecdysis** or a casting off of the cuticle from the preceding stage.

The nematode life history also can be generalized from the standpoint of the important events related to diagnosis, treatment, and control. Figure 3-61 represents these events as four stages (adult, preinfective, infective, preadult) separated by four transitions (contamination, development, infection, and maturation). In the mastering of the details of any particular nematode life history, the process of integrating these two schemes is a profitable intellectual exercise.

Order Strongylida

The order Strongylida is composed of four superfamilies: (1) Strongyloidea, the large bowel "strongyles" of horses and the nodular worms of ruminants, swine, and primates, (2) Trichostrongyloidea, the abomasal and small intestinal "hairworms" of ruminants, (3) Ancylostomatoidea, the "hookworms" of diverse mammals, and (4) Metastrongyloidea, the "lungworms." One of the most important genera of lungworms falls within the Trichostrongyloidea rather than the Metastrongyloidea, but there are always exceptions to be resolved.

MORPHOLOGY. The strongylid **stoma** presents important diagnostic characters that are the same for both male and female and usually sufficient for generic identification. Strongyloids have well-developed buccal capsules often armed, at the base, with teeth (Figure 3-62). Ancylostomatoids also have well-developed buccal capsules, but these are permanently flexed dorsally and armed on their ventral (leading) edge with formidable pointed **teeth** or rounded **cutting plates** (Figure 3-63). In the

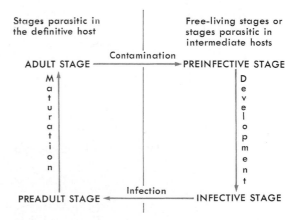

FIGURE 3-61 A generalization of nematode life histories emphasizing the stages and transitions of greatest importance to diagnosis, treatment, and control. As used here, the term preadult stage refers to all stages of parasitic larval development from entry of the parasite into the host to the attainment of sexual maturity. Maturation represents the length of time required for this transition. Similarly, preinfective stage represents all developmental stages leading up to the infective stage, and development represents the time required for that transition.

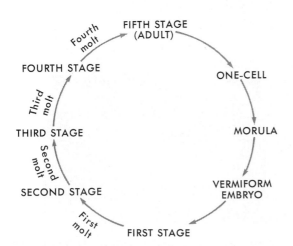

FIGURE 3-60 Stages and transitions in the ontogenetic development of a nematode.

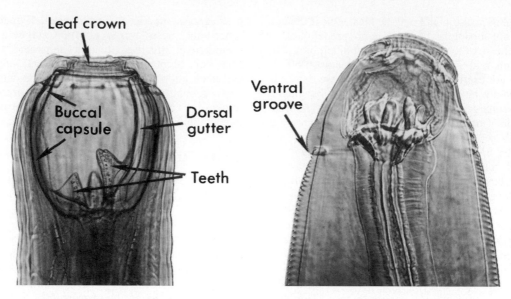

FIGURE 3-62 Superfamily Strongyloidea. Left, *Strongylus equinus* (×45); right, *Ternidens deminutus* (×125).

Trichostrongyloidea, the buccal capsule usually is reduced in size but may be equipped with a tooth or lancet in bloodsucking species (Figure 3-64). In the typical metastrongyloid, the buccal capsule is absent.

Male nematodes of the order Strongylida have a caudal **copulatory bursa** that consists of dorsal, lateral, and ventral expansions of the body cuticle **(lobes)** supported by muscular processes called **rays** (Figure 3-65). The dorsal lobe contains one ray that is usually median in position and variously branched. The lateral lobes each contain an externodorsal ray adjacent to the dorsal lobe and three rays arising in a group: the posterolateral, the mediolateral, and the anterolateral. The ventral lobes

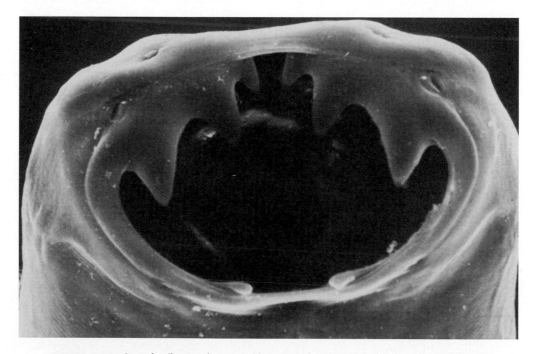

FIGURE 3-63 Superfamily Ancylostomatoidea. Dorsal aspect of the buccal capsule of *Ancylostoma caninum*, the common hookworm of the dog (SEM ×350). The three pairs of pointed teeth are at the ventral margin of the stoma.

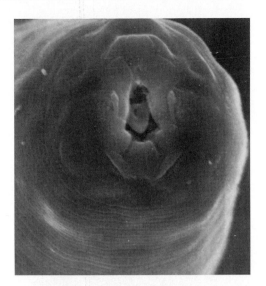

FIGURE 3-64 Superfamily Trichostrongyloidea. *En face* view of the stoma of *Haemonchus contortus*, the stomach worm of sheep (SEM ×1700). This voracious bloodsucking nematode uses its lancet to puncture the mucous membrane of the abomasum.
(Courtesy Dr. Marguerite Frongillo, Cornell University, Ithaca, NY.)

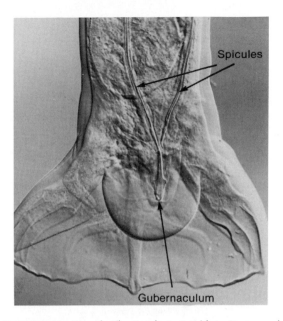

FIGURE 3-66 Superfamily Ancylostomatoidea. Bursa and spicules of *Placoconus lotoris*, a hookworm of the raccoon, *Procyon lotor* (×140).

each contain two rays. The disposition and configuration of these rays are used in classification and identification of strongylids. In typical members of the superfamilies Strongyloidea and Ancylostomatoidea the dorsal and lateral lobes are about equally developed (Figures 3-58 and 3-66); in Trichostrongyloidea, the lateral lobes predominate (see Figure 3-65), and in Metastrongyloidea, the bursa tends to be reduced in size (Figure 3-67). In some metastrongyloids (e.g., *Filaroides* spp.), the bursa is completely absent (Figure 3-68).

The **spicules** of males of the superfamilies Strongyloidea and Ancylostomatoidea tend to be long, thin, and flexible (see Figures 3-58 and 3-66), whereas those of the Trichostrongyloidea tend to be shorter and substantially stouter (see Figures 3-65 and 3-69). In the Metastrongyloidea, spicules vary so widely in size and shape that generalization is unprofitable.

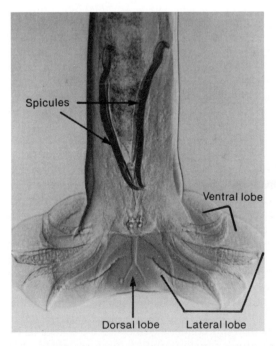

FIGURE 3-65 Superfamily Trichostrongyloidea. Bursa and spicules of *Teladorsagia circumcincta*, an abomasal parasite of sheep (×150).

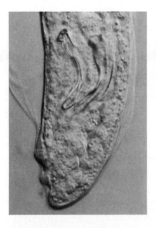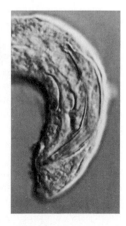

FIGURE 3-67 Superfamily Metastrongyloidea. Bursa and spicules of *Protostrongylus rufescens* (×168).

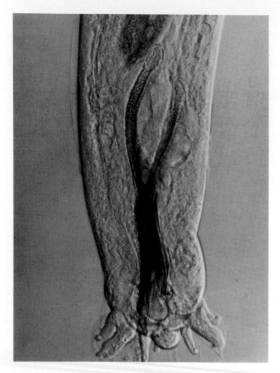

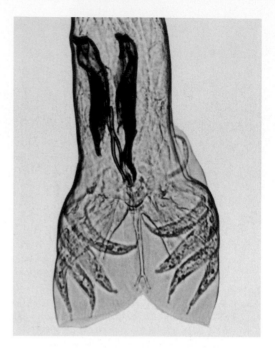

FIGURE 3-69 Superfamily Trichostrongyloidea. Bursa and spicules of *Trichostrongylus axei*, a parasite of the abomasum of ruminants and of the stomach of horses (×375).

FIGURE 3-68 Superfamily Metastrongyloidea. Caudal ends of male *Filaroides hirthi (left)* and *Filaroides milksi (right)*, showing reduction of bursal structures to mere papillae (×1050). The spicules of *F. hirthi* are shorter, are broader in relation to their length, and have broader knobs for the attachment of the retractor muscles than the spicules of *F. milksi.*

The strongylid uterus has two horns and is equipped with a well-developed muscular **ovijector** (see Figure 3-59). In typical trichostrongyloids and ancylostomatoids, the vulva is located near the middle of the body, and the two horns of the uterus extend in opposite directions (amphidelphic). In strongyloids and metastrongyloids, the vulva is typically located close to the anus, and both horns of the uterus extend anteriorly (prodelphic).

LIFE HISTORY. The life histories of superfamilies Strongyloidea, Trichostrongyloidea, and Ancylostomatoidea are typically direct, with free-living microbivorous first and second larval stages and an infective third larval stage (Figure 3-70). Females of all three superfamilies lay typical "strongyle eggs" (i.e., eggs with smooth-surfaced, ellipsoidal shells that contain an embryo in the morula stage of development when laid and passed out with the feces). Such eggs are produced by all members of the order Strongylida, except certain genera in the superfamily Metastrongyloidea, and are therefore properly termed *strongylid eggs.* However, "strongyle" conveys the same meaning to most and is commonly used. The morula develops into a first-stage larva that hatches from the egg within a day or two. After feeding, this larva undergoes its first molt to become a second-stage larva. Both first- and second-stage larvae remain in the feces, where they feed on bacteria. In the second molt, the cuticle of the second stage is temporarily retained as a protective "sheath" about the infective third-stage larva and will not be shed until this larva enters a suitable host. In about a week, these "sheathed" third-stage larvae begin to migrate out of the fecal mass and into the water film covering the surrounding soil particles and vegetation. Infection occurs when these "sheathed larvae" are ingested by grazing animals. Variations on this basic life history pattern are discussed below in connection with the several genera.

Various representatives of the superfamily Metastrongyloidea lay eggs in all stages of development from a single cell (e.g., *Aelurostrongylus* spp.) to an egg containing a first-stage larva (e.g., *Filaroides* spp.). However, sufficient development occurs within the host so that the form found in the feces is either a first-stage larva or an egg containing a first-stage larva. Metastrongyloids typically require a molluscan or annelid intermediate host for development from the first stage to the infective third stage, and infection of the definitive host occurs through ingestion of snails, slugs, or earthworms containing infective third-stage larvae. *Filaroides osleri* and *Filaroides hirthi,* both directly infective to the dog in the first larval stage, form important exceptions to this rule.

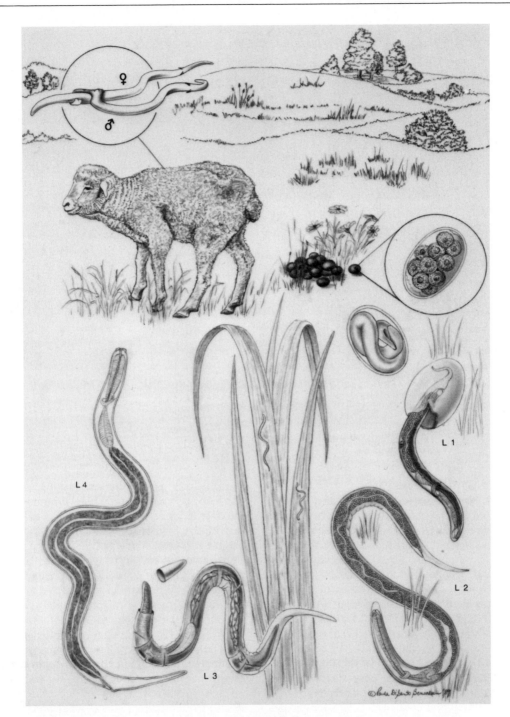

FIGURE 3-70 Life history of a typical strongylid nematode, *Haemonchus contortus*. Eggs are shed in the feces in the morula stage of development. First-stage larvae develop and hatch in a day or two to feed on microorganisms in the feces. After a molt, the resulting second-stage larva also feeds on microorganisms. The second molt is started but not completed in the external environment, so the infective third-stage larva remains encased in the cuticle of the second stage until it is ingested by a sheep. The sheath is cast off in the abomasum of the sheep and the now parasitic third-stage larva undergoes a molt to the fourth stage. The fourth stage sooner or later molts to the fifth or adult stage, depending on whether it enters a period of arrested development.

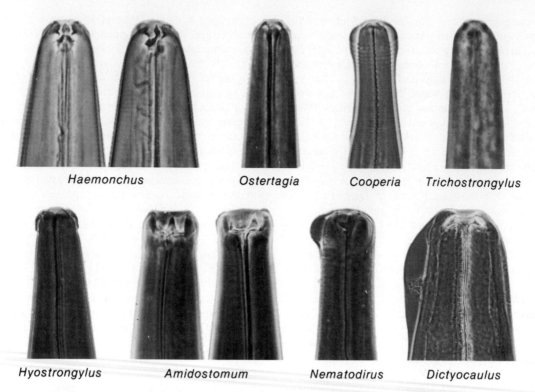

Haemonchus   Ostertagia   Cooperia   Trichostrongylus

Hyostrongylus   Amidostomum   Nematodirus   Dictyocaulus

FIGURE 3-71 Stomas of eight genera of the superfamily Trichostrongyloidea. *Amidostomum* is a parasite of geese and ducks but not of mammals; its large, toothed buccal capsule is not typical of trichostrongyloids.
(From Whitlock JH: *Diagnosis of veterinary parasitisms*, Philadelphia, 1960, Lea & Febiger.)

Superfamily Trichostrongylidae

Trichostrongyloid nematodes are especially common and pathogenic in grazing ruminants, but swine, horses, cats, and birds also host important species. The abomasum and small intestine are the usual locations in ruminants, but one aberrant genus, *Dictyocaulus*, reaches maturity in the air passages. It is sufficient, for practical purposes of effective treatment and control, to identify trichostrongyloids at the generic level of the older classification schemes (Yorke and Maplestone, 1926).

Trichostrongylus

IDENTIFICATION. These are very small, hairlike worms less than 7 mm long, without cephalic inflations, and virtually without buccal capsule; spicules are short, twisted, and usually pointed (see Figures 3-69 and 3-71). *Trichostrongylus axei* parasitizes the simple stomach or abomasum of a wide range of hosts including ruminants, horses, and leporids. Other species are parasites of the small intestine of ruminants and display a higher order of host specificity. Even heavy infections with *Trichostrongylus* will be overlooked on necropsy examination unless care is taken to thoroughly examine washings or scrapings of the stomach and the first six meters of

the small intestine, preferably with a hand lens or stereoscopic microscope. *Trichostrongylus* spp. are most likely to be confused with *Strongyloides* spp. or with the smaller species of *Cooperia*.

LIFE HISTORY. *Trichostrongylus* spp. infective third-stage larvae survive the winter on pasture, and ruminants are exposed to infection when they are turned to pasture in spring. As the weather becomes warmer, the infective larvae die off, and by summer the overwintering generation is essentially gone. However, egg production from new infections rapidly recontaminates the pasture and continues well into fall to produce the next season's overwintering population of *Trichostrongylus* spp.

IMPORTANCE. Although *Trichostrongylus* infections are often asymptomatic, when present in large numbers (10,000 to 100,000 or more), these parasites are capable of producing protracted and debilitating watery diarrhea, especially in stressed or malnourished sheep, cattle, and goats. At first, the feces remain semisolid but soon become watery and dark green in color ("black scours"), staining the fleece of the hindquarters. Some of the feces accumulate in pea- to egg-sized masses ("dingle berries," "dags") that dangle from the fleece and grow by accretion as fluid feces continue to pour over and dry on their surfaces. The resulting foul condition tends to attract blowflies such as *Lucilia cuprina* and result in myiasis. Egg counts rarely exceed 5000 eggs per gram because *Trichostrongylus* sp. is a very small worm that lays few eggs and because the feces are greatly diluted with water. Necropsy examination reveals a wasted carcass without obvious lesions even in the affected small intestine; the parasites themselves are easy to overlook because they are so small. Protracted diarrhea is sufficient to account for the weakness and emaciation typically observed in trichostrongylosis, but it is important to remember that less than massive burdens of *Trichostrongylus* spp. do not usually cause serious illness in well-nourished, unstressed ruminants. Therefore it may be important to consider the quality of the environment and animal husbandry in identifying the ultimate causes of particular outbreaks.

Ostertagia and Teladorsagia

IDENTIFICATION. *Ostertagia* and *Teladorsagia* spp. are indistinguishable by the criteria outlined as follows. However, *Teladorsagia* spp. are parasites of sheep and goats (e.g., *Teladorsagia circumcincta*), and *Ostertagia* spp. are parasites of cattle (e.g., *Ostertagia ostertagi*). Usually less than 14 mm long and brownish in color, with a short, broad buccal

cavity (see Figure 3-71) and short, two- or three-pronged spicules (see Figures 3-65 and 3-72), these genera are found in the abomasum of ruminants. The tip of the mature female's tail is usually annulated (Figure 3-73); the eggs in the amphidelphic ovijector are typical strongylid eggs; and the vulva is guarded by a cuticular expansion called a **vulvar flap.**

LIFE HISTORY. *Ostertagia-* and *Teladorsagia-*infective third-stage larvae resemble those of *Trichostrongylus* spp. in overwintering on northern pastures and in thus infecting ruminants during the early grazing season. However, arrested development of parasitic larvae is also very well developed in *Ostertagia* spp., and this is of both epidemiological and pathological importance. "Type I," or "summer" ostertagiosis, usually occurs in pastured young cattle, the worms maturing without first passing through a developmental arrest (i.e., hypobiotic or latent phase). By contrast, "Type II," or "winter" ostertagiosis, typically occurs in late winter when larvae that have remained in arrested development since fall once again become metabolically active and proceed to develop into adults. Such behavior is part and parcel of the normal mechanism used by *Ostertagia* spp. and certain other trichostrongyloids for overwintering. However, when mistimed or overdone to such an extent as to overcome the compensatory mechanisms of the host, it leads to winter ostertagiosis.

IMPORTANCE. *O. ostertagi* causes chronic abomasitis in young cattle, a disease marked by profuse watery diarrhea, anemia, and hypoproteinemia manifested clinically as submaxillary edema. The animal is typically hidebound and emaciated. The

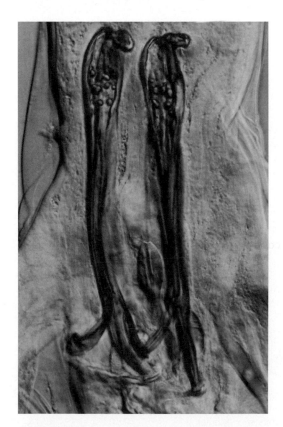

FIGURE 3-72 Spicules of *Ostertagia ostertagi* (×450).

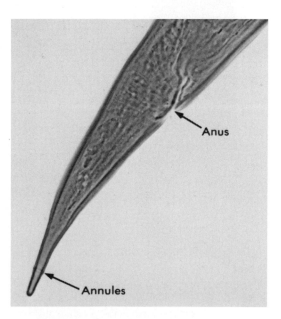

FIGURE 3-73 Tail of female *Ostertagia* (×425).

appetite remains intact, which seems paradoxical in view of the advanced pathological changes taking place in the abomasum. The hydrogen ion concentration of the gastric juice approaches neutrality. Necropsy examination reveals a wasted carcass with depletion of fat deposits typical of extreme malnutrition. The rumen, reticulum, and omasum may be full of good feed, but the alimentary tract from the cardia onward is virtually empty owing to malfunction of the abomasums—the animal has starved to death in the midst of plenty. The "Morocco leather" appearance of the abomasal mucosa is pathognomonic; the whole mucosa is studded with grayish white, pinhead- to pea-sized nodules with a worm protruding from a small opening at the summit of each. *O. ostertagi* is the most important helminth parasite of cattle in the United States. Young cattle infected with large numbers of this parasite waste away and die in a matter of weeks. Those infected with sublethal arasite burdens fail to achieve their full potential for growth and development or require substantially more time to do it. Either is economically disadvantageous. *Telador sagia* spp. of sheep and goats may also cause serious endemic disease in certain localities

Haemonchus

IDENTIFICATION. Up to 30 mm in length, these parasites of the abomasum of ruminants have a

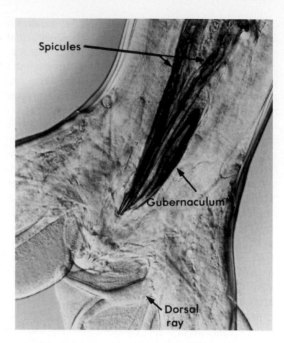

FIGURE 3-74 Spicules of *Haemonchus* spp. (×140).

buccal cavity armed with a lancet (see Figure 3-71). The male has an asymmetrical dorsal ray in its bursa (Figure 3-74) and short, wedge-shaped spicules. The white, egg-filled uterus of the female spirals

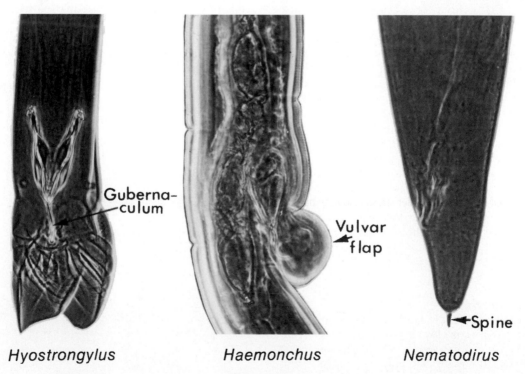

Hyostrongylus *Haemonchus* *Nematodirus*

FIGURE 3-75 Three genera of the superfamily Trichostrongyloidea. (From Whitlock JH: *Diagnosis of veterinary parasitisms,* Philadelphia, 1960, Lea & Febiger.)

around the blood-filled gut, giving rise to the so-called barber pole appearance. The vulva is located about a quarter body length from the tail and may or may not be guarded by variously shaped cuticular inflations ("vulvar flaps"). The prevalence of various vulvar flap configurations varies among species and subspecies of *Haemonchus* (Figure 3-75).

IMPORTANCE. At peak infection, naturally acquired populations of *Haemonchus contortus* may remove one fifth of the circulating erythrocyte volume per day from lambs and may remove an average of one tenth of the circulating erythrocyte volume per day over the course of nonfatal infections lasting two months. These are round figures drawn from observations of a flock of 100 to 175 lambs with erythrocyte loss estimated by the whole-body radioiron retention technique (Georgi, 1964; Georgi and Whitlock, 1965). The pathogenic effects of *H. contortus* result from the inability of the host to compensate for blood loss. If the amount of loss is small and restitution by the host complete, no measurable illness results. "It is doubtful, indeed, whether in such circumstances (i.e., satisfactory nutrition) infection with up to 500 worms has any effect on growth or wool production" (Clunies Ross and Gordon, 1936). However, if the rate of blood loss exceeds the host's hematopoietic capacity, because either the challenge is overwhelming or the response is handicapped by poor nutrition, defective phenotype, or stress, a progressive anemia leads rapidly to death. The cardinal sign of haemonchosis is pallor of the skin and mucous membranes. A hematocrit reading of less than 15% is always accompanied by extreme weakness and shortness of breath and warrants a grave prognosis. Loss of plasma protein results in anasarca frequently manifested externally as submaxillary edema ("bottle jaw"). The appetite typically remains good and, in acute outbreaks, affected animals may not lose appreciable weight. Feces are well formed, diarrhea occurring only in infections complicated by the presence of such species as *Trichostrongylus* and *Cooperia*. Lambs are often the most seriously affected members of a flock, but older sheep under stress also may have fatal anemia. Individual older ewes may succumb in late spring to the overwhelming challenge imposed by hordes of larvae simultaneously emerging from developmental arrest. High egg counts, 10,000 eggs per gram or higher, are typical of haemonchosis.

Mecistocirrus

IDENTIFICATION. Like *Haemonchus* spp., except that the vulva is close to the anus and the spicules are long and thin (Figure 3-76), *Mecistocirrus* spp. are parasites of the abomasum of ruminants and the stomach of pigs in Central America, India, and the Far East.

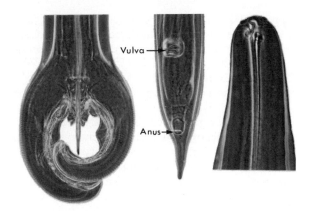

FIGURE 3-76 *Mecistocirrus* spp. (From Whitlock JH: *Diagnosis of veterinary parasitisms*, Philadelphia, 1960, Lea & Febiger.)

Cooperia

IDENTIFICATION. Parasites of the small intestine of ruminants, species of *Cooperia* are less than 9 mm long. The cuticle of the stomal region is transversely striated and slightly inflated, the buccal cavity is very small, the spicules are short and blunted at their tips, and the dorsal ray of the bursa is lyre-shaped (see Figures 3-71, 3-77, and 3-78). *Cooperia* spp. are most likely to be confused with *Trichostrongylus* spp. or *Strongyloides* spp. because of similarity in size and location in the host.

IMPORTANCE. The relationship of *Cooperia* spp. to disease production is similar to that presented for *Trichostrongylus* spp. earlier.

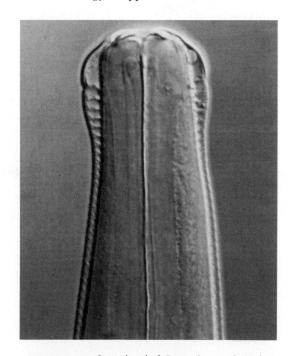

FIGURE 3-77 Stomal end of *Cooperia* spp. (×690).

TABLE 3-3 ■ Some Nematode Prepatent Periods*

Parasite	Prepatent period	Comments
RHABDITIDA		
Strongyloides stercoralis	$\frac{1}{2}$ month	Transmammary infection
Strongyloides papillosus	$\frac{1}{4}$ to $\frac{1}{2}$ month	Transmammray infection
TRICHOSTRONGYLOIDEA		
Trichostrongylus	$\frac{3}{4}$ month	Arrested larvae
Ostertagia	$\frac{3}{4}$ month	Arrested larvae
Haemonchus placei	1 month	
Haemonchus contortus	$\frac{3}{4}$ month	
Cooperia	$\frac{1}{2}$ month	
Nematodirus	$\frac{3}{4}$ month	
Hyostrongylus	$\frac{3}{4}$ to 1 month	
Dictyocaulus	1 to $1\frac{1}{4}$ month	
STRONGYLOIDEA		
Cyathostominae	$2\frac{1}{2}$ to 4 months	Arrested larvae
Strongylus vulgaris	6 to 7 months	
Strongylus equinus	9 months	
Strongylus edentatus	11 months	
Triodontophorus	3 to 6 months	
Chabertia	$1\frac{1}{4}$ months	Arrested larvae
Oesophagostomum	$1\frac{1}{2}$ months	Arrested larvae
Stephanurus dentatus	9 to 16 months	
ANCYLOSTOMATOIDEA		
Ancylostoma caninum	$\frac{1}{2}$ month	Arrested larvae/transmammary infection
Ancylostoma tubaeforme	$\frac{1}{2}$ month	Arrested larvae
Uncinaria stenocephala	$\frac{1}{2}$ month	Arrested larvae
Unicinaria levcas	$\frac{1}{2}$ month	Arrested larve/ transmammary infection
Bunostomum	$1\frac{1}{2}$ to $2\frac{1}{4}$ months	
METASTRONGYLOIDEA		
Crenosoma	$\frac{3}{4}$ month	
Filaroides hirthi	$1\frac{1}{4}$ months	Potential autoinfection
Filaroides osleri	6 months	Potential autoinfection
Aelurostrongylus abstrussus	$1\frac{1}{4}$ to $1\frac{1}{2}$ months	
Protostrongylus	$1\frac{1}{4}$ to $1\frac{1}{2}$ months	
Metastrongylus	$\frac{3}{4}$ to 1 month	
Muellerius	$1\frac{1}{2}$ months	
Parelaphostrongylus tenuis	$2\frac{3}{4}$ to 3 months	Not patent in most domestic animal hosts

Continued

TABLE 3-3 ■ Some Nematode Prepatent Periods*—cont'd.

Parasite	Prepatent period	Comments
OXYURIDA		
Oxyuris equi	4 to 5 months	
ASCARIDIDA		
Ascaris suum	2 months	
Parascaris equorum	$2\frac{1}{2}$ months	
Toxocara vitulorum	$\frac{3}{4}$ month in calves	Transmammary infection
Toxascaris leonina	2 months	
Toxocara canis	1 to 2 months	Transplacental infection
Toxocara cati	2 months	Transmammary infection
SPIRURIDA		
Gongylonema	2 months	
Draschia	2 months	
Habronema	2 months (?)	
Thelazia	$\frac{3}{4}$ to 1 month	
FILARIDS		
Setaria	8 to 10 months	
Onchocerca	10+ months	
Elaeophora	$4\frac{1}{2}$ months	
Dirofilaria	$6\frac{1}{2}$ to 7 months	
ADENOOPHOREAN NEMATODES		
Trichuris vulpis	$2\frac{1}{2}$ to 3 months	
Trichinella spiralis	$\frac{1}{4}$ to $\frac{1}{2}$ month	Find adults in diarrheic feces

*All periods are presented as months postinfection in a naïve animal.

Nematodirus

IDENTIFICATION. Species of *Nematodirus* vary considerably in size; the largest grows to a length of 25 mm. The cuticle of the stomal region is transversely striated and may be inflated; the stoma is armed with a dorsal, triangular tooth (see Figure 3-71). The neck is usually coiled, the spicules are long and thin, the uterus contains very large eggs, and the female has a spine at the tip of her tail (see Figure 3-75).

LIFE HISTORY. The life history and epidemiology of *Nematodirus* species infecting domestic ruminants are distinctly different from those of most other trichostrongyloids. The larva develops to the infective third stage within the eggshell, and hatching depends on extrinsic stimuli, at least in certain species. For example, the infective larva of *Nematodirus battus* must usually be subjected to freezing followed by warmer weather before it will hatch. This property tends to concentrate hatching of infective larvae in the spring, to limit reproduction to one generation per year, and to generate a single wave of infection and disease in late spring. As a result, the severity of infection is typically directly proportional to the previous year's pasture contamination, and timing of the outbreak depends on weather favorable for mass hatching of eggs. However, a second wave of larvae on pasture and consequent infection of sheep has been observed to occur in the fall (Gibson and Everett, 1981; Rodger, 1983; McKellar et al, 1983; Hollands, 1984; Hosie, 1984). Development and hatching of *Nematodirus spathiger* and *Nematodirus fillicollis*–infective larvae tend not to be seasonally constrained in this manner and are common parasites of sheep.

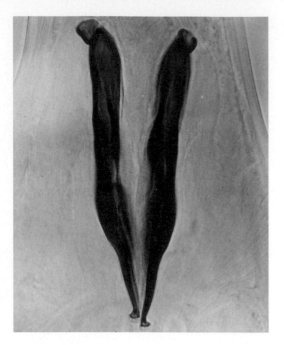

FIGURE 3-78   Spicules of *Cooperia* spp. (×380).

IMPORTANCE. Although *Nematodirus* spp. infections usually are not associated with clinical disease, *N. battus* causes a specific strongylosis characterized by very restricted seasonal incidence and by extremely severe and debilitating diarrhea. Most of the lamb flock display a sudden loss of thrift quickly followed by profuse diarrhea. Deaths begin from 2 days to 2 weeks after onset of clinical signs and continue for several weeks, after which survivors gradually recover; mortality may reach 30%. Egg counts average 600 and rarely exceed 3000 eggs per gram of feces. Necropsy reveals a dehydrated carcass, enlarged pale edematous mesenteric lymph glands, and mild catarrhal enteritis, but very little else in the way of lesions. A count of 10,000 *N. battus* worms is considered significant (Thomas and Stevens, 1956). Originally described from Great Britain (Crofton and Thomas, 1951, 1954), *N. battus* appeared in Oregon in 1985 (Hoberg et al, 1986) and has since been identified in sheep fecal samples from Washington, New York, Vermont, and Maryland (Zimmerman et al, 1986).

Hyostrongylus

IDENTIFICATION. A parasite of the stomach of swine, *Hyostrongylus rubidus* is less than 9 mm long and has a small, annular buccal collar, short spicules with two points, and a long narrow gubernaculum (see Figures 3-71 and 3-75). *Hyostrongylus kigeziensis* is a parasite of the mountain gorilla (Durette-Desset et al, 1992).

LIFE HISTORY AND PATHOGENESIS. *H. rubidus* is a typical trichostrongyloid nematode somewhat resembling *Ostertagia* spp. in its habits. The adult worms parasitize the stomach and produce typical strongylid eggs that closely resemble those of the *Oesophagostomum* spp. infecting swine. Ensheathed third-stage larvae develop within a week under optimum conditions; these are infective when swallowed by swine. Like *Ostertagia* spp., *H. rubidus* invades the gastric glands where the third and fourth molts take place. *H. rubidus* evokes a catarrhal, sometimes diphtheritic, gastritis with ulceration and secretion of a tenacious mucus. Clinical signs include anemia and inappetence with occasional melena as evidence of gastric hemorrhage. Hyostrongylosis is mainly a disease of adult pigs at pasture, but transmission can be markedly reduced during dry summers (Roepstorff and Murrell, 1997). It has been shown, however, that transmission can occur under confinement conditions (Bladt-Knudsen et al, 1994).

ANTHELMINTIC MEDICATIONS. Fenbendazole, ivermectin, and doramectin are approved for or have been shown to successfully treat infections of pigs with *H. rubidus*.

Ollulanus

IDENTIFICATION. A parasite of the stomach of the pig, cat, and other felids including the cougar and tiger, *Ollulanus tricuspis* is minute (less than 1 mm long). The anterior end is rolled up, the vulva is near the anus, the female tail terminates in three or more sharp points, and the spicules are short, equal, and bifurcated (Figure 3-79).

LIFE HISTORY. *O. tricuspis* is ovoviviparous, and the larvae develop to maturity in the stomach. It is a rare example of a nematode capable of completing its life history within a single host. Ingestion of vomitus from an infected host is the most likely means of transmission of *O. tricuspis*.

IMPORTANCE. These worms are capable of causing chronic gastritis in cats that can prove fatal (Hänichen and Hasslinger, 1977). Chronic gastritis also has been observed in a tiger (Breuer et al, 1993) and in captive cheetahs (Collett et al, 2000). In stomachs of infected cats, there is a significant increase in mucosal fibrous tissue and mucosal lymphoid aggregates (Hargis et al, 1983).

ANTHELMINTIC MEDICATION. It has been reported that tetramisole (a 2.5% formulation administered at 5 mg/kg) has proved efficacious and without side effects (Hasslinger, 1984).

Dictyocaulus

IDENTIFICATION. Up to 80 mm long, white adult *Dictyocaulus* worms are found in the respiratory passages of ruminants and horses. The buccal cavity is small, the bursa somewhat reduced, the spicules

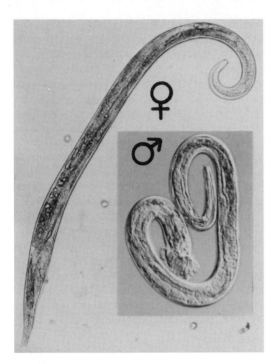

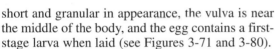

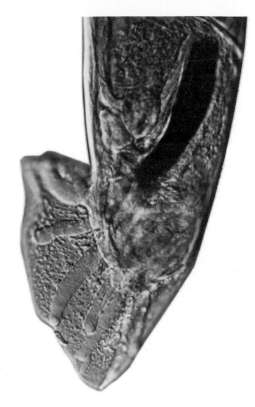

FIGURE 3-79 *Ollulanus tricuspis* from a leopard (×140). Diagnosis is usually based on finding adult specimens of this viviparous species in vomitus.

FIGURE 3-80 Bursa and spicules of *Dictyocaulus* spp. (×168).

short and granular in appearance, the vulva is near the middle of the body, and the egg contains a first-stage larva when laid (see Figures 3-71 and 3-80).

LIFE HISTORY. Adult *Dictyocaulus* spp. live in the lumen of the bronchial tree, where they cause chronic bronchitis and localized occlusion of the bronchial tree with atelectasis. *Dictyocaulus viviparus* is the only nematode that reaches maturity in the lungs of cattle. The freshly laid egg contains a vermiform embryo that usually hatches before being eliminated in the feces. The free-living stages probably derive their energy from stored food materials instead of ingested bacteria because they can develop to the doubly ensheathed infective stage in aerated clean water and because the characteristic "food granules" in the intestinal cells of the first-stage larva become less conspicuous and finally disappear as development proceeds. Development to the infective stage requires about 5 days under optimum conditions. When ingested, the infective larvae migrate by way of the mesenteric lymph nodes and thoracic duct and arrive in the lungs about 5 days later (Jarrett et al, 1957). Egg-laying starts about 4 weeks after infection.

IMPORTANCE. As a group, the lungworms are well-adapted parasites and, in reasonable numbers, impose only a mild burden on their hosts. Light infections with *D. viviparous* are borne without

obvious physiological embarrassment; calves cough occasionally and may breathe slightly faster than normal. Heavier infections lead to partial or complete obstruction of the air passages, and clinical disease develops in proportion to the degree of obstruction. A progressive increase in respiration rate starts at about the fifth day after ingestion of several thousand infective larvae, and the animal coughs occasionally. During the third week, respirations become forced and reach a rate of 100 per minute. Auscultation reveals harsh bronchial sounds and occasional crepitation. Until the fourth week, no larvae are shed in the feces, and the diagnosis rests entirely on the history and clinical signs. During the fourth week, first-stage larvae appear in the feces, and the severity of the clinical signs reaches a maximum. The respiratory rate exceeds 100 per minute, coughing is frequent, crepitation and harsh bronchial sounds can be heard, and air hunger becomes acute. The calves do not feed because they cannot spare the time needed for breathing. Clinical improvement can be noted in survivors after the fifth week.

Dictyocaulus filaria has a life history similar to that of *D. viviparus* (Daubney, 1920). However, unless unusually large infections are acquired, the clinical signs are usually mild. Most cases of

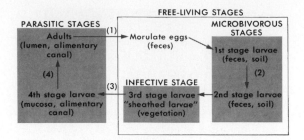

FIGURE 3-81 A typical strongyloid life history. Stages 1 through 4 are explained in the text.

severe clinical illness associated with *D. filaria* are complicated by the presence of less obvious but more pathogenic parasites in the alimentary tract.

Dictyocaulus arnfieldi is a relatively well-adapted parasite of donkeys *(Equus asinus)* but tends to be quite pathogenic in horses. Where this parasite is endemic, it is hazardous to pasture horses and donkeys together.

Ecology and Epidemiology of Strongylid Infections of Ruminants

The following discussion refers principally to ruminants because the ecology and epidemiology of ruminant strongylids have been subjects of intensive research for the best part of a century. The lessons learned from sheep can be applied at least qualitatively to horses. The typical strongylid life history as outlined in Figure 3-81 is generally applicable to members of the superfamilies Trichostrongyloidea, Strongyloidea, and Ancylostomatoidea. Important embellishments on this scheme, such as the skin penetration of hookworm infective larvae and the atypical larval development of *Dictyocaulus* spp., do not significantly alter the qualitative ecological and epidemiological relationships portrayed:

1. The rate of environmental contamination with eggs is in direct proportion to the degree of infection of the host population with adult worms.
2. Development and survival of the infective stage depend on the prevailing conditions of temperature and moisture. Optimum requirements vary distinctly among worm species.
3. Host resistance varies as a function of age, vigor, genetic constitution, presence or absence of an already established infection, and in some instances, acquired immunity.
4. The maturation of the fourth-stage larvae may be held temporarily in abeyance by as yet poorly understood influences. Populations of arrested larvae may be harbored for months before some unknown stimulus restarts their final development.

Adult Worm Populations

Although some infective larvae may survive for weeks or months under suitable environmental conditions, it is the carrier host that often perpetuates strongylid infections from year to year. The infection may be maintained as a small population of adult worms, as a latent population of histotrophic larvae, or as both. Strongylids, like cold viruses and daffodils, display marked seasonal variations. The worm population normally is regulated in a way that spares the host and perpetuates the parasite. Only when this regulation breaks down do outbreaks of disease occur.

During their first season at pasture, calves, lambs, and kids acquire strongylid burdens rapidly by ingesting third-stage larvae as they graze. If the vegetation is heavily contaminated with pathogenic species (e.g., *O. ostertagi* or *H. contortus*), disease and deaths may occur among these young and inexperienced hosts. The accumulation of infection is manifested by a corresponding increase in fecal egg output and by further contamination of the pasture. Provided with sufficient warmth and moisture for larval development, the number of infective stages on vegetation will tend to increase exponentially, at least during the early part of the grazing season. However, the hosts now begin to develop resistance to further infection. The principal component of this developing resistance is a peculiar phenomenon called **premunition:** "a state of resistance to infection which is established after an acute infection has become chronic and which lasts as long as the infecting organisms remain in the body" (*Dorland's Illustrated Medical Dictionary*, ed 27, Philadelphia, 1988, WB Saunders Co). The mechanism of premunition is unknown, but the phenomenon can be readily demonstrated by a variety of simple experiments. For example, if we decide to impose a severe *H. contortus* burden on a sheep that is already harboring a moderate population of these parasites, we must first remove the already established population by anthelmintic medication. Otherwise, part or all of the dose of larvae that we administer experimentally will fail to take. As premunition and other forms of host resistance develop, individual strongylid burdens reach a peak and then begin to decline. Normally, the calf, lamb, or kid enters its first winter with a substantially reduced population of adult strongylids.

What becomes of the infective larvae that the now-premunized host continues to ingest as it grazes? There are three possibilities: such larvae may be rejected, replace established adult worms, or become arrested in their development as fourth-stage larvae, but the total number of adult worms tends to remain at a plateau. The **arrested larvae** (also referred to as **latent, inhibited,** or **hypobiotic** larvae) remain in the alimentary mucous membranes until some stimulus related to the coming of spring, to the reproductive cycle of the host, or to both, restarts their development. For example, in spring a substantial increase in the output of strongylid eggs is observed in the feces of ewes, rams, and wethers. A more pronounced rise also commonly occurs in lambing ewes from 2 weeks before until 8 weeks after parturition at any season. Both **"spring rise"** and **"periparturient rise"** (Crofton, 1954) in fecal egg counts are related principally to the maturation of the larvae that have overwintered as arrested fourth stages in the alimentary mucosae of adult sheep (Herd et al, 1983). "The production of a large number of eggs about two months after parturition ensures that infective stages will be available in large numbers at a time when the sheep population is not only enlarged by lambing but also has a high proportion of susceptible individuals which have not been exposed to infection previously" (Crofton, 1963). The periparturient rise in fecal egg counts can be abrogated by protein supplementation of the ewe (Donaldson et al, 1997).

In summary, calves, lambs, and kids tend to carry large parasite burdens, whereas adult cattle, sheep, and goats usually harbor lighter infections. One peak of strongylid reproductive activity is observed during the grazing season. This occurs in both mature and growing ruminants but tends to be more marked and pathogenic in the latter. A second peak occurs in mature females a few weeks after parturition and is marked by the "postparturient rise" in egg output. This increase is most marked in ewes lambing in spring, at which season a modest spring rise also is observed in wethers and barren ewes.

The **biotic potential** or reproductive capacity of strongylids depends jointly on the rate of production of fertile eggs and on the **generation time** (i.e., the time required for these eggs to develop into egg-producing adults). The normal degree of realization of the biotic potential tends to maintain stable worm populations that display marked periodicity but neither explode nor fade away to extinction. Normally, the probability of any individual strongylid egg reaching reproductive age is only one in thousands, so the worms must compensate by producing enormous numbers of eggs. *Haemonchus* spp. are the most fecund, with *Oesophagostomum* spp., *Chabertia* spp., *Bunostomum* spp., *Ostertagia* spp., *Cooperia* spp., *Trichostrongylus* spp., and *Nematodirus* spp. following roughly in that order. The species with low per-individual reproduction rates tend to compensate either by maintaining larger adult populations (*Trichostrongylus* spp. and *Cooperia* spp.) or by producing eggs more resistant to inclemencies of the external environment (*Nematodirus* spp.).

Development and Survival of the Infective Stage

Most strongylids are capable of developing and maintaining significant populations of infective larvae over considerable ranges of temperature and moisture. Minimum conditions are of interest because they dictate the point at which the environment ceases to harbor significant infection, and optimum conditions are of interest because it is during periods favorable for the development and survival of preparasitic stages that outbreaks of clinical strongylosis usually occur.

No strongylid life history can be completed in totally arid environments, and parasitism with strongylids is correspondingly rare in desert regions. Even under apparently dry conditions, however, microhabitats may exist that contain enough moisture to allow survival if not development of eggs and larvae.

The temperature necessary for development varies with the species, and in each case the rate of development varies with the temperature. With the very significant exceptions of *N. filicollis*, *N. battus*, and *Ostertagia* spp., which appear to be well adapted to cold climates, the egg and larva populations of most strongylids suffer marked reductions or even disappear from northern pastures during winter. Such pastures become recontaminated in spring. *Nematodirus*-infective larvae develop and remain viable in the eggshell during winter in climates about as harsh as possible for the profitable practice of cattle, sheep, or goat husbandry. *Ostertagia* overwinters both as infective larvae on pasture and as arrested larvae in the host population; the pasture larvae begin to die off as warmer and dryer conditions supervene.

Host Resistance

AGE. A general increase in resistance to strongylid infection with age is well marked in cattle, slightly less so in sheep, and least in goats. Age resistance may break down in the face of overwhelming challenge or as a secondary result of malnutrition or disease. Old ewes may succumb to strongylidosis when their teeth fail them, and limited milk production by ewes predisposes their nursling lambs (Whitlock, 1951). Examination of the teeth and udders of ewes should accompany any investigation of parasitic disease in sheep (Love and Biddle, 2000).

PHENOTYPE. Whitlock (1955a, 1958) reported an inherited resistance to trichostrongylidosis in sheep. The progeny of a ram called Violet harbored smaller populations of worms and suffered less reduction in hematocrit than did the progeny of other rams. Unfortunately, one dark and stormy night the electric transmission lines fell on Violet and blew him to glory. Years later, when he retired and turned over his Zeiss photomicroscope, Dr. Whitlock had a brass plate engraved in Violet's memory and mounted on the microscope. Currently, the process has been used in Australia and New Zealand, whereby the resistance status of rams is included in their records. Thus this aspect of genetics is currently being applied on a regular basis to aid in preventing nematode related disease in sheep.

PREMUNITION. The presence of a stable population of adult strongylids in the alimentary canal tends to inhibit further infection or, at least, further maturation of larvae. One ecological explanation of premunition might be kin selection; that is, worms once established exploit the chosen niche and somehow directly or with the manipulation of the host make the niche inhospitable to other worms from different parental stocks. When sheep are infected first with one group of worms and then infected with brothers and sisters or cousins after the first group has matured, there is some evidence that the genetic relatedness of the existing and incoming populations have an effect on the number of worms that will develop to adulthood (Ketzis et al, 2001). Removal of this stable adult population by anthelmintic medication vacates an ecological niche that is promptly filled through maturation of arrested larvae, uninterrupted development of recently ingested infective larvae, or both. For this reason, a ruminant with a subclinical strongylid infection should not be treated with anthelmintics unless an uncontaminated environment can be provided after treatment. The loss of premunition resulting from removal of the stable and established infection will permit rapid reinfection, perhaps with a heavier parasite load than before.

The following seeming paradox lends a measure of symmetry to this argument. If sheep are removed during peak exposure from a *H. contortus*–infested pasture to a parasite-free environment, they will develop more serious infections than if left on the pasture. Interrupting the flow of larvae apparently throws the regulation out of balance in some way. The inhibition of larval development by adult worms is manifested as premunition. It appears that the larvae in turn exercise a measure of control over the adults. At any rate, the practical advice to be gleaned from this is as follows: Be sure to administer an anthelmintic to *H. contortus*–infected sheep before transferring them to an uncontaminated environment, at least during the parasites' normal period of rapid population growth.

SELF-CURE. There are few examples showing the kind of immunity that persists to protect the host against reinfection after the initial strongylid population is gone. Stoll (1929) reported an experiment "in which two helminth-free lambs, upon fenced-in pasturage permitting natural repeated infection, during the summer developed, following an initial dose of *Haemonchus contortus* larvae, first an accumulation of parasites and then a self-cure which expelled the worms and protected the animals thereafter against any significant amount of further infestation with this stomach worm." Thus was born the celebrated phenomenon called **self-cure.**

Stewart (1950) observed seven periods of self-cure within 18 months in a flock of grazing sheep, demonstrated that an identical response could be elicited by giving large doses of infective *H. contortus* larvae, and concluded that self-cure taking place after periods of rain could be attributed to the intake of large numbers of *H. contortus*–infective larvae. He subsequently related the rejection of the previously established adult worm population to an acute hypersensitivity reaction in the alimentary mucous membrane.

An edematous change was evident in the mucous membrane of the abomasum or small intestine, depending upon the site of attachment of the adults, on the day on which a rise of blood histamine occurred after the administration of larvae. The intake of *H. contortus* larvae produced this change only in the abomasum of a sheep which had been infested with *H. contortus* and only in the small intestine of a sheep which had been infested with *Trichostrongylus* spp. (Stewart, 1953).

The lack of permanent protection against reinfection observed by Stewart does not necessarily invalidate Stoll's observations, but examples of functional acquired sterile immunity are rare where *H. contortus* is concerned. We had no difficulty reinfecting lambs of the New York State Veterinary College flock with *Haemonchus contortus cayugensis* after their naturally acquired worm burdens had been removed by anthelmintic therapy. Similar results are commonly observed in other parts of the world with other subspecies of this parasite.

There is at least one definite practical consequence of self-cure. Sheep or goats may die in the throes of evicting their worms and confuse the diagnosis by being found "uninfected" at necropsy when the clinical signs and history correctly pointed to haemonchosis. Profound anemia in grazing sheep or goats is haemonchosis unless positive evidence of another cause (e.g., acute radiation sickness) can be produced. The absence of *H. contortus* worms from the abomasum of an anemic sheep or goat in no way rules out the diagnosis of haemonchosis.

Active Immunity

A durable sterile immunity is conferred in cattle by infection with the lung nematode *D. viviparus*, and considerable success has been achieved by means of artificial immunization with irradiated larval vaccines (see the review by Poynter, 1963). The practical application of vaccines is of course limited to areas of endemic dictyocaulosis, and although *D. viviparous* infection is cosmopolitan in distribution, clinical parasitic disease tends to be sporadic. Clinical dictyocaulosis is common in the British Isles, and that is where the vaccine has found ready acceptance and effective application.

Delayed Maturation of Larvae

Arrested development of larvae not only helps perpetuate certain strongylids from one year to the next but spares the host during the period of winter (or dry season) stress when energy invested in the reproduction of worms with free-living larvae would be a losing proposition biologically. Normally, these larvae mature the following spring. However, outbreaks of severe strongylidosis may result from the unseasonable maturation of arrested larvae during winter and early spring. It is important to recognize the parasitic etiology of such outbreaks despite their unseasonable incidence.

Treatment and Control of Strongylid Infections in Ruminants

The first step in dealing with an outbreak of strongylidosis in a herd of cattle, sheep, or goats is to identify the source of infection and to separate the animals from it. For purposes of observation and nursing, it is usually more convenient to confine the herd in a barn or drylot, and restriction of activity may help prevent losses precipitated by exertion. Never hurry patients acutely ill with haemonchosis; they may drop dead at your feet. Segregate all animals showing anemia, diarrhea, weakness, or depression to facilitate therapy and to prevent their being bullied to death by their stronger fellows, but do not separate nurslings from their dams unless the owner is willing and able to cosset them.

Administration of an anthelmintic may hasten the death of very sick animals, and the owner should be forewarned of possible further losses precipitated by drenching. However, the benefit of an effective anthelmintic drench in primary haemonchosis is usually dramatic. Strongylid nematodes continue to infect our cattle, sheep, and goats despite the plethora of safe and efficacious anthelmintic drugs. The use of anthelmintic drugs should be based on thorough knowledge of the biology of the worms and the area's climatic conditions. The entire herd may be treated at regular "strategic" intervals in the hope of preventing the buildup of infective larvae in the pastures and thus preventing outbreaks of clinical strongylosis. When contamination is particularly severe, strategic treatments preceding parturition and turnout to pasture, at midsummer and in fall,

may need to be supplemented by "tactical" treatments at times when infection pressure may be particularly severe, as for example after a period of moist, warm weather particularly favorable for larval development.

STRONGYLIDS OF THE ALIMENTARY CANAL. Ruminant anthelmintics include thiabendazole, fenbendazole, albendazole, ivermectin, doramectin, levamisole, and morantel. All of these drugs are available in a variety of pharmaceutical forms to suit all types of farm and feedlot management systems.

Abomasal parasites such as *Haemonchus* spp., *Ostertagia* spp., and *Trichostrongylus axei* tend to be more susceptible to anthelmintic medication than related parasites of the small intestine such as *Trichostrongylus* spp., *Cooperia* spp., and *Nematodirus* spp. Normally, these latter genera tend to concentrate in the first quarter of the small intestine, and only a few specimens are found lower down. It is thought that poisoned small intestinal parasites have a greater opportunity to recover and reestablish infection lower down in the small intestine, whereas poisoned abomasal parasites have left the abomasum before they have had a chance to recover. Therefore unless experiments designed to evaluate the efficacy of anthelmintics against parasites of the small intestine are based on postmortem examination of the entire small intestine, the results reported are likely to be biased in favor of the anthelmintic (Bogan et al, 1988).

Fall or early winter treatment ideally should be carried out with anthelmintic drugs active against the immature, arrested parasitic stages of *Ostertagia* spp. (Duncan et al, 1976; Williams et al, 1977; Armour et al, 1978). In northern temperate, nonarid areas of the United States, treatment of ewes with a larvicidal anthelmintic at the time they are put indoors in fall prevents periparturient rise, at least in fall- and early spring–lambing ewes (Herd et al, 1983).

A population of parasites under more or less continuous chemical attack must alter its genetic composition through selection or mutation or be driven to extinction. Increased resistance of the parasites to the chemical, the more frequent outcome, is most common when antiparasitic chemicals are most needed and therefore most frequently used. Purchased livestock also may introduce resistant strains of parasites. However, it must be borne in mind that most cases of apparent anthelmintic failure are due either to continued exposure to infective larvae or to errors in selection and administration of an appropriate anthelmintic chemical (Coles, 1988). *H. contortus, T. circumcincta,* and *Trichostrongylus colubriformis* of sheep and goats in widely scattered parts of the world have displayed resistance to ivermectin, benzimidazoles, and levamisole/morantel. Resistance to anthelmintics has been slower to appear in relation to cattle parasites, but it seems that sporadic cases of resistance to benzimidazoles or macrolides may occur (Vermunt et al, 1995; McKenna, 1996). The genus most typically incriminated in the case of cattle is *Cooperia,* but it appears that *Ostertagia* and *Trichostrongylus* may also sometimes be involved.

Resistance to ivermectin was first reported in the United States for *H. contortus* in Angora goats (Craig and Miller, 1990). Resistance of this same parasite has also been observed in cattle in Texas (DeVaney et al, 1992). *H. contortus* resistance to ivermectin also is present in South Africa and Brazil. In goats in Britain, *Teladorsagia* spp. have manifested a resistance to ivermectin (Jackson et al, 1992). Moxidectin has been shown to remove ivermectin-resistant *H. contortus* in some cases (Craig et al, 1992). However, when effective dosages between susceptible and resistant strains are compared, it would appear that ivermectin resistance is reflected in cross-resistance to the other products with the same modes of action (Shoop, 1992).

A number of reports have indicated that thiabendazole is not as effective against *H. contortus* and *T. colubriformis* as it was when first introduced. The thiabendazole-resistant strains of *H. contortus* show cross-resistance to many other benzimidazole anthelmintics (Drudge et al, 1964; Smeal et al, 1968; Hotson et al, 1970; Theodorides et al, 1970; Kates et al, 1971; Colglazier et al, 1972, 1975; Berger, 1975; Holgarth-Scott et al, 1976; Kelly et al, 1977).

O. circumcincta and *T. colubriformis* resistant to morantel tartrate and levamisole also have been reported (Le Jambre et al, 1977, 1978a,b; Santiago et al, 1977, 1978). A levamisole-resistant *O. circumcincta* isolate was very susceptible to albendazole and oxfendazole (Le Jambre, 1979). Because sheep and goats serve as hosts for similar or identical species of parasites, it is logical to assume that a drug that works well in sheep should work equally well in goats. However, such is not the case. Many anthelmintics are far less effective in goats than in sheep and may require that substantially increased dosages be administered to obtain satisfactory results (Coles, 1986).

LUNGWORMS. Clinical outbreaks of dictyocaulosis are treated with fenbendazole, ivermectin, dormectin, levamisole, oxfendazole, or albendazole. These are highly efficacious against both adult and immature stages of *Dictyocaulus* spp.

SUBCLINICAL PARASITISM OF ADULT DAIRY CATTLE. In light of the development and approval of Ivomec Eprinex, the macrolide eprinomectin, which can be administered to lactating dairy cows with no milk withholding, the question of whether the treatment of adult dairy cows is a profitable enterprise becomes a question of practical importance for the first time. Herd et al (1983) compared 26 trials in which milk production was examined and found that in 14 trials there was no change, in 7 trials there was an increase after treatment, and in 5 trials there was an increase in the control group. In a large trial of 9721 lactations examined in Britain over a 305-day lactation, there was a 42-kg gain in milk production (Michel et al, 1982). The authors thought that this was not a cost-effective increase, whereas others interpreted the gain as cost effective (Theodorides and Free, 1983).

In a New Zealand trial, half of 5556 cows on 47 dairies were treated twice with oxfendazole when dry (Bisset et al, 1987). During the next 251-day lactation, the treated cows produced an average of 2.24 kg more butterfat or 52.9 kg more milk. A positive response was seen in 36 of the 47 treated herds, but only one herd had a significant increase. The authors noted a greater response to treatment in cows that had been grazed previously on pastures that had been occupied with calves and with cows that were historically higher milk producers.

Two trials were performed in the Netherlands (Ploeger et al, 1989, 1990). In the first trial, 285 of 527 dry cows were treated with ivermectin. The milk yield over a hypothetical 305-day lactation increased an average of 205 kg in the treated cows. In this trial, 17 of the 31 treated herds had a positive response, and again greater responses were noted in cows that had historically higher milk yields. In the second trial, 676 of 1385 cows in 81 herds were treated with albendazole within a week of calving. The milk yield during the hypothetical 305-day lactation of the treated cows increased 133 kg, and 49 of the 81 herds had a positive response.

In an Australian trial, half of 498 cows in five pasture-fed herds were treated with ivermectin when dry (Walsh et al, 1995). The milk yield increased 74 L during the first 100 days of lactation, whereas the yield over the entire lactation was 86 L. All of the herds had a positive response, but the increase was significant in only one herd. No increased response was observed among cows that previously had been noted to have a high lactation production index. There was no difference in the cows as to time from calving to first service, but the calving to conception time was reduced in the treated cows by 2 to 8 days. As is typical of lactating dairy cows, there were few eggs present in the feces of the Australian cows, and there was no correlation between egg reduction and the observed increases in milk production (see the excellent review by Reinemeyer, 1995).

In none of these large trials was the product delivered to the cows during lactation. Thus we still have no data on what to expect from the treatment of cows with eprinomectin and, in a sense, are comparing apples with oranges. These studies on the treatment of dry cows do strongly suggest that increased milk yields are to be expected, but whether these will be great enough to offset the cost of the treatment is yet to be shown.

There is no doubt among parasitologists that the treatment of yearlings and 2-year-olds is a profitable undertaking (see a second excellent review by Reinemeyer, 1990). These are the ages of cattle that tend to suffer significantly from parasitism. Parasitized replacements grow more slowly and often fail to reach their full growth potential. Such performance results in real financial loss of which the producer may well be completely unaware.

SUBCLINICAL PARASITISM OF SHEEP. The effects of moderate parasitism in lambs were investigated by administering 5000, 10,000, or 20,000 infective *T. colubriformis* larvae and comparing weight gains and feed efficiency of these artificially infected lambs with the performance of uninfected controls. Although about one half of the larvae administered became adult worms and group average fecal egg counts of 536 to 2236 eggs per gram were observed, these levels of infection apparently caused no significant differences in average daily gain or feed efficiency (Bergstrom et al, 1975).

INTEGRATED CONTROL OF RUMINANT STRONGYLID INFECTIONS. Much has been written about prevention and control of strongylidoses. Every scheme has its proponents and detractors, but there is no unique formula that applies in all situations.

Parasitism should be considered as a year-round game between the livestock, the strongylids, and the stockman. Certain moves at propitious times are capable of biasing the game in the stockman's favor, but these moves must not violate the rules of the game or the results may be disappointing or even disastrous. The ultimate criterion for success in any control effort is the net profit that accrues, not the number of worms fatally poisoned. The purchase of a livestock scale, as suggested by Whitlock (1955b) and the maintenance of adequate production records provide objective measures of success.

Control efforts may be classified under selective breeding for resistant stock, rotational grazing, and anthelmintic medication. The first of these has been used the longest. Long before worms were recognized as disease agents, shepherds selected productive livestock for breeding, and worms claimed the lives of weaklings (against the shepherd's wishes perhaps, but to his eventual benefit) (Whitlock, 1966). There exist, in many parts of the world and under certain systems of husbandry, cattle, sheep, and goats capable of

thriving without help from science and technology. These animals have parasites and handle them effectively as a population. Individual animals occasionally die of parasitism just as individuals occasionally get killed by predators, hung up in fences, or drowned in watering places, but the effect of minor losses such as these on the general population is minimal. On the other hand, there are also parts of the world and systems of husbandry in which the economic production of food and fiber requires intelligent intervention to suppress strongylid populations. Host resistance continues to be of paramount importance here, even though conscious selection of resistant stock is seldom part of the breeding program. The reason is that resistant hosts contribute less to the growth of the parasite populations than do more susceptible animals and their presence thus tends to benefit the flock as a whole.

In theory, rotational grazing seeks to prevent or limit the intake of infective larvae by permitting animals to graze on a particular area of pasture no longer than a week so that eggs passed in their feces do not have time to develop into infective larvae, and then not allowing the animals to return until all the larvae have died off. The considerable investment in fence construction required by rotational grazing schemes usually discourages strict observance of the rules, so the theoretical ideal is seldom realized in practice. However, any practicable rotation scheme undoubtedly increases the productivity of the pasture and may prolong the parasite generation, if only slightly (Levine and Clark, 1961).

Modern anthelmintics are efficient and comparatively nontoxic. There are places in the world where efficient livestock production is virtually impossible without them, and they are of undoubted benefit in increasing productivity wherever significant parasite losses occur. However, there are limitations, hazards, and expenses that we cannot afford to ignore. No anthelmintic can overcome excessive exposure to infection just as no amount of bailing can overcome too large a leak. Crofton (1958) concluded that periodic treatment with interim reinfection merely delayed attainment of the full parasite potential. He suggested concentrating treatments early in the pasture season to obtain maximum delay in the parasite population increase because an adult worm in spring is a potential forebear of a whole series of generations that season.

Currently, it is widely believed that, at least in temperate climates, only one generation of ruminant trichostrongylids capable of causing disease is produced (Herd et al, 1984). However, Crofton's basic premise is supported by Herd, Parker, and McClure, (1984), who found that "prophylactic treatments in the spring were just as effective as suppressive treatments throughout the entire grazing season and resulted in significant ($P < 0.001$) increases in weight gain." The prophylactic treatments used by Herd, Parker, and McClure (1984) consisted of four doses of ivermectin (0.02 mg/kg) administered 3, 6, 9, and 12 weeks after spring turnout. In New York State, we freely admit, 12 weeks after turnout is getting pretty close to fall.

Probably the most important type of host resistance is premunition. The development of premunition in a grazing flock tends to truncate the growth curve of the parasite population by preventing the maturation of new waves of larvae and thus in effect, to prolong the generation time. Although interference with the development of premunition is obviously to be avoided, periodic anthelmintic medication may have precisely this effect.

Superfamily Strongyloidea

MORPHOLOGY. Strongyloids tend to be larger and stouter-bodied than trichostrongyloids, and most of them have a large buccal cavity surrounded by a sclerotized wall (buccal capsule) that is usually rigid but may be jointed or thin and flexible. The stomal structures of strongyloids are sufficiently distinct to permit identification of species with occasional reference to other characters. Greater dependence must be placed on these other characters when it is impossible to examine both dorsal and lateral aspects of the stoma, as is the case with permanently mounted specimens.

The **buccal cavity** of strongyloids is large and directed anteriorly (see Figure 3-62). The stomal opening is surrounded by a row or two of what appear to be leaves or palings of a stockade, depending on the imagination of the observer. These are called **leaf crowns,** and much is made of them in the taxonomy of strongyloids. In some species, the duct of the dorsal esophageal gland is carried to the rim of the buccal capsule in a sclerotized ridge (dorsal gutter; see Figure 3-62) on the inner wall of the buccal capsule. In other species, the dorsal gutter is absent (Figure 3-82). Teeth, when present, lie at the base of the buccal cavity, where they lacerate the plug of mucous membrane that is drawn into the buccal cavity by the sucking action of the muscular esophagus. The copulatory bursa is well developed, the spicules long and thin. The vulva is close to the anus, and the uterus is prodelphic in most strongyloids.

LIFE HISTORY. Strongyloid life histories are typical of the order, but significant variations occur in certain groups. For example, *Syngamus* sp., the "gapeworm" of domestic and wild birds, and *Stephanurus* sp., the "kidney worm" of swine, use earthworms as paratenic hosts.

Family Strongylidae
Subfamily Strongylinae

IDENTIFICATION. Members of the subfamily Strongylinae, often referred to as "large strongyles," are chiefly parasites of the large intestine of equines (*Strongylus, Triodontophorus, Oesophogodontus,* and *Craterostomum*), elephants (*Decrusia, Equinurbia,* and *Choniangium*), macropodid marsupials (*Macropicola* and *Hypodontus*), and ostriches (*Codiostomum*). Identification of genera and species of strongylin parasites of horses is a matter of comparing the microscopic appearance of the stomal region of specimens with the series of illustrations of equine parasites found in Chapter 5. There are two leaf crowns, but because the elements of each are similar in size and number, the two crowns appear as one.

IMPORTANCE. *Strongylus vulgaris, Strongylus edentatus,* and *Strongylus equinus* are among the most destructive parasites of the horse. All three are bloodsuckers as adult worms in the cecum and colon, but even more important, their larvae undergo migrations that inflict even greater damage, especially in foals and yearlings. *Triodontophorus* spp. appear, by the ferocious teeth at the base of their buccal cavities (see Figure 5-49), to be bloodsucking parasites. Clusters of *Triodontophorus tenuicollis* worms cause localized ulceration of the colonic mucous membrane.

LIFE HISTORY OF *STRONGYLUS VULGARIS*. The extrahost development of *S. vulgaris* is typical of strongylids in general (see Figure 3-70). Development to the infective stage requires adequate moisture and temperatures in the range 8° to 39° C; the time required is inversely related to temperature (e.g., about 8 to 10 days at 18° C, 16 to 20 days at 12° C). In arid regions, scattering the droppings with a tractor and harrow reduces strongylid larva populations by breaking up the manure and causing it to dry out before the larvae have reached the desiccation-resistant third stage. However, in more humid regions, the interior of even scattered manure remains sufficiently moist long enough for development to the third stage. Once *S. vulgaris* larvae have arrived at the third stage, they are very resistant to cold and desiccation and can survive on pasture through a northern winter or in stored dry hay for many months. The longevity of *S. vulgaris* third-stage larvae depends mainly on the food reserves in their intestinal cells; the greater the activity of the larvae, the more rapidly these reserves become exhausted. However, it is imprudent to depend on *S. vulgaris* to wear itself out no matter how warm and humid the weather may be. Any pasture that has held a horse within a year can be assumed to be contaminated with *S. vulgaris* infective larvae.

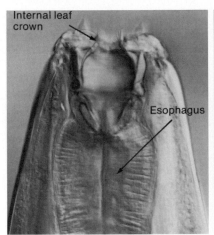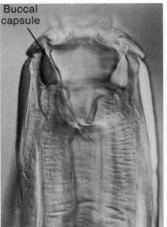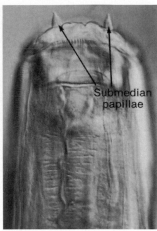

FIGURE 3-82 *Murshidia dawoodi* (Strongylidae: Cyathostominae) from an African elephant (×100).

In 1870 Otto Bollinger hypothesized that occlusion of the intestinal arteries by verminous thrombi and emboli could account for most equine colic cases, both fatal and nonfatal. Since then, the etiological relationship between *S. vulgaris* and colic has been extensively debated and somewhat investigated, although not to an extent commensurate with its scientific and practical importance.

The meticulous experimental observations and well-thought-out conclusions of Enigk (1950b, 1951) provide the basis for the following outline. For the reader interested in greater detail than can be presented here, Dr. Georgi has published an English translation of Enigk's papers (Georgi, 1973), and all serious students of equine medicine and pathology should study the review by Ogbourne and Duncan (1977).

When ingested by a horse, the infective third-stage larvae of *S. vulgaris* cast off their sheaths in the lumen of the small intestine and enter the wall of the cecum and ventral colon. Here the larvae penetrate to the submucosa, where they undergo the third molt, which is completed by the seventh to eighth day after infection. Leaving their third-stage cuticles surrounded by round cells, the fourth-stage larvae penetrate nearby small arterioles that lack an internal elastic lamina and wander in the intima of these vessels and progressively larger branches of the cranial mesenteric artery.

Enigk observed that *S. vulgaris* cannot penetrate the internal elastic lamina, which thus confines the larvae to the intima and helps keep them on their proper course. Thus constrained, the rapidly migrating larvae reach the colic and cecal arteries by the eighth to the fourteenth day after infection and the cranial mesenteric artery by the eleventh to the twenty-first day (Enigk, 1950b; Duncan and Pirie, 1972). Some of the larvae push on into the aorta and its branches, where they may cause important pathological changes. However, larvae proceeding beyond the cranial mesenteric artery are probably lost to their species because of the improbability of their finding their way back to the cecum and ventral colon to breed.

After 2 to 4 months of migrating in the intima, the fourth-stage larvae that have not gone astray or become trapped deep in thrombi are carried away by the bloodstream to the small arteries in the subserosa of the intestinal wall. The larvae, now grown large, occlude these small arteries, whose walls then become inflamed and, in due course, are destroyed. The larvae thus liberated from the arterial tree then enter the surrounding tissue and become encapsulated in pea- to bean-sized nodules wherein the final molt occurs. Some larvae complete the final molt even before returning to the intestinal wall. According to Duncan and Pirie (1972), most of the larvae found in the cranial mesenteric lesions at 4 months after infection have molted to the fifth stage, although the fourth-stage cuticle is still retained as a sheath. This sheath is cast off before these immature adults return to the intestinal wall. Finally, the immature adults enter the lumen of the cecum and ventral colon, mature, and commence reproductive activity at about 6 months after infection. It is rare to find more than 100 or 200 adult *S. vulgaris* worms in a horse, and their egg production usually constitutes 10% or less of the total strongylid output.

The migrations of fourth-stage *S. vulgaris* larvae cause arteritis, thrombosis, and embolism of the cranial mesenteric artery and its branches. Although these arterial lesions exist to some degree in almost every horse, and principal branches are frequently completely occluded by them, fatal infarction of the bowel wall is relatively infrequent. This seeming paradox suggests a Darwinian interpretation. Of all domestic animals, the horse has by far the most elaborate system of anastomoses in the arterial supply to the large intestine. The colic vessels are particularly well supplied with the means for rapidly establishing effective collateral circulation (Dobberstein and Hartmann, 1932). In an evolutionary context, this may be interpreted as evidence that *S. vulgaris,* which has no direct counterpart in other domestic animals, has probably been occluding horses' intestinal arteries and thus exerting selection pressure for ages.

However, despite this exceptional adaptation, obstruction of the intestinal arteries does occasionally lead to fatal infarction of the bowel. Even temporary curtailment of blood flow pending establishment of collateral circulation may account for a high proportion of clinical colic cases from which the patient recovers. Furthermore, the fatal intestinal displacements often interpreted at necropsy examination to be the cause of colic symptoms are more likely to be the result of abnormalities of intestinal tone and motility brought about by verminous thromboembolism and the horse's violent efforts to obtain relief.

After the larvae have migrated back to the intestinal lumen, the arterial lesions heal (Duncan and Pirie, 1975; Pauli et al, 1975). These lesions also heal dramatically after destruction of the larvae by medication with any of several newer anthelmintics, including ivermectin (Holmes et al, 1990). Development and resolution of verminous arteritis can be studied radiographically in young foals by injecting contrast medium through a catheter that has been introduced into the aorta by way of a peripheral artery (Slocombe et al, 1977). Two such radiographs comprise Figure 3-83. The upper radiograph of a 2-month-old pony foal was taken 1 month after 500 *S.vulgaris* larvae were administered through a nasogastric tube. The cranial mesenteric and ileocecal arteries are enlarged, and blood flow through the colic arteries is greatly diminished, as evidenced by the lack of contrast medium flowing through them. The lower radiograph of the same foal was taken 1 month after albendazole therapy. Now the stem arteries have returned to nearly normal size, and the contrast medium clearly outlines the colic arteries, indicating a greatly increased flow through those vessels (Rendano et al, 1979a).

LIFE HISTORIES OF *STRONGYLUS EDENTATUS* AND *STRONGYLUS EQUINUS*. Adult *S. edentatus* and *S. equinus* are about twice as large as *S. vulgaris,* probably twice as bloodthirsty, and considerably more difficult to remove with anthelmintic drugs,

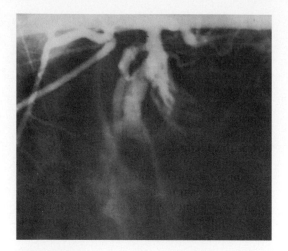
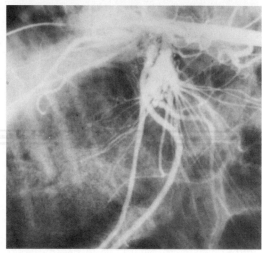

FIGURE 3-83 Resolution of equine verminous arteritis after larvicidal therapy with albendazole. The ramifications of the cranial mesenteric artery are made visible by contrast arteriography. The upper radiograph was taken 1 month after infection with 500 *Strongylus vulgaris* larvae, and albendazole therapy was started immediately afterward. The lower radiograph was taken 1 month after albendazole therapy.

but their larvae are not quite as pathogenic. The migration routes followed by larvae of *S. edentatus* and *S. equinus* have been elucidated by Wetzel (1940a), Wetzel and Kersten (1956), and McCraw and Slocombe (1974, 1978).

The third-stage larvae of *S. edentatus* burrow into the wall of the large intestine and reach the liver through the portal veins. Enclosed in nodules in the hepatic parenchyma, they molt to the fourth stage in about 2 weeks. The fourth-stage larvae then wander about in the hepatic tissue for about 2 months, growing larger as they go. Leaving the liver by way of the hepatic ligaments, the larvae wander for months in the parietal retroperitoneal tissues and eventually make their way to the base of the cecum and thence to the bowel lumen. The prepatent period usually is cited as 11 months but may be as short as 6 months (McCraw and Slocombe, 1978).

The third-stage larvae of *S. equinus,* like those of *S. vulgaris,* undergo their third molt in nodules in the wall of the cecum and colon. About 11 days after infection, the newly molted fourth-stage larvae leave their intestinal nodules, cross the peritoneal space, and enter the right half of the liver, which, in the living horse, lies in contact with the cecum. These larvae wander about in the hepatic tissue for 2 months or longer before emerging and entering the pancreas or abdominal cavity, where they complete their development to the fifth stage. The fourth molt occurs about 4 months after infection. Finally, these adult worms penetrate the wall of the large intestine and reenter the lumen to mate. The prepatent period of *S. equinus* is 9 months.

Triodontophorus

Triodontophorus spp. (and the 40-odd species of cyathostomes) do not migrate far beyond the mucous membrane of the colon; therefore the pathogenic effects of their larvae are considerably less dramatic than those inflicted by larvae of *Strongylus* spp. However, *T. tenuicollis* adults are frequently observed clustered in ulcerated areas in the large intestine.

Subfamily Cyanthostominae

IDENTIFICATION. These "small strongyles" are parasites of the large intestine of horses, elephants, pigs, marsupials, and turtles, and there is a multitude of them. About 40 species of cyathostomes parasitize the cecum and colon of horses, and it is commonplace to find as many as 15 to 20 of these species infecting an individual host at the same time. Cyathostomins have somewhat smaller buccal cavities than strongylins. All have distinct inner and outer leaf crowns, the elements of which differ in size and number (see Figure 3-82). In some species, the inner leaf crown elements are inconspicuous and can be seen only in well-cleared specimens. Identification of species of equine cyathostomes can be accomplished by comparing dorsal and lateral aspects of the buccal regions of fresh or cleared, fixed specimens with the photomicrographs of strongylins and cyathostomins portrayed in Chapter 5. All of the more common species are represented in that collection.

IMPORTANCE. From 75% to 100% of the eggs passed in the feces of naturally infected horses are produced by the small strongyles (Cyathostominae) because these greatly outnumber the large strongyles (Strongylinae) both in numbers of species and in numbers of individuals. Cyathostomin larvae do not migrate beyond the mucous membrane

of the cecum and colon, so their pathogenic effects are usually less dramatic than those inflicted by the larvae of *Strongylus* spp. However, infection by large numbers of arrested cyathostomin larvae causes a distinctive clinical disease that usually is observed in late fall, winter, or early spring. Affected horses display persistent diarrhea, progressive emaciation, and marked hypoalbuminemia sometimes attended by anasarca. The feces may be negative for strongylid eggs, and the history often includes regular and vigorous anthelmintic medication; there is no response to anthelmintic medication (Jasko and Roth, 1984; Church et al, 1986). Lesions consist of granulomatous colitis, and masses of cyathostomin larvae are embedded in the mucous membrane (Figure 3-84). Massive invasions of the bright red fourth-stage larvae of *Cylicocyclus insigne* riddling the mucosa of the large intestine are particularly impressive in this regard. Mirck (1977) described verminous enteritis in young horses and ponies in which large numbers of fourth- and early fifth-stage cyathostomins are discharged in the feces. This form of **cyathostominosis** occurs

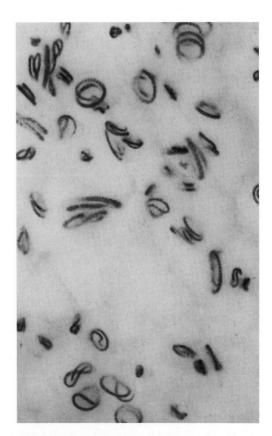

FIGURE 3-84 Fourth-stage larvae and juvenile adult "small strongyles" (Cyathostominae) in the colonic mucosa of a horse (×16). Massive invasions such as this usually cause severe diarrhea.

in the Netherlands from November to May, is characterized by watery diarrhea associated with severe inflammation of the mucous membrane of the cecum and colon, and often terminates fatally. Most of the worms are immature, and egg counts are therefore misleadingly low. Anthelmintic therapy has no influence on the course of the disease or on the number of worms being passed in the feces. Apparently, the larvae encysted in the mucosa are basically unaffected by any currently available anthelmintic drugs, including oral ivermectin at 0.2 or 1.0 mg/kg and moxidectin at 0.3 or 0.4 mg/kg (Klei et al, 1993; Xiao et al, 1994). There are many more larvae than can be accommodated as adult parasites, and as they mature, many are swept out with the manure. Church et al (1986) diagnosed their two cases heroically by taking full-thickness biopsies of the jejunum and cecum or ventral colon, and cured them both with steroid therapy directed at the inflammatory reaction. In one case, dexamethasone (20 mg) was administered intramuscularly each day for 4 days and on alternate days thereafter with the dose reduced by 4 mg every fourth day. In the second case, dexamethasone (20 mg) was administered intramuscularly for 10 days. In both cases, response to steroid therapy was dramatic, with improvement in fecal consistency noted within 24 hours and return to normal serum albumin levels within 1 week.

Development of Strongylid, Ascarid, and Strongyloides Infections in Foals

Ann F. Russell (1948) studied the sequential changes in the composition of worm populations in 26 foals from seven different thoroughbred studs. She performed fecal egg counts and identified infective larvae developing in fecal cultures of samples collected from these foals every week from the age of 4 weeks to at least 6 months and, in a few cases, to more than 1 year.

In Figure 3-85, egg counts are plotted against age for *Strongyloides westeri,* for *Parascaris equorum,* and for the family Strongylidae collectively. Note that *S. westeri* infection reached a maximum early in life, then rapidly dropped to a low level, and finally disappeared at about 5 months of age. This accords perfectly with what we now know about the mammary transmission of *S. westeri.*

P. equorum eggs first appeared at about 12 weeks of age, after which egg counts rose steeply to a peak and then rapidly fell but, instead of disappearing completely, persisted at a low level indefinitely. The 12-week delay in appearance of *P. equorum* eggs corresponds closely to the prepatent period of this parasite, and we may deduce from this that the infection was acquired soon after birth. Thus, anthelmintic medication of the pregnant mare,

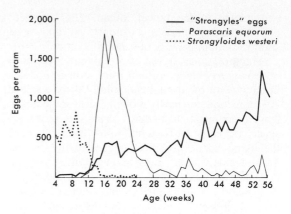

FIGURE 3-85 Average number of eggs of *Parascaris equorum,* "strongyles," and *Strongyloides westeri* counted per gram of manure. Data obtained from weekly observations of 26 foals. (Modified from Russell, 1948; reproduced from Evans JW, Barton A, Hintz HF, et al: *The horse,* New York, 1977, WH Freeman & Co.)

careful bathing of her udder and teats, and thorough cleaning of the foaling box are logical measures for the prevention of significant infection of foals with *P. equorum.* The persistence of infection at a low level in horses of all ages and the extraordinary resistance of the egg to the rigors of the external environment make *P. equorum* a difficult parasite to control.

The third and most important curve shown in Figure 3-85 represents a gradual increase in the composite strongylid egg counts during the first year of life. To interpret this curve, one must take into account the relative abundances of *S. vulgaris, S. edentatus,* and the "small strongylids" as determined by fecal culture and identification of the infective larvae. These findings are portrayed in Figure 3-86, which shows that the eggs of the small strongylids always predominated, representing, at various ages, between 80% and 100% of the total strongylid eggs shed in the feces of these foals. This is to be expected in view of the 6- to 11-month prepatent periods of *Strongylus* spp. and the general predominance of cyathostomes in horses. It is curious, therefore, that small numbers of *S. vulgaris* and *S. edentatus* eggs appear in fecal samples of foals up to 12 weeks of age. Russell (1948) observed this phenomenon in every one of 26 foals studied and interpreted it as evidence of coprophagia. This ingestion of feces by foals is probably related to the normal process of "seeding" the cecum and colon with beneficial microorganisms essential for the digestion of cellulose, but it also presents a clear opportunity for invasion by parasites.

As Figures 3-85 and 3-86 show, strongylid egg output increases steadily, and *S. vulgaris* and *S. edentatus* eggs appear on schedule at 6 months and

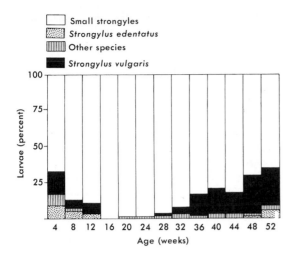

Small strongles
Strongylus edentatus
Other species
Strongylus vulgaris

FIGURE 3-86 Percentage of larvae of different species of strongyles in fecal cultures. Data obtained from weekly observations of 26 foals.
(Modified from Russell, 1948; reproduced from Evans JW, Barton A, Hintz HF, et al: *The horse,* New York, 1977, WH Freeman & Co.)

11 months, respectively. This clearly indicates that strongylid infection begins shortly after birth of the foal and proceeds without interruption thereafter. Because young foals are much more susceptible to the pathogenic effects of these parasites than are older horses, it follows that the greatest efforts should be directed toward preventing excessive exposure, especially during the first months of life.

Treatment and Control of Strongylid Infections in Horses

Horses, asses, and mules host a far greater variety of strongylid parasites than ruminants and other domestic animals do. Even an apparently healthy horse may be infected with tens or even hundreds of thousands of small strongylid worms (Cyathostominae). Most equine parasites are distributed wherever horses are kept all over the world. The relative abundances of individual species may vary from place to place, but the group as a whole seems well adapted to a wide range of climates. In fact, the conditions under which horses are kept and the uses to which they are put seem to have far more influence on the mix of strongylid parasites they harbor than does the part of the world they happen to inhabit. This is in stark contrast to the situation in ruminants. For example, two sheep farms lying a few miles apart but at substantially different altitudes may have completely different parasite problems because the ecological conditions at pasture favor development and survival of the infective larvae of different species of trichostrongylids at different elevations.

With horses, it is a case of management more than of weather. Backyard ponies, livery horses, show and race horses, and horses kept for breeding purposes follow distinctly different careers and therefore present distinctly different problems for parasite control. "Because management of horses is so variable and the uses to which horses are put are so different, recommendations as far as control of horse parasites should be tailored to the particular horse establishment rather than to a set of universal recommendations" (Craig and Suderman, 1985). "What's a good worming schedule for horses?" is a common but naive question.

About the most strongylid-contaminated environment ever devised for a horse is the neat little paddock which, in wealthy neighborhoods at least, is surrounded by a white board fence. There is rarely enough grass in such an enclosure to satisfy the horse's nutritional needs for more than a few weeks each year, so hay and grain must be fed to make up the difference. Great masses of horse manure accumulate, and thriving hordes of strongylid infective larvae develop in them and spread out onto the surrounding grass. The horse enjoys nibbling whatever grass is available and is capable of cutting it closer than a lawnmower. In such a situation a horse cannot fail to ingest large numbers of infective strongylid larvae.

A sensible solution to this problem might be to provide horses the exercise and fresh air they need in bare paddocks containing no green plants at all. However, the almost universally adopted "solution" is to keep the horses in their green exercise lots and try to trim the worm population to subclinical levels by periodic administration of anthelmintic drugs. This program has been pursued so energetically that the strongylid parasites of horses excel those of all other hosts relative to benzimidazole resistance, at least in North America.

On many breeding farms, all horses older than 2 months are routinely dewormed every 4 to 8 weeks (Drudge and Lyons, 1965). The objective of this program is to prevent contamination of the pasture with strongylid eggs, and that is why it is essential that all horses on the premises be treated. Piperazines are effective against both ascarids and cyathostomes and are thus the logical choice for worming foals aged up to 6 months. Thereafter, drugs effective against *Strongylus* spp. should be substituted. On the basis of epidemiological evidence, the most essential of all strategic treatments is that administered in spring, around foaling time. It is during this period that the adult worm population is greatly augmented through maturation of arrested and migrating larvae. The fecundity of these worms is also increased, and larger numbers of larvae reach the infective stage, thus posing a threat to young, susceptible horses. Elimination of these egg-laying worms in spring thus renders the pastures safer for grazing horses (Duncan, 1974).

Adult *S. vulgaris, S. edentatus, S. equinus,* cyathostomes, *Oxyuris* spp., and *Parascaris* spp. are susceptible to febantel, fenbendazole, ivermectin, levamisole with piperazine, mebendazole, oxfendazole, oxibendazole, pyrantel pamoate, and thiabendazole alone or with piperazine. Administration of a macrolide in fall and early spring affords control of ascarids and stomach bots.

Larvae of *S. vulgaris* migrating in the cranial mesenteric artery and its ramifications are accessible to attack by several anthelmintics. Ivermectin is highly effective in a single dose at 0.2 mg/kg (Slocombe and McCraw, 1980, 1981; Lyons et al, 1982; Slocombe et al, 1983; Klei et al, 1984). Fenbendazole may be administered in a single dose of 30 to 60 mg/kg (Duncan et al, 1977) or in five daily doses of 7.5 to 10 mg/kg (Duncan et al, 1980). Oxfendazole is effective at the dose of 10 mg/kg (Duncan et al, 1980; Kingsbury and Reid, 1981; Slocombe et al, 1986).

ANTHELMINTIC RESISTANCE. Phenothiazine, thiabendazole, cambendazole, mebendazole, fenbendazole, oxfendazole, and febantel are no longer as effective against small strongylids as they were when first introduced (Drudge and Elam, 1961; Drudge and Lyons, 1965; Drudge et al, 1977, 1979; Slocombe et al, 1977; Hagan, 1979). Drudge et al (1979) identified five species (*Cyathostomum catinatum, Cyathostomum coronatum, Cylicocyclus nassatus, Cylicostephanus goldi,* and *Cylicostephanus longibursatus*) that exhibited cross-resistance to cambendazole, fenbendazole, mebendazole, oxfendazole, and thiabendazole. However, all of these worms were highly susceptible to 10 mg/kg of oxibendazole, a 2-amino substituted benzimidazole. Later trials after repeated dosing of the herd for 14 years with oxibendazole showed that these five species of worms were resistant to other benzimidazoles but still affected by ivermectin and piperazine (Lyons et al, 1997a). Resistant populations also may be controlled with pyrantel pamoate, ivermectin, or by a benzimidazole administered with piperazine. The selection of populations of these five cyathostome species resistant to benzimidazole anthelmintics has been rather rapid. Duncan (1982) suggested that in any worm control program, drugs of different chemical structures should be alternated every 6 to 12 months to reduce the likelihood of development of resistant worm populations, but there is no experimental evidence to support this recommendation. The benzimidazole anthelmintics continue to retain excellent potency against the large strongylids and other nematode parasites of horses.

Because resistance is the inevitable result of frequent, regular anthelmintic medication, a better course might be to worm only those horses with significant fecal egg counts (e.g., 100 eggs per gram). Such a process of selective chemotherapy has been tried with horses in a polo string (Hamlen-Gomez and Georgi, 1991). This work showed that certain horses may have had a predisposition to infection, and that by strategic deworming of chronic egg shedders, there was a significant savings over regular, routine deworming. The possible combination of selective chemotherapy with the use of a daily deworming product such as Strongid-C (pyrantel tartrate) could possibly lead to significant improvements in parasite management in certain herds of horses.

Coles et al (1991) reported on the discovery of large strongyles that were resistant to pyrantel. Strongyle eggs were collected from the feces of the three horses that had high numbers of eggs after treatment, and they were found by in vitro methods to apparently be resistant. A second treatment of one horse had very little effect on the fecal egg counts after treatment. Culture of the larvae to the infective stage allowed it to be determined that all three horses were shedding some eggs of *S. edentatus* and one horse was shedding mainly the eggs of *S. edentatus.* This appears to be the first report of large strongyle resistant to any anthelminthic.

Subfamily Oesophagotominae

IDENTIFICATION. There is a transverse fold of cuticle ("ventral groove," see Figure 3-62) on the ventral side of the body just posterior to the buccal cavity. The buccal cavity varies in size from small (e.g., *Oesophagostomum columbianum,* Figure 3-87) to very large (e.g., *Chabertia ovina,* Figure 3-88). Oesophagostomins are parasites of the large intestines of ruminants (*O. columbianum, Oesophagostomum venulosum, Oesophagostomum radiatum,* and *C. ovina*), swine (*Oesophagostomum dentatum, Oesophagostomum brevicaudum*), and primates (*Conoweberia* spp. and *Ternidens deminutus*).

IMPORTANCE. Oesophagostomins are called *nodular worms* because their parasitic larvae tend to become encapsulated by a somewhat excessive reactive inflammation on the part of the previously sensitized host. Acute inflammation may lead to clinical disease characterized by fetid diarrhea that may be fatal. The nodules later caseate and calcify, and severe involvement may interfere mechanically with normal intestinal motility. Clinical signs in ruminants and swine usually are associated with these reactions to the larval stages in the wall of the bowel and not to adult worms in the lumen. Therefore clinical disease is likely to be associated with nonpatent infection, and diagnosis must depend on correct interpretation of clinical signs or parasitic enteritis but may occasionally cause intussusception or other mechanical abnormality.

The most important effect of *Oesophagostomum* spp. in swine is the formation of nodules in the gut wall by developing third-stage larvae. The fourth-stage larvae emerge from these nodules as early as 2 weeks after infection, or they remain for several months. Nodule formation may be accompanied by catarrhal enteritis, spoils sausage casings, and probably interferes with maximum growth of young swine. A rise in egg output by sows peaks at 6 or 7 weeks after farrowing and then drops off rapidly. This could be an important epidemiological factor in situations favorable for the development of infective larvae.

Conoweberia apiostomum, Conoweberia stephanostomum, and *T. deminutus* are pathogenic, especially in recently captured primates with the unaccustomed stresses of confinement and transportation. Acute and chronic disease syndromes caused by *C. stephanostomum* occurred in gorillas from the thirteenth to fortieth days after capture (Rousselot and Pellissier, 1952). The chronic syndrome consisted of intermittent diarrhea, paleness

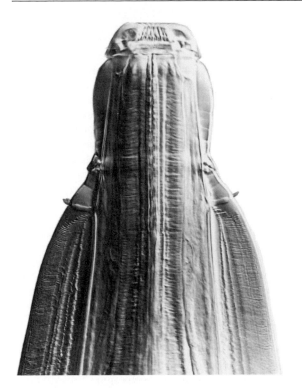

FIGURE 3-87 *Oesophagostomum columbianum*, dorsoventral view of buccal and anterior esophageal regions (×168).

postmortem findings. The feces are watery, dark, and very fetid. Weakness is marked and emaciation rapid. Necropsy examination conducted during an outbreak of nodular worm disease reveals an inflamed intestine studded with active nodules filled with creamy pus, each containing a living larva (Figure 3-89). Caseated and calcified nodules should not be held accountable for current acute

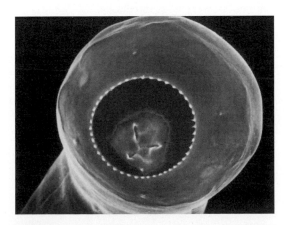

FIGURE 3-88 *Chabertia ovina*, head-on. The oral end of the esophagus with its triradiate lumen is visible at the base of the buccal cavity (SEM ×100).

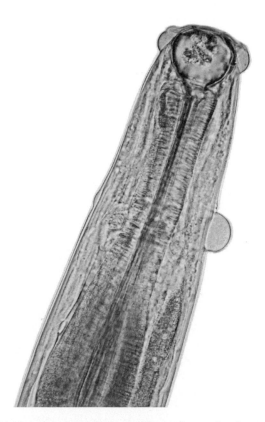

FIGURE 3-89 *Oesophagostomum radiatum* fourth-stage larva from a nodule in the intestinal wall of a calf (×250). *Oesophagostomum* spp. fourth-stage larvae are unusual in having buccal cavities relatively larger than those in the adult stage.

of the mucous membranes, and the presence of eggs in the feces. In the acute form, the gorilla refuses to eat or nibbles a little and suffers some diarrhea but very soon passes only small quantities of glairy mucus streaked with blood, much like that observed in acute amebic dysentery of humans. The gorilla remains either lying down or sitting with both hands on its head in an attitude of human desperation.

ANTHELMINTIC MEDICATION. There are many different products approved for treating the adults of *Oesophagostomum* and *Chabertia* spp. in cattle and sheep and *Oesophagostomum* spp. in swine.

Family Stephanuridae

IDENTIFICATION. *Stephanurus dentatus*, the kidney worm of swine, is a stout (up to 2 by 40 mm) parasite of the hepatic, renal, and perirenal tissues, axial musculature, and spinal canal of swine and sometimes of cattle. The buccal cavity is cup shaped and directed straightforward with 6 to 10 triangular teeth at its base (Figure 3-90). The gut is convoluted, the spicules equal and short, and the bursa reduced.

Earthworms serve as intermediate hosts. The life history may be direct or could involve earthworms as facultative intermediate hosts, infection occurring by ingestion or skin penetration of third-stage larvae or by ingestion of infected earthworms. Once in the body of the pig, the larvae enter the liver and spend 4 to 9 months wandering destructively there. Some are trapped by an encapsulating tissue reaction, but the rest migrate to the retroperitoneal tissues surrounding the kidneys and ureters. Eggs appear in the urine 9 to 16 months after infection and persist for 3 years or longer. Piglets may become infected in utero (Batte et al, 1960, 1966).

S. dentatus larvae migrate abortively in other hosts (e.g., cattle) and frequently lose their way in pigs. Not only liver and kidney but also choice loin chops are frequently condemned because of these destructive larvae. Although migration of *S. dentatus* larvae in the spinal cord may cause posterior paralysis, otherwise the clinical signs of infection are not distinctive. Extensive liver damage may lead to emaciation and death.

ANTHELMINTIC MEDICATION. Levamisole and fenbendazole are the approved anthelmintics for the treatment of *S. dentatus* infections. Ivermectin in a mixture as a feed additive designed to deliver a dosage of approximately 0.1 mg/kg daily for 7 days is also approved for the treatment and control of *S. dentatus*. Ivermectin (0.3 mg/kg body weight subcutaneously) has a marked effect on *S. dentatus* infections (Becker, 1986). Albendazole is very active against both adult and immature *S. dentatus*, but is not approved for use in swine in the United States.

Family Syngamidae

The family Syngamidae includes the genera *Syngamus* and *Cyathostoma* (not *Cyathostomum*) in birds and *Mammomonogamus* in mammals. All three have large buccal capsules (Figure 3-91), and all are parasites of the upper respiratory tract. Males and females of *Syngamus* spp. and *Mammomonogamus* spp. are fused permanently in copula. *Syngamus trachea* infections have caused the deaths of farmed rheas, and in these birds, treatment with fenbendazole at 25 mg/kg was successful therapy (deWitt, 1995). Earthworms serve as intermediate hosts. Ivermectin also is highly effective in the treatment of *Syngamus* infections.

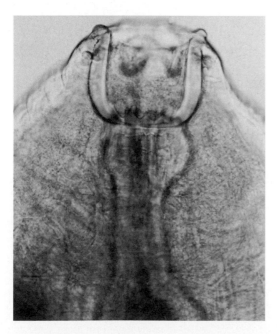

FIGURE 3-90 *Stephanurus dentatus* (×108).

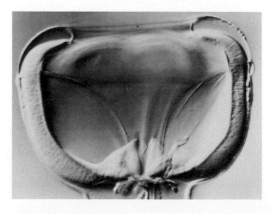

FIGURE 3-91 *Cyathostoma* (family Syngamidae) buccal capsule (×110).

Superfamily Ancylostomatoidea
Family Ancylostomatidae

IDENTIFICATION. Adult hookworms are parasites of the small intestine. Some species such as *Ancylostoma caninum* cause the loss of large quantities of blood from their hosts, whereas others such as *Uncinaria stenocephala* remove very little. Fresh specimens of *A. caninum* tend to be dark in color, whereas those of *U. stenocephala* are quite pale. All hookworms have a large buccal cavity directed obliquely dorsally, so the anterior end of the worm is more or less "hooked," but, again, this trait is variably developed as can be appreciated from a comparison of *Bunostomum* spp. (Figure 3-92) and *Globocephalus* spp. (Figure 3-93). The male hookworm, provided with well-developed bursa, is often found in copula with the female, the two worms forming a T because the vulva is located some little distance from the caudal extremity. The female lays typical strongylid eggs, and these appear in the feces during the morula stage of development.

Two subfamilies are distinguished: Ancylostomatinae and Bunostominae. "Carnivorous hosts are parasitized only by the Ancylostomatinae, herbivorous hosts by the Bunostominae, and omnivorous hosts by both subfamilies" (Lichtenfels, 1980).

The subfamily Ancylostomatinae includes the genera *Ancylostoma, Uncinaria, Globocephalus,* and *Placoconus.*

The most common hookworms of the dog and cat are species of *Ancylostoma* and *Uncinaria stenocephala.* Species of *Ancylostoma* have buccal cavities

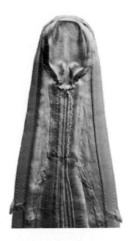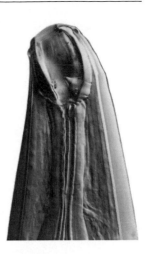

FIGURE 3-93 *Globocephalus urosubulatus,* a hookworm of swine; dorsal (*left*) and lateral (*right*) aspects (×100). (Specimen courtesy Dr. E. I. Braide.)

with sharp teeth while those of *Uncinaria* have cutting plates (Fig. 3-94). The ventral margin of the stoma of Ancylostoma is armed by one (*Ancylostoma braziliense*), two (*Ancylostoma duodenale*), or three pairs of sharp teeth (*A. caninum, Ancylostoma tubaeforme*). *A. braziliense* matures in dogs and cats, *A. duodenale* in humans, *A. caninum* in dogs (see Figures 3-63 and 3-94), and *A. tubaeforme* in cats (Figure 3-95). The ventral margin of the stoma of *Globocephalus urosubulatus* of swine has neither plates nor teeth (see Figure 3-93). The buccal capsule of *Placoconus lotoris* of raccoons is formed of five articulating plates (Figure 3-96).

The subfamily Bunostominae includes the genera *Bunostomum* of ruminants (see Figure 3-92), *Necator* of humans, *Bathmostomum* of elephants, and *Grammocephalus* of elephants and rhinoceroses.

LIFE HISTORY. Infection occurs through either ingestion or skin penetration by infective larvae, which then undergo more or less extensive migrations through the tissues of the host before developing into adult hookworms in the small intestine (Figure 3-97).

Hookworm Disease of Dogs

The principal importance of hookworms attaches to their ability to cause anemia, especially in humans and dogs. Hookworm disease varies in severity from asymptomatic infection to rapidly fatal exsanguination, depending on the magnitude of the challenge and the resistance of the host.

Magnitude of challenge is determined by the virulence and number of hookworms. Virulence depends on the species of hookworm involved. *A. caninum* is much more pathogenic for dogs than *A. braziliense* or *U. stenocephala* because it sucks much more blood. The number of hookworms

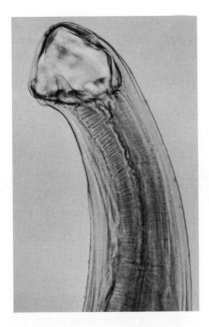

FIGURE 3-92 *Bunostomum* sp. (×100).

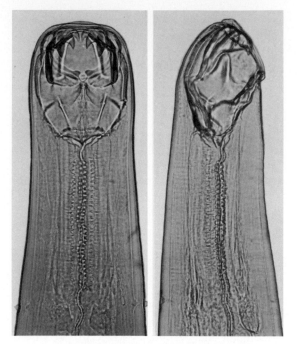
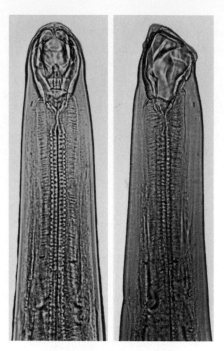

Ancylostoma caninum   *Uncinaria stenocephala*

FIGURE 3-94   Dorsoventral and lateral aspects of the buccal and esophageal regions of *Ancylostoma caninum* (×100) and *Uncinaria stenocephala* (×160).

infecting a particular host depends very heavily on the degree of exposure to infective larvae. Exposure, in turn, depends on the extent to which infected hosts have contaminated the environment by shedding eggs in their feces, and on the suitability of the substrate (gravel and sand are ideal), temperature, and moisture for development and survival of infective larvae.

Host resistance is resolvable into two abilities: (1) The ability to limit the number of hookworms maturing in the small intestine is influenced by age, premunition, and acquired immunity. As dogs grow older, they become more resistant to hookworms whether or not they experience infection. Immunity acquired from previous infection confers increased resistance, but this is difficult to disentangle from

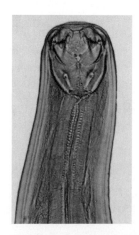
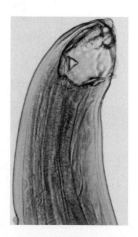
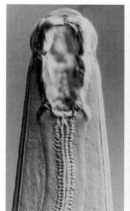
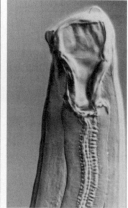

FIGURE 3-95   *Ancylostoma tubaeforme.* At the left is the dorsoventral aspect of the stoma and at right, its lateral aspect (×78).

FIGURE 3-96   *Placoconus lotoris,* hookworm of the raccoon; dorsoventral *(left)* and lateral *(right)* aspects of the buccal and esophageal regions (×140).

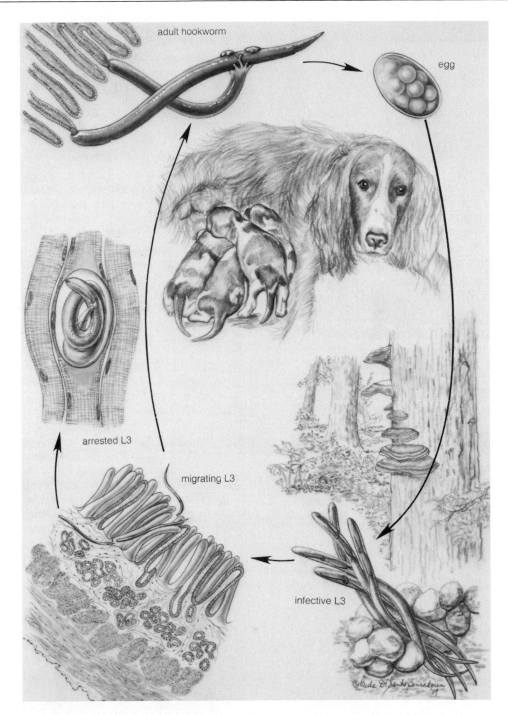

FIGURE 3-97 Life history of *Ancylostoma caninum*. The actively motile sheathed larva develops in 2 to 8 days. Shaded, well-drained soils, warmth, and humidity provide optimum conditions for development and survival of this stage, which may infect the host either on being swallowed or by penetrating its skin. Eggs are shed in the feces about 2 weeks after ingestion of larvae and about a month after penetration of skin by larvae. However, not all larvae mature. Some invade skeletal muscle cells (Little, 1978) or gut wall (Schad, 1974, 1979) and enter an arrested state of development. Arrested larvae later become reactivated in response to obscure cues and migrate either to the small intestine where they mature or to the mammary glands where they are shed in the milk and infect the pups. Arrested larvae are regularly reactivated during the last 2 weeks of pregnancy.

the influences of advancing age and from the marked inhibition of further infection exerted by a residual population of hookworms (premunition). (2) The ability to compensate for blood loss caused by hookworms is influenced by the hematopoietic capacity and state of nutrition of the individual and by the presence or absence of other stresses.

Because hookworm infection is common and the females are prodigious egg layers, populations of infective larvae are likely to bloom whenever the weather becomes favorable for their development and survival. Therefore most frank hookworm disease cases occur during late spring, summer, and early autumn in temperate climates, particularly when mild weather is accompanied by adequate rainfall. The infective challenge may become overwhelming in carelessly managed kennels and pet shops where feces are allowed to accumulate long enough to permit infective larvae to develop. Unpaved runs are particularly favorable for the perpetuation of the parasite because the feces mixes with the soil. This not only makes sanitation difficult, but provides more favorable cultural conditions, especially when the soil is light, open textured, and well drained.

The following clinical forms of canine hookworm disease may be distinguished:

Peracute hookworm disease results from the passage of infective larvae from dam to nursing pups in the milk. Transmammary infection of very young pups with as few as 50 to 100 adult *A. caninum* may prove fatal. Typically, the pups appear healthy and sleek the first week, then sicken and deteriorate rapidly the second week. The visible mucosae are very pale, and the soft to liquid feces are very dark in color because the blood shed by the hookworms in the small intestine has been partially digested on the way out. The worms do not lay eggs until the sixteenth day of infection, so diagnosis must rest on the clinical signs of disease. Prognosis is guarded to poor with or without treatment.

Acute hookworm disease results from sudden exposure of susceptible older pups to large numbers of infective larvae. Even mature dogs may be overwhelmed if exposure is sufficiently great. Usually, many eggs will be found in the feces of affected animals, but clinical signs may precede the appearance of eggs by about 4 days in particularly heavy infections.

Chronic (compensated) hookworm infection is usually asymptomatic. Diagnosis rests on the presence of hookworm eggs in the feces and measurable reductions in erythrocyte count, blood hemoglobin, or packed cell volume. Occasionally, however, incomplete adjustment between parasite and host produces a state of chronic ill health.

Secondary (decompensated) hookworm disease usually involves older dogs that have more ailing them than just hookworms. The cardinal sign again is profound anemia, usually in a malnourished or even emaciated animal. The hookworms may indeed kill the dog, but it is important in this case to recognize that they play a secondary role. An accurate diagnosis, for example, of "malnutrition with secondary hookworm infection" logically leads to effective therapy.

Control of Hookworm Infections
Sources of Infection

CONTAMINATED ENVIRONMENT. From 2 to 8 days are required for the morula in the hookworm egg to develop into an infective third-stage larva. Shirt-sleeve temperatures (23° to 30° C) and a moderately moist, well-aerated medium are optimal. Thus hookworm larvae develop well in shaded areas of well-drained soils but not in heavy, water-logged soils or where they are exposed to direct sunlight and desiccation. *Ancylostoma* eggs and larvae are destroyed by freezing, whereas those of *Uncinaria* are very resistant to cold. *A. caninum* larvae will not develop to the infective stage at temperatures consistently below 15° C. Above the optimum temperature for development (30° C), larvae rapidly develop to the infective stage. It can be reached in 48 hours at 37° C, the highest temperature compatible with development (McCoy, 1930). Thus compared with *Toxocara* eggs, soil pollution by hookworm infective larvae may be viewed as a temporary problem that a good hard freeze will probably solve. During mild weather, sodium borate, broadcast at the rate of 10 lb/100 sq ft (0.5 kg/m^2) and raked in, will destroy hookworm larvae in gravel- or loam-surfaced runs. This treatment destroys vegetation as well as hookworm larvae and is therefore unsuitable for lawns. Resinated dichlorvos was reported to interfere with the development of first- and second-stage larvae of *A. caninum* (Kalkofen, 1971).

Paved surfaces, cages, and the like should first be cleaned thoroughly and then mopped or sprayed with 1% sodium hypochlorite solution (Clorox). This solution kills the larvae or at least induces them to cast off their sheaths, after which they are more susceptible to drying and other unfavorable environmental stresses.

Large commercial dog-rearing operations make extensive use of wire-bottomed cages and pens to effect the physical separation of the dogs from the bulk of their feces. Anthelmintic medication may be used to reduce the output of hookworm eggs in the feces and thus limit the degree of contamination of the environment with infective larvae. Therapeutic dosages may be administered periodically or when indicated by positive fecal examinations, or suitable medication at lower dosage may be administered continuously mixed with feed.

ARRESTED LARVAE IN TISSUES. Currently available anthelmintics administered at dosages to treat and control adult hookworm infections appear to lack significant efficacy against hookworm larvae arrested in the tissues. The arrested larvae of *A. caninum* in the intestinal wall and skeletal muscle tissue of the adult dog population are thus a relatively inaccessible reservoir of infection. This reservoir "leaks" larvae directly or through the lungs to the intestinal lumen of the adult dog and through the mammary gland to the intestines of the nursling pups (see Figure 3-97).

Little (1978) obtained evidence that larvae are continually migrating from the muscles to the intestine through the lungs. When adult worms were already present in the intestine, few if any of these larvae developed to maturity, but when the adult worms were eliminated by disophenol therapy, these larvae from the muscles were able to mature and start producing eggs in about 4 weeks. A second course of disophenol then eliminated the new adults, and these in turn were replaced by more larvae from the muscles. Why these reactivated larvae from the muscles should require twice as long as newly ingested larvae to mature is unclear. Schad's experiences with arrested *A. caninum* larvae differ from those of Little. Infective larvae were chilled before being administered orally to dogs. These larvae became arrested in the gut wall instead of the muscle tissue and when reactivated were able to become established in the intestine in the presence of adults. Neither removal of adult worms with anthelmintic nor treatment with the corticosteroid drug prednisolone initiated resumed development of arrested *A. caninum* larvae (Schad, 1974, 1979; Schad and Page, 1982).

The findings of both investigators led to similar practical consequences, however. Practicing veterinarians frequently encounter dogs with hookworm infections that refuse to "clean up" even after repeated wormings with a variety of drugs over the course of many months. This "larva leak" phenomenon provides a plausible explanation for such refractory cases.

Infection of nursling pups occurs through the mammary gland (Kotake, 1929a, 1929b; Stone and Girardeau, 1966, 1968). Formerly, prenatal infection by migration of larvae across the placenta was supposed to account for the occurrence of peracute hookworm disease in 2- or 3-week-old pups. However, meticulous experimentation by Stoye (1973) has demonstrated that transplacental infection, if it occurs at all, is overshadowed by transmammary infection in the case of the hookworm. A bitch exposed to only one substantial oral or percutaneous infection will shed hookworm larvae in her milk for the next three lactations, although the larval output will diminish with each lactation.

Anthelmintic Medication

Pyrantel pamoate, dichlorvos, mebendazole, febantel, fenbendazole, milbemycin oxime, and nitroscanate are effective against hookworms and several other important helminth parasites of the intestinal tract. Two older drugs, *N*-butyl chloride and toluene, are still available in several commercial preparations and retain their original efficacy, but in light of the safety of the newer products, it is hard to recommend their use. Filaribits Plus, Heartgard Plus, Interceptor, and Sentinel are heartworm preventatives that also provide control of canine hookworm infections. ProHeart6, injectable moxidectin, will clear dogs of their existing hookworm infections, but at this time, it is not known if it will prevent further infections during the six months in which heartworm infection is prevented. Drontal Plus is a combination of pyrantel pamoate, febantel, and praziquantel, which has good activity against hookworms.

Feline hookworm infections may be treated with pyrantel pamoate, and pyrantel pamoate formulated with praziquantal in Drontal, and with ivermectin in Heartgard Plus. Particular attention should be paid to ridding young kittens of hookworms.

PRIMARY HOOKWORM DISEASE. Treatment is often to little avail in peracute neonatal hookworm disease. Blood transfusion is essential to keep affected pups alive long enough for anthelmintic medication to take effect, and anthelmintic medication must be administered immediately to stop the loss of blood as soon as possible. On no account should anthelmintic therapy be delayed. It is impracticable to attempt replacement of hookworm blood losses by transfusion for any appreciable length of time.

In acute hookworm disease and in chronic (compensated) hookworm infection, response to simple anthelmintic therapy is usually dramatic. Supportive therapy beyond provision of an adequate diet is unnecessary.

SECONDARY HOOKWORM DISEASE. The efficacy of mebendazole and fenbendazole was dramatically reduced in iron- and protein-deficient rats infected with *Nippostrongylus brasiliensis* (Duncombe et al, 1977a, 1977b). Clinical experience indicates that protein sufficiency is also essential to efficient anthelmintic action against hookworms and other parasites. Cases of malnourished dogs that have secondary hookworm disease and dogs that seem adequately nourished but fail to respond to anthelmintic medication should first be given a course of supportive therapy (e.g., high protein diet, ferrous sulfate orally or parenteral iron injections, vitamins, and, if necessary, blood transfusion) and then remedicated with a suitable anthelmintic (e.g., mebendazole, pyrantel pamoate, disophenol).

PREVENTING PERACUTE NEONATAL HOOKWORM DISEASE. Routine cage, pen, and run sanitation and periodic anthelmintic medication of all adult dogs are essential to reduce the level of environmental contamination with hookworm larvae. When neonatal losses have already been experienced, it is essential to examine the visible mucosae of each pup daily from about the seventh day of life until weaning and to administer an anthelmintic at the first sign of anemia. Alternatively, antihookworm therapy should begin 2 weeks after pups are whelped and continue weekly for 3 months (Kelly, 1977).

Bitches that have lost litters may be treated with fenbendazole, 50 mg/kg per day, from the fortieth day of gestation to the fourteenth day of lactation, to prevent further losses (Düwel and Strasser, 1978; Burke and Roberson, 1983). This treatment attacks the reactivated larvae and is effective but rather expensive. It also has been shown that ivermectin treatment of the bitch (0.5 mg/kg body weight administered 4 to 9 days before whelping followed by a second treatment 10 days later) can also prevent puppies from being infected by larvae passed in the milk (Stoye et al, 1987). Treatment of four bitches with a single 1 mg/kg subcutaneous injection of doramectin failed to prevent transmammary infection of all their puppies, with 5 of the 23 puppies, representing three of the four litters, becoming infected (Schnieder et al, 1996).

THE REFRACTORY HOOKWORM EGG-SHEDDER. Despite excellent supportive therapy and flawless anthelmintic medication, the larva leak phenomenon provides a few highly persistent cases of hookworm infection. Prevention of somatic larval burdens is the key to prevention of such refractory clinical problems because, at present, there seems to be no satisfactory way of handling the dog that persists in shedding hookworm eggs after months of treatment. The intracellular location and metabolic quiescence of arrested *A. caninum* larvae should, it would seem, shelter them from even the most effective anthelmintics. Stoye (1973), however, showed that estrogens stimulate the reactivation of arrested larvae. This author induced an outpouring of larvae in the milk of lactating bitches by treatment with estradiol and progesterone. Perhaps a way can be found to combine hormonal and anthelmintic therapy effectively in attacking the somatic burden of *A. caninum* larvae.

Cutaneous Larva Migrans

"Creeping eruption" (human cutaneous larva migrans) is a linear, tortuous, erythematous, and intensely pruritic eruption of the human skin usually caused by migration of a nematode larva (Kirby-Smith et al, 1926). *A. braziliense* larvae are most frequently involved in the typical protracted cases,

especially in the coastal regions of the southeastern United States (White and Dove, 1926). Accidental sporadic or experimental cases involving *A. caninum, U. stenocephala, Bunostomum phlebotomum, Strongyloides stercoralis,* and *Gnathostoma* spp. have also been reported, and the larvae of those species that normally mature in man (*A. duodenale, A. ceylonicum,* and *Necator americanus*) produce a transient but otherwise typical creeping eruption in previously sensitized individuals. It should also be noted that larvae of *Gasterophilus* spp. and *Hypoderma* spp. also migrate in human skin (James, 1947), producing a clinical condition properly termed *cutaneous larva* migrans.

Probably no nematode larva capable of penetrating the skin is above suspicion in individual cases, but the epidemiological importance of any particular species depends on many influences beyond its intrinsic capabilities. For example, the etiological prominence of *A. braziliense* may have much to do with the defecation behavior of dogs and cats, as may be surmised from the following description of circumstances surrounding infection, lesions, and symptoms by Kirby-Smith and colleagues (1926).

At least 50 percent of the cases of creeping eruption seen by the senior author are believed to have originated at the beach, the probable origin being traced to the soft damp sand in front of the beach buildings at points slightly above the high water mark. Such patients reported with lesions varying in numbers. They were not the most extensively infected ones. Persons with hundreds of lesions definitely attributed the origin of their infection to contact with damp sand when they were wet with perspiration while working: repairing an automobile, doing brick work, or making plumbing connections underneath houses, and the like.

The most recent visible lesion is a very narrow erythematous formation along the course traveled by the worm. Soon a slightly raised line representing the location of the burrow can be palpated. This line becomes visibly elevated, more or less continuous and vesicular. Sometimes bullae are formed. The surface of the lesion dries, resulting in a thin crust. When the parasite travels it moves from a fraction of an inch to several inches a day, advancing, as a rule, more rapidly at night.

To some patients the itching sensation resulting from infection is almost intolerable, while others endure it with less suffering. The severity of the lesions, too, is more pronounced in some than in others.

The severity and persistence of the lesions are at least partly related to hypersensitivity resulting from previous exposure. The lungs may be invaded, but intestinal infection with mature worms ensues only in cases involving those species that are normal parasites of humans.

Human Enteric Infections with *Ancylostoma caninum*

Prociv and Croese (1996) reported on a series of human cases with **eosinophilic enteritis** from northern semitropical Queensland, Australia. Most of these cases came from typical suburban housing developments. An adult *A. caninum* was recovered at colonoscopy from the terminal ileum of one patient, and an unidentifiable adult hookworm was found on a portion of ileum resected from a second patient. There have since been additional cases reported from Australia and the United States in which adult *A. caninum* have been recovered and cases that have signs and serology suggestive of *A. caninum* infection (Vikram-Khoshoo et al, 1995; Prociv and Croese, 1996). Signs of infection have included obscure abdominal pain that may or may not be associated with an increased level of circulating eosinophils. Worms are not observed in most seropositive patients. It appears that these people became infected with infective-stage larvae by the cutaneous route as they went about parks and yards without shoes and socks. These cases provide yet another good reason why veterinary practitioners must insist that clients submit fecal samples from their pets for annual evaluation and work with their clients to practice hookworm prevention and control.

Superfamily *Metastrongyloidea*

Metastrongyloids are parasites of the respiratory, vascular, and nervous systems of mammals. Most species whose life histories have been investigated require a snail or slug intermediate host. However, *Metastrongylus* spp. develop to the infective stage in earthworms, and *F. osleri* and *F. hirthi* infect their definitive hosts directly. The copulatory bursa is of the basic strongylid pattern but has suffered varying degrees of reduction in the evolution of different families. For example, the bursa is best developed in the family Metastrongylidae (Figure 3-98) but reduced to mere papillae in the family Filaroididae. The vulva is close to the anus except in the family Crenosomatidae, in which it is located in the midregion of the body. The diversity of structure and biology displayed by members of the superfamily Metastrongyloidea makes further generalization precarious. It seems doubtful that this superfamily is monophyletic.

Family Metastrongylidae

The family Metastrongylidae contains only one genus, *Metastrongylus*, all species of which are large white parasites of the bronchi and bronchioles of swine.

IDENTIFICATION. The mouth is flanked by a pair of trilobed lips. The spicules are long and thin, the

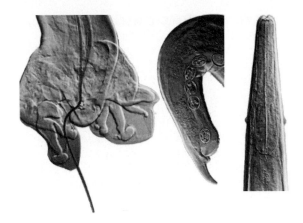

FIGURE 3-98 *Metastrongylus apri* (×168).

bursa is well developed, and the vulva is near the anus (see Figure 3-98). When passed in the feces of infected swine, the egg contains a larva.

LIFE HISTORY. Oviparous females lay eggs containing first-stage larvae. The standard view is that these eggs do not hatch or develop into infective larvae unless they are ingested by an earthworm. However, continued high prevalence (50%) in Iowa swine despite confinement rearing and improved sanitation indicates that the earthworm may not be an obligatory intermediate host of *Metastrongylus* spp. (Ledet and Greve, 1966).

Metastrongylus spp. are of only modest pathological and economic importance. It was once supposed that they acted as vectors of swine influenza virus, but substantial proof for this idea is lacking (Wallace, 1977).

ANTHELMINTIC MEDICATION. Fenbendazole, levamisole, and ivermectin are approved anthelmintics with activity against swine lungworms.

Family Protostrongylidae

IDENTIFICATION. Protostrongylids have a well-developed bursa, spicule, and spicule guide, and the vulva is near the anus (Figures 3-99 and 3-100).

LIFE HISTORY. The oviparous protostrongylid females deposit unsegmented eggs in the surrounding lung, vascular, or neural tissues. These eggs develop into first-stage larvae before they appear in the feces. If these first-stage larvae are ingested by any of a wide range of snails and slugs, they develop in these intermediate hosts into doubly ensheathed third-stage infective larvae. The protostrongylids considered here are all parasites of sheep and goats.

Protostrongylus

Protostrongylus rufescens lives in the smaller bronchioles where they may cause localized lesions.

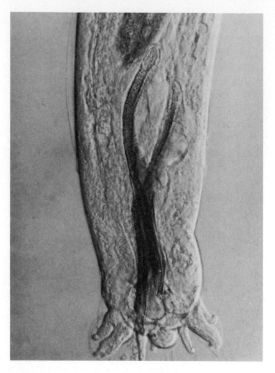

FIGURE 3-99 *Protostrongylus rufescens*, bursa and spicules of male (×168).

Males of this brownish red species can be distinguished from *D. filarial* by their longer, comblike spicules (see Figure 3-99). The female *Protostrongylus* sp. is prodelphic, whereas the female *Dictyocaulus* sp. is amphidelphic. Fenbendazole-medicated salt has been used successfully to control protostrongylid lungworms in free-ranging Rocky Mountain bighorn sheep in Montana (Jones and Worley, 1997).

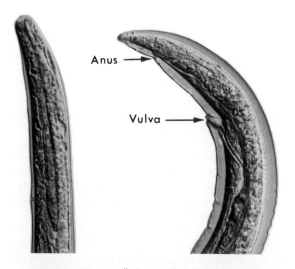

FIGURE 3-100 *Muellerius capillaris* female (×425).

Muellerius

Muellerius capillaris (see Figure 3-100) is a tiny species so deeply embedded in lung tissue or reactive nodules that specimens are extremely difficult to dissect out intact. Antemortem diagnosis is less difficult because the active first-stage larvae are easily separated from the host's feces by the Baermann technique and are not difficult to distinguish from those of *Protostrongylus* spp. and *Dictyocaulus* spp. Unfortunately however, the larvae of *Muellerius* spp. cannot be reliably distinguished from those of *Parelaphostrongylus* spp. (see later). *Muellerius* spp. are usually nonpathogenic at the levels of infection normally encountered in nature and agriculture, but heavy infections may have serious consequences, especially in goats.

TREATMENT. A single dose of cambendazole (60 mg/kg) eliminated larvae from the feces of 10 of 13 chronically infected goats (Bliss and Greiner, 1985). Levamisole, fenbendazole, albendazole, tetramisole, and ivermectin have been used to treat *M. capillaris* infections in sheep and goats, but results have been less than would be hoped for all these products.

Parelaphostrongylus

Parelaphostrongylus tenuis is normally a parasite of the meninges of the white-tailed deer, *Odocoileus virginianus*, in which species it rarely if ever causes disease. However, in abnormal hosts such as sheep, goats, llama, camel, moose, caribou, reindeer, wapiti, fallow deer, and mule deer, *P. tenuis* tends to invade the nervous tissue proper, causing serious or fatal neurological disease (Mayhew et al, 1976; Baumgärtner et al, 1985; Nichols et al, 1986; Krogdahl et al, 1987). Because *P. tenuis* rarely matures in these hosts, larvae are not shed in the feces. Therefore diagnosis is presumptive and based on the appearance of neurological signs in ruminants that share their pastures with white-tailed deer. Cattle are now known to also succumb to infection with this parasite, and at least two cases have been reported (Duncan and Patton, 1998). Recently, six horses have presented with neurological signs of parelephostrongylosis, and worms have been seen in the nerve tissue of two of these animals (Dr. de Lahunta, personal communication, Cornell University, 2002).

Family Crenosomatidae

IDENTIFICATION. Crenosomatids have well-developed bursac with a large dorsal ray, the uterus is amphidelphic with a prominent ovijectoral sphincter, and the cuticle is thrown into crenated folds, especially anteriorly (Figure 3-101). *Crenosoma vulpis* is less than 16 mm long and found in the bronchi and bronchioles of foxes

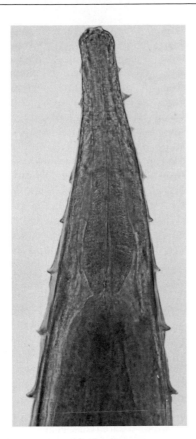

FIGURE 3-101 *Crenosoma* sp. from the lung of a bear (×250).

(Vulpes fulva), wolves *(Canis lupus),* raccoons *(Procyon lotor),* and dogs. *Troglostrongylus* spp. are parasites of Felidae.

LIFE HISTORY. The ovoviviparous females deposit first-stage larvae or thin-shelled eggs containing first-stage larvae. These ascend the trachea and descend the alimentary tract to exit in the host's feces and develop into infective third-stage larvae in snails and slugs. The definitive host becomes infected by ingesting infected molluscs; the prepatent period is 19 days (Wetzel, 1940b).

TREATMENT. Stockdale and Smart (1975) treated *C. vulpis*–infected dogs with a single oral dose of 8 mg/kg of levamisole. Fenbendazole (50 mg/kg daily for 3 days) was apparently successful in curing an infection of *C. vulpis* in a Labrador retriever (Peterson et al, 1993).

A survey of 55 afebrile dogs with chronic cough in Prince Edward Island, Canada, revealed that 15 (27.3%) were infected with *C. vulpis* (Bihr and Conboy, 1999). The dogs were successfully treated with a course of fenbendazole therapy (50 mg/kg daily for 3 to 7 days). The high percentage of positive dogs with the only sign being chronic cough indicates the need to carefully consider this worm in the differential for such a sign in regions where this worm is prevalent. As foxes become more and more abundant in North America because of reduced amounts of hunting, it is expected that this infection will become more prevalent.

Crenosoma spp. require a molluscan intermediate host. Control depends on preventing the dog's access to these intermediate hosts.

Family Angiostrongylidae

The angiostrongylid bursa may be somewhat reduced, but the rays conform to the typical strongylid pattern and are well defined. The vulva is near the anus, and the uterus is prodelphic. *Aelurostrongylus abstrusus* is a parasite of the lung parenchyma in cats, *Gurltia paralysans* is a parasite of the leptomeningeal veins in South American cats, and *Angiostrongylus* spp. are parasites of the lungs and blood vessels of canids and rodents.

Aelurostrongylus abstrusus

LIFE HISTORY. The oviparous female of *A. abstrusus* deposits unsegmented eggs in "nests" in the lung parenchyma. These appear as small, grayish white subpleural nodules. In histological sections or squash preparations of such nodules (see Figure 5-108), all degrees of development from one-celled eggs to hatched first-stage larvae are in evidence. The first-stage larvae are carried up the tracheobronchial tree and swallowed, appearing later in the cat's feces (see Figure 5-19). These larvae are very active and can be readily demonstrated by the Baermann technique, which was found to detect 18 of 20 cases of infection with this parasite (Willard et al, 1988). Further development occurs only if these first-stage larvae enter any of a wide variety of snails and slugs (Hobmaier and Hobmaier, 1935; Blaisdell, 1952). Two molts without cuticle shedding occur in the mollusc's foot tissues so that the infective larvae, which develop in 2 to 5 weeks, are enclosed in two sheaths. Cats may be infected experimentally by being fed snails containing third-stage larvae, but the natural mode of infection is probably through predation of paratenic hosts that normally eat snails. Mice and possibly birds may serve as paratenic hosts. The third-stage larvae merely encyst in their tissues and undergo no further development until they are ingested by a cat. Larvae appear in the cat's feces 5 to 6 weeks after infection.

Infection with *A. abstrusus* usually involves individual rural cats that like to hunt. Control consists of preventing the cat's access to infected intermediate hosts. Unfortunately, we cannot specify what these might be, except for a wide range of snails and slugs that few cats would deign to eat anyway. Probably the cats get their *A. abstrusus* infective larvae from paratenic hosts such as mice and voles, but our knowledge of the epidemiology of *A. abstrusus* and other carnivoran metastrongyloids is incomplete.

IMPORTANCE. Although many animals with *A. abstrusus* infection are free of clinical signs, coughing and anorexia may be associated with moderate infections. Severe infections are manifested by cough, dyspnea, and polypnea, all of which may terminate fatally (Blaisdell, 1952).

TREATMENT. Levamisole administered orally to cats at the rate of 8 mg/kg 3 times at 2-day intervals is usually effective in stopping the output of *A. abstrusus* larvae in the feces. Kirkpatrick and Megella (1987) successfully treated a case of *A. abstrusus* infection with a single parenteral dose of ivermectin (0.40 mg/kg). Fenbendazole (50 mg/kg daily for 3 days) also has been proved efficacious in the treatment of a cat infected with *A. abstrusus* (Schmid and Düwel, 1980). Prednisone (1 mg/kg orally twice a day for 5 days) may help alleviate many of the clinical signs during recovery.

Other Angiostrongylus Species

LIFE HISTORY. *Angiostrongylus vasorum* is a widely distributed parasite of the pulmonary arterial tree of dogs in western Europe. Recently, this worm was found for the first time to occur in dogs in North America in Newfoundland, Canada (Conboy et al, 1997). First-stage larvae shed in the feces of infected dogs resemble those of *A. abstrusus*. These larvae invade a wide range of molluscan intermediate hosts and develop there to the infective third stage, but the practical epidemiology of canine angiostrongylosis has yet to be worked out in detail. A fatal case in a greyhound imported from Ireland was marked by extensive pulmonary thrombosis and interference with clotting leading to multiple subcutaneous hemorrhages (Williams et al, 1985b). *A. vasorum* has been treated with ivermectin at 0.2 mg/kg (Migaud et al, 1992; Martins et al, 1993), fenbendazole at 20 mg/kg twice daily for 2 or 3 weeks (Migaud et al, 1992; Patteson et al, 1993), or levamisole at 7.5 mg/kg for 2 consecutive days, followed by 10 mg/kg for 2 days. If the infection does not clear, the regimen is repeated (Bolt et al, 1994).

Angiostrongylus cantonensis, a lungworm of the rat, causes eosinophilic meningitis and encephalomyelitis in humans. During the past few decades, it has spread across the Pacific with one of its intermediate hosts, the giant African snail *Achatina fulica*. Infection is acquired by eating infected raw snails or slugs or freshwater prawns, which serve as paratenic hosts (Alicata, 1988). A series of 55 natural cases of canine neural angiostrongylosis from Brisbane, Australia were characterized by ascending paresis involving the tail and urinary bladder and lumbar hyperalgesia. Three grades of clinical illness were characterized. Grade 1 consisted of caudal paresis and ataxia of one or both pelvic limbs and pain on deep pressure over the lumbar muscles. Grade 2 began as Grade 1, but posterior paresis and inability to stand unaided developed quickly. Manual expression of urine was necessary. Dogs with both Grade 1 and Grade 2 illness responded satisfactorily to nursing care and immunosuppressive corticosteroid therapy. However, when the anthelmintics levamisole and mebendazole were administered in Grade 1 and Grade 2 cases, either alone or in combination with corticosteroids, a death rate of 75% ensued. Clearly, anthelmintic medication is contraindicated in canine neural angiostrongylosis. Grade 3 illness was characterized by rapidly developing ascending paralysis and extreme hyperalgesia. The prognosis was very poor, and all seven dogs were euthanized (Mason, 1987).

In 1986 and 1987, rats in New Orleans, Louisiana, were found to be infected with *A. cantonensis* (Campbell and Little, 1988) A few years later, a howler monkey in the New Orleans zoo had fatal cerebral disease and was ultimately diagnosed as having been infected with this worm (Gardiner et al, 1990). In 1995 a nonfatal case was reported from New Orleans in an 11-year-old boy who ate a snail on a dare (New et al, 1995). In 1996 a miniature horse in Baton Rouge, Louisiana, had meningoencephalitis and was euthanized (Costa et al, 2000). At necropsy, the horse was found to be infected with *A. cantonensis*. As of 1997, around one quarter of rats, *Rattus norvegicus*, examined in Baton Rouge were found to be infected with this parasite. It is expected that additional cases will begin to turn up in dogs and possibly cats.

Family Filaroididae

IDENTIFICATION. The bursal lobes are reduced to mere papillae (Figure 3-102). The spicules are short and arcuate, the vulva is preanal, the uterus is prodelphic, and the body cuticle is inflated to form a diaphanous teguminal sheath (see Figure 3-102). (Do not confuse the family Filaroididae with the very distantly related superfamily Filarioidea.) The canine parasites, *F. osleri* and *F. hirthi* occur in nodules within the epitehlium of the trachea and bronchi or within the lung parenchyma, respectively.

LIFE HISTORY. The ovoviviparous females deposit delicate, thin-shelled eggs containing first-stage larvae that hatch before being voided in the host's fcces (Figure 3-103). Unlike other metastrongyloids, most or all of which require a molluscan or annelid intermediate host to develop into the infective third-larval stage, *Filaroides* spp. are directly infective as first-stage larva, and development through all five stages is completed in the lung tissue of the dog.

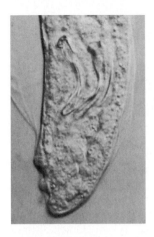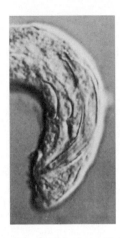

FIGURE 3-102 *Filaroides hirthi* (*left*) and *Filaroides milksi* (*right*); caudal ends of male worms ((1050). The spicules of *F. hirthi* are shorter, are broader in relation to their length, and have broader knobs for the attachment of the retractor muscles than the spicules of *F. milksi*.

Infection is acquired through the ingestion of regurgitated stomach contents, lung tissue, or feces of infected dogs.

Adult *F. osleri* worms occur in nodules in the trachea and bronchi of dogs and certain wild canids such as the Australian dingo (Figure 3-104). The first clue to the transmission of *F. osleri* was reported by Urquhart et al (1954), who isolated 300 larvae from feces, fed them to a 6-week-old pup, then euthanized the pup (prematurely, as will be seen) at 60 days after infection. Although they found only one worm with developing eggs immediately exterior to a tracheal cartilage, they correctly concluded that the life history was direct. Later, John Dorrington, a South African veterinary practitioner, reported success in transmitting *F. osleri* infection to dogs by feeding them first-stage larvae obtained from female worms (Dorrington, 1968).

Like so many original observations in science, these reports were credited by very few parasitologists, so firm was the belief that all metastrongyloids must develop to the infective stage in an intermediate host. However, the infectivity of first-stage *F. osleri* larvae for dogs was eventually confirmed by other investigators (Dunsmore and Spratt, 1976; Polley and Creighton, 1977) and demonstrated to hold true for *F. hirthi* as well (Georgi, 1976a). It has been postulated that transmission of *F. osleri* occurs directly from parent dingoes to their pups during the period of regurgitative feeding (Dunsmore and Spratt, 1976) and from bitches to their pups by salivary contamination during licking (Dorrington, 1968).

F. hirthi, like *F. osleri*, is infective in the first larval stage and requires no period of development outside the host (Georgi, 1976a; see Figure 3-103).

Transmission has been shown to occur among cagemate puppies through the ingestion of first-stage larvae in freshly passed feces, and it has been hypothesized that transmission from brood bitches to their litters occurs by the same mechanism after the fourth or fifth week of the nursing period (Georgi et al, 1979a). First-stage larvae arrive in the lungs as early as 6 hours after oral infection, traveling by way of the hepatic portal circulation, the mesenteric lymphatic drainage, or both. Molts occur at 1, 2, 6, and 9 days in the lung tissue, and larvae can be demonstrated in the feces by zinc sulfate flotation (specific gravity = 1.18) at 32 to 35 days after infection (Georgi et al, 1977; Georgi et al, 1979b).

IMPORTANCE. *F. osleri* infection develops slowly. Nodule formation can be detected with the bronchoscope at about 2 months, and larvae can first be demonstrated in the feces by zinc sulfate flotation (S.G. 1.18) at 6 to 7 months after experimental feeding of larvae. Milks (1916) summarized the clinical signs manifested in his three cases of *F. osleri* infection as follows:

> The only common symptom … was the spasmodic attack of a hard, dry cough which could be started by exercise or exposure to cold air. These attacks could not be started by pressure upon the larynx as in most cases of bronchitis. The dogs would cough several times and finally retch after which the attack would usually cease … the disease runs a very chronic course and does not materially interfere with the health of the animal until the knots become so numerous as to seriously obstruct the air passages.

F. osleri displays rather low prevalence in spite of its worldwide distribution. It tends to become entrenched in breeding stock and resists all efforts to expel it. Public knowledge that *F. osleri* is present in a kennel can destroy its reputation.

F. hirthi is important because the lesions it induces in the lungs of dogs used in toxicological research interfere with the interpretation of experiments (see Figures 3-104, 5-107, and 5-108). In 1973, Hirth and Hottendorf described pathological changes in commercially reared beagle dogs that were associated with *F. hirthi*. The presence of these minute lungworms in the alveoli and bronchioles evoked a focal granulomatous reaction and other pulmonary changes, including some that resembled drug-induced and neoplastic lesions. As Hirth (1977) has indicated more recently, "It is possible that some reports of toxic and carcinogenic effects of test substances in Beagle dogs may have been based on false interpretation of the lesions caused by this lungworm."

Usually, *F. hirthi* infection is not attended by clinical signs of disease, and antemortem diagnosis is based on demonstrating first-stage larvae in the

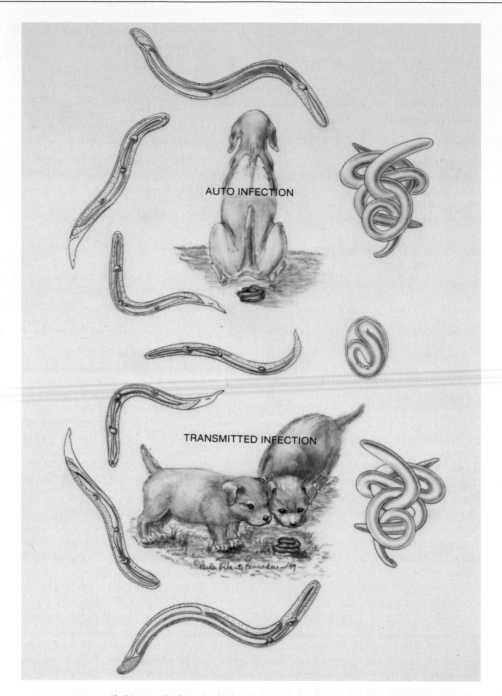

FIGURE 3-103 Life history of *Filaroides hirthi*. The female worm in the lung parenchyma of the dog lays eggs containing infective first-stage larvae. Because these larvae are released within the host, autoinfection is inevitable and the degree of resulting infection is apparently governed solely by the host's immune reactions. First-stage larvae pass up the trachea and out with the feces, and transmission of *F. hirthi* infection occurs principally by coprophagy. Cannibalism and regurgitative feeding provide other mechanisms.

feces (see Figure 5-8), although very severe infections may be suspected from radiographical changes (Rendano et al, 1979b). However, fatal cases of hyperinfection with this parasite have developed in severely stressed and immune-deficient animals (Craig et al, 1978; August et al, 1980). Massive hyperinfection with *F. hirthi* was observed in two beagle pups experimentally treated

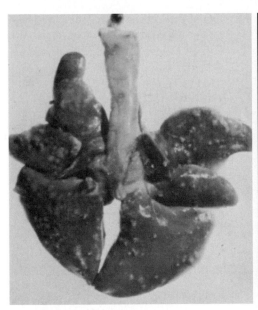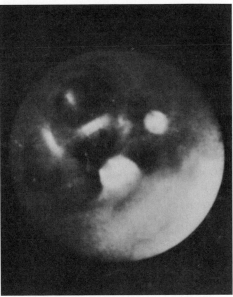

FIGURE 3-104 Lesions of *Filaroides* spp. At left, the lung of a dog with *Filaroides hirthi* infection. Foci of inflammatory reaction to dead and dying worms are scattered over the lungs. Live *F. hirthi* worms excite little if any tissue reaction and, because they are so very small, are scarcely visible to the unaided eye. At right, early *Filaroides osleri* nodules near the tracheal bifurcation of a dog photographed through a fiber-optic endoscope. (Courtesy Dr. James Zimmer.)

with prednisolone at a dosage rate of 4 mg/kg/day for more than 4 months (Genta and Schad, 1984). Dr. Georgi encountered several other cases of fatal *F. hirthi* hyperinfection in dogs experimentally maintained on corticosteroids for long periods. However, because these occurred in commercial pharmaceutical laboratories observing strict proprietary secrecy, the particulars were unavailable.

TREATMENT AND CONTROL. For treatment of *F. hirthi* infection, albendazole administered orally at a dosage of 25 mg/kg of body weight twice daily for 5 days is highly effective (Georgi et al, 1978). Fenbendazole, 50 mg/kg daily for 2 weeks, did not clear a dog of its *F. hirthi* infection, whereas a single subcutaneous injection of ivermectin (0.05 mg/kg) given at a later time appeared to clear the dog of its infection (Bourdeau and Ehm, 1992). Treatment of 40 dogs with subcutaneously administered ivermectin once at 1 mg/kg or ivermectin twice at 1 mg/kg a week apart reduced infections with *F. hirthi* by 44.8% and 74.1%, respectively, as revealed by necropsy (Bauer and Bahnemann, 1996). Fecal examination of these treated dogs revealed that only 5% to 10% of the dogs were shedding larvae in their feces, although higher percentages of the dogs still had worms in their lungs.

The principal objective of *F. hirthi* control is to produce experimental dogs whose lungs are free of worms and tissue reactions to them. Such infections still occur today despite markedly improved husbandry in most animal facilities (Bahnemann and Bauer, 1994). Therefore medication of the prospective experimental animals themselves is contraindicated. Recall that the infective stage of *F. hirthi* is the first-stage larva in the freshly passed feces of the infected host and that dogs become infected by eating these feces. One sure way to raise *F. hirthi*–free pups from an infected dam is to remove them by cesarean section and raise them artificially out of contact with all infected dogs, but this is obviously impracticable on a large scale. For *F. hirthi*–free experimental dogs to be produced, two large research Beagle-breeding colonies with initial infection rates among marketed dogs of 65% to 100% cooperated in the following experiment: All stud dogs and all nonpregnant, nonlactating brood bitches were given two courses of albendazole 2 to 4 weeks apart, each course consisting of 25 mg albendazole suspension per kilogram body weight orally, twice daily for 5 days with the objective of eliminating infective first-stage larvae from the feces of the bitches. In addition, puppies of treated dams were isolated from puppies of nontreated dams to exclude that source of infection. By the beginning of 1981 the infection rate among marketed dogs had dropped to 0.2% for one of the colonies and 24% for the other (Erb and Georgi, 1982).

Infection with *F. osleri* can virtually destroy the reputation of a kennel. This situation will continue until an effective anthelmintic or practicable control measures can be devised. As with *F. hirthi*, infection is passed from dog to dog as first-stage larvae in fresh feces, so transmission is easy to prevent except in the case of bitches and their litters. Because there is no really effective anthelmintic against *F. osleri*, there is no convenient way of interrupting the flow of infective first-stage larvae from feces of the bitch to stomachs of her offspring. The only sure way of raising *F. osleri*–free pups from infected bitches is to remove the pups by cesarean section and raise them artificially and in isolation from all infected dogs. Such expensive and laborious measures might be appropriate in the case of extraordinarily valuable breeding stock, but only when the kennel managers and staff are people who have great affection for their dogs and exceptional patience and perseverance, because only such people can succeed in raising more than a litter or two on the bottle.

Criteria for successful chemotherapy of *F. osleri* infection include (1) disappearance of cough and air hunger on exercise, (2) resolution of tracheal and bronchial nodules as demonstrated by bronchoscopy, and (3) cessation of fecal larval output. These criteria have rarely been satisfied, and authors disagree as to the efficacy of various treatments. Thiacetarsemide injected intravenously at 2.2 mg/kg daily for 21 days has led to resolution of nodules in some but not in all cases (Dietrich, 1962; Dorrington, 1963, 1968). Thiabendazole administered orally at 32 mg/kg twice daily for 21 days resulted in resolution of nodules in three dogs but left one of them with a mild cough (Bennett and Beresford-Jones, 1973; Bennett, 1975). Levamisole also showed promise in a clinical trial when administered orally at 7.5 mg/kg daily for 10 to 30 days (Darke, 1976). Fenbendazole (50 mg/kg daily for 7 days) was reported to stop coughing in a dog with an *F. osleri* infection (Lamb, 1992). Also, ivermectin has been reported to clear dogs of the signs of *F. osleri* infections (Boersema et al, 1989, Valet-Picavet, 1991).

Unfortunately, in none of these trials were the numbers of animals sufficient or the opportunities for prolonged observation subsequent to medication adequate to meet the standards of experimental proof. Despite the high anthelmintic efficacy displayed by albendazole against the closely related *F. hirthi*, this drug proved disappointing against *F. osleri* in an experiment described as follows: Three pups received 25 mg albendazole suspension per kilogram body weight orally twice daily for 5 days 10 to 12 months after artificial infection with *F. osleri*. When the pups underwent necropsy 39 to 66 days later, all were found still infected with reproductively active *F. osleri* worms. At this writing, there appears to be no documented report of satisfactory anthelmintic medication for *F. osleri* infection.

Order Rhabditida

The order Rhabditida is a very large group of small nematodes with **rhabditoid** or **rhabditiform esophagus** consisting of **corpus, isthmus,** and **bulb** (Figure 3-105). Many species are free-living inhabitants or parasites of lower vertebrate or invertebrate animals. Only three genera of the order Rhabditida, *Rhabditis* (syn., *Pelodera*), *Halicephalobus (Micronema)*, and *Strongyloides*, parasitize domestic animals.

Rhabditis (Pelodera)

Rhabditis (Pelodera) strongyloides is a free-living inhabitant of decaying organic matter but occasionally produces a pruritic, hyperemic dermatitis of cattle, swine, dogs, horses, and rodents that have been exposed to an excess of the nematode's normal habitat. Damp straw bedding has been incriminated repeatedly in canine dermatitis caused by this parasite. Diagnosis is based on finding nematode larvae with a rhabditiform esophagus in skin

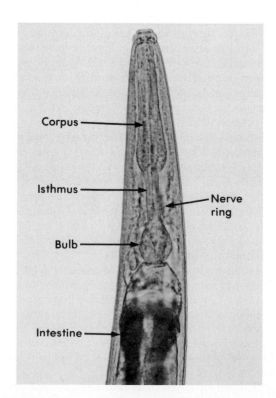

FIGURE 3-105 Anterior end of a *Strongyloides papillosus* free-living adult with a typical rhabditiform esophagus (×430).

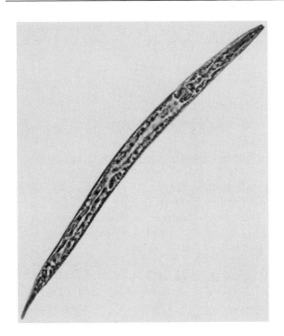

FIGURE 3-106 *Rhabditis strongyloides* rhabditiform larva from a nutrient agar culture. The culture was grown from scrapings of an acute erythematous dermatitis affecting a dog (×250).

scrapings (Figure 3-106); sometimes adults are also present. If *R. strongyloides* larvae are placed on nutrient agar, they will develop into adults in a day or so. These adults are 1 to 2 mm long and will promptly fill the Petri dish with their offspring.

In cattle, especially in the tropics, a parasitic otitis externa can develop that is caused by a nematode described as *Rhabditis bovis*. Once the infection is established in the ear canal, there appears to be a destruction of the ear epithelium resulting in ulcerations (Msolla, 1989). These ulcerations predispose the ears to secondary bacterial infection. The cattle have a condition that appears as chronic wasting. There is some indication that treatment of cattle with ivermectin may help with these infections, but typically, they are treated by the topical application of various agents.

Halicephalobus (Micronema)

Halicephalobus deletrix (syn. *Micronema deletrix*) is tiny (250 to 450 by 15 to 20 µm), has a rhabditoid esophagus and only one egg in its uterus. A male of this species has yet to be reported. The other seven species of *Halicephalobus* apparently are all free-living in soil, manure, or humus, but *H. deletrix* is a highly pathogenic parasite of horse and man. *H. deletrix* also has been seen in a section of skin from the scrotum of a bull. *H. deletrix* was first observed in a nasal swelling in a horse (Anderson and Bemrick, 1965) and from the nasal and maxillary

sinuses, gums, jaws, kidneys, heart, brain, spinal cord, and meninges in 12 equine cases reported subsequently (Blunden et al, 1987). The paper by Blunden et al deserves recognition as a model case report, which students and clinicians would do well to emulate. There have been three fatal human infections with this nematode (Gardiner et al, 1981). The first reported human case of fatal meningoencephalomyelitis caused by *H. deletrix* involved a 5-year-old boy who sustained extensive injuries heavily contaminated with manure when he fell into a running manure spreader and passed through its mechanism (Hoogstraten et al, 1976).

Strongyloides

Strongyloides is a very aberrant genus in terms of morphology and life history. Be careful not to confuse the genus name *Strongyloides* with the species name of *R. strongyloides* or with the superfamily name Strongyloidea. Also be warned that the adjective "strongyloid," as used by many authors, is more likely to refer to properties of members of the superfamily Strongyloidea than to those of the genus *Strongyloides*. The ubiquitous prefix derives from the Greek word "*strongylos*," meaning round and compact and apparently has great appeal to taxonomists of every stripe. "Strongyl-" has not been restricted to the christening of worms but has been applied to such diverse animals as sponges (*Strongylophora*), bugs (*Strongylodemas*), and fishes (*Strongyliscus*), among as many as eight others.

LIFE HISTORY. Many parasites have free-living stages in their life histories, but *Strongyloides* spp. is unique among parasites of domestic animals in having alternate free-living and parasitic *generations*. Parasitic males do not exist, and parasitic females contain no male gonads. The filariform parasitic female produces eggs by mitotic parthenogenesis, and the larvae that hatch from these eggs are termed **homogonic** rhabditiform larvae to distinguish them from the **heterogonic** offspring of the free-living, sexual generation. Homogonic rhabditiform larvae in the external environment may develop through two molts into infective filariform larvae or through four molts into free-living males and females. If the filariform larva enters a suitable host, usually by penetrating its skin, development proceeds through third and fourth molts to the filariform parasitic female. Thus there are five stages separated by four molts in both parasitic and free-living generations. The free-living rhabditiform males and females mate to produce heterogonic rhabditiform larvae that, with minor exceptions, develop only into infective filariform larvae (Basir, 1950; Triantophyllou and Moncol, 1977). The life history of *Strongyloides* spp. is portrayed in Figure 3-107.

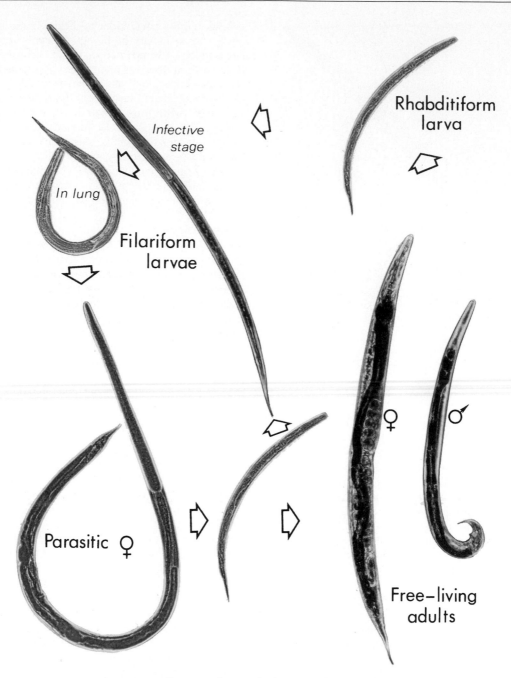

Infective stage

In lung

Filariform larvae

Rhabditiform larva

♀

♂

Parasitic ♀

Free-living adults

FIGURE 3-107   Life stages of *Strongyloides stercoralis*. Not to same scale.

The major mode of transmission of *Strongyloides* spp. in mammals would appear to be transmammary. This occurs in dogs, horses, pigs, and ruminants. After an initial infection has been established, additional larvae tend to migrate to deeper body tissues, from which they are then passed to offspring in the colostrum and milk. This mode of transmission has important implications for disease induction and control and is discussed in this context in the following section.

IDENTIFICATION. The tiny parasitic female lies deep in the mucosal crypts of the alimentary tract, particularly the small intestine. The esophagus is nearly cylindrical and at least one fourth as long as the body (Figure 3-108). Other small nematodes in this location include members of the superfamily Trichostrongyloidea, which have a very much shorter esophagus, and *Trichinella* spp. and *Capillaria* spp., both of which have a stichosome esophagus (see the section on Trichuroidea, near

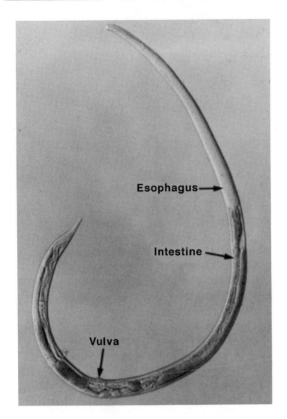

Esophagus →

Intestine →

Vulva
↑

FIGURE 3-108 *Strongyloides stercoralis* parasitic female (×95).

the end of this chapter). The egg, rhabditiform larva, and infective filariform larva are the stages most important in diagnostic procedures. Of the significant species of *Strongyloides* in veterinary medicine, only those of dogs and cats (also humans) produce eggs that routinely hatch before leaving the body such that first-stage larvae rather than embryonated eggs are found in the feces. The free-living adults (see Figures 3-105 and 3-107) frequently develop in cultures of feces from *Strongyloides*-infected animals.

Prominent species of *Strongyloides* parasitizing domestic animals and humans include *Strongyloides stercoralis* of humans, dogs, and cats; *Strongyloides papillosus* of ruminants; *Strongyloides ransomi* of swine; *Strongyyloides westeri* of horses; *Strongyloides fuelleborni* of African and Asian primates and of humans; *Strongyloides cebus* of American primates; and *Strongyloides ratti* and *Strongyloides venezuelensis* of rats. Thus all species of domestic animals have a species of *Strongyloides*, as do many species of wild mammals and birds (Little, 1966a, 1966b).

IMPORTANCE. *Strongyloides* infections are moderate and asymptomatic in most individuals of all domestic species, and when disease does occur, it usually is confined to massively challenged neonates

and nurslings. *S. papillosus*, although almost universally prevalent in ruminants, has been considered to only rarely cause detectable illness even though the newborn calves, lambs, and kids acquire infective larvae at a tender age in their dam's milk. Transmammary infection also occurs with *S. ransomi* of swine and *S. westeri* of horses. Piglets heavily infected with *S. ransomi* have debilitating dysentery, rapid emaciation, anemia, and stunting, starting only a few days after birth (Moncol and Batte, 1966). In like manner, foals begin to shed *S. westeri* eggs about 2 weeks after birth and may have diarrhea at this time (Lyons et al, 1969; Enigk et al, 1969).

S. stercoralis infection in dogs may be asymptomatic, or it may cause any grade of clinical illness. Serious cases involve signs of bronchopneumonia and severe watery or mucous diarrhea that may easily be confused with the generalized viral diseases of puppyhood. In massive invasions, the lungs of young pups may be sprinkled with petechial and ecchymotic hemorrhages caused by migrating larvae breaking out of the alveolar capillaries. The prepatent period is about 1 week. The epidemiological role of the dog in human *S. stercoralis* infection has actually been documented by only one report of natural transmission from dog to man (Georgi and Sprinkle, 1974). However, the potential hazard to human health should always be taken into account in dealing with infected dogs.

S. stercoralis infection in man is unique in its chronicity. Once contracted, this infection may persist for decades or for life, now as a slumbering asymptomatic and nonpatent infection, again as a bout of abdominal pain with diarrhea or of intensely pruritic "creeping eruption," and sometimes as a catastrophic terminal illness precipitated by massive infection. In at least some cases of human *S. stercoralis* infection, development to the infective filariform larval stage occurs within the patient's digestive tract. These infective larvae may reinvade the host by penetrating either the wall of the bowel **(internal autoinfection)** or the perianal skin **(external autoinfection).** Autoinfection accounts for the extreme chronicity of strongyloidiasis in man and, in part, for the explosive development of massive disseminated infection **(hyperinfection)** that may overwhelm patients with depressed cell-mediated immunity. Hyperinfection with *S. stercoralis* has caused the deaths of many persons who have immune deficiency diseases or are undergoing immunosuppressive therapy (Dwork et al, 1975). *S. stercoralis* also appears to cause disseminated disease in some AIDS patients and can lead to death if not diagnosed (Cahill and Sheuchuk, 1996). Dogs also have been shown capable of developing autoinfection when immunosuppressed

(Schad et al, 1984). The ability of *S. tercoralis* to cause internal autoinfection is probably due in part to the passage of larvae rather than eggs as occurs with the other species of *Strongyloides* parasitic in domestic animals. The larvae in the fecal stream are then capable of developing to the infective stage before leaving the body.

No invariable statement of fact can be made about the infectivity or virulence of *S. stercoralis* because geographic strains exist that differ greatly in their infectivity and virulence for different hosts. For example, Galliard (1951b) had no difficulty producing durable infections in dogs by using 19 strains of *S. stercoralis*, 11 obtained from Europeans infected in different regions of French Indochina (Vietnam) and 8 from natives of Tonkin, but he found dogs to be quite refractory to strains imported from the West Indies and Africa. Therefore the actual threat to human health posed by any particular *S. stercoralis*–infected dog is unpredictable, and the introduction or emergence of highly virulent strains is always at least a theoretical possibility. Clearly it is best to play it safe and handle infected dogs with extraordinary caution until it is quite certain that their *S. stercoralis* burdens have been eliminated. For further details, see Georgi, 1982.

S. westeri of horses, as with other members of the genus, develops rapidly in passed feces to the infective filariform stage, which usually enters the host by penetrating its skin or oral mucous membranes. A remarkable fact about *S. westeri* is that the adult worms are encountered principally in suckling and weanling foals; the dam of an infected foal sheds no *S. westeri* eggs even though she is the source of infection. Infection is transmitted from the dam to the foal by way of the mammary gland (Lyons et al, 1969, 1973), and the foals begin to shed eggs in their feces at 10 days to 2 weeks after birth. Diarrhea rather frequently afflicts foals between the ninth and thirteenth day of life, thus occurring coincidentally with the first postparturient estrus of the mare. Enigk et al (1974) presented convincing evidence that this so-called foal-heat diarrhea is caused by *S. westeri* and is not related to any alteration in the chemical composition of the mare's milk. Heavy infections in foals persist for 10 weeks; lighter infections may last 2 or 3 times as long. Occasionally, very light infections are observed in yearlings and older horses. These may represent percutaneous infections in hosts that were not exposed as sucklings (Enigk et al, 1974).

S. papillosus of ruminants has long been considered to behave typically as a commensal or at the least causing significant disease only when present in very large numbers. In a recent report on a series of studies performed in the late 1960s and early 1970s, it was shown that even relatively light infections with this parasite can cause severe disease in goats (Pienaar et al, 1999). In these studies with 89 goats infected with various dosing regimens, some kids died after three infections with as few as 2000 to 5000 larvae per exposure. The most susceptible age group was kids 6 weeks to 6 months of age, although older goats, 6 to 12 months of age, would also succumb. Death would typically occur within 9 to 30 days of receiving 75,000 larvae. The clinical signs included dehydration, inappetence, emaciation, weakness, cachexia, diarrhea, anemia, respiratory distress, and abnormal stools. Fever was not seen in any of the animals. Nervous signs were exhibited from Day 43 after exposure onward, and about 22% of the goats that died had histopathological lesions in the brain and spinal cord. Sudden death from hepatic rupture occurred in 6% of the goats. In a different set of studies (Nakamura et al, 1994), it was shown that the inoculation of live parthenognetic females into the duodenum of susceptible lambs produced continuous sinus tachycardia immediately after inoculation with the result being death due to cardiac arrest. Thus the effects of adults in the one study and the numerous lesions seen in varied tissues of the goats in the other set of studies would suggest that *S. pappilosus* may be more pathogenic than previously considered.

In swine, the tiny parthenogenetic *S. ransomi* female lies deeply embedded in the mucous membrane of the small intestine. The eggs shed in the feces contain first-stage rhabditiform larvae that develop into infective third-stage filariform larvae in 2 or 3 days, or slightly longer if a generation of free-adults is included in the cycle. Infection occurs by penetration of the skin or oral mucosae by filariform larvae. These may follow a tracheal migration route to maturation in about 6 days or a somatic migration route to accumulate as arrested larvae in the adipose tissues, especially those of the mammary area. Tracheal migration and maturation is the usual outcome in piglets and occurs to some extent in older pigs. Mature gilts tend instead to store *S. ransomi* larvae in their adipose tissues and to shed them later in the colostrum and milk. The third-stage larvae shed in the colostrum and milk are said to be "advanced" as compared with the third-stage larvae that originally infected the gilt because they are slightly larger and their genital primordia longer, wider, and more conspicuous, and because they mature in suckling pigs in only 2 to 4 days instead of 6 days. Transmammary infection is the key to the epidemiology of *S. ransomi* infection. Piglets separated at birth from their dam and reared artificially were free of *S. ransomi* infection, whereas piglets allowed to nurse began to shed eggs in their feces 2 to 4 days after birth

(Moncol and Batte, 1966). This initial transmammary infection thus serves to contaminate the environment of the sow and litter, thereby augmenting the mature worm burdens of the piglets and rebuilding the sow's tissue store of arrested larvae for subsequent litters (Moncol, 1975).

Strongyloidosis of piglets is an acute enteritis with bloody diarrhea (dysentery), rapid emaciation, anorexia, anemia, and stunting. There may be death losses but, from an economic standpoint, these may be economically less significant than the retarded growth of the survivors.

TREATMENT. Ivermectin administered subcutaneously at 0.2 mg/kg seems to be the treatment of choice for naturally infected dogs and humans (Mansfield and Schad, 1992; Lindo et al, 1996). However, it appears that in some cases a second treatment may be necessary. In dogs with experimental infections of *S. stercoralis*, treatment with 0.8 mg/kg body weight failed to remove larvae from the tissues of the dogs (Mansfield and Schad, 1992). Kelly (1977) recommended 100 to 150 mg thiabendazole per kilogram body weight for 3 days, repeated weekly until larvae disappear from the feces. Continuous feeding of 250 ppm of thiabendazole prevented establishment of *S. stercoralis* in puppies (Yakstis et al, 1968).

Any dog or cat infected with *S. stercoralis* should be isolated from other animals, and care should be taken to avoid human infection. Chronic strongyloidiasis tends to be refractory and recurrent, so fecal specimens from recognized cases should be examined monthly for *S. stercoralis* larvae for at least 6 months after apparently successful therapy. In no case should a single negative fecal specimen be accepted as proof of cure because the numbers of larvae shed in the feces of infected animals may oscillate drastically from day to day (Galliard, 1951a).

S. ransomi can be treated in neonatal pigs with ivermectin, levamisole resinate, or thiabendazole. Doramectin and ivermectin can also be used to treat adult *S. papillosus* in cattle and sheep. *S. westeri* in horses can be treated with oxibendazole, thiabendazole, and ivermectin. It has also been shown that the treatment of mares at foaling with ivermectin can prevent the infection of suckling foals (Ludwig et al, 1983).

CONTROL MEASURES. The epidemiological importance of the heterogonic cycle depends on the degree of contact between the host and the soil, but *S. stercoralis* is able to achieve and maintain high morbidity rates even in colonies that are housed on wire-bottom cages. Homogonic filariform infective larvae can develop from freshly passed rhabditiform larvae within 24 to 36 hours, so cages and pens must be cleaned and sanitized at less than 24-hour intervals to break the cycle. Development of

somatic arrested larval burdens and transmammary infection of offspring have not been specifically demonstrated as applying to *S. stercoralis* infection in dogs but are well established for several other species of *Strongyloides*. We have observed *S. stercoralis* infection in dam-reared pups but not in their hand-reared littermates, indicating that infection is acquired after birth either from dam's milk, dam's fecal contamination, or both.

The rigor of measures adopted to control *S. stercoralis* infection in populations must, as always, be consonant with the objectives of control and the resources of the client. For example, to reliably produce *S. stercoralis*–free experimental pups from infected breeding stock, it is necessary to deliver pups by cesarean section or separate them from their dam immediately at natural birth and rear them artificially on canine milk substitute. This procedure requires 24-hour attendance and a strong maternal instinct; it can seldom be applied under practical kennel conditions.

Reduction of the infection level in a breeding colony from the point of sporadic deaths to the point of asymptomatic infection probably can be accomplished by rigorous daily disinfection of cages and pens and monthly or bimonthly administration of a suitable anthelmintic drug. However, *S. stercoralis* will probably not be driven from the scene either completely or permanently by these measures, thanks to its exceedingly rapid development and the accumulation of arrested larvae in the tissues of bitches. Continued reliance on anthelmintics eventually produces resistant strains. Usually the next step is to switch to a different anthelmintic, invariably a more expensive one.

To prevent transmission of *S. stercoralis* from an infected pet to its master requires appropriate anthelmintic medication and monthly Baermann fecal examination of the dog for 6 months to a year to ensure that larval output has been terminated.

Order Oxyurida

Although the order Oxyurida is named for *Oxyuris equi,* the common and unusually large pinworm of the horse, most pinworms are very much smaller than *O. equi.* The oxyurid esophagus has a more or less spherical bulb immediately anterior to its junction with the intestine; this bulb often has a valve in its lumen (Figure 3-109). One or both sexes have a long, tapering tail, and it is for this that they are called pinworms. All oxyurids are highly host-specific parasites of the large intestine.

Oxyuris equi

Adult *O. equi* (Figure 3-110) are found principally in the small colon, although occasional specimens

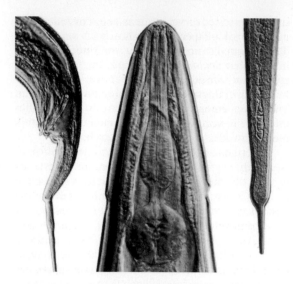

FIGURE 3-109   *Passalurus ambiguus* (a pinworm of the rabbit) tail of male *(left),* stomal end *(center),* and tail of female *(right)* (×168).

may be found in the large colon. Instead of simply discharging her eggs in the fecal stream, the gravid female *O. equi* migrates down the colon and rectum and out through the anus to cement her eggs in masses to the skin of the anus and its immediate surroundings. These egg masses consist of a tenacious yellowish gray fluid containing 8000 to 60,000 eggs. The eggs develop to the infective stage in 4 or 5 days, during which the cementing fluid dries, cracks, and detaches from the skin in flakes.

These flakes, which contain large numbers of infective eggs, adhere to mangers, water buckets, walls, and the like, thus contaminating the environment of the stable. Paper towels or disposable cloths are to be preferred for cleansing the perineum of horses because any nondisposable object, such as a sponge or towel, will inevitably become heavily contaminated with *O. equi* eggs. Then when the sponge or towel is applied to a horse's muzzle after a workout or used to clean the bit, the future brightens up for *O. equi*. The prepatent period is 5 months.

Severe infection with third- and fourth-stage *Oxyuris equi* (Figure 3-111) may produce significant inflammation of the cecal and colonic mucosa manifested by vague signs of abdominal discomfort. However, the most common affliction perpetrated by *O. equi* on the horse is *pruritus ani* caused by the adhesive egg masses deposited on the perianal skin by the female worm. In its efforts to relieve the itching, the horse will persistently rub its tail against posts, mangers, and the like until the tail head becomes disheveled, bare of hair, or even scarified.

TREATMENT. *O. equi* is an easy parasite to control. All of the available equine anthelmintics are highly effective against both immature and adult large pinworms. Ivermectin appears to continue to work very well (Klei et al, 2001). Pinworms also are controlled by the daily administration of pyrantel tartrate.

Probstmayria vivipara

This tiny (less than 3 mm long) pinworm gives birth to infective larvae and is therefore capable of

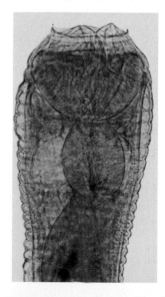

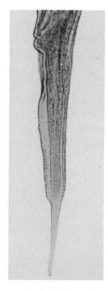

FIGURE 3-110   *Oxyuris equi* anterior end showing the esophageal bulb (×25).

FIGURE 3-111   *Oxyuris equi* fourth-stage larva. At left, the anterior end shows the temporary buccal capsule-like modification of the esophageal corpus that permits attachment to the mucous membrane and at right, the tail (×168).

completing its life history within the confines of its host's large intestine (Figure 3-112).

Skrjabinema

Skrjabinema ovis and *Skrjabinema caprae,* harmless parasites of sheep and goats, respectively, are 8 to 10 mm long. The genus name is pronounced "Skreeyabinema."

Enterobius vermicularis

This small (up to 13 mm long) pinworm of humans and great apes still has an extensive distribution among civilized man despite cooking and washing, the nemeses of many of his other parasites (see Figure 5-68). Infection rates vary up to 40%, depending on age and race. White elementary school children display the greatest intensity and prevalence of infection. The gravid *E. vermicularis* female migrates through the anal opening to cement her eggs to the host's perianal skin. The eggs develop to the infective stage within hours and are ready to reinfect the host by contamination of the hands, to infect other individuals by contamination of bedclothing or other fomites, or to become airborne on dust particles.

Infection may be suspected in children who have *pruritus* ani and insomnia. Diagnosis is reached by observing the female worm in the act of depositing her eggs on the perianal skin or by demonstrating the eggs. This can best be accomplished by momentarily pressing the adhesive side of a piece of cellophane tape against the anus and then sticking the tape to a slide to prepare it for microscopic examination. Conventional fecal examination techniques almost uniformly fail to demonstrate the eggs of *Enterobius* spp. and many other pinworms (e.g., *Oxyuris* spp.). The important practical point for veterinarians is that *E. vermicularis* is a parasite of humans and apes (apes have other species of *Enterobius* as well), but never of dogs or cats. Occasionally, a physician prescribes euthanasia of the family pet to help control pinworms. The finest degree of tact is required in dealing with this situation.

Infection of apes with species of *Enterobius* spp. is usually asymptomatic. However, sporadic cases of fatal ulcerative enteritis with extensive invasion of the intestinal submucosa and even of the mesenteric lymph nodes by the adult pinworms have been reported in chimpanzees (Schmidt and Prine, 1970; Keeling and McClure, 1974; Holmes et al, 1980). Both *Enterobius anthropopitheci,* a natural parasite of apes, and *E. vermicularis* of humans have been implicated.

Order Ascaridida

Ascarids are among the largest and most familiar of nematode parasites infecting the intestinal tract of domestic animals. The worms found in domestic animals range from several inches up to 2 feet in length. The mouth is surrounded by three fleshy lips, one dorsal and two subventral (Figure 3-113), and the tail of the male is usually curved ventrally. Some genera have lateral cervical alae that make the anterior end of the worm resemble an arrowhead, thus such generic names as *Toxocara* and *Toxascaris.*

Development to the infective stage differs only in detail for the various ascarid genera. The single cell develops into an infective larva inside the eggshell within several days or weeks, depending on the species of worm and the ambient temperature. There are many genera of ascaridoid nematodes that parasitize aquatic vertebrates (e.g., fish, crocodilians, birds, and sea mammals), and these genera typically have free-swimming larval stages initially and various required intermediate hosts. The ascaridoids found in domestic animals have adapted to their terrestrial existence by changing the typical life history pattern. Thus the life cycles of the ascaridoids in domestic animals are direct with or without various migrations in the body of the host or through transplacental or transmammary pathways. Another adaptation to the terrestrial environment has been the development of an eggshell capable of withstanding the extremes of harsh environments. Ascarid eggs are remarkably resistant to chemical and physical insults, especially after they have arrived at the infective stage. The single most important fact to remember in relation to the epidemiology of ascariasis is that the eggs

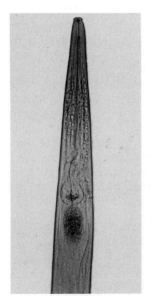
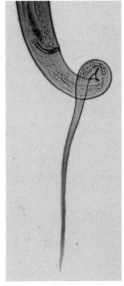

FIGURE 3-112 *Probstmayria vivipara* adult male anterior end *(left)* and tail *(right)* (×108).

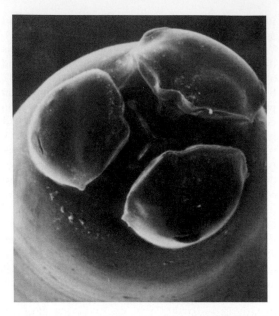

FIGURE 3-113   *Ascaris suum* lips and stoma (SEM ×125).

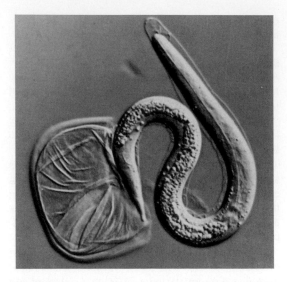

FIGURE 3-114   *Ascaris suum* mechanically hatched infective larva with retained cuticle of previous stage (×520).

remain infective in soil for many years. Various ascarid genera display remarkable differences in patterns of intrahost development; however, for the terrestrial species, almost without exception it is now accepted by most that part of the adaptation to the terrestrial environment has been the incorporation of two molts within the eggshell so that the larval stage hatching from the egg of these ascaridoids is a third-stage larva.

IDENTIFICATION. For the purposes of practical identification, adult ascarids are quite host-specific. Thus *Ascaris suum* infects swine, *Parascaris equorum* infects horses, *Toxocara vitulorum* infects cattle, *Toxocara canis* infects dogs, and *Toxocara cati* infects cats. Dogs and cats also share a second ascarid, *Toxascaris leonina*, which must be distinguished from their respective species of *Toxocara* (see Figures 5-23 to 5-26).

Ascarid eggs are relatively thick walled, contain a single cell when passed in the feces, and are usually sufficiently distinctive to permit identification of the species (see Figures 5-7, 5-8, 5-9, 5-28, 5-41, and 5-58).

Ascaris

A. suum is a ubiquitous and pathogenic parasite of swine. The adult worms are about 30 cm long, white to cream colored, with three large lips typical of the ascaridoids (Figure 3-113). Long considered a variety of the morphologically indistinguishable human ascarid *Ascaria lumbricoides*, *A. suum* is considered a distinct species by most contemporary authors. However, *A. lumbricoides* can mature in swine, and *A. suum* can mature in humans. Typi-

cally, however, these two species maintain separate cycles, with the swine species staying in swine and the human species in humans even when both hosts live very closely together (Anderson et al, 1993; Anderson, 1995).

Although the eggs of both species will hatch and their larvae will migrate extensively in a wide range of hosts, the infective egg in polluted soil or stuck to the mammary skin of the sow is the key element in the epidemiology of *A. suum* infection. The infective egg hatches in the stomach and small intestine (Figure 3-114), releasing the third-stage larva (Geenen et al, 1999), which enters the wall of the cecum and colon and proceeds to the liver, arriving there in a matter of hours by way of the portal vein (Murrell et al, 1997). After tunneling about in the liver for several days, the larva arrives in a pulmonary capillary by way of the caudal vena cava, heart, and pulmonary artery. At this point, the larva either may remain in the circulation to be carried to the somatic tissues or may lodge temporarily in the pulmonary capillary and then break out into an alveolus. In the case of *A. suum*, the latter course appears to be much more probable because the larva will typically proceed up the bronchial tree and trachea to the pharynx, there to be swallowed, then will arrive once again in the small intestine, where it will mature.

In their migrations through various tissues, ascarid larvae at first inflict only mechanical damage, but hypersensitivity rapidly develops, and allergic inflammation with eosinophilic inflammation characterizes the host reaction to subsequent invasions. In pig livers, the inflammation heals by fibrosis, giving rise to the so-called **milk spot** lesions that cause the organ to be condemned by meat inspectors as unfit for human consumption. Contrary to the teachings of histologists who argue that because the interlobular septa appear formidable under the microscope, pig liver must necessarily be tough, pig liver is in fact very tender, and the losses caused by *A. suum* larvae must be measured in gastronomic as well as economic terms.

The lesions of early migrations in the lungs are likewise mechanical in nature and once again, the initial focal hemorrhages are followed by hyperemia, edema, and eosinophilic infiltration as hypersensitivity develops. In young pigs, extensive lung lesions give rise to severe respiratory embarrassment. Breathing is rapid, shallow, and marked by audible expiratory efforts ("thumps") and coughing; pigs may die.

The pathological effects of adult *A. suum* infections in the small intestine are less dramatic than those of the larval migrations, but they are undoubtedly significant. There may be diarrhea, but the most important effect is interference with proper nutrition and normal growth. Heavily infected pigs fail to make economically profitable gains. Occasional bizarre accidents such as occlusion of the bile duct or perforation of the bowel wall result from the tendency of ascarids to wander.

Diagnosis of clinical ascarosis frequently depends on clinical and necropsy findings because the main pathological events occur during the prepatent stage. Clinical signs of severe respiratory distress in a group of growing pigs and the discovery of extensive petechial and ecchymotic pulmonary hemorrhages and edema contribute to a diagnosis of acute ascarosis. Pieces of lung tissue should be minced and placed in a Baermann apparatus to demonstrate the migrating larvae. Less acute cases are marked by respiratory distress, varying degrees of malnutrition, and lesions of interstitial pneumonia. Chronic ascarosis is marked by stunting, emaciation, a copious outpouring of *A. suum* eggs in the feces, and lesions of chronic interstitial pneumonia and hepatic fibrosis. Such pigs are hopeless from an economic point of view.

ANTHELMINTIC MEDICATION. *A. suum*, the economically most important nematode of swine, continues to menace the swine industry despite its susceptibility to piperazines, hygromycin B, dichlorvos, fenbendazole, levamisole, ivermectin, and pyrantel tartrate. It is obvious that drugs alone are not successful in controlling this ubiquitous parasite. However, treating and cleaning sows with soap and warm water 2 weeks before moving them to the farrowing crates will materially reduce the contamination to which the piglets will be exposed. Treating again at weaning with continuing attention to the hygienic conditions of the premises should keep the growing pigs reasonably free of *A. suum*. Continuous

provision of feeds containing pyrantel tartrate prevents the migration and establishment of *A. suum*. Pyrantel tartrate is the only approved drug that kills the infective larva immediately after it hatches in the small intestine. Continuous administration of thiabendazole prevents the migration of larvae through the lungs but not through the liver.

In summary, control efforts should be directed at preventing infection of pigs during the first few weeks of life. Anthelmintic medication of the sow before farrowing, careful sanitation at farrowing time, and avoidance of exposure of young pigs to contaminated soils all serve to limit early infection.

Parascaris

Parascaris equorum, the very large ascarid parasite of the horse, resembles *A. suum* both epidemiologically and with respect to the route adopted by its larvae in migrating through the tissues. When the infective egg of *P. equorum* is swallowed by a foal, the larva hatches, burrows into the wall of the small intestine, and is carried to the liver by the portal vein. After migrating about in the hepatic tissues, the larva enters a hepatic vein and is carried by the caudal vena cava, heart, and pulmonary artery to the lung, where it enters an alveolus. After completing a molt in the lungs, the larva ascends in the expectorant mucus of the tracheobronchial tree and returns by way of the lumen of the esophagus and stomach to the intestine, where it completes a final molt and matures.

The first waves of invading larvae inflict mainly mechanical injury, and little more than petechial hemorrhages can be observed. However, as the host becomes sensitized to *Parascaris* antigens, the tissues respond to the presence of larvae with infiltrations of eosinophilic leukocytes and other inflammatory cells. The damage done to the liver and lungs eventually heals, but the chronic reduction in functional capacity suffered during what normally is a period of rapid growth leaves its mark on the yearling. It never will be what it could have been.

The durable infective egg is the key element in the epidemiology of *P. equorum* infection. These eggs accumulate as a growing reservoir of infection in polluted soils, and they adhere by their sticky shell covering to the teats and udder of the brood mare and wait there for the foal to be born.

Heavy infection with adult ascarids causes moderate enteritis and subnormal growth through interference with digestion and absorption of nutrients. Ascaridosis produces a malnourished, undersized, sickly individual with little stamina and reduced resistance to disease: its haircoat is dull, its skin dry and leathery, and its abdomen too large for its frame. It is not unusual to find a half-full pail of *P. equorum* in the small intestine of a foal, a sufficient mass of parasites actually to compete with the host for nutrients. Occasionally, adult *P. equorum* perforate the bowel wall and cause fatal peritonitis. Administration of anthelmintics that tend to paralyze ascarids (e.g., pyrantel pamoate, piperazine, and ivermectin) to a foal with a heavy *P. equorum* may occasionally cause impaction or complete obstruction of the bowel (Schusser et al, 1988.)

CONTROL. The thick outer proteinaceous layer of the *P. equorum* eggshell is very sticky and enables the eggs to adhere to stall walls, mangers, water buckets, mares' teats, and other objects. The epidemiology of *P. equorum* infection therefore differs considerably from that of strongylids with their free-living infective larvae, and from that of the carnivoran ascarids with their paratenic hosts and perinatal transmission of infection from dam to offspring. Unfortunately, most chemical disinfectants available in the United States have no appreciable effect on ascarid eggs. Therefore effective stall sanitation for the control of ascarids involves weekly removal of all manure and bedding and thorough cleaning of all surfaces with a high-pressure cleaner or steam jenny. Most horsemen find such a program excessively laborious and rely instead on anthelmintics to suppress production and environmental contamination with the eggs of *P. equorum*. However, because of the extraordinary longevity and hardihood of ascarid eggs, contamination, however gradual, tends to be cumulative, and thorough cleaning at least of the foaling stall and of the mare's udder and teats before foaling is well worth the effort.

ANTHELMINTIC MEDICATION. Piperazine compounds (100 mg/kg), fenbendazole (10 mg/kg), pyrantel (6.6 mg/kg), ivermectin (0.2 mg/kg), and a number of other anthelmintics both current and obsolete are highly effective against the intestinal stages of *P. equorum*. Pyrantel tartrate used as a feed additive prevents ascarid infections in horses much as it does in swine.

Toxascaris

Toxascaris leonina is a parasite of cats and dogs in the cooler climates of the world. The life cycle of *T. leonina* is such that this ascaridoid often becomes a problem of felids housed in zoological gardens. Because of the direct life cycle of this parasite, the worm tends to be found in animals older than the hosts of *T. canis* or *T. cati*.

The simplest form of ascarid life history is displayed by *T. leonina*. The egg of *T. leonina* develops rapidly, usually reaching the infective stage in about a week. When the infective egg is ingested by a suitable definitive host, it hatches in the stomach, and the larva invades the mucosa of the small intestine. There it develops and molts

before returning to the lumen of the intestine to mature. If the egg is ingested by a rodent or other unsuitable animal, the larva hatches and invades the wall of the intestine, where it remains for about a week before proceeding to other tissues, where it encysts and remains arrested in the infective stage. Cats and dogs can thus acquire *T. leonina* infection by ingesting infective eggs or rodents with infective larvae encysted in their tissues. These relationships are presented diagrammatically in Figure 3-115.

The restricted mucosal migration of *T. leonina* in dogs and cats precludes the development of somatic larval burdens and the transmission of infection by way of the placenta and mammary gland. Ingestion of infective eggs and paratenic hosts seems to be the only means by which cats and dogs acquire *T. leonina* infection; however, *T. leonine* possesses one advantage: its eggs develop to the infective stage in only 1 week as compared with 4 weeks for *Toxocara* spp. This rapid development might explain the persistence of *T. leonina* infection in reasonably well-sanitized cage colonies of dogs. Of course, there is always the possibility that mice or other paratenic hosts are to blame.

Toxocara

Toxocara is a genus of rather large ascaridoids that as adults are parasites in the small intestine of various mammals. The worms have three large lips and a glandular esophageal bulb (the **ventriculus**) located at the junction of the esophagus and intestine. They tend to have cervical alae, and their eggs have pitted surfaces. *T. canis* and *T. cati* are two of the most commonly observed parasites of the dog and cat, respectively. *Toxocara vitulorum* of calves is commonly seen in developing parts of the world, and the egg still can be observed occasionally in feces from calves in the United States. Other species of *Toxocara* include those

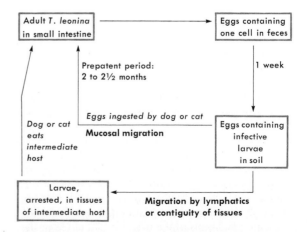

FIGURE 3-115 Alternative life histories of *Toxascaris leonina*.

found in elephants, hippopotami, bats, civet cats, rats, coati mundis, and mongooses.

TOXOCARA CANIS. This worm is commonly seen in puppies during the few months after birth. The adults tend to be 10 to 15 cm long and cream colored, with the internal reproductive organs appearing white when viewed through the cuticle in fresh worms. Sometimes when worms are passed in the feces, the gut tends to appear rather gray or black, and the worms appear darker than when still quite lively. When looked for, adult dogs infected with this parasite can be found that are shedding the eggs in their feces.

Heavy prenatal *T. canis* infections cause severe abdominal discomfort in nursling pups. The pups whimper and shriek almost continuously and adopt a peculiar straddle-legged posture of the hind limbs when standing or walking. Alarming numbers of immature and adult worms may appear in the feces or vomitus. Death may result from rupture or obstruction of the intestine as the ascarids, reacting to some irritant, thrash about and become tangled into knots. Obstruction of the bile or pancreatic duct occasionally provides prize exhibits for pathology museums.

LIFE HISTORY. The adolescent wanderings of nematode larvae are influenced not only by their intrinsic capabilities for penetrating tissues and responding to various chemical and physical stimuli, but also by the suitability of the host invaded. If a *T. canis* egg hatches in a dog's stomach, the larva invades the bowel wall and arrives in a pulmonary capillary by the same route outlined earlier for *A. suum*. Unlike *A. suum*, however, the *T. canis* larva is considerably more prone to remain in the circulation than to break into the alveolus, especially if its host is a mature dog. If the larva fails to enter the alveolus, it will be returned to the heart by the pulmonary veins and carried away by the systemic circulation, perhaps to lodge in a kidney or some other somatic tissue where it will encyst as an arrested infective larva.

The direction taken at the alveolus is crucial in determining whether the larva will undergo a **tracheal migration** and develop to sexual maturity or a **somatic migration** to remain arrested as an infective larva in that particular dog. The probability of tracheal migration is high in a newborn puppy. However, by the time the pup is 1 or 2 months old, the probability that a newly hatched *T. canis* larva will develop into an adult ascarid in that particular pup has fallen to a very low level and remains so indefinitely. During the same period of the pup's life, the probability of somatic migration progressively increases, and arrested infective larvae accumulate in the tissues.

Somatic migration also accounts for the accumulation of arrested infective *T. canis* larvae in

the tissues of a wide range of other paratenic intermediate hosts, including rodents, sheep, pigs, monkeys, humans, and earthworms. If a mouse with arrested infective larvae in its tissues is eaten by a dog, somatic migration is not observed, and in some instances at least, development proceeds to maturity in the alimentary tract (Sprent, 1958). The mouse not only has saved the larvae but apparently changed them, too. Migration and encystment in paratenic hosts and exploitation of the prey-predator relationship is an epidemiological norm for carnivoran ascarids in general. Both *T. cati* and *T. leonine* can be transmitted in this manner, as can ascarid parasites of certain wild carnivorans such as *Baylisacaris procyonis* of the raccoon *Procyon lotor* (see later).

As important as infected intermediate hosts may be to the epidemiology of carnivoran ascarids, the most important arrested *T. canis* larvae are those to be found in the tissues of the female of the definitive host species itself. Transmission of infection from bitch to pups occurs by way of both placenta and mammary gland. During the last trimester of pregnancy, arrested larvae are reactivated and migrate from the tissues of the bitch to the pups in utero (Fülleborn, 1921). After parturition, small numbers of reactivated larvae also may be shed in the milk. The alternative life histories of *T. canis* are summarized in Figure 3-116.

TOXOCARA CATI. This worm is slightly smaller than *T. canis* and has very elegant cervical alae (Figure 3-117). When the fresh worm is observed, the ventral curvature of the anterior end along with the large cervical alae gives the front end of the worm a pythonlike appearance. These worms are commonly delivered to practitioners after they have been observed in vomitus by owners. If in doubt about the worm's identity, the practitioner can always break the worm open about one third of the body length behind the head and look for the more familiar *Toxocara* eggs with a microscope. This will work, of course, only if the worm presented is a female.

LIFE HISTORY. The migration patterns of *T. cati* differ qualitatively from those of *T. canis* in that (1) prenatal infection through the placenta does not occur and (2) the probability of tracheal migration in egg infections remains high throughout the cat's life. Neonatal infection through the mammary glands is an important route of infection in kittens (Swerczek et al, 1971), and infected paratenic hosts unquestionably represent an important reservoir of infection for adult cats, at least those with well-developed predatory habits. In both of these latter cases, the infective larvae adopt a much more conservative migration pattern than when they first hatched. Migration and arrested development in the

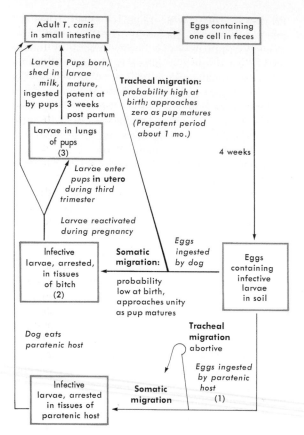

FIGURE 3-116   Alternative life histories of *Toxocara canis*. *1*, A *paratenic host* is any in which a larval parasite may survive and remain infective for its definitive host without undergoing development. Any of a wide range of animal species including rodents, sheep, pigs, monkeys, humans, earthworms, and adult dogs may serve as paratenic host for *T. canis* larvae. *2*, Arrested infective larvae are also found in the tissues of male dogs, but these are supposed to be of little if any epidemiological importance. *3*, The larvae that have entered the pups through the placenta molt once in the fetuses but defer further development until after birth (From Sprent JFA: *Parasitology* 48[1–2]:184–209, 1958.)

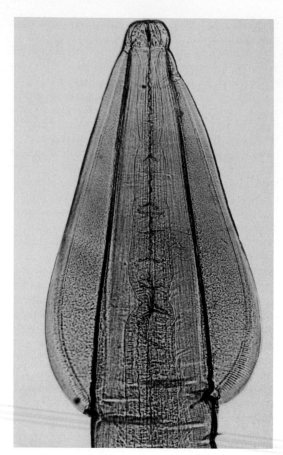

FIGURE 3-117   *Toxocara cati* stomal end showing the broad cervical alae (×40).

paratenic host appear in some way to satisfy the larval wanderlust and, although a small proportion of the larvae may wander as before, most develop to maturity after a sojourn in the wall of the stomach (i.e., a **mucosal migration;** Sprent, 1956).

It follows from these considerations that somatic migration with accumulation of arrested larvae of *T. cati* in the tissues of cats must occur only, or at least principally, in egg infections. Because cats ordinarily display little tendency to ingest soil, many authors have discounted the significance of egg infections in the epidemiology of *T. cati*. However, when one reflects on the perpetual self-grooming in which cats indulge, it is plain enough how infective *T. cati* eggs might be conveyed to their stomachs from time to time. The

alternative life histories of *T. cati* are summarized diagrammatically in Figure 3-118.

Control of Canine and Feline Ascarid Infections
Sources of Infection

SOIL POLLUTION. *Toxocara* and *Toxascaris* eggs are very resistant to environmental adversity and remain infective for years, especially in poorly drained clay and silt soils, hence their accumulation in soil and filth and the threat they pose to successful dog rearing progress with time. A reasonable explanation for the heavy ascarid infections so frequently encountered in hound pups might be sought in the common practice of chaining the hounds almost permanently to doghouses, a practice particularly conducive to soil pollution. Because the infective eggs are virtually immune to any reasonable measures taken to destroy them, the most effective measure is to entomb them under a concrete or bituminous asphalt slab. Once the slab is installed and provided that feces are not allowed to accumulate for more than a week at a time, the

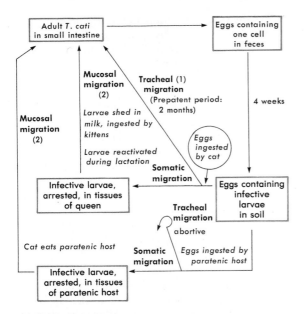

FIGURE 3-118 Alternative life histories of *Toxocara cati. 1,* The probability that ingestion of infective eggs will lead to patent infection remains substantial throughout the life of the cat. *2,* Larvae that have already undergone somatic migration in a paratenic host, including the queen, satisfy their histotrophic requirements with a mucosal migration. The relative epidemiological importance of these alternatives will depend on the kind of environment, the abundance of suitable paratenic hosts, and the sex and habits of the cats. (From Sprent JFA: *Parasitology* 46[1–2]:54–58, 1956; Swerczek TW, Nielsen SW, and Helmbolt CF: *Am J Vet Res* 32:89–92, 1971.)

probability of the confined dog ingesting infective ascarid eggs becomes quite small. The next best way of decontaminating polluted soil is to replace the top foot or so with fresh gravel.

CONTAMINATED KENNEL AREAS. All surfaces must first be made physically clean. High-pressure washers like those in car washes are very effective, and inexpensive mobile units are quite satisfactory. Wood and wire construction is difficult to clean properly with any kind of equipment or amount of effort. After surfaces are physically clean, they may be mopped or sprayed with 1% sodium hypochlorite (three cups Clorox per gallon of cool water) to strip off the outer protein coat of the ascarid eggs so they will not stick to surfaces and can be rinsed away. The preliminary cleaning is absolutely essential because any appreciable amount of residual organic matter will neutralize the sodium hypochlorite and render it ineffective in stripping the ascarid eggs. Notice that nothing has been said about killing the ascarid eggs. The preceding treatment does not kill ascarid eggs; it just knocks them loose.

ARRESTED LARVAE IN TISSUES OF BITCHES AND QUEENS. Arrested larvae are immune to anthel-

mintics because they are metabolically inactive. When reactivated, these larvae become moderately susceptible to a few anthelmintics administered frequently and in high dosage (see the section on dogs later), but there is still no easy, inexpensive way to get rid of somatic larval burdens.

PARATENIC HOSTS. Mice and other small paratenic hosts may play a significant role in the epidemiology of *Toxocara* and *Toxascaris* infection, especially as regards predacious cats. If you dissect the mice, voles, moles, shrews, and snakes that your cat drags in, you will probably find *Toxocara* larvae encysted in most of them. In a rural setting, there is probably little that can be done about this source of infection except to confine the dogs and cats indoors. Rodents are attracted to the abundance of food in kennels and catteries and are not put off by the presence of their ferocious predators; a mouse is quite willing to risk its life for a kibble. There seems to be little information about the importance of rodents in transmitting ascarids and other parasites to dogs and cats confined to buildings and outdoor enclosures. However, considering the facts gathered here, an investment in rodent control could be partly written off against the cost of controlling parasites.

Anthelmintic Medication

YOUNG PUPS. Piperazine compounds are practically nontoxic yet highly effective against ascarids in the lumen of the alimentary tract. Therefore they are ideally suited to removing *T. canis* as they arrive and develop in the intestinal lumens of perinatally infected pups. Unless heroic measures have been taken to prevent infection, pups may be assumed to be infected. Medication should start routinely as early as the second week of life and be repeated every 3 weeks until the pup is 3 months old. The standard therapeutic dose is 110 mg piperazine base per kilogram body weight, but substantially lower dosages appear on the labels of many proprietary preparations. The reason for this is not clear. If the ascarids receive too little piperazine, they may recover their motility and their place in the small intestine before peristalsis has had a chance to eliminate them. It is better to give the full dose. Special preparations of dichlorvos are also available for pups, but these are more expensive and therefore might be applied more economically to mixed infections of *Toxocara* and *Ancylostoma*. Milbemycin oxime is highly efficacious in treating mixed infections of *Toxocara* and *Ancylostoma*, as is pyrantel formulated with ivermectin for heartworm prevention. These combination products are not approved for dogs younger than 4 weeks. Pyrantel and febantel in combination with praziquantel also can be used if the puppies are over 2 pounds and 3 weeks of age. Selamectin will remove roundworms from dogs although it has not received a claim for this use in the United States (McTier et al, 2000a).

In breeding situations, the role of the bitch in the epidemiology of *T. canis* is paramount because she harbors the better part of the reservoir of infection not contained in the soil. Clients should be advised that bitches bestowing pathogenic *T. canis* burdens on their litters will likely repeat the performance once or twice again, even after the uptake of infective eggs has ceased. Clients should also be made aware that the environment of a bitch with a litter of nurslings is likely to contain veritable clouds of eggs from 3 weeks postpartum onward, and it is during this period that anthelmintic medication and sanitation can be applied most effectively and efficiently. Rather heavy patent infections are regularly observed in nursing bitches for a short period beginning about 1 month after parturition. This has been explained as follows (Sprent, 1961). Some reactivated larvae fail to establish themselves in the pups' intestines and are passed with their feces. Brood bitches eat their pups' feces to clean the nest and, in so doing, afford these jettisoned larvae a second chance to mature.

DOGS. *T. canis*–free dogs imply that the dogs are devoid of both adult and larval parasites. However, it is nearly impossible to detect small numbers of arrested larvae in the tissues of even a small pup, so the status "*T. canis*–free" is always to be taken with a grain of salt. The sort of measures required to produce *T. canis*–free dogs are usually beyond the resources (and requirements) of commercial breeders.

Griesemer and Gibson (1963) obtained *T. canis*–free pups from colostrum-deprived bitches raised in isolation and given daily therapeutic doses of diethylcarbamazine for many months. In addition, three beagle bitches that had been maintained on wire through several gestations yielded *T. canis*–free litters without anthelmintic medication. In the latter case, the somatic larval burden apparently was eliminated through the placenta over the course of several pregnancies, whereas in the former case, somatic contamination of the bitches was precluded by preventing their access to infective eggs from birth.

Bitches with *T. canis* and *A. caninum* infections were medicated daily with fenbendazole from the fortieth day of gestation to the fourteenth day of lactation at a dosage rate of 50 mg/kg. Their pups were found free of both parasites (Düwel and Strasser, 1978). Burke and Roberson (1983) obtained 89% fewer ascarids and 99% fewer hookworms in pups from dams subjected to the same regimen. The timing of medication coincided with the period of reactivation and migration of arrested *T. canis* larvae in these parturient females.

Thiabendazole administered orally at 150 mg/kg for 20 to 25 days starting when the pups were 5 days old controlled prenatal *T. canis* infections (Congdon and Ames, 1973).

Ivermectin administered during gestation has been shown to cause marked reductions in the number of *T. canis* in puppies born to experimentally infected bitches (Shoop et al, 1988). Treatments of 1.0 mg/kg body weight on Days 20 and 42, or 0.5 mg/kg body weight on Days 38, 41, 44, and 47 of gestation both caused marked reductions in the number of worms recovered from puppies of treated bitches. These dosages are well above the level of ivermectin used in heartworm prophylaxis.

CATS. Somatic migration of *T. cati* larvae occurs principally in egg infections. Because cats are such ardent self-groomers, infective eggs adhering to fur gain easy access to their interiors, and arrested larvae accumulate in the tissues. When reactivated during lactation, these larvae pass to the nurslings, undergo a mucosal migration, and mature, somatic migration in the queen apparently having satisfied their wanderlust (Sprent, 1956; Swerczek et al, 1971). Because *T. cati* larvae do not cross the placenta, it is theoretically possible to raise *T. cati*–free kittens for experimentation by removing them from their dam by cesarean section or at natural birth but before they have nursed, and raising them artificially. However, if less than absolute *T. cati*–free status is required, administration of an anthelmintic at intervals of 3 weeks for the first 3 or 4 months of life should suffice.

Piperazine compounds and pyrantel formulated with praziquantel (Drontal) are the preferred anthelmintics for the control of ascarid infections in cats. Milbemycin oxime is highly effective in the removal of *T. cati*. Selamectin is labeled for the removal of roundworms from cats (McTier et al, 2000b). The role of paratenic hosts in the epidemiology of *T. cati* infection should always be taken into account in planning control measures.

Human Toxocarosis (Visceral Larva Mirgrans)

The widespread distribution of dog feces and the prevalence of *T. canis* eggs therein led Fülleborn (1921) to wonder about the pathological significance in man of nodules containing larvae of this parasite. These nodules occurred principally in the liver, lungs, kidneys, and brain. Beaver et al (1952) recognized the etiological role of *T. canis* larvae in cases of sustained eosinophilia (above 50%), pneumonitis, and hepatomegaly in children younger than 3 years and dubbed the condition *visceral larva migrans*. As a horrible sequela occurring at 3 to 13 years, the larvae may produce granulomatous retinitis. Misdiagnosis of *T. canis*–induced granulomatous retinitis as retinoblastoma has prompted the unnecessary enucleation of children's eyes in at least 36 reported cases.

The typical epidemiological situation involves a toddler eating soil heavily contaminated with infective *T. canis* eggs. Such soil is likely to be found wherever dogs habitually defecate and, in particularly high concentration, in the nests of maternal bitches and their litters. The soil of public parks in cities tends to be heavily contaminated with infective *T. canis* eggs (Woodruff and Burg, 1973; Dubin et al, 1975).

Although dirt eating is often considered to be a manifestation of depraved appetite (i.e., pica) resulting from dietary deficiency or emotional insecurity, even well-nourished, well-adjusted babies should not be trusted to forgo whatever delicacies may be at hand. Children must not be allowed to play where dogs habitually defecate, and dog feces must never be used to fertilize vegetable gardens. Because ascarid eggs remain infective in soils for years, *T. canis* contamination and the hazard of visceral larva migrans tends to be cumulative. *T. cati* is only somewhat less important than *T. canis* as a cause of human visceral larva migrans. Cases have been reported of children infected with adult *T. cati* (Eberhard and Alfano, 1998), but it is believed that these children may have ingested intact adult worms recovered from litter boxes. The veterinary profession has a clear responsibility to identify and eliminate *T. canis* and *T. cati* infection at every opportunity and to provide the public with objective scientific information about the epidemiology and prevention of human toxocarosis.

Baylisascaris

Species of *Baylisascaris* common in North American wildlife include *Baylisascaris procyonis* of the raccoon, *Baylisascaris columnaris* of the skunk, and *Baylisascaris laevis* of the woodchuck. *B. procyonis* causes a particularly serious form of visceral larva migrans in a wide range of hosts including man (Kazacos, 1983). Unlike *Toxocara* larvae, the larvae of *B. procyonis* grow larger as they migrate. However, they resemble *T. canis* larvae in that they tend to invade the central nervous system of intermediate hosts and, because they grow as they migrate, only one to three *B. procyonis* larvae in the brain may prove fatal. These properties render them very pathogenic to woodchucks, rabbits, ground squirrels, chickens, turkeys, partridges, pigeons, cockatiels, chuckar partridges, emus, quail, and humans (Roth et al, 1982; Kazacos, 1983; Kazacos et al, 1983; Myers et al, 1983). Unfortunately, human cases continue to occur (Park et al, 2000), and it is imperative that

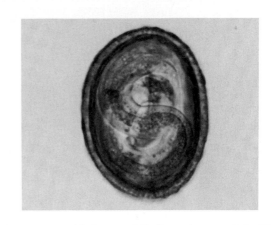

FIGURE 3-119 Infective egg of *Baylisascaris procyonis* (×600).

veterinarians be aware of the risk posed by raccoons either being held in captivity or within a community.

Hay, straw, and other feedstuffs and bedding materials contaminated with raccoon feces are often found to be the source of infective eggs (Figure 3-119) of this parasite. Haylofts and attics may be attractive places for children to play during inclement weather, but such areas should be inspected beforehand to make sure that raccoons have not been nesting in them. Ground-feeding birds such as doves, pigeons, and robins are particularly at risk when they feed on nondigested seeds in dried raccoon feces (Evans and Tangredi, 1985). Greve and O'Brien (1989) diagnosed infection with adult *B. procyonis* in a 5-month-old Labrador retriever (patent) and a 6-month-old golden retriever (nonpatent) by administering piperazine and identifying the adult and juvenile worms when these were passed in the feces. Eggs of this worm also have been observed in the feces of dogs in Minnesota, Indiana, Michigan, and Prince Edward Island. The raccoon has been introduced into Europe, where it has proliferated quite successfully. Unfortunately, the raccoon roundworm is also now present in Europe, and zoonotic infections occur there as well (Kuchle et al, 1993). Raccoons infected with *B. procyonis* can be treated with most of the anthelmintics active against *T. canis* (Bauer and Gey, 1995).

Order Spirurida

The order Spirurida contains two suborders: Camallanina and Spirurina. Members of both suborders require either an insect or a crustacean intermediate host for development to the infective stage. The definitive host acquires spirurid infection by ingesting infected arthropods or paratenic hosts

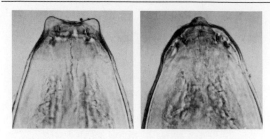

FIGURE 3-120 *Dracunculus insignis* from the axillary connective tissue of a dog. *Left*, The lateral aspect of the stomal end; *right*, the dorsoventral aspect (×150).

that have fed on such arthropods. The suborder Spirurina also includes the superfamily Filarioidea for which the intermediate host is a blood-feeding arthropod that becomes infected while taking its blood meal and that vectors the parasite when taking another blood meal.

Suborder Camallanina
Dracunculus

The suborder Camallanina contains only one genus of veterinary significance, *Dracunculus*, a parasite of the subcutaneous tissues of carnivorans and man (Figure 3-120). The female *Dracunculus* is very large (up to 120 cm), and the male is smaller (up to 40 mm). When a female has been fertilized, the anus and vulva atrophy, and a shallow ulcer forms in the host's skin at the location of the anterior end of the worm. When water wets this ulcer, the female projects her body and prolapses a length of uterus, which then bursts to discharge a horde of larvae (Figure 3-121). Then she retires to await the next wetting.

A primitive technique for extracting *Dracunculus* spp. consists of wetting the ulcer to lure the worm out far enough to grasp it and then winding it up on a stick a little at a time. The winding takes days because if the worm is broken in the process, a severe reaction may develop. Surgical excision is the modern treatment of choice. If they are ingested by a copepod of the genus *Cyclops*, the larvae discharged into the water develop to the infective third larval stage in about 3 weeks. The definitive host becomes infected by ingesting these *Cyclops* in the drinking water. Two species of *Dracunculus* are *Dracunculus insignis*, a parasite of the raccoons and other carnivorans, including the dog and cat in North America, and *Dracunculus medinensis*, a parasite of man in the Middle East and India. It appears that in the case of *D. insignis* that frogs can serve as paratenic hosts (Eberhard and Brandt, 1995), which increases the chance of dogs becoming infected by the ingestion of frogs.

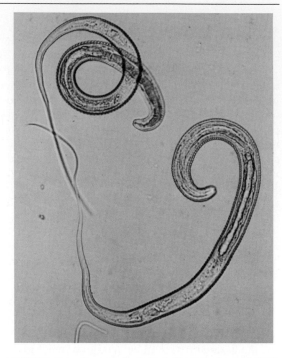

FIGURE 3-121   *Dracunculus insignis* first-stage larvae (×250).

Suborder Spirurina

The suborder Spirurina contains 10 superfamilies. Six are of interest as parasites of domestic animals. The stoma and surrounding structures of spirurins are distinctive. Comparison of specimens with the illustrations of this section should suffice for generic identification. The one exception here are the Filarioidea, which for the most part have very plain and simple stomas.

Superfamily Gnathostomatoidea

Gnathostoma spp. have a doughnut-shaped collar of spines surrounding their oral opening (Figure 3-122). Adult specimens are found in cystic nodules in the stomach walls of wild and domestic carnivores. Eggs are passed in the one- to two-cell stage and develop to the second larval stage in water. These larvae hatch and develop to the infective third stage only if ingested by copepods (*Cyclops*). A variety of amphibians, snakes, and fishes may serve as paratenic hosts to convey the gnathostome from the copepod to the definitive host. The migrations of gnathostome larvae in the liver and other organs of the definitive host are destructive. The cystic nodules housing adult *Gnathostoma spinigerum* may break open into the peritoneal cavity with fatal outcome. Larvae of *G. spinigerum* ingested by human beings tend to wander aimlessly without maturing.

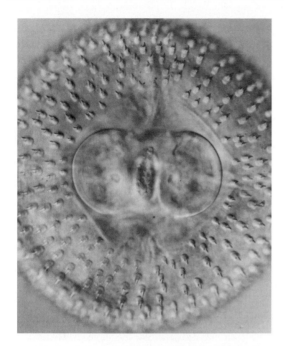

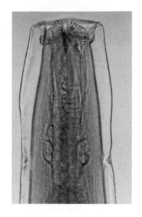
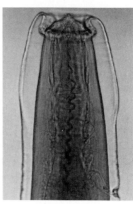

FIGURE 3-123 *Physaloptera* sp. *Left,* The dorsoventral aspect of the anterior extremity; *right,* the lateral aspect of the anterior extremity (×100).

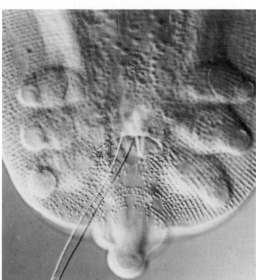

FIGURE 3-122 *Gnathostoma* stomal end *(upper)* and caudal extremity of the male *(lower)* (×140).

Superfamily Physalopteroidea

Physaloptera spp. are parasites of the stomach of carnivorans. The female worm lays thick-walled eggs that develop to the infective stage in various coprophagous beetles. The mouth is flanked by pseudolabia and surrounded by a cuticular collar (Figures 3-123 and 3-124).

The adult worms are white or pinkish in color and tend to live with the anterior end embedded in the mucosa. In the dog, the adult worms often are present also in the very anteriormost portion of the

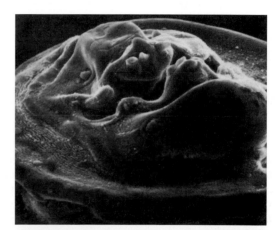

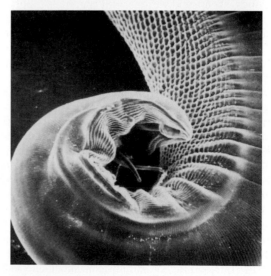

FIGURE 3-124 *Physaloptera* sp. stoma *(upper,* ×400) and caudal extremity of male *(lower,* ×80).

duodenum at the level of the gastric valve. Infections with these worms in dogs and cats often are associated with vomiting, and the adults are viewed often during endoscopy (Jergens and Greve, 1992). Treatment in dogs has been performed with fenbendazole at 50 mg/kg for 3 days (Jergens and Greve, 1992). Infected cats have been treated with ivermectin at 0.2 mg/kg (Gustafson, 1995) and with two doses of pyrantel pamoate at 5 mg/kg given 3 weeks apart (Santen et al, 1993). The recent summary of *Physaloptera* infections in 29 dogs and 6 cats in Iowa concludes with the recommendation that animals be given a trial course of pyrantel pamoate at 20 mg/kg that may be repeated if signs of vomiting do not cease (Campbell and Graham, 1999). These authors also suggest that the different anthelmintics used in their series of cases (fenbendazole, pyrantel pamoate, dichlorvos, and pyrantel pamoate, praziquantel, and febantel) all appeared efficacious, but some required elevated doses or longer treatment times that suggested for typical labeled use.

Superfamily Thelazioidea
Family Pneumospiruridae
Pneumospirurids are parasites of the lungs of wild carnivorans and appear occasionally in domestic dogs and cats. *Pneumospirura* and *Metathelazia* are representative genera.

Family Thelaziidae
Thelazia spp. (Figure 3-125) are parasites of the conjunctival and lacrimal sacs of domestic animals. North American species include *Thelazia lacrymalis* in horses, *Thelazia skrjabini* in cattle and horses, *Thelazia gulosa* in cattle, and *Thelazia californiensis* in dogs, sheep, and various wild mammals. Slightly less than half of the horses surveyed in Kentucky were found infected with *T. lacrymalis* (Lyons et al, 1986). Thelazia spp. apparently do little harm to cattle and horses in North America, but exceptional cases requiring treatment may arise.

The female *Thelazia* worm deposits thin-shelled eggs containing larvae that develop to the infective stage in the face fly, *Musca autumnalis*. The Oriental face fly, *Musca hervei*, serves as intermediate host of *Thelazia* spp. in Japanese cattle (Shinonaga et al, 1974).

TREATMENT. Doramectin at 0.2 mg/kg given either subcutaneously or intramuscularly has been approved for the treatment and control of *Thelazia* infections in cattle. A single dose of tetramisole subcutaneously at 12.5 to 15 mg/kg produced rapid clinical recovery in infected cattle. Levamisole at a dosage rate of 5 mg/kg administered subcutaneously or 1% aqueous solution as an eye lotion was also effective (Corba et al, 1969; Aruo, 1974; Vassiliades

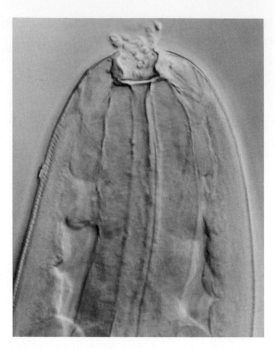

FIGURE 3-125 *Thelazia* sp. from the conjunctival sac of a horse (×365).

et al, 1975). *Thelazia* infections in dogs have been successfully treated by subcutaneous injections of 0.2 mg ivermectin per kilogram body weight (Rossi and Peruccio, 1989). Brooks et al (1983) successfully treated conjunctivitis in a Senegal parrot caused by *Thelazia* sp. by instilling one drop of a 0.125% demecarium bromide, a cholinesterase inhibitor, into the conjunctival sac and subsequently flushing three paralyzed worms with sterile saline solution.

Superfamily Spiruroidea
Gongylonema spp. (see Figure 5-68) are covered with wartlike cuticular bosses, especially near the anterior end, and can usually be found woven into a remarkably regular sinusoidal tract in the mucous membrane of the host's esophagus (*Gongylonema pulchrum*) or rumen (*Gongylonema verrucosum*) (Figure 3-126). Eggs containing first-stage larvae are passed on the host's feces and, if ingested by a dung beetle or a cockroach, develop to the infective stage in about a month. The definitive host becomes infected by ingesting the infected insect. *Gongylonema* spp. are usually harmless.

Spirocerca lupi is found in fibrous nodules in the wall of the esophagus or stomach (see Figures 5-118, 5-119, and 5-120). The very small (12 × 30 µm) egg contains a vermiform embryo when shed in the feces (see Figures 5-6 and 5-121). If ingested by a coprophagous beetle, this vermiform embryo develops into a larva capable of infecting dogs and a broad range of paratenic hosts, including lizards,

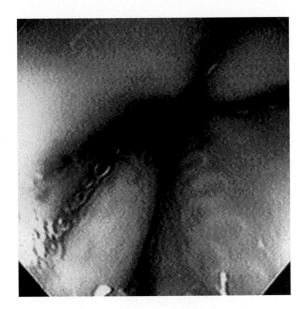

FIGURE 3-126 *Gongylonema* pulchrum. Sinusoidal worm under esophageal mucosa as viewed with an endoscope. (Photo courtesy Dr. Thomas Divers, College of Veterinary Medicine, Cornell University, Ithaca, New York.)

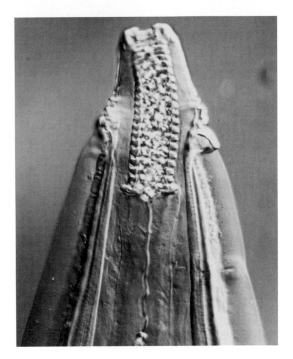

FIGURE 3-127 *Physocephalus sexalatus* (×168).

chickens, and mice. When infective larvae are ingested by a dog, they migrate in the adventitia of the visceral arteries and aorta to the walls of the esophagus and stomach. Some go astray and encyst in ectopic locations, but reproductive adults are normally found in cystic nodules that communicate with the lumen of the esophagus or stomach through fistulas. Dysphagia and vomiting, esophageal neoplasia, aortic aneurysm or rupture, and secondary pulmonary osteoarthropathy may be associated with chronic *S. lupi* infection.

Disophenol, 10 mg/kg, administered twice at an interval of 1 week was very effective against adult *S. lupi* (Seneviratna et al, 1966; Chhabra and Singh, 1972).

Other examples of spiruroids are *Ascarops* and *Physocephalus* spp. (Figure 3-127), parasites of swine, and *Streptopharagus* spp. (see Figure 5-68), parasites of primates.

Superfamily Habronematoidea

Draschia megastoma, Habronema muscae, and *Habronema microstoma* are parasites of the equine stomach, where the adult worms stay remarkably close to the margo plicatus. *D. megastoma* is about 13 mm long and has a funnel-shaped buccal cavity, whereas *Habronema* spp. are larger (22 to 25 mm) and have cylindrical buccal cavities (Figure 3-128). The left spicule of *H. muscae* is five times as long as the right one, whereas only a twofold disparity exists between the spicules of *H. microstoma*. *D. egastoma* excites the formation by the host of

fibrous nodules riddled with intercommunicating galleries filled with a creamy puslike material in which the worms live. *Habronema* spp. are not associated with nodules. Larvae hatch from the tiny eggs (see Figure 5-31) soon after they are laid. If ingested by maggots (*Musca domestica* for *D. megastoma* and *H. muscae*; *Stomoxys calcitrans* for *H. microstoma*), these develop to the infective third-stage larvae in a little more than a week.

The infective larvae migrate to the head of the fly and collect in the labium. When a fly alights on a warm, moist surface such as the muzzle, ocular conjunctiva, or cutaneous wounds of a horse, the

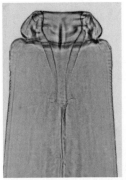
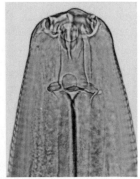

FIGURE 3-128 *Draschia megastoma* (*left,* ×150) and *Habronema muscae* (*right,* ×250).

larvae change hosts. Those larvae that are swallowed presumably complete their life histories, whereas those that enter wounds have probably reached an impasse. However, from a veterinary standpoint, these aberrant larvae are extremely important because of the granulomas they induce.

Although *Draschia* spp. and *Habronema* spp. are unimportant as stomach parasites, their larvae are responsible for persistent **cutaneous granulomas** called cutaneous habronemiasis and a variety of colloquial names ("swamp cancer," "bursatti," "summer sores," "esponja"). These granulomas develop in minor wounds and in areas of skin subjected to more or less continuous wetting. In pastured horses, the skin adjacent to the medial canthus of the eye may be drenched in tears stimulated by the presence of flies and also very attractive to them. Typical cutaneous habronemiasis lesions are characterized by an initial rapid production of granulation tissue that steadfastly refuses to resolve during fly season, by the subsequent appearance of caseocalcareous nodules in this granulation tissue, and by the presence of *Draschia* or *Habronema* larvae. Pruritus is intense, and secondary injury may result from the horse's efforts to find relief. Habronemic conjunctivitis usually assumes the form of an ulcerated nodule containing caseocalcareous foci and situated near the medial canthus. Such nodules tend to abrade the cornea and must be removed surgically to prevent or alleviate keratitis (Underwood, 1936; Rebhun et al, 1981).

TREATMENT AND CONTROL. Ivermectin is the treatment of choice for *Habronema* spp., and probably *Draschia* spp., adults. Ivermectin is also approved for the treatment of summer sores caused by larvae of *Habronema* spp. and *Draschia* spp. Other older products also can be used. Carbon disulfide, when administered with large amounts of 2% sodium bicarbonate, afforded excellent efficacy against *Draschia* spp. and *Habronema* spp. (Wright et al, 1931). Ronnel administered dosages of 100 mg/kg every 2 weeks until the lesions are healed, reportedly has been effective when combined with local treatment (Wheat, 1961). Intralesional injection of 2 to 3 ml of 10% solution of fenthion promotes healing of habronemic granulomas (Rossoff, 1974). The gritty masses on conjunctival membranes must be excised to prevent injury to the cornea.

Superfamily Filarioidea

The dog heartworm, *Dirofilaria immitis,* is probably the filarioid of most importance in veterinary medicine. The filarioids also include some of the most important nematode parasites of man in tropical climates. *Wuchereria bancrofti* and *Brugia malayi* cause the acute lymphangitis and chronic elephantiasis of bancroftian filariasis, and *Onchocerca volvulus* causes the ophthalmitis of "river blindness."

Filarioids tend to be rather long and thin white- to cream-colored worms. They are found typically in tissue spaces and body cavities, or sometimes within the vasculature or lymphatic system. They tend to be without marked cuticular ornamentation or lips and have almost no buccal capsule. Often the tail of the male has a spiral flexure. All filarioids are transmitted by bloodsucking insects in which vermiform embryos called **microfilariae** develop into infective third-stage larvae. The microfilariae either circulate in the blood of the definitive host (e.g., *Wuchereria, Brugia, Dirofilaria, Dipetalonema,* and *Setaria* spp.) or accumulate in the dermal connective tissues (e.g., *Onchocerca, Elaeophora* spp.). In either case, the microfilariae are ingested and the infective larvae deposited when the insect feeds on the definitive host.

Dirofilaria

D. immitis, the canine heartworm, is by far the most important filarioid parasite of domestic animals in North America. The dog and its close relatives are the natural hosts, but infection also occurs in cats (Calvert and Mandell, 1982; Dillon et al, 1982) and ferrets *(Mustela putorius furo).* As few as five adult *D. immitis* may prove lethal to a ferret (Campbell and Blair, 1978; Miller and Merton, 1982; Parrot et al, 1984; Moreland et al, 1986). Human infection is abortive and results in radiographic changes referred to as "coin lesions," which have been misinterpreted as representing neoplasia and can lead to unnecessary thoracic surgery.

Adult heartworms normally are found in the pulmonary arteries. In heavy infections worms may be found in the right heart. Worms probably are more common in the right heart at necropsy than in living dogs because of the reduced pressure that occurs as the blood stops flowing into the

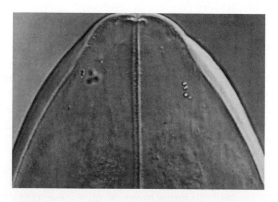

FIGURE 3-129 *Dirofilaria immitis,* stomal end (×150).

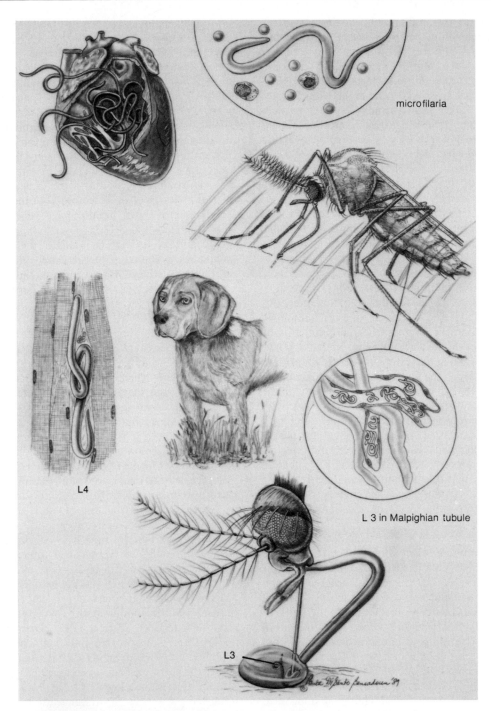

FIGURE 3-130 Life history of *Dirofilaria immitis*, the canine heartworm. Adult heartworms may survive and produce microfilariae for as long as 5 years. Microfilariae circulate in the blood, where they may be ingested by a feeding mosquito. About half of the species of North American mosquitoes are possible intermediate hosts, but significant vector roles have been demonstrated for only a few. Larval development occurs in the malpighian tubules, after which infective third-stage larvae migrate to the salivary glands of the mosquito. The third-stage larvae enter the bite wound when the mosquito feeds on a dog. The molt from third-stage larva to fourth-stage larva occurs within 3 days after the bite of the infecting mosquito. Fourth-stage larvae remain in the connective tissues for several months, with the molt from fourth-stage larva to young adult occurring 2 to 3 months after infection. After the final molt, the immature adults (fifth stage) migrate to the pulmonary arteries, apparently by way of the venous circulation. After reaching the right side of the heart, the young adults mature and start producing microfilariae at 6 to 9 months after infection.

pulmonary arteries. When defunct, the worms are carried deeper into the lungs where they occlude the pulmonary arterial branches and produce infarcts. The faces of these large (up to 30 cm long) white worms are very plain indeed (Figure 3-129). Endemic areas exist in all parts of the United States (Rothstein, 1963). Heartworm infection is particularly common along the Atlantic and Gulf Coasts where salt marsh mosquitoes are prevalent, and in some localities half the dogs examined will be found infected. There is also an increased prevalence along the course of the Mississippi River and its major tributaries such as the Ohio and the Missouri Rivers. A lower prevalence is encountered in the Midwest and north-central states. Even Minnesota contains endemic areas.

LIFE HISTORY. The life history, as outlined in Figure 3-130, may involve several species of mosquitoes as intermediate hosts. Today, mosquito-borne diseases such as malaria and filarial infections are popularly viewed as tropical diseases, but not too long ago malaria accompanied every summer in the United States. Malaria disappeared when the population density of suitable mosquitoes fell below the level necessary for transmission of the malarial plasmodia. Reduction in mosquitoes came with the drainage of swamps for agricultural purposes, with the construction of roads, and to some extent with intentional efforts at mosquito abatement. Heartworm manages to remain endemic and even to spread to regions where malaria has disappeared, possibly because this parasite is less discriminating in its choice of mosquito hosts. In any case, only when mosquito populations are sufficiently reduced will heartworm disappear.

The life cycle of *D. immitis* is initiated when the dog is bitten by an infected mosquito. The cycle is summarized in detail in the excellent review of Abraham (1988). The third-stage larva enters the bite wound and takes up residence in the skin. The third-stage larva that enters the bite wound molts to a fourth-stage larva within 3 days after infection. The young fourth-stage larvae are about 1.5 mm long at this time. The fourth-stage larvae reside in the subcutaneous connective tissues and muscles of the abdomen or thorax for the next 2 to 3 months after infection. Orihel (1961) reported that the molt from the fourth-stage to adult occurred 60 to 70 days after infection. Lichtenfels et al (1985) reported that the molt occurred at 50 to 58 days after infection.

The worms are 12 to 15 mm long when they molt to become juvenile adults. The worms enter the pulmonary arteries and heart after being in the dog for 70 days (Kotani and Powers, 1982). When worms first reach the right heart and pulmonary arteries, they are 20 to 40 mm (about an inch) long (Orihel, 1961). By 85 to 120 days after infection

they reach lengths of up to 3.2 to 11 cm (Kume and Itagaki, 1955).

Fertilized females appear by 120 days after infection of the dog, and they contain fully developed microfilariae within the sixth month after infection (Orihel, 1961). Microfilariae typically are not found in the peripheral blood for several more weeks. Thus the prepatent period (i.e., the period between the infection and the first appearance of microfilariae in the blood) is between 6 and 9 months' long. Once worms begin to produce microfilariae, they can continue to do this for over 5 years. The microfilariae circulate in the blood of the dog and are capable of living for up to $2\frac{1}{2}$ years (Underwood and Harwood, 1939).

Mosquitoes are infected when they bite an infected dog. The microfilariae, after remaining in the midgut of the mosquito for a day, make their way to the malpighian tubules where they penetrate the cytoplasm of the primary cells. Under optimal conditions, the larvae reenter the lumen of the malpighian tubules about 5 days after infection and molt to second-stage larvae about 10 days after infection and to third-stage larvae by 13 days after infection. The infective third-stage larvae then migrate through the body of the mosquito to the cephalic spaces in the head and proboscis where they await the chance of gaining entry into a new canine host.

The 6- to 7-month prepatent period is free of any evidence of infection, and the developing and migrating worms cause no disturbance. The patent period, when microfilariae (see Figure 5-40) may be detected in the circulating blood, is the time of clinical illness. In the conventional view, the physiological burden imposed on the host is attributed in part to the physical obstruction of vessels, heart chambers, and valves by the adult worms and in part to the development of a progressive pulmonary endarteritis and obstructive fibrosis leading to pulmonary hypertension and right heart failure (Adcock, 1961). There is also a remarkable villous proliferation that occurs on the endothelium of the pulmonary arteries that grossly causes the surface of the vessel to appear as though it is covered with a lawn of villi (Figure 3-131). Repeated embolisms of the finer arterial branches by defunct adults with infarction and inflammatory response eventually lead to permanent damage of the vascular bed. However, obstruction of capillaries by microfilariae may also play a part in the pathogenesis of heartworm disease.

Jackson et al (1966) found that dogs with no signs of disease harbored an average of 25 worms, and that about 50 worms were associated with moderate-to-severe heartworm disease. In dogs with signs of acute hepatic failure, about 100

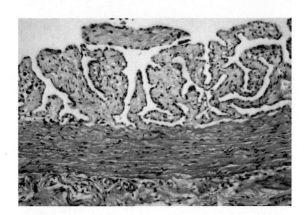

FIGURE 3-131 Histological section (hematoxylin and eosin [H&E] stained) of the pulmonary artery of a dog infected with *Dirofilaria immitis* showing the villous proliferation present on the endothelium (×40).

worms were concentrated in the venae cavae and right atrium. Dogs with typical heartworm disease fatigue easily, cough, and appear unthrifty. Decompensation of the right heart leads to chronic venous congestion, with hepatic cirrhosis and ascites. Pulmonary embolism precipitates acute episodes of respiratory distress during which blood and worms from ruptured vessels may be coughed up. Postcaval occlusion causes sudden collapse followed by death within a few days from acute hepatic insufficiency. A surgical procedure has been devised for relieving the caval occlusion by way of a jugular vein (Jackson et al, 1962, 1977).

DIAGNOSIS. The monthly preventatives, ivermectin and milbemycin oxime, are capable of suppressing circulating microfilariae in dogs that have patent heartworm infections (Bowman et al, 1992). It seems that the effect is on the microfilariae and on the reproductive systems of the adult worms. Thus the American Heartworm Society (*AHS* Bulletin, 1993) has developed recommendations for the diagnosis of heartworm infection that differ depending on whether the screening is for primary diagnosis (before a dog is placed on a chemoprophylactic regimen) or for the retesting of a dog that is already receiving a preventative (i.e., diethylcarbamazine or a macrolide [ivermectin, milbemycin oxime, selamectin, or moxidectin]).

In the case of primary screening, if microfilariae are found in the blood of a North American dog, it can be assumed that they belong to either *D. immitis* or *Dipetalonema reconditum*. (Differentiation of microfilariae of these two species is discussed in Chapter 5.) In the normal course of events, microfilariae of *D. immitis* first appear in the circulation about 6 months after exposure of the dog to the bites of infected mosquitoes. Thus during the rather long prepatent period, no

microfilariae can be detected in blood samples from an infected dog. Microfilariae also fail to appear if the adult worms are all of one sex or have been sterilized by medications administered to the dog, or if microfilariae are being produced only to be destroyed by host immune responses (Rawlings et al, 1982). These so-called occult cases represent a significant proportion of naturally occurring infections with *D. immitis* (Grieve et al, 1986), and diagnosis of such cases must rest on radiographical and serological evidence.

Radiography is valuable when characteristic radiographic changes are present, but negative findings do not rule out the possibility of a low level of infection. There are currently numerous tests marketed for the detection of antigen from adult worms in serum, plasma, or whole blood. These tests should be performed in compliance with the manufacturer's instructions. It should be remembered that false negative tests can occur when dealing with prepatent infections and small numbers of female worms. There also appear to be dogs that may have circulating microfilariae, perhaps very high numbers, but no antigenemia as detected by the different tests. False positive results will be most likely when dealing with large percentages of truly negative dogs.

For dogs receiving prophylaxis, the choices are different depending on whether the dog is receiving the daily product, diethylcarbamazine, or an avermectin in the form of a monthly product, ivermectin, milbemycin oxime, and selamectin, or one designed to be administered every 6 months, moxidectin. Testing for microfilariae is mandatory before dogs are restarted on diethylcarbamazine prophylaxis because of the high microfilaricidal nature of this compound, which can cause serious side effects if dogs with patent infections are treated. In the case of ivermectin and milbemycin oxime, it is unlikely that a dog receiving either of these products will develop a patent infection. Thus the test of choice when retesting these dogs is an antigen test.

It must be remembered when performing an antigen test on a large population of dogs without infection (by definition, all dogs on preventive regimens should be without infection) that there are going to be false-positive results no matter how good the test is (sensitivity and specificity of 99.9% translate to one false-positive test in every 1000 tests performed). Thus if a dog on a preventive regimen tests positive for heartworm, it should be retested and carefully examined for any clinical signs of infection before the initiation of adulticide therapy.

How often dogs on a preventive program are tested for heartworm infection depends in part on the program administered to each dog. If the dog is receiving a daily product for only part of the year, it must be retested before the initiation of therapy each year. If the dog is receiving a monthly product for only a portion of the year, it probably should also be tested once each year or every other year. In both of these cases, it must be remembered that the antigen tests typically will not be optimal for detecting infection until 4 or 5 months after the infection was initiated. Thus testing must occur some time after the transmission season has ended.

If a dog is on a preventive regimen the year around, testing can be performed yearly or more infrequently. In cases of year-round prevention, there is no reason why testing cannot be performed any time during the year, and in these cases and with puppies that started year-round prevention soon after birth, heartworm testing can just become part of the annual examination. It must be remembered that macrolide products are anthelmintics, and there is always the potential of resistance. Because of the relatively long life cycle of *D. immitis*, it seems unlikely that resistance will occur, but the threat remains. Only by the regular checking of dogs on a preventive program can a vigilance be guaranteed that would identify and prevent the spread of a resistant form of the parasite if one ever did appear.

TREATMENT. Different anthelmintics are used to attack three different parasitic stages of *D. immitis*: microfilariae in the circulating blood, larvae migrating through the tissues on their way to the heart, and adult worms in pulmonary arteries and the right heart. Treatment of a dog with patent heartworm infection consists of first removing the adult parasites with arsenamide and then eliminating the circulating microfilariae with ivermectin or milbemycin oxime later. Drugs targeting the larvae migrating through the tissues are used for prevention.

Melarsomine dihydrochloride has been approved for the treatment of dogs infected with adult heartworms. In dogs infected with mild-to-moderate clinical signs, the treatment consists of two intramuscular injections (2.5 mg/kg) given 24 hours apart. This treatment can be repeated 4 months later if necessary. Dogs with more severe disease should receive a single intramuscular injection of (2.5 mg/kg) followed 1 month later by two such treatments 24 hours apart. Melarsomine dihydrochloride treatment seems to be more effective than thiacetarsemide without any increase in the severity of posttreatment hypertension and thromboembolism (Rawlings et al, 1993).

Thiacetarsamide (arsenamide), the other approved adulticide, is administered intravenously at the rate of 0.1 ml of 1% buffered solution per pound of body weight (e.g., 2.2 mg/kg) twice a day for 2 days to remove adult heartworms. Some veterinarians think that the therapeutic efficiency is more consistent if this regimen is extended to 3 days. The anthelmintic efficiency of arsenamide was observed to vary with the duration of infection. Efficiency was highest at 2 months, lowest at 4 months, and thereafter gradually increased (Blair et al, 1982). These observations suggest that in the case of poor response to arsenamide therapy it might be wise to wait a few months before trying again.

After arsenical therapy has been used, heartworms die slowly over a period of days or weeks and are carried by the pulmonary arteries to the lungs, where they lodge and obstruct the circulation temporarily. Eventually, the dead worms are removed by phagocytosis. Probably, if the worms were killed rapidly and simultaneously, treatment would prove more lethal than the heartworms. However, even with the slow kill, the lungs are gravely insulted during the 4 to 6 weeks after arsenical therapy, and the dog must not be subjected to stress during this period. Occasionally a dog vomits or has fever and respiratory distress after treatment. If these reactions are more than transitory, arsenical medication should be discontinued and supportive therapy, administration of steroids, and enforced rest initiated.

For the removal of microfilariae from the circulation after adulticide therapy, dogs can be given either a microfilaricidal dose of ivermectin (0.05 mg/kg body weight), ivermectin at the preventative dose of 0.006 mg/kg, or milbemycin oxime at the prophylactic dose of 0.5 mg/kg body weight. These products are not "labeled" for this use, but because of the lack of drugs approved for the removal of circulating microfilariae, the American Heartworm Society has included these treatments in its recommendations.

Ivermectin displays remarkable activity against migrating larvae up to 30 days after infection but no significant activity against adult *D. immitis* (Blair et al, 1983).

PREVENTION. Prevention of heartworm infection currently involves the daily administration of diethylcarbamazine, monthly administration of a macrolide, or the every-6-month injection of a slow-release macrolide (moxidectin) to all dogs exposed to attacks of infectious mosquitoes. Prevention of canine heartworm infection can be achieved by daily oral administration of diethylcarbamazine at 6.6 mg/kg from the beginning until 2 months after the end of mosquito activity (Kume et al, 1962a, 1962b, 1964, 1967). Diethylcarbamazine must not be administered to dogs with microfilaremia because severe or fatal shocklike reactions may ensue (Levine and Diamond, 1967; Kume, 1970). Dogs with patent heartworm infections must therefore be treated for the underlying infection and then undergo the ivermectin or milbemycin oxime therapeutic sequence outlined earlier before being placed on the diethylcarbamazine prophylactic regimen. Ivermectin (Heartgard) tablets are administered at a minimum dosage of 0.006 mg/kg to dogs once per month starting 1 month from first exposure to mosquitoes and ending within 1 month after last exposure. Milbemycin oxime tablets (Interceptor) are administered at a minimum dosage of 0.5 mg/kg to dogs once a month. Selamectin (Revolution) is applied to dogs topically each month at a minimum dosage of 6.0 mg/kg. The injectable form of moxidectin (ProHeart6) is given as an injection at a dose of 0.17 mg/kg. Collies genetically predisposed to macrolide sensitivity may have adverse neurological reactions to 10 times the approved preventive dose of these macrolides but tolerate the much lower prophylactic doses without any negative effect.

Oxibendazole combined with diethylcarbamazine citrate in the daily preventive Filaribits-Plus will also control intestinal helminth infections with *Ancylostoma* spp., *T. canis, Trichuris vulpis,* and probably *U. stenocephala* and *T. leonina.* Milbemycin oxime (Interceptor) at the dose chosen for heartworm prevention will also control intestinal helminth infections with *Ancylostoma* spp., *T. canis, T. leonina,* and *T. vulpis.* Ivermectin in its presentation with pyrantel pamoate (Heartgard Plus) will also control intestinal helminth infections with *Ancylostoma* spp., *U. stenocephala, T. canis,* and *T. leonina.* Milbemycin oxime has also now been combined with lufenuron (Sentinel), and this product will prevent heartworm infection, control most intestinal helminth infections, and provide the client and pet with flea control. Selamectin (Revolution) will also treat and control flea infestations and ear mites, and can be used to treat sarcoptic mange at the same dosage level. The injectable form of moxidectin (ProHeart6) will also treat any existing larval or adult infections with *A. caninum.*

A commonly asked question is whether dogs should undergo a heartworm prevention program year-round, for 6 months, or for even shorter periods in regions where the potential transmission cycle may be less than 6 months. Dr. Slocombe and colleagues (Slocombe et al, 1995) and Drs. Knight and Lok (1995) have presented isolines for the mean start and end dates of heartworm transmission in Canada and the United States. These isolines are based on a model that includes the average life of a mosquito, the times when mosquitoes are likely to take their first and last blood meals each year, the amount of time required at different temperatures for an ingested microfilaria to become an infectious third-stage larva, and temperature data collected at different national weather collection stations. Thus by examination of the maps presented, the period of transmission for the locale in which they practice can be determined. The model proposed by Knight and Lok (1995) indicates that there are probably no parts of the continental United States where transmission occurs throughout the year. Thus treatment might be given for 3 months in parts of Canada and 10 months in parts of Florida with different starting and stopping dates in various locations from south to north. This model has received support recently by work done in Florida and Louisiana where mosquitoes (a total of 109,597) were examined year-round with a polymerase chain reaction assay for *D. immitis* DNA (Watts et al, 2001). No infected mosquito heads were detected in Gainesville, Florida, or Baton Rouge, Louisiana, in the months of December, January, February, and March.

The practical advantage of applying this model is a reduction in the prescriptions for unnecessary preventive treatment in areas where it is not required. If the model is to be applied, other factors must be taken into consideration. First, there are likely to be microclimatic fluctuations (large bodies of water that stabilize temperatures, decaying manure or vegetable matter that raises temperatures, heated industrial effluents, or heat-absorbing natural and artificial surfaces) that allow mosquitoes to feed longer, perhaps much longer, in certain areas within given isolines. Second, it is likely that many dogs will travel with their owners, with the effect that isolines will be crossed by many pets during the course of a year. It also is unlikely that most patients will see their veterinarian often enough for the discovery and initiation of preventive therapy to work in all cases. Third, the availability of products that control infections or have been combined with anthelmintics active against intestinal helminths complicates the desire to stop therapy for the pets of some clients during periods when there may be no heartworm transmission. *T. canis, T. leonina,* and *T. vulpis* are all capable of being transmitted even in the coldest months of the year if soil containing infective eggs is disturbed, and *A. caninum* larvae in sequestered sites in the body are known to migrate periodically back to the intestine where they develop. Finally, the addition of a flea-control product to the heartworm preventive adds another reason for considering year-round prevention. In a household, it is highly possible that the temperatures will remain such that fleas can continue to cycle throughout the year, even if they are worse in the summer.

With the currently available products, there is no good reason why any dog under the care of a veterinarian should become infected with heartworm.

Thus it is imperative that the practitioner carefully consider the area in which the practice is located, the individual client, and the stated and suspected behavior of the pet when formulating a plan for each individual going on a preventive program. However, in the design of specific programs for individuals, it is important to remember that clients do converse with each other, and difficulties will arise when all clients and pets are not treated equally if the reasons behind the specific recommendations are not made very clear.

Feline Heartworm

Infection with *D. immitis* in cats has received increasing awareness, and in 1995 the American Heartworm Society published *Guidelines for the Diagnosis, Treatment, and Prevention of Heartworm (Dirofilaria immitis) Infection in Cats*, which can be obtained from the American Heartworm Society, P.O. Box 667, Batavia, IL 60510–0667. The cat differs from the dog in several major respects relative to heartworm infection. First, cats tend to harbor very few adult worms and to remain amicrofilaremic. Thus examination of blood with concentration methods usually is not a reliable detection method, and there may not be sufficient circulating antigen for detection by the different antigen detection assays. Heska Corporation (Fort Collins, Colorado) has developed antibody testing methods that can be used as aids in making a diagnosis in a potentially infected cat. Second, it seems that cats have heartworms more commonly in ectopic sites and fall victims to sudden death as a result of aberrantly migrating heartworms. Third, because cats often have very few worms, adulticide therapy in cats usually is reserved for those cases in stable condition that nevertheless continue to have clinical signs not controlled by empirical therapy. Fourth, thiacetarsamide now is considered to be the treatment of choice for infected cats. There is now a heartworm preventive available for cats that contains ivermectin (Heartgard for cats). This product prevents feline heartworm infections and also controls infections with *Ancylostoma* spp. in the cat. Also, selamectin (Revolution) has been approved for preventing heartworm infections in cats, and this product will also treat and control flea and treat ear mites, and will treat and control intestinal infections with *T. cati* and *A. caninum*.

Setaria

Setaria labiatopapillosa (Figure 3-132) and *Setaria equina* (Figure 3-133) are large white parasites of the serous membranes of cattle and horses, respectively. Microfilariae of *Setaria* spp. show up on blood smears, and the adult parasites are likely to be encountered during abdominal

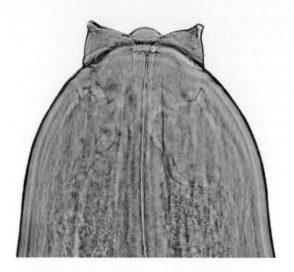

FIGURE 3-132 *Setaria labiatopapillosa*, stomal end (×225).

surgery or on the killing floor or necropsy table. Migrating *Setaria* larvae occasionally invade the central nervous system and cause serious neurological disease, especially when they find themselves in other than their normal host species.

Actively motile *Setaria* spp. adult worms are occasionally observed in the anterior eye chamber of horses. Jemelka (1976) described surgical removal of a 4.38-cm-long *Setaria digitata* adult from the anterior eye chamber of a horse suffering from corneal opacity and hypopion.

Onchocerca

Onchocerca spp. adults, although large, are likely to escape notice because they are intricately woven into the deep connective tissues. Once found, they

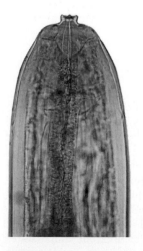
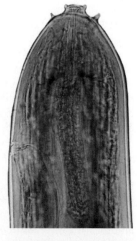

FIGURE 3-133 *Setaria equina*, dorsoventral *(left)* and lateral *(right)* aspects of the stomal end (×50).

are virtually impossible to isolate intact, so specimen bottles tend to contain many fragments of midsection and very few ends.

Onchocerca cervicalis adults are found in the nuchal ligament of the horse, and the microfilariae are widely distributed in the dermis and other connective tissues including those of the ocular conjunctivae. In a random survey of pastured horses in Tompkins County, New York, 8 of 12 horses yielded from 1 to 3000 *O. cervicalis* microfilariae per biopsy specimen, a piece of skin weighing about 15 mg (Georgi, 1976b). **Microfilarial pityriasis**, summer mange, equine dhobie itch, and plica polonica are colloquial names for an intensely pruritic dermatitis conventionally ascribed to microfilariae of *O. cervicalis*.

In North American cattle, *Onchocerca gutterosa* adults are found in connective tissues about the nuchal ligament, and *Onchocerca lienalis* are found in the connective tissue between the spleen and rumen. Both species also may be found in other connective tissue locations on occasion. Microfilariae of both species are found in the dermis. The intermediate hosts of bovine *Onchocerca* species have not been identified with certainty but may involve simuliid or heleid (ceratopogonid) flies.

A species of *Onchocerca* found in African cattle, *Onchocerca ochengi,* like many other filariid nematodes is host to an enosymbiotic bacterium of the genus *Wohlbachia*. These bacteria are also present in *D. immitis, Onchocerca volvulus,* and in the species causing lymphatic filariasis in humans. The bacterium is passed transovarially from the female to her offspring (Kozek, 1977). It has been suspected that if these endosymbionts are required for survival or if their breakdown products were toxic for the nematode host that they might be used as targets for chemotherapy. Recent work with the *O. ochengi* model in cattle has shown that treating cattle with ocytetracycline cleared the cattle of their infections with adult worms in nodules, which suggests that similar strategies may be useful in other systems (Langworthy et al, 2000).

MICROFILARICIDAL TREATMENT. Herd and Donham (1983) successfully treated 40 horses with dermatitis, alopecia, and pruritus in association with microfilariae of *O. cervicalis* with a single intramuscular injection of 0.2 mg ivermectin per kilogram body weight. Twenty-four hours after medication, the ventral abdomens of four of the horses became edematous. However, this reaction to dead microfilariae subsided over the next few days, and marked clinical improvement followed in all horses 2 to 3 weeks after treatment. Moxidectin at 0.3 to 0.5 mg/kg also will eliminate these microfilariae from the blood of infected horses (Monahan et al, 1995).

Parafilaria

"Summer Bleeding." This condition is caused by *Parafilaria multipapillosa* in horses and *Parafilaria bovicola* in cattle. These parasites live in the subcutaneous and intermuscular connective tissues and when sexually mature, produce crops of pea-sized nodules that bleed through a tiny pore. The blood escapes in fine drops, runs off in streaks along the hairs, and dries in brown crusts. Eggs and microfilariae of *Parafilaria* spp. may be demonstrated in this material but never in samples from the circulation. Active bleeding occurs only during daylight hours and especially when horses are exposed to direct sunshine. Baumann (1946) reported that bleeding in affected horses would, as a rule, immediately stop when they were brought into the stable, only to start again when led back out into the sunshine. He rarely observed bleeding during cool weather. The activity of the lesions observed by Baumann suggests an adaptation on the part of *Parafilaria* spp. to the habits of flies that feed on blood; they are active in warm weather and avoid shade. It has been shown that *P. multipapillosa* develops in the fat body of *Haematobia atripalpis* (Gnedina and Osipov, 1960).

P. bovicola causes dermal bleeding and subcutaneous bruiselike lesions in cattle in the Philippines, India, Tunisia, Morocco, the former Soviet Union, Rwanda, Burundi, Romania, Bulgaria, South Africa, and Sweden (Bech-Nielsen et al, 1982). The subcutaneous lesions result in substantial trim losses at slaughter. In South Africa, three vectors have been identified: *Musca lusoria, Musca fasciata,* and a third as yet undescribed species. Transmission probably occurs there throughout the year (Nevill, 1975, 1985). These dung-breeding *Musca* spp. ingest the first-stage larvae in the bloody discharge from skin perforations made by the adult *P. bovicola* female worms lying in the subcutaneous tissues. The larvae develop to the infective third stage in the body of the fly and are probably deposited in the eyes of cattle when the infected fly feeds on the lacrimal secretions (Nevill, 1975).

Dipetalonema

Adult specimens of *Dipetalonema* spp. are most likely to be encountered as parasites of the peritoneal cavity of monkeys, in which they are very common (Figure 3-134).

The canine parasite *Dipetalonema reconditum* has, as its species name suggests, been viewed by few human beings because it is small, usually few in number, and lies inconspicuously in the connective tissues. The microfilariae, on the other hand, are rather commonly seen (see Figure 5-40) and easy to confuse with those of *D. immitis*. *D. reconditum* is nonpathogenic to dogs. Its clinical importance

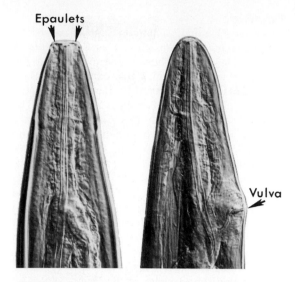

Epaulets

Vulva

FIGURE 3-134 *Dipetalonema* sp. from the peritoneal cavity of a monkey. *Left*, The dorsoventral aspect of the stomal end; *right*, the lateral aspect of the stomal end (×110).

attaches only to confusion of its microfilariae with those of *D. immitis* (Lindeman et al, 1983).

LIFE HISTORY. *D. reconditum* develops to the infective stage in the flea *Ctenocephalides felis* and in the amblyceran louse *Heterodoxus spiniger.* Microfilariae taken in with the blood meal develop into infective third-stage larvae in 7 to 14 days. When injected into a dog, these third-stage larvae develop into adult worms in 2 to 3 months (Farnell and Faulkner, 1978; Lindemann and McCall, 1984).

DIAGNOSIS. The small adults of *D. reconditum* cause no pathological changes to betray their presence, but may be demonstrated in a sufficiently lean cadaver by scanning the loose subcutaneous fascia of the limbs and back with a stereoscopic microscope (Nelson, 1962). About 90% of the adults are located in subcutaneous tissues, but a small percentage can be found in the peritoneal cavity (Mello et al, 1994). The microfilariae circulate in the blood, usually at low densities. However, substantial microfilaremias are occasionally observed. It is not safe to assume that because many microfilariae are present, it must necessarily follow that their parents are heartworms. The microfilariae of *D. reconditum* are distinguished from those of *D. immitis* by the more slender body, lack of taper at the anterior extremity, and presence of a very much larger **cephalic hook** in the former species. (Differentiation of these two species of microfilaria is considered in detail in Chapter 5.)

Patton and Faulkner (1992) found that the microfilariae in about 50% of 805 microfilarial-positive dogs in eastern Tennessee were the microfilariae of *D. reconditum*, and these authors

warn practitioners concerning the need of making an accurate diagnosis before initiating heartworm adulticide therapy. Most of the antigen detection tests used for diagnosing *D. immitis* infections are capable of distinguishing between infections with these two parasites.

Elaeophora

Microfilariae of *Elaeophora schneideri,* the arterial worm of deer, elk, and domestic sheep, produce patches of moist, exudative dermatitis with crust formation on the polls and faces of sheep sent to summer range above 6000 feet (1828 m) in New Mexico, Arizona, and Colorado. Adults up to 120 mm long are found in the carotid, iliac, and mesenteric arteries. Tabanids are cyclodevelopmental hosts.

Stephanofilaria

Adults and microfilariae of *Stephanofilaria stilesi,* a very small (less than 6 mm long) filariid, are found in dermatitic lesions on the ventral abdomen of cattle. The infective larvae of *S. stilesi* develop in the horn fly *Haematobia irritans.*

In India, *Stephanofilaria assamensis* causes a serious dermatitis called *humpsore* in cattle *(Bos indicus).* Lesions may occur on other parts of the body, but the major sites are the hump, neck, and legs. Pal et al (1989) reported recovery in 100 cases of humpsore within 10 to 20 days after treatment with diethylcarbamazine citrate, either as an ointment or as a 10% injectable solution. Both medications were compounded by the authors, and their report should be consulted for details. Ten milliliters of the injectable solution was infiltrated subcutaneously all around the wound, with treatment repeated on the fifth day. The diethylcarbamazine ointment was applied once daily until the wound healed.

Order Enoplida
Superfamily Dioctophymatoidea

Dioctophyme

Dioctophyme renale, the "giant kidney worm" of carnivorans, swine, and sometimes man, is one of the largest species of nematodes (Figure 3-135). Mink are the principal definitive hosts. The female *D. renale,* which may reach 1 m in length and 1 cm in diameter, produces brownish, thick-shelled eggs (68 × 44 μm) with bipolar plugs. Males are somewhat smaller (less than 400 mm) and have a terminal bell-shaped copulatory bursa and one spicule. The eggs are passed in the urine in the one- or two-cell stage and develop, in water, to the first larval stage in a month or longer. Larvated eggs are infective to oligochaete annelid worms in which they develop to the infective third larval stage. If infected oligochaetes are ingested by fish or frogs, the larvae invade the tissues of these paratenic hosts but do not undergo development. However, if the infected oligochaete (or paratenic host) is ingested by a dog, the *D. renale* larvae mature and complete the cycle (Karmanova, 1968). In the dog, *D. renale* may be found in the pelvis of the right kidney or free in the abdominal cavity. The latter type of infection is nonpatent.

Superfamily Trichinelloidea

The superfamily Trichuroidea contains some very common parasites of domestic animals. Members of this superfamily are distinguished by their **stichosome esophagus,** which consists of a capillary tube surrounded by the bodies of a single-file column of gland cells called **stichocytes** (Figure 3-136). There are five genera of interest: *Trichinella, Trichuris, Capillaria, Trichosomoides,* and *Anatrichosoma*.

Trichinella

IDENTIFICATION. The tiny adults of *Trichinella spiralis* are found embedded in the mucosa of the small intestine of swine, carnivorans, and man. The male is 1.4 to 1.6 mm long, lacks spicule or spicular sheath, and presents two small knobs over the cloaca. The female is 3 to 4 mm long with vulva and anus terminal in the midesophageal region. She deposits **prelarvae** directly into the host's intestinal mucosa (Figure 3-137). Males of other trichuroid genera have a single spicule or at least a spicular sheath, which is often spinate, and the females lay eggs with bipolar plugs (see Figures 5-9, 5-28, and 5-32).

LIFE HISTORY. Predation has provided an efficient channel for the evolutionary development of many parasites. In most instances, the larval parasite lies encysted in the tissues of the prey, and the

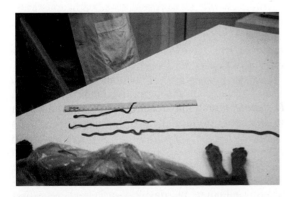

FIGURE 3-135 Three specimens of *Dictyphyme renale* recovered at necropsy from the abdominal cavity of a dog in Brazil. The ruler in the figure is 30 cm long. (Courtesy Dr. Suzanne Wolfson.)

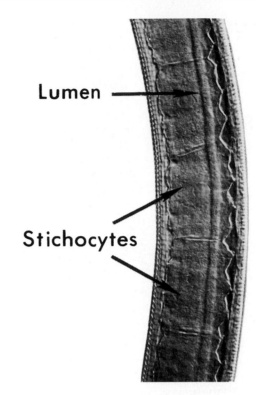

Lumen

Stichocytes

FIGURE 3-136 A portion of the stichosome esophagus of *Trichuris giraffae* (×168).

reproductive adults inhabit the alimentary tract of the predator. Thus in most systems, the predator becomes infected by eating the prey, and the prey becomes infected by ingesting eggs passed in the feces of the predator. However, in the unique life history of *Trichinella spiralis*, both adult and larval stages occur in sequence in the same host, the tiny adults lying among the villi of the small intestine and the larvae curled up in cysts in the striated muscle.

First-stage larvae of *T. spiralis,* liberated from their cysts by digestive enzymes of the host, invade the intestinal mucosa. Both sexes reach maturity about 2 days after the infected meat is eaten. The male dies after copulation. At 5 days after infection, the viviparous females are giving birth to prelarvae (Figure 3-138), which enter the lymphatics and later the bloodstream to be transported to the muscles (Ali Kahn, 1966). After these prelarvae invade striated muscle cells, they at first lie parallel to the long axes of the fibers and are quite easily overlooked. After 2 or 3 weeks they have developed into first-stage larvae and roll up in spirals, or like pretzels become enveloped in cysts and are then infective (Figures 3-139, 5-59, and 5-125). Old cysts containing defunct larvae calcify.

The intestinal (adult) phase of *T. spiralis* infection varies in duration from a little more than a week in a dog to 3 or 4 months in man. Immunosuppressant

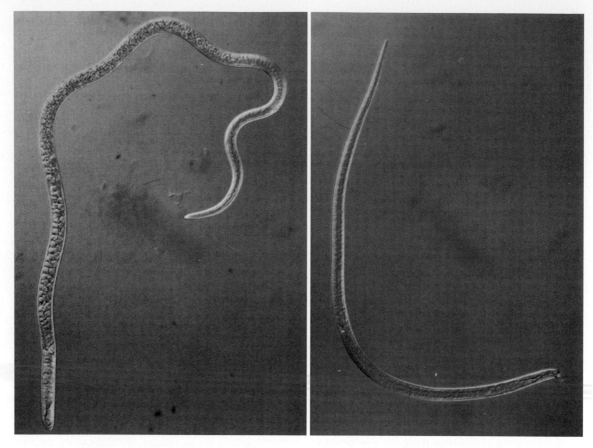

FIGURE 3-137   *Trichinella spiralis* adult female *(left)* and male *(right)* from the small intestine of an experimentally infected rat (×100).
(Specimens courtesy Dr. Judy Appleton.)

therapy, often instituted to ameliorate the tissue reaction to invading larvae, may prolong the lives of the adult female worms. Fortunately, these are accessible to anthelmintic attack. Almost all mammals can be experimentally infected with *T. spiralis*, but carnivores and omnivores are more likely to become naturally infected. Infection occurs through predation, cannibalism, and carrion feeding. The larvae encysted in muscles are exceptionally resistant to external conditions, including extreme putrefaction. Madsen (1976) considered that *T. spiralis* larvae in the decomposing carcass represent a free-living stage in a special biotope whose function is analogous to that of the species-dispersing, free-living eggs and larvae of other nematodes. Madsen attached paramount importance to the rotting carcass of carnivores in the epidemiology of *T. spiralis*.

IMPORTANCE. Human **trichinosis** usually results from eating raw or undercooked pork, bear, or seal. Properly cooked trichinae are quite harmless, but a sojourn in the oven does not guarantee that the parasites in the center of a large roast will be made more than uncomfortable unless raised to a uniform internal temperature of 77° C. The cut surface of cooked fresh pork should be "white"; any trace of pink demands its return to the oven or frying pan. Some methods of rapid cooking in microwave ovens do not kill all of the encysted *T. spiralis* at 77° C or even at 82° C, apparently because the meat does not heat uniformly (Kotula et al, 1983). Even roasts that appear to be well done may contain live larvae when prepared in a microwave oven (Zimmermann, 1983).

Freezing of pork products for several weeks (e.g., at −15° C for 20 days) has long been considered adequate to kill *T. spiralis*. However, this cannot safely be applied to the sylvatic sibling species, *Trichinella nativa*, found in bears and other holarctic wildlife, which can withstand storage at −20° C for 6 months (Pozio et al, 1992). In certain countries (e.g., Germany) where the public demands uncooked pork products, meat inspection includes microscopic examination for trichinae in diaphragm muscle squash preparations of every carcass. In the United States, the

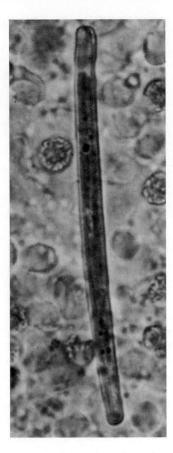

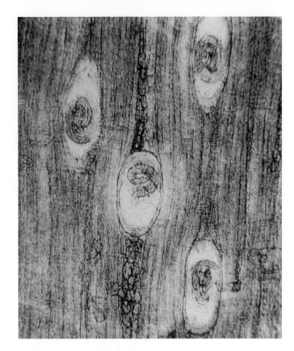

FIGURE 3-139 *Trichinella spiralis*, larvae in muscle press (×60).

FIGURE 3-138 *Trichinella spiralis* prelarva demonstrated in the blood of a cat by the Knott technique (×1000).

traditional policy has been instead to persuade the public to cook fresh pork thoroughly and to require manufacturers of "ready-to-eat" products to cook or freeze them according to specifications that ensure the destruction of trichinae.

Outbreaks of human clinical trichinosis most often involve small groups of people that have shared uncooked sausage or an undercooked roast from a locally slaughtered pig. However, in one Illinois outbreak, in which 23 of 50 members of an extended Dutch-German family became ill, the source of the *T. spiralis* larvae in the homemade sausage was USDA-inspected pork (Potter et al, 1976).

Occasionally, individuals perversely eat completely raw ground meat ("cannibal sandwich"), a habit more prevalent among beef lovers than pork lovers. However, neither is safe. Hamburger often contains a considerable amount of ground pork whether it is supposed to or not. Outbreaks of trichinellosis in France and other European countries have been traced to consumption of horse-meat. A plausible explanation for paradoxical *T. spiralis* infection in the strictly herbivorous horse

was proposed by Gretillat (1985). Severe parasitism of rats could lead to widespread contamination of equine feed with adult *T. spiralis* expelled by diarrheal rats. Adult female *T. spiralis* are packed full of larvae capable of infecting virtually any warm-blooded animal.

It has been estimated that for humans, ingestion of 5 trichina larvae per gram of body weight is fatal, for hogs 10, and for rats 30 (Chandler and Read, 1961). Human trichinosis sufferers may display periorbital edema, myalgia, fever, gastroenteritis, conjunctivitis, pruritus, and skin eruption. Eosinophilia usually exceeds 20%.

Clinical trichinosis in domestic animals may result from both insult inflicted on the intestinal mucosa by the adult worms and the host's reaction to invasion of skeletal muscles by the larvae. A case of trichinosis in a rural Massachusetts cat caused transient hemorrhagic enteritis, during which adult *T. spiralis* worms were found in the feces, and prelarvae were identified in the blood (Figure 3-140). The phase of muscle invasion was without clinical signs, but eosinophilia persisted for 3 months (Holzworth and Georgi, 1974). A second case in a 3-month-old kitten is typical of the phase of muscle invasion: The kitten was lying helplessly on its side with limbs extended, showed pain on handling, salivated, breathed superficially, and cried constantly (Hemmert-Halswick and Bugge, 1934). Case reports of trichinosis in dogs and cats

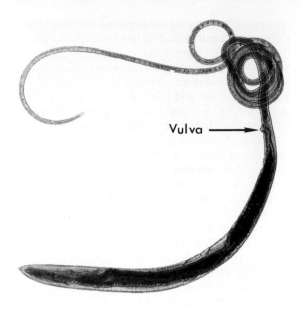

FIGURE 3-140   *Trichuris* sp. from a cat from Puerto Rico (×11).

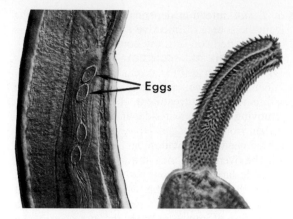

FIGURE 3-141   *Trichuris discolor* (×84). *Left,* Four eggs are seen in the vagina of a female; *right,* the spinate spicular sheath of the male is protruded.

are few, but it is a question how often it may be overlooked or misdiagnosed.

TREATMENT. *T. spiralis* infection is infrequently diagnosed in cats and dogs, but because both of these hosts frequently consume uncooked meat in the form of scraps and prey and because the dog displays such a predilection for eating carrion, it stands to reason that canine and feline *Trichinella* infection must in fact be rather common. Treatment is experimental. Cats and dogs experimentally infected with *T. spiralis* have been found to have reduced numbers of muscle-stage larvae after treatment with albendazole, 50 mg/kg body weight twice daily for 7 days (Bowman et al, 1993).

Trichuris

IDENTIFICATION. The adult body is whip-shaped, the anterior end fine, hairlike, and embedded in the wall of the large intestine, and the posterior end stout and lying free in the lumen (see Figure 3-140). The egg is lemon-shaped with a distinct plug at each pole and contains a single cell when passed in the feces (see Figures 3-139, 5-9, 5-28, and 5-32); the male has a spinate spicular sheath (Figure 3-141).

LIFE HISTORY. An infective first-stage larva develops inside the egg in about 1 month but does not hatch unless swallowed by a suitable host. The infective egg is very resistant, so animals confined in contaminated environments tend to become reinfected after treatment. Once eggs are ingested, all development occurs within the epithelium of the intestine (i.e., there is no extraintestinal migration). The prepatent period of *Trichuris vulpis* in the dog

is slightly less than 3 months, in cattle about 3 months, and in swine about 45 days.

IMPORTANCE. Most canine whipworm infections are symptom-free, but heavy infections cause bouts of diarrhea alternating with periods during which normal stools are passed. The diarrheal feces often contain much mucus and may be flecked with blood. *Trichuris* infection is rare and unimportant in North American cats but interesting for its novelty (see Figures 3-140 and 5-28).

Ruminants are frequently infected but only occasionally made ill by their respective species of *Trichuris.* Individual young cattle with extraordinarily heavy *Trichuris discolor* infections may suffer massive, sometimes fatal hemorrhages into the lumen of the cecum (Georgi et al, 1972). Such cases tend to be isolated and rare. When a bona fide case of bovine whipworm disease is diagnosed, all other members of the herd may be free of clinical signs. Possibly, clinically affected individuals are those that practice peculiar habits favoring ingestion of soil containing *T. discolor* eggs, or perhaps they are afflicted with a hemorrhagic diathesis that magnifies the cost of the minor trauma inflicted on the cecal wall by the parasites.

Very severe *Trichuris suis* infections in young swine cause catarrhal enteritis with clinical signs of diarrhea, dehydration, anorexia, and retardation of growth (Batte et al, 1977). It has been shown that pigs experimentally infected by the feeding of *T. suis* eggs in the presence of antibiotics will have significantly reduced lesions compared with pigs that are simply infected with the whipworms (Mansfield and Urban, 1996). The authors suggest that the complex pathogenesis of necrotic proliferative colitis in pigs may be linked to worm-induced suppression of mucosal immunity to resident bacteria. The control of *T. suis* infection depends on separating swine from the source of infective eggs, which usually is contaminated soil or filthy housing.

TREATMENT AND CONTROL. Infective *T. vulpis* eggs survive in soil for a long time, and dogs kept in contact with contaminated soils tend to become reinfected after treatment. Lasting success in removing these parasites depends on separating the patient from these eggs. However, in the emphasis for the need for sanitation, an important possibility may be overlooked. Assuming that the developing parasitic larvae are more resistant to anthelmintic action than are the adult worms, it follows that patent infection is almost certain to recur through maturation of immature forms that have survived a dose of anthelmintic. Most common canine intestinal nematode parasites require only a few weeks to mature, so a second dose of anthelmintic administered 2 or 3 weeks after the first theoretically rids the host of the worms that were unaffected by the first treatment. *T. vulpis* differs from the others in requiring about 3 months to mature, so medication should be routinely repeated three times at monthly intervals to destroy the worms as they mature and prevent them from contaminating the environment.

In the United States, the preferred drugs for treatment of *T. vulpis* infection are fenbendazole (Panacur), milbemycin oxime (Interceptor or Sentinel), febantel (with praziquantel and pyrantel pamoate in Drontal Plus), dichlorvos, and oxibendazole (with diethylcarbamazine citrate in Filaribits Plus). The rare case of *Trichuris* infection in the cat must be handled on an experimental basis because no drug has been cleared specifically for this purpose, although febantel is probably suitable.

Trichuris infections in beef cattle can be treated with ivermectin pour-on with 5 mg/10 kg body weight, or with injectable doramectin with 0.2 mg/kg body weight. Ivermectin can be used as a drench in sheep for treatment of *Trichuris ovis* at 0.2 mg/kg body weight.

T. suis infections in swine are susceptible to hygromycin B (Hygromix) when fed for at least 3 weeks at 12 g per ton of feed, and to dichlorvos (Atgard) fed in meal-type feed at 11.2 to 21.6 mg/kg body weight. *T. suis* infections are also susceptible to fenbendazole (9 mg/kg for 3 to 12 days).

Capillarids

The genus *Capillaria* has been divided by taxonomists into a number of genera on several occasions (Moravec, 1982; Moravec et al, 1987). The capillarids comprise a very large group of worms parasitic in all classes of vertebrates, and it would seem that differences in morphology and life cycles would warrant such a division of the group, although not all systematists working in the field agree with some or all the divisions that have been made. Because it is such a large group, the genus *Capillaria* has been divided into quite a large number of smaller genera with names unfamiliar to most (e.g., *Eucoleus, Hepaticola, Skrjabinocapillaria, Thominx,* and upward of a dozen others), and most of us would be incapable of distinguishing the adults of the different genera.

The adult worms typically are associated with certain epithelial surfaces of their hosts. The veterinary practitioner almost never sees the worms themselves, that is, unless the worms are associated with visible epithelia allowing their tracts to be observed, as when the worms are in the skin of the African clawed frog (Wade, 1982) or the frontal sinuses of the fox (Supperer, 1953). Thus in most cases, the practitioner sees only eggs passed in the feces. The species found in the dog and cat have been placed in three genera: (1) *Eucoleus* for those found in the airways, (2) *Aonchotheca* for the worms found in the intestinal tract, and (3) *Pearsonema* for those that occur in the bladder. The worms found in the liver of rats and a few other hosts have been placed in the genus *Calodium*. It is possible to differentiate these eggs with relative ease, and it seems that this division, at least, is workable.

IDENTIFICATION. The adult body is small and although not whip-shaped, otherwise somewhat resembles *Trichuris* spp. and lies partially embedded in mucous membranes (e.g., bronchial, alimentary, vesical) or buried in tissue (e.g., liver; see Figure 5-127). The eggs differ from those of *Trichuris* spp. only in detail, and are described well by Campbell (1991).

NASAL CAPILLARIASIS. *Eucoleus (= Capillaria) böhmi* was described as a parasite of the frontal sinus mucosae of the fox (Supperer, 1953). This report has been largely overlooked by American authors, including us, who have tended to assume that capillarids found in the nasal and paranasal sinuses are the same as those found in the bronchi (i.e., *Eucoleus aerophilus*). The eggs of *E. böhmi* can be distinguished from those of *Eucoleus aerophilus* by careful microscopic inspection of their surfaces. The surface of *E. böhmi* is covered with tiny pits like those of a thimble, whereas the surface of *E. erophilus* is a network of branching and anastomosing ridges (Supperer, 1953). A fecal specimen from a dog that had been treated repeatedly over a period of a year for purported intractable whipworm infection was found to contain the eggs of *E. böhmi*, not *T. vulpis*, and the reason for the repeated therapeutic failures became clear.

BRONCHIAL CAPILLARIASIS. The life history of *E. (= Capillaria) aerophilus* may be direct or it may involve earthworms as facultative intermediate hosts. Infection of dogs and cats is rarely responsible for more than a slight cough, but foxes on fur farms may harbor pathogenic burdens. Hanson (1933) described the disease in foxes as insidious and chronic, characterized by a rattling and wheezy respiration with spells of coughing and weakness, and by poor growth, unthrifty fur, failure to shed properly, and death due to bronchopneumonia in heavy infections. Low-grade *E. aerophilus* infection is common in cats and dogs. Diagnosis is based on identifying the rather plump, often asymmetrical bipolar eggs in the feces or tracheal mucus (see Figure 5-19). However, cats and dogs infrequently develop the severe degree of infection observed in captive foxes confined to earthen runs.

INTESTINAL CAPILLARIASIS. *Aonchotheca (=Capillaria) putorii*, a parasite of the small intestine of bears, hedgehogs, raccoons, swine, bobcats, and various mustelids, is occasionally found in the domestic cat, in which it causes little if any harm. However, the eggs present a differential diagnostic problem with respect to those of other capillarid species found in cats (Greve and Kung, 1983). Ruminants also host several species of capillarids, none of which are of importance in producing disease in these hosts.

HEPATIC CAPILLARIASIS. Adult *Calodium (=Capillaria) hepaticum* worms live in the livers of rats, muskrats, woodchucks, other rodents, and a wide range of occasional hosts, including humans. Eggs deposited by the female worms are trapped in the hepatic tissues (see Figure 5-127) where, for lack of sufficient oxygen, they remain undeveloped until the host is eaten or otherwise dies and disintegrates. Only then do the eggs develop to the infective first larval stage.

URINARY CAPILLARIASIS. *Pearsonema (=Capillaria) plica* adults weave the anterior portions of their bodies into the mucous membrane of the urinary bladder and other parts of the urinary tract of dogs, cats, foxes, and wolves. The eggs contain one cell when passed in the urine. The first-stage larva develops in a little more than a month but does not hatch unless ingested by an earthworm, which serves as paratenic host. The definitive host becomes infected by eating earthworms with first-stage larvae in their tissues, and eggs first appear in the urine about 2 months later. Enigk (1950a) claimed that *P. plica* infection caused growth impairment in young foxes, but dogs and cats appear to bear their usually modest worm burdens without inconvenience. *Pearsonema (= Capillaria) feliscati* is a parasite of the urinary bladder of the cat and resembles *P. plica* in its biological properties (see Figure 5-19).

TREATMENT. Capillariasis, whether nasal, bronchial, urinary, or intestinal, is usually asymptomatic. Nevertheless, having identified *Capillaria* eggs in the feces or urine sediment or on a bronchial swab, the veterinarian usually feels compelled to medicate. There is no known specific drug for the treatment of *Capillaria* infections. Kelly (1977) suggested levamisole at 2.5 mg/kg for 5 days or a single oral dose of fenbendazole at 50 mg/kg as potentially useful for the treatment of these parasitisms in dogs and cats. Evinger et al (1985) reported success in treating nasal capillariasis with a single oral dose of ivermectin, 0.2 mg/kg Kirkpatrick and Nelson (1987) reported apparent success in treating a case of symptomatic urinary capillariasis in a border terrier with a single dose of ivermectin, 0.2 mg/kg, injected subcutaneously.

Trichosomoides

Trichosomoides crassicauda is a parasite of the urinary bladder of rats. The tiny male *T. crassicauda* lives inside the uterus of its mate (Figure 3-142). Infection usually is transmitted from mother rats to their offspring before weaning. *T. crassicauda* has been treated in rats with ivermectin subcutaneously at 0.2 mg/kg or orally at 3 mg/kg (Findon and Miller, 1987; Summa et al, 1992).

Anatrichosoma

Anatrichosoma spp. are 25×0.2-mm trichuroids of that burrow in the stratified squamous epithelium of the nasal passages of African monkeys and the buccal mucosa of the American opossum, *Didelphis virginiana*. The female worms deposit 76×58-μm bipolar eggs in these burrows. The fully embryonated eggs reach the surface in the normal course of regeneration and desquamation. Antemortem diagnosis is based on demonstrating the eggs on nasal swabs (see Figure 5-67). *Anatrichosoma cutaneum* gives rise to subcutaneous nodules and edema about the joints of the extremities and serpiginous blisters of the palms and soles of monkeys.

■ MISCELLANEOUS WORMS

Thorny-headed worms and leeches are not related to the nematodes, nor are they related to each other. They are lumped together here for want of a logical and convenient alternative.

Phylum Acanthocephala

The Acanthocephala, or thorny-headed worms, are a small phylum of highly specialized parasites of the vertebrate digestive tract (Figures 3-143 and 3-144). The body is normally flattened in situ but becomes more or less cylindrical when placed in water, which is the indispensable first step in preparing specimens for identification. The resulting osmotic turgor forces the retractable, spiny attachment organ or **proboscis** out of the body so that the

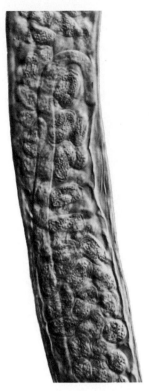

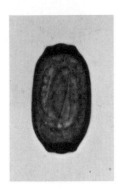

FIGURE 3-142 *Trichosomoides crassicauda* male in the uterus of a female *T. crassicauda* (*left*, ×168). S. H. Weisbroth, who provided this specimen, has described a Millipore filtration procedure for demonstrating the eggs of *T. crassicauda* (*right*, ×425) in rat urine.

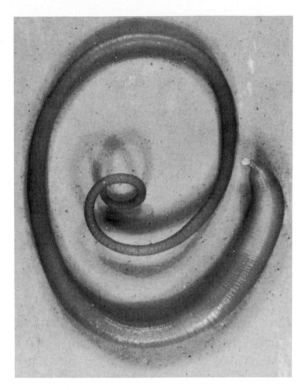

FIGURE 3-143 *Macracanthorhynchus hirudinaceus* (three fourths natural size).

shape and number of spines can be ascertained and the specimen thereby identified (see Figure 3-144). Once the proboscis (and male copulatory bursa) is well protracted, the specimen can be fixed in hot alcohol-formaldehyde-acetic acid (AFA) solution (85 parts of 85% ethanol, 10 parts of stock formalin, 5 parts of glacial acetic acid). These technical details are stressed here because, unless specimens are properly prepared, even a specialist may not be able to identify them.

IDENTIFICATION. Acanthocephalans consist of a body and a retractable spiny proboscis by which the parasite attaches itself to the intestinal wall of its host. There is no digestive tract. Nutrients are absorbed through the tegument.

LIFE HISTORY. When the egg is laid, it contains a fully developed larva called an **acanthor** (Figure 3-145). If the egg is ingested by a suitable arthropod intermediate host, the acanthor develops through an **acanthella** stage (Figure 3-146) into an encysted infective larva called a **cystacanth** (Figure 3-147). The cystacanth is capable of reencysting in a range of vertebrate paratenic hosts should they ingest the infected arthropod. Frequently, the

cystacanth even reencysts in its normal definitive host instead of developing to maturity. For example, *Prosthenorchis elegans* adults may be found in the intestinal lumen of a monkey, and cystacanths of the same parasite may be found encysted in the peritoneal membranes.

Macracanthorhynchus

Macracanthorhynchus hirudinaceus is a parasite of the small intestine of swine (see Figure 3-143). The

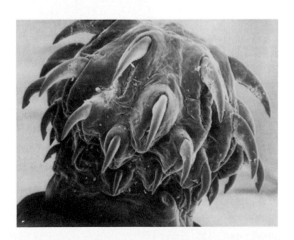

FIGURE 3-144 *Macracanthorhynchus ingens* proboscis (×125).

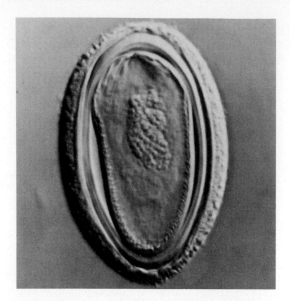

FIGURE 3-145 *Macracanthorhynchus ingens* egg containing acanthor larva (×660).

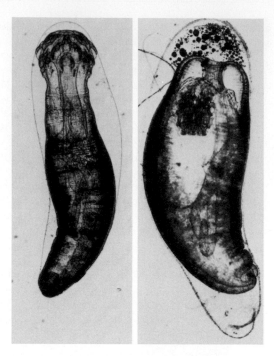

FIGURE 3-147 *Macracanthorhynchus ingens* cystacanth infective larvae from a *Narceus* millipede (×20).

body is flattened and transversely wrinkled, which occasionally causes this parasite to be mistaken for a tapeworm. Development to the **cystacanth** stage infective for pigs occurs in May beetles, dung beetles, or water beetles in about 3 months. Pigs acquire *M. hirudinaceus* infection when rooting for beetle grubs, but the infected adult beetle is also a source of cystacanths. The prepatent period is 2 or

3 months. Pigs may display no outward sign of *M. hirudinaceus* infection, or there may be diarrhea and emaciation with evidence of acute abdominal pain, depending on how deeply the proboscis is embedded in the intestinal wall.

TREATMENT. There is no effective treatment for *M. hirudinaceus* infection. Benzimidazole anthelmintics may be tried. An in-feed formulation of ivermectin (0.1 or 0.2 mg/kg body weight for 7 days) resulted in 100% removal of adult *M. hirudinaceus* from pigs (Alva-Valdes et al, 1989).

Macracanthorhynchus ingens (see Figure 3-144), even larger than *M. hirudinaceus*, is a parasite of the raccoon *(Procyon lotor)* and uses millipedes of the genus *Narceus* as intermediate hosts. These parasites occasionally infect dogs that eat the infected millipedes. To eat a millipede requires extraordinary cunning, frightful taste, great excitement, or utter boredom on the part of the dog because the millipedes give off a potent defensive secretion. The raccoon gets around the problem by rolling the millipede about in the dust to exhaust its supply of defensive secretion, but few dogs have learned that trick.

Prosthenorchis

Prosthenorchis spp. are up to 55 mm long, pink acanthocephalan parasites of primates. *Prosthenorchis* spp. propagate very successfully in monkey colonies by using cockroaches and certain beetles as intermediate hosts. Monkeys become

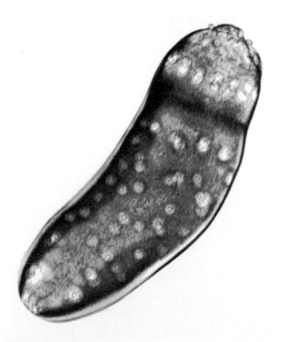

FIGURE 3-146 *Macracanthorhynchus ingens* acanthella from a *Narceus* millipede (×27).

infected when they eat a cockroach containing the cystacanth larvae of *Prosthenorchis* spp.

Both chronic and acute disease syndromes have been described for *Prosthenorchis* infection. The chronic course is marked by watery diarrhea of several months' duration with weakness and progressive emaciation. The appetite remains normal until a day or so before death. The acute course is of less than one day's duration and caused by acute bacterial peritonitis resulting from perforation of the intestinal wall by the proboscis.

Treatment of caged marmosets *(Saguinus mystax)* infected with *P. elegans* has shown that fenbendazole (20 mg/kg body weight for 7 days) was effective in removing these parasites (Demidov et al, 1988).

Moniliformis
The great length (up to 32 cm) and pseudosegmentation of the body invite misidentification of this acanthocephalan as a tapeworm. A common parasite of wild rodents, *Moniliformis* spp. use cockroaches as intermediate hosts.

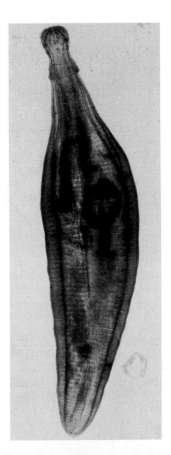

FIGURE 3-148 *Oncicola* sp. from an Arizona coyote *Canis latrans* (×14).
(Specimen courtesy Dr. Frances Phillips.)

Oncicola
Oncicola canis (Figure 3-148), less than 14 mm long, is a parasite of the dog, coyote, and other canids. It uses the armadillo as paratenic host for cystacanths.

Phylum Annelida
Class Hirudinea

Leeches are predatory or parasitic worms of the phylum Annelida, which includes the free-living earthworms. Leeches have terminal suckers for locomotion and attachment and move by looping movements like those of an inchworm. They usually are dark or black in color. Bloodsucking species fasten to the skin or oropharyngeal mucous membrane by means of their powerful suckers, pierce the epidermis, and suck blood. A salivary enzyme, hirudin, acts as an anticoagulant and ensures a copious flow of blood. In some localities, surface waters abound with bloodsucking leeches that attach to the oropharyngeal or laryngeal mucous membrane when imbibed by the unwary person or animal. Their presence in these locations may cause severe bouts of coughing and choking, during which blood is ejected by the victim. Infection may last several weeks and occasionally causes death. Treatment consists of mechanically removing the leech.

■ REFERENCES
Abraham D: Biology of *Dirofilaria immitis*. In Boreham, PFL, Atwell RB, editors: *Dirofilariasis*, Boca Raton, Fla, 1988, CRC Press, pp 29–46.

Adcock JL: Pulmonary arterial lesions in canine dirofilariasis, *Am J Vet Res* 22(89):655–662, 1961.

Alicata JE: Angiostrongyliasis cantonensis (eosinophilic meningitis): historical events in its recognition as a new parasitic disease of man, *J Wash Acad Sci* 78:38–46, 1988.

Ali Kahn Z: The postembryonic development of *Trichinella spiralis* with special reference to ecdysis, *J Parasitol* 52:248–259, 1966.

Alva-Valdes R, Wallace DH, Foster AG, et al: Efficacy of an in-feed formulation against gastrointestinal helminths, lungworms, and mites in swine, *Am J Vet Res* 50:1392–1395, 1989.

American Heartworm Society: American Heartworm Society recommended procedures for the diagnosis and management of heartworm *(Dirofilaria immitis)* infections. *American Heartworm Society Bulletin* 19:1–8, 1993.

Anderson FL, Conder GA, Marsland WP: Efficacy of injectable and tablet formulations of praziquantel against mature *Echinococcus granulosus, Am J Vet Res* 39:1861–1862, 1978.

Anderson RV, Bemrick WJ: *Micronema deletrix* n. sp.: a saprophagus nematode inhabiting a nasal tumor of the horse, *Proc Helminthol Soc Wash* 32:74–75, 1965.

Anderson TJC: *Ascaris* infection in humans from North America: molecular evidence for cross infection, *Parasitology* 110:215–219, 1995.

Anderson TJC, Romero-Abal ME, Jaenike J: Genetic structure and epidemiology of *Ascaris* populations: patterns of host affiliation in Guatemala, *Parasitology* 107:319–334, 1993.

Anderson WI, Georgi ME, Car BD: Pancreatic atrophy and fibrosis associated with *Eurytrema procyonis* in a domestic cat, *Vet Rec* 120:235–236, 1987.

Araujo FP, Schwabe CW, Sawyer JC, Davis WG: Hydatid disease transmission in California: a study of the Basque connection, *Am J Epidemiol* 102:291–302, 1975.

Armour J, Duncan JL, Reid JFS: Activity of oxfendazole against inhibited larvae of *Ostertagia ostertagi* and *Cooperia oncophora*, *Vet Rec* 102:263–264, 1978.

Arru E, Garippa G, Manger BR: Efficacy of epsiprantel against *Echinococcus granulosus* infections in dogs, *Res Vet Sci* 49:378–379, 1990.

Arundel JH: *Cysticercosis in sheep and cattle*, Australian Meat Research Committee Review No 4, 1972.

Aruo SK: The use of "Nilverm" (tetramisole) in the control of clinical signs of *Thelazia rhodesii* (eyeworm) infections in cattle, *Bull Epizoot Dis Afr* 22:275–277, 1974.

August JR, Powers RD, Bailey WS, et al: *Filaroides hirthi* in a dog: fatal hyperinfection suggestive of autoinfection, *J Am Vet Med Assoc* 176:331–334, 1980.

Bahnemann R, Bauer C: Lungworm infection in a beagle colony: *Filaroides hirthi*, a common but not well-known companion, *Exp Tox Pathol* 46:55–62, 1994.

Ballard NB, Vande Vusse FJ: *Echinococcus multilocularis* in Illinois and Nebraska, *J Parasitol* 69:790–791, 1983.

Bankov D: *Efficacy of praziquantel against* Stilesia globipunctata *and other cestodes in sheep,* International Conference, Pathophysiology of Parasitic Infections, Thessaloniki, Greece, 1975, p 46.

Bankov D: Opiti za diagnostika i terapiya na stileziozata po ovtsete, *Vet Nauki* 13:28–36, 1976.

Barclay WP, Phillips TN, Foerner JJ: Intussusception associated with *Anoplocephala perfoliata* infection in five horses, *J Am Vet Med Assoc* 180:752–753, 1982.

Basir MA: The morphology and development of the sheep nematode, *Strongyloides papillosis* (Wedl, 1856), *Can J Res* 28:173–196, 1950.

Batte EG, Harkema R, Osborne JC: Observations of the life cycle and pathogenicity of the swine kidney worm *(Stephanurus dentatus)*, *J Am Vet Med Assoc* 136:622–625, 1960.

Batte EG, McLamb RD, Muse KE, et al: Pathophysiology of swine trichuriasis, *Am J Vet Res* 38:1075–1079, 1977.

Batte EG, Moncol DJ, Barber CW: Prenatal infection with the swine kidney worm *(Stephanurus dentatus)* and associated lesions, *J Am Vet Med Assoc* 149:758–765, 1966.

Bauer C, Bahnemann R: *Filaroides hirthi* infections in beagle dogs by ivermectin, *Vet Parasitol* 65:269–273, 1996.

Bauer C, Gey A: Efficacy of six anthelmintics against luminal stages of *Baylisascaris procyonis* in naturally infected raccoons *(Procyon lotor)*, *Vet Parasitol* 60:155–159, 1995.

Baumann R: Beobachtungen beim parasitären Sommerbluten der Pferde, *Wien Tierärtzl Monatschr* 33:52–55, 1946.

Baumgärtner W, Zajac A, Hull BL, et al: Parelaphostrongylosis in llamas, *J Am Vet Med Assoc* 187:1243–1245, 1985.

Beaver PC, Snyder CH, Carreara GM, et al: Chronic eosinophilia due to visceral larva migrans, *Pediatrics* 9:7–19, 1952.

Bech-Nielsen S, Sjogren U, Lundquist H: *Parafilaria bovicola* (Tubangi 1934) in cattle: epizootiology-disease occurrence, *Am J Vet Res* 43:945–947, 1982.

Becker HN: Efficacy of injectable ivermectin against natural infections of *Stephanurus dentatus* in swine, *Am J Vet Res* 47:1622–1623, 1986.

Bennett D: The diagnosis and treatment of *Filaroides osleri* infestation in the dog, *Vet Ann* 15:256–260, 1975.

Bennett D, Beresford-Jones WP: Treatment of *Filaroides osleri* infestation in a 16-month-old male Yorkshire Terrier with thiabendazole, *Vet Rec* 93:226–227, 1973.

Berger J: The resistance of a field strain of *Haemonchus contortus* to five benzimidazole anthelmintics in current use, *J South Afr Vet Assoc* 46:369–372, 1975.

Bergstrom RC, Maki LR, Kercher CJ: Average daily gain and feed efficiency of lambs with low level trichostrongylid burdens, *J Anim Sci* 41(2):513–516, 1975.

Bergstrom RC, Taylor RF, Presgrove T: Fitting fenbendazole into the treatment plan for sheep with fringed tapeworms, *Vet Med* 83:846–847, 1988.

Beroza GA, Barclay WP, Phillips TM, et al: Cecal perforation and peritonitis associated with *Anoplocephala perfoliata* infection in three horses, *J Am Vet Med Assoc* 183:804–806, 1983.

Bihr T, Conboy GA: Lungworm *(Crenosoma vulpis)* infection in dogs on Prince Edward Island, *Can Vet J* 40:555–559, 1999.

Bisset SA, Marshal ED, Morisson L: Economics of a dry-cow anthelmintic drenching programme for dairy cows in New Zealand. I. Overall response in 47 herds, *Vet Parasitol* 26:117–118, 1987.

Bladt-Knudsen TS, Fossing EC, Bjorn H, et al: Transmission of *Hyostrongylus rubidus* in housed pigs, *Bull Scand Soc Parasitol* 4:117–122, 1994.

Blair LS, Malatesta PF, Ewanciw DV: Dose response study of ivermectin against *Dirofilaria immitis* microfilariae in dogs with naturally acquired infections, *Am J Vet Res* 44:475–477, 1983.

Blair LS, Malatesta PF, Jacob L, et al: *Efficacy of thiacetarsamide in experimentally infected dogs at 2 months, 4 months, 6 months, or 12 months postinfection with* Dirofilaria immitis, Proceedings of the twenty-seventh annual meeting of the American Association of Veterinary Parasitolologists, 14–15, 1982.

Blaisdell KA: A study of the cat lungworm, *Aelurostrongylus abstrusus*, doctoral thesis, Cornell University, 1952.

Bliss EL, Greiner EC: Efficacy of fenbendazole and cambendazole against *Muellerius capillaris* in dairy goats, *Am J Vet Res* 46:1923–1925, 1985.

Blunden AS, Khalil LF, Webbon PM: *Halicephalobus deletrix* infection in a horse, *Equine Vet J* 19:255–259, 1987.

Boersema JH, Baas JJM, Schaeffer F: Een harnekking geval van "Kennelhoest" veroorzaakt door *Filaroides osleri*, *Tidschrft. Diergenskd* 114:10–13, 1989.

Bogan JA, McKellar QA, Mitchell ES, et al: Efficacy of ivermectin against *Cooperia* curticei infection in sheep, *Am J Vet Res* 49:99–100, 1988.

Boisvenue RJ, Hendrix JC: Studies on location of adult fringed tapeworms, *Thysanosoma actinoides,* in feeder lambs, *Proc Helm Soc Wash* 54:204–206, 1987.

Bollinger O: Die Kolik der Pferde und das Wurmaneurysma der Eingeweidearterien. Eine pathologische und Klinische Untersuchung. *Beitr. Vergleich. Path. u. Path. Anat. Hausth. München*, Heft I, 1870.

Bolt G, Monrad J, Koch J, et al: Canine angiostrongylosis: a review, *Vet Rec* 135:447–452, 1994.

Boray JC, Strong MB, Allison JR, et al: Nitroscanate, a new broad-spectrum anthelmintic against nematodes and cestodes of dogs and cats, *Austr Vet J* 55:45–53, 1979.

Bourdeau P, Ehm JP: Cas original de Filaroïdose due à *Filaroïdose* sp. chez le chien. Données actuelles sur la Filaroïdose à *Filarïdose hirthi* Georgi et Anderson 1975, *Rec Med Vet* 168:315–321, 1992.

Bowman DD, Darrigrand RA, Frongillo MK, et al: Treatment of experimentally induced trichinosis in dogs and cats, *Am J Vet Res* 54:1303–1305, 1993.

Bowman DD, Frongillo MK, Johnson RC, et al: Evaluation of praziquantel for treatment of experimentally induced paragonimiasis in dogs and cats, *Am J Vet Res* 52:68–71, 1991.

Bowman DD, Johnson RC, Ulrich ME, et al: *Effects of long-term administration of ivermectin and milbemycin oxime on circulating microfilariae and parasite antigenemia in dogs with patent heartworm infections,* Proceedings of the 1992 Heartworm Symposium, March 27, 1992, Austin, TX, pp 151–158.

Breuer W, Hasslinger MA, Hermanns W: Chronische Gastritis durch Ollulanus tricuspis (Leuckart, 1865) bei einem, *Tiger Berl Munch Tierärztl Wochenschr* 106:47–49, 1993.

Brooks DE, Greiner EC, Walsh MT: Conjunctivitis caused by *Thelazia* sp. in a Senegal parrot, *J Am Vet Med Assoc* 183:1305–1306, 1983.

Burke TM, Roberson EL: Fenbendazole treatment of pregnant bitches to reduce prenatal and lactogenic infections of *Toxocara canis* and *Ancylostoma caninum* in pups, *J Am Vet Med Assoc* 183:987–990, 1983.

Cahill KM, Sheuchuk M: Fulminant systemic strongyloidiasis in AIDS, *Ann Trop Med Parasitol* 90:313–318, 1996.

Calvert CA, Mandell CP: Diagnosis and management of feline heartworm disease, *J Am Vet Med Assoc* 180:550–552, 1982.

Campbell BG: *Trichuris* and other trichinelloid nematodes of dogs and cats in the United States, *Comp Cont Educ Pract Vet* 13:769–778, 1991.

Campbell BG, Little MD: The finding of *Angiostrongylus cantonensis* in rats in New Orleans, *Am J Trop Med Hyg* 38:568–573, 1988.

Campbell KL, Graham JC: *Physaloptera* infection in dogs and cats, *Comp Cont Ed Pract Vet* 21:299–314, 1999.

Campbell WC, Blair LS: *Dirofilaria immitis:* experimental infection in the ferret *(Mustela putorius furo), J Parasitol* 64:119–122, 1978.

Chandler AC, Read CP: *Introduction to parasitology*, ed 10, New York, 1961, John Wiley and Sons.

Chhabra RC, Singh KS: Diagnosis, treatment and control of spirocercosis in dogs, *Ind J Anim Sci* 42:203–207, 1972.

Chung NY, Miyahara AY, Chung G: The prevalence of feline liver flukes in the City and County of Honolulu, *J Am Anim Hosp Assoc* 13:258–262, 1977.

Church S, Kelly DF, Obwolo MJ: Diagnosis and successful treatment of diarrhoea in horses caused by immature small strongyles apparently insusceptible to anthelmintics, *Equine Vet J* 18:401–403, 1986.

Clunies Ross I, Gordon HMcL: *The internal parasites and parasitic diseases of sheep,* Sydney, 1936, Angus and Robertson Ltd.

Coles GC: Strategies for control of anthelmintic-resistant nematodes of ruminants, *J Am Vet Med Assoc* 192:330–334, 1988.

Colglazier ML, Kates KC, Enzie FD: Activity of cambendazole and morantel tartrate against two species of *Trichostrongylus* and two thiabendazole-resistant isolates of *Haemonchus contortus* in sheep, *Proc Helminthol Soc Wash* 39:28–32, 1972.

Colglazier ML, Kates KC, Enzie FD: Cross-resistance to other anthelmintics in an experimentally produced cambendazole-resistant strain of *Haemonchus contortus* in lambs, *J Parasitol* 61:778–779, 1975.

Coles GC, Brown SN, Trembath CM: Pyrantel-resistant large stronglyes in racehorses, *Vet Rec* 145:408, 1999.

Collett MG, Pomroy WE, Guilford WG, et al: Gastric *Ollulanus tricuspis* infection identified in captive cheetahs *(Acinonyx jubatus)* with chronic vomiting, *J S Afr Vet Assoc* 71:251–255, 2000.

Conboy GA, Stromberg BE, Schlotthauer JC: Efficacy of clorsulon against *Fascioloides magna* infection in sheep, *J Am Vet Med Assoc* 192:910–912, 1988.

Conboy GA, Whitney H, Ralhan S: Angiostrongylus vasorum *infection in dogs in Newfoundland, Canada,* Forty-third annual meeting of the American Association of Veterinary Parasitologists, July 25, 1998, Baltimore, Abst. No 78.

Congdon LL, Ames ER: Thiabendazole for control of *Toxocara canis* in the dog, *Am J Vet Res* 34:417–418, 1973.

Corba J, Scales B, Froyd G: The effect of DL-tetramisole on *Thelazia rhodesii* (eye-worm) in cattle, *Trop Anim Health Prod* 1:19–22, 1969.

Costa LRR, McClure JJ, Snider III TG, et al: Verminous meningoencephalomyclitis by *Angiostrongylus (=Parastrongylus) cantonenisis* in an American Miniature Horse, *Eq Vet Ed* 12:2–6, 2000.

Courtney CH, Shearer JK, Plue RE: Efficacy and safety of clorsulon used concurrently with ivermectin for control of *Fasciola hepatica* in Florida beef cattle, *Am J Vet Res* 46:1245–1246, 1985.

Craig TM, Brown TW, Shepstad DK, et al: Fatal *Filaroides hirthi* infection in a dog, *J Am Vet Med Assoc* 172:1096–1098, 1978.

Craig TM, Hatfield TA, Pankavich JA, et al: Efficacy of moxidectin against an ivermectin-resistant strain of *Haemonchus contortus* in sheep, *Vet Parasitol* 41:329–333, 1992.

Craig TM, Miller DK: Resistance by *Haemonchus contortus* to ivermectin in Angora goats, *Vet Rec* 126:580, 1990.

Craig TM, Suderman MT: Parasites of horses and considerations for their control, *Southwestern Vet* 36:211–226, 1985.

Crofton HD: Nematode parasite populations in sheep on lowland farms. I. Worm egg counts in ewes, *Parasitology* 44:465–477, 1954.

Crofton HD: Nematode parasite populations in sheep on lowland farms. IV. The effects of anthelmintic treatment, *Parasitology* 48:235–242, 1958.

Crofton HD: *Nematode parasite populations in sheep and on pasture,* Farnham Royal, Bucks, England, 1963, Commonwealth Agricultural Bureaux.

Crofton HD: *Nematodes,* London, 1966, Hutchinson University Library.

Crofton HD, Thomas RJ: A new species of *Nematodirus* in sheep, *Nature* 168:559, 1951.

Crofton HD, Thomas RJ: A further description of *Nematodirus battus* Crofton and Thomas, 1951, *J Helminthol* 28:119–122, 1954.

Darke PGG: Use of levamisole in the treatment of parasitic tracheobronchitis in the dog, *Vet Rec* 99:293–294, 1976.

Daubney R: The life histories of *Dictyocaulus filaria* (Rud.) and *Dictyocaulus viviparous* (Bloch), *J Comp Pathol Therap* 33(4):225–226, 1920.

Demidov NV, Khrustalev AV, Vibe PP, et al: Use of anthelmintics against helminth infections in monkeys, *Helminthol Abs Ser A* 60:1524, 1988 (abstract).

DeVaney JA, Craig TM, Rowe LD: Resistance to ivermectin by *Haemonchus contortus* in goats and calves, *Int J Parasitol* 22:369–376, 1992.

de Witt JJ: Mortality of rheas caused by *Syngamus trachea* infection, *Vet Quart* 17:39–40, 1995.

Dey-Hazra A: The efficacy of Droncit (praziquantel) against tapeworm infections in dog and cat, *Vet Med Rev* 2:134–141, 1976.

Dietrich LE: Treatment of canine lungworm infection with thiacetarsamide, *J Am Vet Med Assoc* 140:572–573, 1962.

Dillon R, Sakas PS, Buxton BA, et al: Indirect immunofluorescence testing for diagnosis of occult *Dirofilaria immitis* infection in three cats, *J Am Vet Med Assoc* 180:80–82, 1982.

Dobberstein J, Hartmann H: Über die Anastomosenbildung im Bereich der Blind- und Grimmdarmarterien des Pferdes und ihre Bedeutung für die Entstehung der embolischen, *Kolik Berl Tierärztl Wochenschr* 48:399–402, 1932.

Donaldson J, van Houtert MFJ, Sykes AR: The effect of protein supply on the periparturient parasite status of the mature ewe, *Proc New Zealand Soc Anim Prod* 57:186–189, 1997.

Dorrington JE: *Filaroides osleri:* the success of thiacetarsamide sodium therapy, *J S Afr Vet Med Assoc* 34:435–438, 1963.

Dorrington JE: Studies on *Filaroides osleri* infestation in dogs, *Onderstepoort J Vet Res* 35:225–286, 1968.

Drudge JH, Elam G: Preliminary observations on the resistance of horse strongyles to phenothiazine, *J Parasitol* 47(suppl): 38–39, 1961.

Drudge JH, Lyons ET: *Newer developments in helminth control and* Strongylus vulgaris *research,* Proceedings of the eleventh annual meeting of the Association of Equine Practioners, Miami Beach, 1965, pp 381–389.

Drudge JH, Lyons ET, Tolliver SC: Resistance of equine strongyles to thiabendazole: critical tests of two strains, *Vet Med Small Anim Clin* 72:433–435, 437–438, 1977.

Drudge JH, Lyons ET, Tolliver SC: Benzimidazole resistance of equine strongyles-critical tests of six compounds against population, *B Am J Vet Res* 40:590–594, 1979.

Drudge JH, Szanto J, Wyant ZN, et al: Field studies on parasite control in sheep: comparison of thiabendazole, ruelene, and phenothiazine, *Am J Vet Res* 25:1512–1518, 1964.

Dubey JP, Miller TB, Sharma SP: Fenbendazole for treatment of *Paragonimus kellicotti* infection in dogs, *J Am Vet Med Assoc* 174:835–837, 1979.

Dubin S, Segall S, Martindale J: Contamination of soil in two city parks with canine nematode ova including *Toxocara canis:* a preliminary study, *Am J Public Health* 65:1242–1245, 1975.

Duncan JL: Field studies on the epidemiology of mixed strongyle infection in the horse, *Vet Rec* 94:337–345, 1974.

Duncan JL: Internal parasites of horses: treatment and control, *In Practice* 4:83–188, 1982.

Duncan JL, Armour J, Bairden K, et al: The successful removal of inhibited fourth-stage *Ostertagia ostertagi* larvae by fenbendazole, *Vet Rec* 98:342, 1976.

Duncan JL, McBeath DG, Best JMJ, et al: The efficacy of fenbendazole in the control of immature strongyle infections in ponies, *Equine Vet J* 9:146–149, 1977.

Duncan JL, McBeath DG, Preston NK: Studies on the efficacy of fenbendazole used in a divided dosage regime against strongyle infections in ponies, *Equine Vet J* 12:78–80, 1980.

Duncan JL, Pirie HM: The life cycle of *Strongylus vulgaris* in the horse, *Res Vet Sci* 13:374–379, 1972.

Duncan JL, Pirie HM: The pathogenesis of single experimental infections with *Strongylus vulgaris* in foals, *Res Vet Sci* 18:82–93, 1975.

Duncan Jr RB, Patton S: Naturally occurring cerebrospinal parelaphostrongylosis in a heifer, *J Vet Diag Invest* 10:287–291, 1998.

Duncombe VM, Bolin TD, Davis AE, et al: *The effect of iron and protein deficiency and dexamethasone on the efficacy of benzimidazole anthelmintics,* Eighth international conference of the World Association for the Advancement of Veterinary Parasitology, Sydney, Australia, 1977a.

Duncombe VM, Bolin TD, Davis AE, et al: *Nippostrongylus brasiliensis* infection in the rat: effect of iron and protein deficiency and dexamethasone on the efficacy of benzimidazole anthelmintics, *Gut* 18:892–896, 1977b.

Dunsmore JD, Spratt DM: The life cycle of *Filaroides osleri* in the dingo. Paper presented at the meeting of the Australian Society of Parasitology, Melbourne, Australia, 1976, (abstract).

Durette-Desset MC, Chabaud AG, Ashford RW, et al: Two new species of Trichostrongylidae (Nematoda: Trichostrongyloidea), parasitic in *Gorilla gorilla beringei* in Uganda, *Syst Parasitol* 23:59–166, 1992.

Düwel D, Strasser H: Versuche zur Geburt helminthenfreier Hundewelpen durch Fenbendazol-behandlung, *Dtsch Tierärztl Wschr* 85:239–241, 1978.

Dwork KG, Jaffe JR, Lieberman HD: Strongyloidiasis with massive hyperinfection, *NY State J Med* 75(8):1230–1234, 1975.

Eberhard ML, Alfano E: Adult *Toxocara cati* infections in U.S. children: report of four cases, *Am J Trop Med Hyg* 59:404–406, 1998.

Eberhard ML, Brandt FH: The role of tadpoles and frogs as paratenic hosts in the life cycle of *Dracunculus insignis* (Nematoda: Dracunculoidea), *J Parasitol* 81:792–793, 1995.

Eckerlin RP, Leigh WH: *Platynosomum fastosum* Kossack, 1910 (Trematoda: Dicrocoeliidae) in South Florida, *J Parasitol* 48(suppl):49, 1962.

Eckert J, von Brand T, Voge M: Asexual multiplication of *Mesocestoides corti* (Cestoda) in the intestines of dogs and skunks, *J Parasitol* 55(2):241–249, 1969.

Ehrenford FA: True parasitism of dogs by *Hymenolepis diminuta, Canine Pract* 4:31–34, 1977.

Enigk K: Die Biologie von *Capillaria plica* (Trichuroidea: Nematodes), *Z Tropenmed Parasitol* 1:560–571, 1950a.

Enigk K: Zür Entwicklung von *Strongylus vulgaris* (Nematodes) in Wirtstier, *Z Torpenmed Parasitol* 2:287–306, 1950b.

Enigk K: Weitere Untersuchungen zür Biologie von *Strongylus vulgaris* (Nematodes) in Wirtstier, *Z Tropenmed Parasitol* 2:523–535, 1951.

Enigk K, Dey-Hazra A, Batke J: Zür klinischen Bedeutung und Behandlung des galaktogen erworbenen *Strongyloides* Befalls der Fohlen, *Dtsch Tierärztl Wochschr* 81:605–607, 1974.

Erb HN, Georgi JR: Control of *Filaroides hirthi* in commercially reared Beagle dogs, *Lab Anim Sci* 32(4):394–396, 1982.

Evans JW, Green PE: Preliminary evaluation of four anthelmintics against the cat liver fluke *Platynosomum concinnum, Austr Vet J* 54:454–455, 1978.

Evans RH, Tangredi B: Cerebrospinal nematodiasis in free-ranging birds, *J Am Vet Med Assoc* 187:1213–1214, 1985.

Evinger JV, Kazacos KR, Cantwell HD: Ivermectin for treatment of nasal capillariasis in a dog, *J Am Vet Med Assoc* 186:174–175, 1985.

Fan PC, Lin CY, Chen CC, et al: Morphological description of *Taenia saginata* asiatica (Cyclophyllidea Taeniidae) from man in Asia, *J Helminthol* 69:299–303, 1995.

Farnell DR, Faulkner DR: Prepatent period of *Dipetalonema reconditum* in experimentally infected dogs, *J Parasitol* 64:565–567, 1978.

Findon G, Miller TE: Treatment of *Trichosomoides crassicauda* in laboratory rats using ivermectin, *Lab Anim Sci* 37:496–499, 1987.

Foreyt WJ, Drawe DL: Efficacy of clorsulon and albendazole against *Fascioloides magna* in naturally infected white-tailed deer, *J Am Vet Med Assoc* 187:1187–1188, 1985.

Foreyt WJ, Gorham JR: Evaluation of praziquantel against induced *Nanophyetus salmincola* infections in coyotes and dogs, *Am J Vet Res* 49:563–565, 1988.

Freeman RS, Stuart PF, Cullen JB, et al: Fatal human infection with mesocercariae of the trematode *Alaria Americana, Am J Trop Med Hyg* 25:803–807, 1976.

Fülleborn F: Askarisinfektion durch Verzehren eingekapselter Larven und ubergelungene intrauterine Askarisinfektion, *Arch Schiffs u Tropenhyg* 25:367–375, 1921.

Galliard H: Recherches sur l'infestation expérimentale à *Strongyloides stercoralis* au Tonkin VIII-X, *Ann Parasitol* 26(1-2):68–84, 1951a.

Galliard H: Recherches sur l'infestation expérimentale à *Strongyloides stercoralis* au Tonkin XII, *Ann Parasitol* 26(3):201–227, 1951b.

Gardiner CH, Koh DS, Cardella TA: *Micronema* in man: third fatal infection, *Am J Trop Med Hyg* 30:586–589, 1981.

Gardiner CH, Wells S, Gutter AE, et al: Eosinophilic meningoencephalitis due to *Angiostrongylus cantonensis* as the cause of death in captive non-human primates, *Am J Trop Med Hyg* 42:70–74, 1990.

Geenen PL, Bresciani J, Boes J: The morphogenesis of *Ascaris suum* to the infective third-stage larvae within the egg, *J Parasitol* 85:616–622, 1999.

Genta RM, Schad GA: *Filaroides hirthi*: hyperinfective lungworm infection in immunosuppressed dogs, *Vet Pathol* 21:349–354, 1984.

Georgi JR: Estimation of parasitic blood loss by whole-body counting, *Am J Vet Res* 25(104):246–250, 1964.

Georgi JR: The Kikuchi-Enigk model of *Strongylus vulgaris* migrations in the horse, *Cornell Vet* 63:220–263, 1973.

Georgi JR: *Filaroides hirthi:* Experimental transmission among Beagle dogs through ingestion of first-stage larvae, *Science* 194:735, 1976a.

Georgi JR: Letter to the Editor: accessions of the Laboratory of Parasitology for 1975, *Cornell Vet* 66(4):604–615, 1976b.

Georgi JR: Strongyloidiasis. In Schultz MG, editor: *Handbook series in zoonoses, section C: parasitic zoonoses*, vol 2, Boca Raton, Fla, 1982. CRC Press.

Georgi JR, de Lahunta A, Percy DH: Cerebral coenurosis in a cat: report of a case, *Cornell Vet* 59:127–134, 1969.

Georgi JR, Fahnestock GR, Bohm MFK, et al: The migration and development of *Filaroides hirthi* in dogs, *Parasitology* 79:39–47, 1979b.

Georgi JR, Georgi ME, Cleveland DJ: Patency and transmission of *Filaroides hirthi* infection, *Parasitology* 75:251–257, 1977.

Georgi JR, Georgi ME, Fahnestock GR, et al: Transmission and control of *Filaroides hirthi,* lungworm infection in dogs, *Am J Vet Res* 40:829–831, 1979a.

Georgi JR, Slauson DO, Theodorides VJ: Anthelmintic activity of albendazole against *Filaroides hirthi* lungworms in dogs, *Am J Vet Res* 39(5):803–806, 1978.

Georgi JR, Sprinkle CL: A case of human strongyloidosis apparently contracted from asymptomatic colony dogs, *Am J Trop Hyg* 23(5):899–901, 1974.

Georgi JR, Whitlock JH: Erythrocyte loss and restitution in ovine haemonchosis: methods and basic mathematical model, *Am J Vet Res* 26(111):310–314, 1965.

Georgi JR, Whitlock RH, Flinton JH: Fatal *Trichuris discolor* infection in a Holstein-Friesian heifer: report of a case, *Cornell Vet* 62:58-–60, 1972.

Gibson TE, Everett G: Ecology of the free-living stages of *Nematodirus battus, Res Vet Sci* 31:323–327, 1981.

Gnedina MP, Osipov AN: The life cycle of *Parafilaria multipapillosa* (Dondamine and Drouilly, 1878) parasitic in the horse, *Doklad Acad Nauk SSSR* 131:1219, 1960.

Goff WL, Ronald NC: Miracidia hatching technique for diagnosis of canine schistosomiasis, *J Am Vet Med Assoc* 117:699–700, 1980.

Greiner EC, Lane TJ: Effects of the daily feeding of pyrantel tartrate on *Anoplocephala* infections in three horses: a pilot study, *J Eq Vet Sci* 14:43–44, 1994.

Gretillat S: Quelques remarques concernant l'infestation de cheval par *Trichinella spiralis* dans les conditions d'engraissement pour le boucherie, *Bull Mensuel Soc Vet Practique de France* 69:653–654, 656–658, 1985.

Greve JH, Kung FY: *Capillaria putorii* in domestic cats in Iowa, *J Am Vet Med Assoc* 182:511-513, 1983.

Greve JH, O'Brien SE: Adult *Baylisascaris* infections in two dogs, *Companion Anim Pract* 19:41–43, 1989.

Griesemer RA, Gibson JP: The establishment of an ascarid-free beagle dog colony, *J Am Vet Med Assoc* 143(9):965–967, 1963.

Grieve RB, Glickman LT, Bater AK, et al: Canine *Dirofilaria immitis* infection in a hyperenzootic area: examination by parasitologic findings at necropsy and by two serodiagnostic methods, *Am J Vet Res* 47:329–332, 1986.

Guilhon J, Graber M: Recherches sur l'activité du G4 à l'égard des principaux cestodes parasites du mouton, *Rev Elev* 13:297–304, 1960.

Gustafson BW: Ivermectin in the treatment of *Physaloptera praeputialis* in two cats, *J Am Anim Hosp Assoc* 31:416–418, 1995.

Hagan CJ: More on febantel and trichlorfon, *Vet Med Small Anim Clin* 74: 6, 1979.

Hamlen-Gomez H, Georgi JR: Equine helminth infections: control by selective chemotherapy, *Equine Vet J* 23:198–200, 1991.

Hänichen T, Hasslinger MA: Chronische Gastritis durch *Ollulamus tricuspis* (Leuckart, 1865) bei einer Katze, *Berl Munch Tierärztl Wochenschr* 90:59–62, 1977.

Hanson KB: Test of the efficacy of single treatments with tracheal brushes in the mechanical removal of lungworms from foxes, *J Am Vet Med Assoc* 82(1):12–33, 1933.

Hargis AM, Prieur DJ, Blanchard JL: Prevalence, lesions, and differential diagnosis of *Ollulanus tricuspis* infection in cats, *Vet Pathol* 20:71–79, 1983.

Hasslinger MA: *Ollulanus tricuspis,* the stomach worm of cats, *Feline Pract* 14:22–35, 1984.

Hayes MA, Creighton SR: A coenurus in the brain of a cat, *Can Vet J* 19:341–343, 1978.

Hemmert-Halswick A, Bugge G: Trichinen und Trichinose, *Ergebn Allgem Path u Path Anat* 28:313–392, 1934.

Herd RP: A practical approach to parasite control in dairy cows and heifers, *Comp Cont Ed Pract Vet* 5:573–580, 1983.

Herd RP, Coman BJ: Transmission of *Echinococcus granulosus* from kangaroos to domestic dogs, *Aust Vet J* 51:591, 1975.

Herd RP, Donham JC: Efficacy of ivermectin against *Onchocerca cervicalis* microfilarial dermatitis in horses, *Am J Vet Res* 44:1102–1105, 1983.

Herd RP, Parker CF, McClure KE: Epidemiologic approach to the control of sheep nematodes, *J Am Vet Med Assoc* 184:680–687, 1984.

Herd RP, Streitel RH, McClure KE, et al: Control of hypobiotic and benzimidazole-resistant nematodes of sheep, *J Am Vet Med Assoc* 184:726–730, 1984.

Herd RP, Streitel RH, McClure KE, et al: Control of periparturient rise in worm egg counts of lambing ewes, *J Am Vet Med Assoc* 186:375–379, 1983.

Hirth RS: *Filaroides hirthi* infection in Beagle dogs used for research, *Bull Soc Pharm Environ Path* 5:11–17, 1977.

Hirth RS, Hottendorf GH: Lesions produced by a new lungworm in Beagle dogs, *Vet Path* 10:385–407, 1973.

Hoberg EP, Alkire NL, de Queiroz A, et al: Out of Africa: origins of the *Taenia* tapeworms in humans, *Proc Roy Soc London Ser B* 268:781–787, 2001.

Hoberg EP, Zimmerman GL, Lichtenfels JR: First report of *Nematodirus battus* (Nematoda: Trichostrongyloidea) in North America: redescription and comparison to other species, *Proc Helminthol Soc Wash* 53:80–88, 1986.

Hobmaier A, Hobmaier M: Intermediate hosts of *Aelurostrongylus abstrusus* of the cat, *Proc Soc Exp Biol Med* 32:1641–1647, 1935.

Hogarth-Scott RS, Kelly JD, Whitlock HV, et al: The anthelmintic efficacy of fenbendazole against thiabendazole-resistant strains of *Haemonchus contortus* and *Trichostrongylus colubriformis* in sheep, *Res Vet Sci* 21:232–237, 1976.

Hollands RD: Autumn nematodirosis, *Vet Rec* 115:526, 1984.

Holmes DD, Kosanke SD, White GL: Fatal enterobiasis in a chimpanzee, *J Am Vet Med Assoc* 177:911–913, 1980.

Holmes RA, Klei TR, McClure JR, et al: Sequential mesenteric arteriography in pony foals during repeated inoculations of *Strongylus vulgaris* and treatment with ivermectin, *Am J Vet Res* 51:661–665, 1990.

Holzworth J, Georgi JR: Trichinosis in a cat, *J Am Vet Med Assoc* 165(2):186–191, 1974.

Hoogstraten J, Connor DH, Neafie RC: Micronemiasis. In *Pathology of tropical and extraordinary diseases,* vol 2, Washington, DC, 1976, Armed Forces Institute of Pathology.

Hoover RC, Lincoln SD, Hall RF, et al: Seasonal transmission of *Fasciola hepatica* to cattle in northwestern United States, *J Am Vet Med Assoc* 184:695–698, 1984.

Hosie BD: Autumn nematodirosis, *Vet Rec* 115:666, 1984.

Hotson IK, Campbell NJ, Smeal MG: Anthelmintic resistance in *Trichostrongylus colubriformis, Austr Vet J* 46:356–360, 1970.

Isseroff H, Sawma JT, Reino D: Fascioliasis: role of proline in bile duct hyperplasia, *Science* 198:1157–1159, 1977.

Isseroff H, Spengler RN, Charnock DR: Fascioliasis: similarities of the anemia in rats to that produced by infused proline, *J Parasitol* 65:709–714, 1979.

Jackson F, Coop RL, Jackson E, et al: Multiple anthelmintic resistant nematodes in goats, *Vet Rec* 130:210–211, 1992.

Jackson RF, Otto GF, Bauman PM, et al: Distribution of heartworms in the right side of the heart and adjacent vessels of the dog, *J Am Vet Med Assoc* 149(5):515–518, 1966.

Jackson RF, Seymour WG, Growney PJ, et al: Surgical treatment of the caval syndrome of canine heartworm disease, *J Am Vet Med Assoc* 171(10):1065–1069, 1977.

Jackson RF, von Lichtenberg F, Otto GF: Occurrence of adult heartworms in the venae cavae of dogs, *J Am Vet Med Assoc* 141(1):117–121, 1962.

James MT: *The flies that cause myiasis in man,* Washington, D.C., USDA Misc Publication 631, 1947, USDA.

Jarrett WFH, McIntyre WIM, Jennings FW, et al: The natural history of parasitic bronchitis with notes on prophylaxis and treatment, *Vet Rec* 69(49; pt I):1329, 1957.

Jasko DJ, Roth L: Granulomatous colitis associated with small strongyle larvae in a horse, *J Am Vet Med Assoc* 185:553–554, 1984.

Jemelka ED: Removal of *Setaria digitata* from the anterior chamber of the equine eye, *VM/SAC* 71:673–675, May 1976.

Jergens AA, Greve JH: Endoscopy case of the month: chronic vomiting in a dog, *Vet Med* 87:872–876, 1992.

Jones LC, Worley DE: Use of fenbendazole for long-term control of protostrongylid lungworms in free-ranging Rocky Mountain bighorn sheep, *J Wildl Dis* 33:365–367, 1997.

Kalkofen VP: Effect of dichlorvos on eggs and larvae of *Ancylostoma caninum, Am J Trop Med Hyg* 20:436–440, 1971.

Kanter M, Mott J, Ohashi N, et al: Analysis of 16S rRNA and 51-kilodalton antigen gene and transmission in mice of *Ehrlichia risticii* in virgulate trematodes from *Elimia livescens* snails in Ohio, *J Clin Microbiol* 38:3349–3358, 2000.

Karmanova EM: *Fundamentals of nematology, vol 20: dioctophymatoidea of animals and man and diseases caused by them,* Moscow, 1968, Nauka Publishers. (Translated from Russian by Amerind Publishing Co Pvt Ltd, New Delhi, 1985.)

Kates KC, Colglazier ML, Enzie FD, et al: Comparative activity of thiabendazole, levamisole, and parbendazole against natural infections of helminths in sheep, *J Parasitol* 57:356–362, 1971.

Kazacos KR: *Racoon roundworms (*Baylisascaris procyonis*): a cause of animal and human disease,* Station Bulletin No. 442, Agricultural Experiment Station, Purdue University, 1983.

Kazacos KR, Reed WM, Kazacos EA, et al: Fatal cerebrospinal disease caused by *Baylisascaris procyonis* in domestic rabbits, *J Am Vet Med Assoc* 183:967–971, 1983.

Keeling ME, McClure HM: Pneumococcal meningitis and fatal enterobiasis in a chimpanzee, *Lab Anim Sci* 24:92–95, 1974.

Kelly JD: *Canine parasitology,* New South Wales, Australia, 1977, Post-Graduate Foundation in Veterinary Science.

Kelly JD, Bain SA: Critical test evaluation of micronized mebendazole against *Anoplocephala perfoliata* in the horse, *N Z Vet J* 23:229–232, 1975.

Kelly JD, Hall CA, Whitlock HV, et al: The effect of route of administration on the anthelmintic efficacy of benzimidazole anthelmintics in sheep infected with strains of *Haemonchus contortus* and *Trichostrongylus colubriformis* resistant or susceptible to thiabendazole, *Res Vet Sci* 22:161–168, 1977.

Ketzis J, Bowman DD, Fogarty EA, et al: *Explaining premunition with kin selection,* Aug. 26, 2001. 18th International Conference of the Wold Association for the Advancement of Veterinary Parasitology, 2001, Abst. No. H5.

Kingsbury PA, Reid JFS: Anthelmintic activity of paste and drench formulations of oxfendazole in horses, *Vet Rec* 109:404–407, 1981.

Kingston N, Williams ES, Bergstrom RC, et al: Cerebral coenuriasis in domestic cats in Wyoming and Alaska, *Proc Helminthol Soc Wash* 51:309–314, 1984.

Kirby-Smith JL, Dove WE, White GF: Creeping eruption, *Arch Dermatol Syphilol* 13:137–173, 1926.

Kirkpatrick CE, Megella C: Use of ivermectin in treatment of *Aelurostrongylus abstrusus* and *Toxocara cati* infections in a cat, *J Am Vet Med Assoc* 190:1309–1310, 1987.

Kirkpatrick CE, Nelson GR: Ivermectin treatment of urinary capillariasis in a dog, *J Am Vet Med Assoc* 191:701–702, 1987.

Klei TR, Chapman MR, French DD, et al: Evaluation of ivermectin at an elevated dose against equine cyathostome larvae, *Vet Parasitol* 47:99–106, 1993.

Klei TR, Rehbein S, Visser M, et al: Reevaluation of ivermectin efficacy against equine gastrointestinal parasites, *Vet Parasitol* 98:315–320, 2001.

Klei TR, Torbert BJ, Chapman MR, et al: Efficacy of ivermectin in injectable and oral paste formulations against 8-week-old *Strongylus vulgaris* in ponies, *Am J Vet Res* 45:183–185, 1984.

Knight DH, Lok JB: *Seasonal timing of heartworm chemoprophylaxis in the United States,* March 30, 1995, Auburn, AL, Proceedings of the 1995 Heartworm Symposium, 1995, pp 37–42.

Kotake M: An experimental study on passing through the mammary gland of ascaris and hookworm larvae, *Osaka, Igakkai Zasshi* 28:1251, 1929a.

Kotake M: Hookworm larvae in the mammary gland, *Osaka, Igakkai Zasshi* 28:2493–2518, 1929b.

Kotani T, Powers KG: Developmental stages of *Dirofilaria immitis* in the dog, *Am J Vet Res* 43:2199–2206, 1982.

Kotula AW, Murrell KD, Acosta-Stein L, et al: Destruction of *Trichinella spiralis* during cooking, *J Food Sci* 48:765–768, 1983.

Kozek WJ: Transovarially-transmitted intracellular microorganizms in adult and larval stages of *Brugia malayi, J Parasitol* 63:992–1000, 1977.

Krogdahl DW, Thilsted JP, Olsen SK: Ataxia and hypermetria caused by *Parelaphostrongylus tenuis* infection in llamas, *J Am Vet Med Assoc* 190:191–193, 1987.

Kuchle M, Knorr HLJ, Medenblik-Frysch S, et al: Diffuse unilateral subacute neuroretinitis syndrome in a German most likely caused by the raccoon roundworm, *Baylisascaris procyonis, Graefe's Arch Clin Exp Ophthalmol* 231:48–51, 1993.

Kume S: Pathogenesis of allergic shock from the use of diethylcarbamazine. In Bradley RE, editor: *Canine heartworm disease,* Gainesville, 1970, University of Florida, pp 7–20.

Kume S, Itagaki S: On the life-cycle of *Dirofilaria immitis* in the dog as the final host, *Br Vet J* 111:16–24, 1955.

Kume S, Ohishi I, Kobayashi S: A new approach to prophylactic therapy against the developing stages of *Dirofilaria immitis* before reaching the canine heart, *Vet Clin North Am* 8(2):353–378, 1962a.

Kume S, Ohishi I, Kobayashi S: Prophylactic therapy against the developing stages of *Dirofilaria immitis, Am J Vet Res* 23:1257–1260, 1962b.

Kume S, Ohishi I, Kobayashi S: Extended studies on prophylactic therapy against the developing stages of *Dirofilaria immitis* in the dog, *Am J Vet Res* 25:1527–1530, 1964.

Kume S, Ohishi I, Kobayashi S: Prophylactic therapy against the developing stages of *Dirofilaria immitis:* supplemental studies, *Am J Vet Res* 28(125):975–978, 1967.

Lamb CR: What is your diagnosis? *J Small Anim Pract* 33:358, 366, 1992.

Langworthy NG, Renz A, Mackenstedt U, et al: Macrofilaricidal activity of tetracycline against the filarial nematode *Onchocerca ochengi:* elimination of *Wolbachia* precedes worm death and suggests a dependent relationship, *Proc Roy Soc Lond Ser B* 267:1063–1069, 2000.

Leathers CW, Foreyt WJ, Fetcher A, et al: Clinical fascioliasis in domestic goats in Montana, *J Am Vet Med Assoc* 180:1451–1454, 1982.

Ledet AE, Greve JH: Lungworm infection in Iowa swine, *J Am Vet Med Assoc* 148:547–549, 1966.

Le Jambre LF: Effectiveness of anthelmintic treatments against levamisole-resistant *Ostertagia, Austr Vet J* 55:65–67, 1979.

Le Jambre LF, Southcott WH, Dash KM: Resistance of selected lines of *Ostertagia circumcincta* to thiabendazole, morantel tartrate, and levamisole, *Int J Parasitol* 7:473–479, 1977.

Le Jambre LF, Southcott WH, Dash KM: Development of a simultaneous resistance in *Ostertagia circumcincta* to thiabendazole, morantel tartrate, and levamisole, *Int J Parasitol* 8:443–447, 1978a.

Le Jambre LF, Southcott WH, Dash KM: Effectiveness of broad-spectrum anthelmintics against selected strains of *Trichostrongylus colubriformis, Austr Vet J* 54:570–574, 1978b.

Levine BG, Diamond SS: Clinical experience with medical treatment for canine heartworms, *Practicing Vet* 39:136–140, 1967.

Levine ND, Clark DT: The relation of weekly pasture rotation to acquisition of gastrointestinal nematodes by sheep, *Ill Vet* 4(4):42–50, 1961.

Lichtenfels JR: *CIH keys to the nematode parasites of vertebrates. VIII. Keys to genera of the superfamilies Ancylostomatoidea, and Diaphanocephaloidea,* Farnham Royal, Bucks, England, 1980, Commonwealth Agricultural Bureaux.

Lichtenfels JR, Pilitt PA, Kotani T, et al: Morphogenesis of developmental stages of *Dirofilaria immitis* (Nematoda) in the dog, *Proc Helminthol Soc Wash* 52:98–113, 1985.

Lienert E: Hexachlorophene (G-11) is extremely efficient in cats and dogs naturally infected with the liver fluke *Opisthorchis tenuicollis* (Rudolphi, 1819) Stiles and Hassall, 1896, *Wien Tierärztl Monatschr* 49:353–359, 1962.

Lindemann BA, Evans TL, McCall JW: Clinical responses of dogs to experimentally induced *Dipetalonema reconditum* infection, *Am J Vet Res* 44:2170–2172, 1983.

Lindemann BA, McCall JW: Experimental *Dipetalonema reconditum* infections in dogs, *J Parasitol* 70:167–168, 1984.

Lindo JF, Atkins NS, Lee MG, et al: Parasite-specific serum IgG following successful treatment of endemic strongyloidiasis using ivermectin, *Trans Roy Soc Trop Med Hyg* 90:702–703, 1996.

Little MD: Comparative morphology of six species of *Strongyloides* (Nematoda) and redefinition of the genus, *J Parasitol* 52:69–84, 1966a.

Little MD: Seven new species of *Strongyloides* (Nematoda) from Louisiana, *J Parasitol* 52:85–97, 1966b.

Little MD: *Dormant Ancylostoma caninum larvae in muscle as a source of subsequent patent infection in the dog,* Fifty-third annual meeting of the American Society of Parasitology, Abstract 75, Chicago, 1978.

Loos-Frank B: One or two intermediate hosts in the life cycle of *Mesocestoides* (Cyclophyllidea, Mesocestoididae), *Parasitol Res* 77:726–728, 1991.

Love S, Biddle A: WormKill 2000, *Agnote—NSW—Agriculture,* No. DAI/118, 12 pp, 2000.

Loveless RM, Anderson FL, Ramsay MJ, et al: *Echinococcus granulosus* in dogs and sheep in central Utah, 1971–1976, *Am J Vet Res* 39:499-502, 1978.

Ludwig KG, Craig TM, Bowen JM, et al: Efficacy of ivermectin in controlling *Strongyloides westeri* infections in foals, *Am J Vet Res* 44:314–316, 1983.

Lyons ET, Drudge JH, Tolliver S: Parasites from the mare's milk, *Blood Horse* 95:2270–2271, 1969.

Lyons ET, Drudge JH, Tolliver S: On the life cycle of *Strongyloides westeri* in the equine, *J Parasitol* 59:780–787, 1973.

Lyons ET, Drudge JH, Tolliver S: Ivermectin: activity against larval *Strongylus vulgaris* and *Trichostrongylus axei* in experimental infections in ponies, *Am J Vet Res* 43:1449–1450, 1982.

Lyons ET, Tolliver SC, Drudge JH, et al: Activity of praziquantel against *Anoplocephala perfoliata* (Cestoda) in horses, *J Helm Soc Wash* 59:1–4, 1992.

Lyons ET, Tolliver SC, Drudge JH, et al: Critical test evaluation (1977–1992) of drug efficacy against endoparasites featuring benzimidazole-resistant small strongyles (population S) in Shetland ponies, *Vet Parasitol* 66:67–73, 1997a.

Lyons ET, Tolliver SC, McDowell KJ, et al: Field test of the activity of the low dose rate (2.64 mg/kg) of pyrantel tartrate on *Anoplocephala perfoliata* in thoroughbreds on a farm in central Kentucky, *J Helm Soc Wash* 64:283–285, 1997b.

Lyons ET, Tolliver SC, Drudge JH, et al: Eyeworms *(Thelazia lacrymalis)* in one- to four-year-old thoroughbreds at necropsy in Kentucky, *Am J Vet Res* 47:315–316, 1986.

Madigan JE, Pusterla N, Johnson E, et al: Transmission of *Ehrlichia risticii*, the agent of Potomac horse fever, using naturally infected aquatic insects and helminth vectors: preliminary report, *Eq Vet J* 32:275–279, 2000.

Madsen H: The life cycle of *Trichinella spiralis* (Owen, 1835) Railliet, 1896 (Syns. *T. nativa* Britov et Boev, 1972, *T. nelsoni* Britov et Boev, 1972, *T. pseudospiralis* [Garkavi, 1972]), with remarks on epidemiology and a new diagram, *Acta Parasitol Pol* 24(14):143–158, 1976.

Malone JB, Loyacano AF, Hugh-Jones ME, et al: A three-year study on seasonal transmission and control of *Fasciola hepatica* of cattle in Louisiana, *Prev Vet Med* 3:131–141, 1984.

Malone JB, Ramsey RT, Loyacano AF: Efficacy of clorsulon for treatment of mature naturally acquired and 8-week-old experimentally induced *Fasciola hepatica* infections in cattle, *Am J Vet Res* 45:851–854, 1984.

Mansfield LS, Schad GA: Ivermectin treatment of naturally acquired and experimentally induced *Strongyloides stercoralis* infections in dogs, *J Am Vet Med Assoc* 201:726–730, 1992.

Mansfield LS, Urban Jr JF: The pathogenesis of necrotic proliferative colitis in swine is linked to whipworm induced suppression of mucosal immunity to resident bacteria, *Vet Immunol Immunopathol* 50:1–17, 1996.

Martinez GMH: Tratamiento con praziquantel en la parasitosis ocasionada por *Thysanosoma actinoides* en borregos, *Vet Mex* 15:230, 1984.

Martins MWS, Aston G, Simpson VR, et al: Angiostrongylosis in Cornwall: clinical presentation of eight cases, *J Small Anim Pract* 34:20–25, 1993.

Mason KV: Canine neural angiostrongylosis: the clinical and therapeutic features of 55 natural cases, *Aust Vet J* 64:201–203, 1987.

Mayhew IG, deLahunta A, Georgi JR, et al: Naturally occurring cerebrospinal parelaphostrongylosis, *Cornell Vet* 66(1):56–72, 1976.

McCoy OR: The influence of temperature, hydrogen-ion concentration and oxygen tension on the development of the eggs and larvae of the dog hookworm *Ancylostoma caninum*, *Am J Hyg* 11:413–448, 1930.

McCraw BM, Slocombe JOD: Early development of and pathology associated with *Strongylus edentatus*, *Can J Comp Med* 38:124–138, 1974.

McCraw BM, Slocombe JOD: *Strongylus edentatus:* development and lesions from ten weeks postinfection to patency, *Can J Comp Med* 42:340–356, 1978.

McKellar Q, Bairden K, Duncan JL, et al: Change in *N. battus* epidemiology, *Vet Rec* 113:309, 1983.

McKenna DB: Anthelmintic resistance in cattle nematodes in New Zealand: is it increasing? *N Z Vet J* 44:76, 1996.

McTier TL, Shanks DJ, Wren JA, et al: Efficacy of selamectin against experimentally induced and naturally acquired infections of *Toxocara cati* and *Ancylostoma tubaeforme* in cats, *Vet Parasitol* 91:311–319, 2000.

McTier TL, Siedek EM, Clemence RG, et al: Efficacy of selamectin against experimentally induced and naturally acquired ascarid (*Toxocara canis* and *Toxascaris leonina*) infections in dogs, *Vet Parasitol* 91:333–345, 2000.

Mello EBF, Maia AAM, Mello LAP: Localizacao do *Dipetalonema reconditum* (Grassi, 1890) (Nematoda: Filariidae) de *Canis familiaris, Braz J Vet Res Anim Sci* 31:9–11, 1994.

Michel JF, Richards M, Altman JFB, et al: Effect of anthelmintic treatment on the milk yield of dairy cows in England, Scotland, and Wales, *Vet Rec* 111:546–550, 1982.

Migaud P, Marty C, Chartier C: Quel es votre diagnostic? *Point Vet* 23:989–991, 1992.

Milks HJ: A preliminary report on verminous bronchitis in dogs, *Cornell Vet* 6(1):50–55, 1916.

Miller WR, Merton DA: Dirofilariasis in a ferret, *J Am Vet Med Assoc* 180:1103–1104, 1982.

Mirck MH: Cyathostominose: een vorm van ernstige strongylidose, *Tijdschr Diergeneesk* 102(15):932–934, 1977.

Monahan CM, Chapman MR, French DD, et al: Efficacy of moxidectin oral gel against *Onchocerca cervicalis* microfilariae, *J Parasitol* 81:117–118, 1995.

Moncol DJ: Supplement to the life history of *Strongyloides ransomi* Schwartz and Alicata, 1930 (Nematoda: Strongyloididae) of pigs, *Proc Helminth Soc Wash* 42:86–92, 1975.

Moncol DJ, Batte EG: Transcolostral infection of newborn pigs with *Strongyloides ransomi, Vet Med/SAC* 61:583–586, 1966.

Moravec F: Proposal of a new systematic arrangement of nematodes of the family Capillariidae, *Folia Parasitol* 29:119–132, 1982.

Moravec F, Prokopic J, Shlikas AV: The biology of nematodes of the family Capillaridae Neveu-Lemaire, 1936, *Fol Parasitol* 34:39–56, 1987.

Moreland AF, Battles AH, Nease JH: Dirofilariasis in a ferret, *J Am Vet Med Assoc* 188:864, 1986.

Msolla P: Bovine parasitic otitis: an up-to-date review, *Vet Ann* 1989:2973–2977, 1989.

Mueller JF: The biology of *Spirometra, J Parasitol* 60:3–14, 1974.

Mueller JF, Coulston F: Experimental human infection with the sparganum larva of *Spirometra mansonoides* (Mueller, 1935), *Am J Trop Med* 2:399–425, 1941.

Murrell KD, Eriksen L, Nansen P, et al: *Ascaris suum;* a revision of its early migratory path and implications for human ascariasis, *J Parasitol* 83:255–260, 1997.

Myers RK, Monroe WE, Greve JH: Cerebrospinal nematodiasis in a cockatiel, *J Am Vet Med Assoc* 183:1089–1090, 1983.

Nakamura Y, Tsuji N, Taira N, et al: Parasitic females of *Strongyloides papillosus* as a pathogenic stage for sudden cardiac death in infected lambs, *J Vet Med Sci* 56:723–727, 1994.

Nelson GS: *Dipetalonema reconditum* (Grassi, 1889) from the dog with a note on its development in the flea, *Ctenodephalides felis* in the louse, *Heterodoxus spiniger, J Helminthol* 36:297–308, 1962.

New D, Little MD, Cross J: *Angiostrongylus cantonensis* infection from eating raw snails, *New Engl J Med* 332:1105–1106, 1995.

Nevill EM: Preliminary report on the transmission of *Parafilaria bovicola* in South Africa, *Onderstepoort J Vet Res* 41:41–48, 1975.

Nevill EM: The epidemiology of *Parafilaria bovicola* in the Transvaal Bushveld of South Africa, *Onderstepoort J Vet Res* 52:261–267, 1985.

Nichols DK, Montali RJ, Phillips LG, et al: *Parelaphostrongylus tenuis* in captive reindeer and sable antelope, *J Am Vet Med Assoc* 188:619–621, 1986.

Ogbourne CP, Duncan JL: *Strongylus vulgaris* in the horse: its biology and veterinary importance, CIH Misc Pub No 4, Farnham Royal, Slough, England, 1977, Commonwealth Agricultural Bureaux.

Orihel TC: Morphology of the larval stages of *Dirofilaria immitis* in the dog, *J Parasitol* 47:252–262, 1961.

Pal RN, Biswas PK, Gupta ID: Effective treatment of stephanofilarial dermatitis in cattle, *Trop Agric (Trinidad)* 66:176–177, 1989.

Palsson PA: Echinococcosis and its elimination in Iceland, *Hist Med Vet* 1:4–10, 1976.

Park SY, Glase C, Murray WJ, et al: Raccoon roundworm *(Baylisascaris procyonis)* encephalitis: case report and field investigation, *Pediatrics* 106:1–5, 2000.

Parrott TY, Greiner EC, Parrott JD: *Dirofilaria immitis* infection in three ferrets, *J Am Vet Med Assoc* 184:582–583, 1984.

Patteson MW, Gibbs C, Wotton PR, et al: *Angiostrongylus vasorum* infection in seven dogs, *Vet Rec* 133:565–570, 1993.

Patton S, Faulkner CT: Prevalence of *Dirofilaria immitis* and *Dipetalonema reconditum* infection in dogs: 805 cases (1980–1989), *J Am Vet Med Assoc* 200:1533–1534, 1992.

Pauli B, Althaus S, Von Tscharner C: Über die Organisation von Thromben nach Arterienverletzungen durch wandernde 4. Larvenstadien von *Strongylus vulgaris* beim Pferd (licht- und elektronmikroscopische Untersuchungen), *Beitr Pathol* 155:357–378, 1975.

Peterson EN, Barr SC, Gould WJ, et al: Use of fenbendazole for treatment of *Crenosoma vulpis* infection in a dog, *J Am Vet Med Assoc* 202:1483–1484, 1993.

Pienaar JG, Basson PA, du Plessis JL, et al: Experimental studies with *Strongyloides papillosus* in goats, *Onderst J Vet Res* 66:191–235, 1999.

Ploeger HW, Kloosterman A, Bargeman G, et al: Milk yield increases after anthelmintic treatment of dairy cattle related to some parameters estimating helminth infection, *Vet Parasitol* 35:103–116, 1990.

Ploeger HW, Schoenmaker GJW, Kloosterman A, et al: Effect of anthelmintic treatment of dairy cattle on milk production related to some parameters estimating nematode infection, *Vet Parasitol* 34:239–253, 1989.

Polley L, Creighton SR: Experimental direct transmission of the lungworm, *Filaroides osleri* in dogs, *Vet Rec* 100:136–137, 1977.

Potter ME, Kruse MB, Matthews MA, et al: A sausage-associated outbreak of trichinosis in Illinois, *Am J Public Health* 66(12):194–1196, 1976.

Poynter D: Parasitic bronchitis, *Adv Parasitol* 1:179–212, 1963.

Pozio E, LaRosa G, Murrell KD, et al: Taxonomic revision of the genus *Trichinella*, *J Parasitol* 78:654–659, 1992.

Prociv P, Croese J: Human enteric infection with *Ancylostoma caninum*: hookworms reappraised in the light of a "new" zoonosis, *Acta Tropica* 62:23–44, 1996.

Proudman CJ, Edwards GB: Are tapeworms associated with equine colic? A case control study, *Eq Vet J* 25:224–226, 1993.

Proudman CJ, French NP, Trees AJ: Tapeworm infection is a significant risk factor for spasmodic colic and ileal impaction colic in the horse, *Eq Vet J* 30:194–199, 1993.

Pugh RE: Effects on the development of *Dipylidium caninum* and on the host reaction to this parasite in the adult flea *(Ctenocephalides felis felis)*, *Parasitol Res* 73:171–177, 1987.

Pusterla N, Johnson E, Chae JS, et al: Molecular detection of an *Ehrlichia*-like agent in rainbow trout *(Oncorhynchus mykiss)* from northern California, *Vet Parasitol* 92:199–207, 2000.

Rawlings CA, Dawe DL, McCall JW, et al: Four types of occult *Dirofilaria immitis* infection in dogs, *J Am Vet Med Assoc* 180:1323–1326, 1982.

Rawlings CA, Raynaud JP, Lewis RE, et al: Pulmonary thromboembolism and hypertension after thiacetarsamide vs. melarsomine dihydrochloride treatment of *Dirofilaria immitis* infection in dogs, *Am J Vet Res* 54:920–925, 1993.

Rebhun WC, Mirro EJ, Georgi ME, et al: Habronemic conjunctivitis in horses, *J Am Vet Med Assoc* 179:469–472, 1981.

Reinemeyer CR: Prevention of parasitic gastroenteritis in dairy replacement heifers, *Comp Cont Ed Pract Vet* 12:761–766, 1990.

Reinemeyer CR: Should you deworm your client's dairy cattle? *Vet Med* 90:496–502, 1995.

Rendano VT, Georgi JR, Fahnestock GR, et al: *Filaroides hirthi* lungworm infection in dogs: its radiographic appearance, *Vet Radiol* 20:2–9, 1979b.

Rendano VT, Georgi JR, White KK, et al: Equine verminous arteritis: an arteriographic evaluation of the larvicidal activity of albendazole, *Equine Vet J* 11:223–231, 1979a.

Rodger JL: Change in *N. battus* epidemiology, *Vet Rec* 112:261, 1983.

Roepstorff A, Murrell KD: Transmission dynamics of helminth parasites of pigs on continuous pasture: *Oesophagostomum dentatum* and *Hyostrongylus rubidus*, *Int J Parasitol* 27:553–562, 1997.

Rolfe PF, Boray JC: Chemotherapy of paramphistomiasis in cattle, *Aust Vet J* 64:328–334, 1987.

Rolfe PF, Boray JC: Comparative efficacy of moxidectin, and ivermectin/clorsulon combination, and closantel against immature paramphistomes in cattle, *Aust Vet J* 70:265–266, 1993.

Rommel M, Grelck H, Hörchner F: Zür Wirksamkeit von Praziquantel gegen Bandwürmer in experimentell infizierten Hunden und Katzen, *Ber Münch Tierärtzl Wochenschr* 89:255–257, 1976.

Ronald NC, Craig TM: Fenbendazole for the treatment of *Heterobilharzia Americana* infection in dogs, *J Am Vet Med Assoc* 182:172, 1983.

Rossi L, Peruccio C: Thelaziosi oculare nel canei aspetti clinici e terapeutici, *Veterinaria* 3:47–50, 1989.

Rossoff IS: *Handbook of veterinary drugs,* New York, 1974, Springer, p 215.

Roth L, Georgi ME, King JM, et al: Parasitic encephalitis due to *Baylisascaris* sp. in wild and captive woodchucks *(Marmota monax)*, *Vet Pathol* 19:658–662, 1982.

Rothstein N: Canine microfilariasis in sentry dogs in the United States, *J Parasitol* 49(5 sect 2):49, 1963.

Roudebush P, Schmidt DA: Fenbendazole for treatment of pancreatic fluke infection in a cat, *J Am Vet Med Assoc* 180:545–546, 1982.

Rousselot R, Pellissier A: III. Oesophagostomose nodulaire à *Oesophagostomum stephanostomum* du gorille et du chimpanzee, *Soc Path Exotique Bull* 45(4):568–574, 1952.

Russell AF: The development of helminthiasis in thoroughbred foals, *J Comp Pathol* 58:107–127, 1948.

Ryff JF, Browne JO, Stoddard HL, et al: Removal of the fringed tapeworm from sheep, *J Am Vet Med Assoc* 117:471–473, 1950.

Sakamoto T: The anthelmintic effect of Droncit on adult tapeworms of *Hydatigera taeniaeformis, Mesocestoides corti, Echinococcus multilocularis, Diphyllobothrium erinacei*, and *D. latum, Vet Med Rev* 1:64–74, 1977.

Santen DR, Chastain CB, Schmidt DA: Efficacy of pyrantel pamoate against *Physaloptera* in a cat, *J Am Anim Hosp Assoc* 29:53–55, 1993.

Santiago MAM, Costa VC, Benevenga SF: *Trichostrongylus colubriformis* resistante ao levamisole, *Rev Centro Ciencias Rurais* 7:421–422, 1977.

Santiago MAM, Costa VC, Benevenga SF: Antivadade anti-helmintica do dl-tetramisole e do thibendazole uma estirpe do *Trichostrongylus colubriformis* resistente ao levamisole, *Rev Centro Cienias Rurais* 8:257–261, 1978.

Schad GA: Experimentally induced arrested development of parasite larvae of hookworms, *Proc 3rd Int Congr Parasitol* 2:772–773, 1974.

Schad GA: *Ancylostoma duodenale:* maintenance through six generations of helminth-naive pups, *Exptl Parasitol* 47:246–253, 1979.

Schad GA, Hellman ME, Muncey DW: *Strongyloides stercoralis:* hyperinfection in immunosuppressed dogs, *Exp Parasitol* 57:287–296, 1984.

Schad GA, Page MR: *Ancylostoma canium:* adult worm removal, corticosteroid treatment, and resumed development of arrested larvae in dogs, *Exptl Parasitol* 54:303–309, 1982.

Schmid K, Düwel D: Zum Einsatz von Fenbendazol (Panacur Tableten ad us. vet.) gegen Helminthenbefall bei Katzen, *Tierartzl Umschau* 45:868–870, 873–875, 1980.

Schmidt RE, Prine JR: Severe enterobiasis in a chimpanzee, *Pathologia Veterinaria (Vet Path)* 7:56–59, 1970.

Schnieder T, Lechler M, Epe C, et al: The efficacy of doramectin on arrested larvae of *Ancylostoma* in early pregnancy of bitches, *J Vet Med B* 43:351–356, 1996.

Schusser G, Kopf N, Prosl H: Dünndarmverstopfung (Obturatio intestini jejuni) bei einem fünf Monate alten Traber-hengstfohlen durch Askariden nach Eingabe eines Anthelmintikums, *Wien Tierärtzl Mschr* 75:152–156, 1988.

Seneviratna P, Fernando ST, Dhanapala SB: Disophenol treatment of spirocercosis in dogs, *J Am Vet Med Assoc* 148:269–274, 1966.

Shinonaga S, Miyamoto K, Kano R, et al: *Musca hervie* Villeneuve, 1922 as an intermediate host of eyeworms (*Thelazia*) in Japan, *J Med Entomol* 11:595–598, 1974.

Shoop WL: Resistance to avermectins and milbemycins, *Vet Rec* 130:563, 1992 (correspondence)

Shoop WL, Corkum KC: Transmammary infection of newborn by larval trematodes, *Science* 223:1082–1083, 1984.

Shoop WL, Egerton JR, Eary CH, et al: *Control of* Toxocara canis *transmission from bitch to offspring with ivermectin*, Sixty-third annual meeting of the American Society of Parasitologists, Program and Abstracts, 1988, pp 59–60.

Slocombe JOD: Prevalence and treatment of tapeworms in horses, *Can Vet J* 20:136–140, 1979.

Slocombe JOD, Bhactendu-Srivastava B, Surgeoner GA: *The transmission period for heartworm in Canada,* March 31, 1995, Auburn, AL, Proceedings of the 1995 Heartworm Symposium, pp 43–48.

Slocombe JOD, McCraw BM: Evaluation of pyrantel pamoate, nitramisole, and avermectin B1a against migrating *Strongylus vulgaris* larvae, *Can J Comp Med* 44:93–100, 1980.

Slocombe JOD, McCraw BM: Controlled tests of ivermectin against migrating *Strongylus vulgaris* in ponies, *Am J Vet Res* 42:1050–1051, 1981.

Slocombe JOD, McCraw BM, Pennock PW, et al: Effectiveness of fenbendazole against later fourth-stage Strongylus vulgaris in ponies, *Am J Vet Res* 44:2285–2289, 1983.

Slocombe JOD, McCraw BM, Pennock PW, et al: Effectiveness of oxfendazole against early and later fourth-stage *Strongylus vulgaris* in ponies, *Am J Vet Res* 47:495–500, 1986.

Slocombe JOD, McCraw BM, Pennock PW, et al: Effectiveness of ivermectin against later fourth-stage *Strongylus vulgaris* in ponies, *Am J Vet Res* 43:1525–1529, 1982.

Slocombe JOD, Rendano VT, Owen RR, et al: Arteriography in ponies with *Strongylus vulgaris* arteriti, *Can J Comp Med* 41(2):137–145, 1977.

Smeal MG, Gough PA, Jackson AR, et al: The occurrence of *Haemonchus contortus* resistant to thiabendazole, *Austr Vet J* 44:108–109, 1968.

Smith MC, Bailey CS, Baker N, et al: Cerebral coenurosis in a cat, *J Am Vet Med Assoc* 192:82–84, 1988.

Sprent JFA: The life history and development of Toxocara cati (Schrank, 1788) in the domestic cat, Parasitology 46(1-2): 54–58, 1956.

Sprent JFA: Observations on the development of *Toxocara canis* (Werner, 1782) in the dog, *Parasitology* 48(1-2):184–209, 1958.

Sprent JFA: Post-parturient infection of the bitch with *Toxocara canis, J Parasitol* 47:284, 1961.

Stewart DF: Studies on the resistance of sheep to infestation with *Haemonchus contortus* and *Trichostrongylus* spp. and on the immunological reactions of sheep exposed to infestation. IV. The antibody response to natural infestation in grazing sheep and the "self-cure" phenomenon, *Aust J Agr Res* 1:427–439, 1950.

Stewart DF: Studies on the resistance of sheep to infestation with *Haemonchus contortus* and *Trichostrongylus* spp. and on the immunological reactions of sheep exposed to infestation. V. The nature of the "self-cure" phenomenon, *Aust J Agr Res* 4:100–117, 1953.

Stockdale PHG, Smart ME: Treatment of crenosomiasis in dogs, *Res Vet Sci* 18:178–181, 1975.

Stoll NR: Studies with the strongyloid nematode *Haemonchus contortus.* I. Acquired resistance of hosts under natural rein-fection conditions out-of-doors, *Am J Hyg* 10:384–418, 1929.

Stone WM, Girardeau MH: *Ancylostoma caninum* larvae present in the colostrum of a bitch, *Vet Rec* 79(24):773–774, 1966.

Stone WM, Girardeau MH: Transmammary passage of *Ancylostoma caninum* larvae in dogs, *J Parasitol* 54:426–429, 1968.

Stoye M: Untersuchungen über die Möglichkeit Pränataler und galaktogener Infecktionen mit *Ancylostoma caninum* Ercolani, 1859 (Ancylostomidae) beim Hund, *Zentralbl Vet Med Series B* 20(1):1–39, 1973.

Stoye M, Meyer O, Schneider T: Zur Wirkung von Ivermectin auf reaktiverte somatische Larven von *Ancylostoma caninum* Ercolani 1858 (Ancylostomatidae) in der graviden Hünden, *J Vet Med B* 34:13–21, 1987.

Stromberg BE, Schlotthauer JC, Seibert BP, et al: Activity of closantel against experimentally induced *Fascioloides magna* infection in sheep, *Am J Vet Res* 46:2527–2529, 1985.

Summa MEL, Ebisui L, Osaka JT, et al: Efficacy of oral ivermectin against *Trichosomoides crassicauda* in naturally infected laboratory rats, *Lab Anim Sci* 42:620–622, 1992.

Supperer R: *Capillaria böhmi* spec. nov., eine neue Haarwurm Art aus den Stirnhöhles des Fuchses, *Zeitschrift für Parasitenkunde* 16:51–55, 1953.

Swerczek TW, Nielsen SW, Helmbolt CF: Transmammary passage of *Toxocara cati* in the cat, *Am J Vet Res* 32:89–92, 1971.

Theodorides VJ, Free SM: Effects of anthelmintic treatment on milk yield, *Vet Rec* 113:248, 1983.

Theodorides VJ, Freeman JF, Georgi JR: Anthelmintic activity of albendazole against *Dicrocoelium dendriticum* in sheep, *Vet Med/SAC* 77:569–570, 1982.

Theodorides VJ, Scott GC, Laderman M: Strains of *Haemonchus contortus* resistant against benzimidazole anthelmintics, *Am J Vet Res* 31:859–863, 1970.

Thomas H, Gönnert R: The efficacy of praziquantel against cestodes in cats, dogs, and sheep, *Res Sci* 24:20–25, 1978.

Thomas RJ, Stevens AJ: Some observations on *Nematodirus* disease in Northumberland and Durham, *Vet Rec* 68:471–475, 1956.

Tindall B: *Fasciola hepatica*, this fluke is no fluke, *Animal Nutrition & Health* 40:6, 10–11, 1985.

Triantophyllou AC, Moncol DJ: Cytology, reproduction, and sex determination of *Strongyloides ransomi* and *S. papillosus*, *J Parasitol* 63(6):961–973, 1977.

Underwood JR: Habronemiasis, *Vet Bull* 30:16–28, 1936.

Underwood PC, Harwood PD: Survival and location of the microfilariae of *Dirofilaria immitis* in the dog, *J Parasitol* 25:23–33, 1939.

Urquhart GM, Jarrett WHF, O'Sullivan JG: Canine tracheobronchitis due to infection with *Filaroides osleri*, *Vet Rec* 66(10):143–145, 1954.

Valet-Picavet S: Une bronchite tres "verminuese" ou filaroidose a *Oslerus osleri chez* un chien, *Action Vet* 1157:19–22, 1991.

Vassiliades G, Bouffet P, Friot D, et al: Traitement de la thelaziose oculaire bovine au Senegal, *Rev Elev Med Vet Pays Trop* 28:315–317, 1975.

Vermunt JJ, West DM, Pomroy WE: Multiple resistance to ivermectin and oxfendazole in *Cooperia* species of cattle in New Zealand, *Vet Rec* 137:43–45, 1995.

Verster A: A taxonomic revision of the genus *Taenia* Linnaeus, 1758, *Onderstepoort J Vet Res* 36:3–58, 1969

Vikram-Khoshoo, Craver R, Schantz P, et al: Abdominal pain, pangut eosinophilia, and a dog hookworm infection, *J Ped Gastroent Nutr* 21:481, 1995.

Wade SE: *Capillaria xenopodis* sp. n. (Nematoda: Trichuroidea) from the epidermis of the South African clawed frog (*Xenopus laevis*, Daudin), *Proc Helm Soc Wash* 49:86–92, 1982.

Wallace GW: Swine influenza and lungworms, *J Infect Dis* 135:490–492, 1977 (editorial).

Walsh TA, Younis PJ, Morton TM: The effect of ivermectin treatment of late pregnant dairy cows in southwest Victoria on subsequent milk production and reproductive performance, *Aust Vet J* 72:201–207, 1995.

Wardle RA, McLeod JA: *The zoology of tapeworms*, Minneapolis, 1952, University of Minnesota Press.

Watts KJ, Reddy GR, Holmes RA, et al: Seasonal prevalence of third-stage larvae of *Dirofilaria immitis* in mosquitoes from Florida and Louisiana, *J Parasitol* 87:322–329, 2001.

Wetzel R: Zür Entwicklung des grossen Palisadenwurmes (*Strongylus equinus*) im Pferde, *Arch für Wissench Tierheilk* 76:81–118, 1940a.

Wetzel R: Zür Biologie des Fuchslungenwurmes *Crenosoma vulpis*, *Archiv fur Wissenschaftl und Praktische Tierheilk* 75:445–460, 1940b.

Wetzel R, Kersten W: Die Leberphase der Entwicklung von *Strongylus edentatus, Wien Tierztl Monatsch* 43:664–673, 1956.

Wheat JD: Treatment of equine summer sores with a systemic insecticide, *Vet Med* 56:477–478, 1961.

White GF, Dove WE: *Dogs and cats concerned in the causation of creeping eruption,* Official Record, vol 5, No 43, 1926, USDA, Beltsville, MD.

Whitlock JH: The relationship of the available natural milk supply to the production of the trichostrongylidoses in sheep, *Cornell Vet* 41:299–311, 1951.

Whitlock JH: *Trichostrongylidosis in sheep and cattle,* Proceedings of the ninety-second annual meeting of American Veterinary Medical Association, 1955a, pp 123–131.

Whitlock JH: A study of the inheritance of resistance to trichostrongylidosis in sheep, *Cornell Vet* 45(3):422–439, 1955b.

Whitlock JH: The inheritance of resistance to trichostrongylidosis in sheep. I. Demonstration of the validity of the phenomenon, *Cornell Vet* 48(2):127–133, 1958.

Whitlock JH: *Diagnosis of veterinary parasitisms,* Philadelphia, 1960, Lea & Febiger.

Whitlock JH: Biology of a nematode. In Soulsby, EJL, editor: *Biology of parasites,* New York, 1966, Academic Press.

Willard MD, Roberts RE, Allison N, et al: Diagnosis of *Aelurostrongylus abstrusus* and *Dirofilaria immitis* infections in cats from a humane shelter, *J Am Vet Med Assoc* 192:913–916, 1988.

Williams JC, Knox JW, Sheehan D, et al: Efficacy of albendazole against inhibited early fourth-stage larvae of *Ostertagia ostertagi*, *Vet Rec* 101:484–486, 1977.

Williams JF, Keahey KK: Sudden death associated with treatment of three dogs with bunamidine hydrochloride, *J Am Vet Med Assoc* 168:689–691, 1976.

Williams JF, Lindemann B, Padgett GA, et al: Angiostrongylosis in a greyhound, *J Am Vet Med Assoc* 10:1101–1102, 1985b.

Williams JF, Lindsay M, Engelkirk P: Peritoneal cestodiasis in a dog, *J Am Vet Med Assoc* 186:1103-1104, 1985a.

Williams JF, Shearer AM: *Taenia taeniaeformis* in cats, *J Am Vet Med Assoc* 181:386, 1982.

Woodruff AW, Burg OA: Prevalence of infective ova of *Toxocara* species in public places, *Br Med J* 4:470–472, 1973.

Wright WH, Bozicevich J, Underwood PC: Critical experiments with carbon bisulphide in the treatment of habronemiasis, *J Roy Army Vet Corps* 2:66–70, 1931.

Xiao LH, Herd RP, Majewski GA: Comparative efficacy of moxidectin and ivermectin against hypobiotic and encysted cyathostomes and other equine parasites, *Vet Parasitol* 53:83–90, 1994.

Yakstis JJ, Egerton JR, Campbell WC, et al: Use of thiabendazole-medicated feed for prophylaxis of four common roundworm infections in dogs, *J Parasitol* 54:359–369, 1968.

Yazwinski TA, Kilgore RL, Presson BL, et al: Efficacy of oral clorsulon in treatment of *Fasciola hepatica* infections in calves, *Am J Vet Res* 46:163–164, 1985.

Yorke W, Maplestone PA: *The nematode parasites of vertebrates,* Philadelphia, 1926, P. Blakiston's Son & Co.

Zimmerman GL, Hoberg EP, Rickard LG, et al: *Broadened geographic range and periods of transmission for Nematodirus battus in the United States,* Proceedings from the eighty-ninth annual meeting of the U.S. Animal Health Association, Louisville, Ky, 1986.

Zimmermann WJ: Evaluation of microwave cooking procedures and ovens for devitalizing trichinae in pork roasts, *J Food Sci* 48:856–860, 1983.

CHAPTER 4

ANTIPARASITIC DRUGS

RANDY CARL LYNN

A parasiticide is a poison that is more toxic to parasites than to their hosts. The degree of discrimination is sometimes small, sometimes considerable, but never complete, so that application of parasiticides always entails some hazard to the host. As a matter of fact, it is sometimes easier to explain the deleterious effects that parasiticides frequently exert on the host than to explain how they kill parasites.

Stages in the development of a typical insecticide or anthelmintic proceed approximately as follows. First, many thousands of compounds usually must be screened before one is found that shows promise. The screening procedure, in the case of an anthelmintic, could require the demonstration of in vivo activity against some convenient parasite (e.g., *Nematospiroides dubius, Nippostrongylus brasiliensis, Syphacia obvelata,* or *Hymenolepis nana* of laboratory rodents; *Ascaridia galli* or *Heterakis gallinarum* of chickens). Recently, in vitro assays have been developed that allow rapid screening of large numbers of potential agents (Londershausen, 1996). A preliminary estimate of mammalian toxicity is also obtained from experiments on rats and mice.

The activity screening tests and preliminary toxicity studies greatly reduce the list of suitable candidates, but are of little value in predicting the effect of a particular drug either on a particular species of domestic animal or on its customary assemblage of parasites. Responses of various species and strains of parasites and their hosts to antiparasitic agents are sometimes quite selective. Thus ascarids are very sensitive to piperazines, whereas hookworms are quite refractory. Most breeds of cattle and dogs tolerate judicious applications of organophosphate insecticides, whereas Brahman cattle, greyhounds, and whippet dogs are likely to be fatally intoxicated by such treatment. The necessary information can be obtained only through experiments on domestic animals and the parasites for which the anthelmintic is intended.

When a manufacturing firm files a New Animal Drug Application with the Food and Drug Administration (FDA), it must submit complete information on its chemistry, process of manufacture, and quantitative assay methods. Results of all experiments conducted to establish the safety and efficacy of the new product and all relevant published reports must also be submitted. Drugs intended for food animals must be accompanied by data on tissue residues and the route and rate of excretion of the parent compound and its major metabolites. The amount and the structures of the longest-lasting tissue residue also must be determined, and if the substance has similarities to known carcinogenic chemicals, a 2-year toxicity experiment is then required in rats and mice.

The Environmental Protection Agency (EPA) requires an environmental impact analysis of the new compound. Phytotoxicity and the effects on fish and other lower animals also must be vigorously studied. A thorough analysis must be conducted to establish any potential effects on workers who apply the product. Worker safety must also be addressed, so that the appropriate safety measures (e.g., gloves, safety glasses) can be written into the instructions.

Before a new anthelmintic or any new parasiticide can be approved, well-controlled experiments must be carried out involving slaughter of the test animals and determination of residual worm burdens after treatment. Confirmation experiments must be conducted by several independent laboratories as a series of field tests in different geographic regions of the United States.

The package label is required by law to bear all the necessary cautions and to notify the user about all adverse reactions that have been discovered. Six months after a product enters the market and at regular intervals thereafter, the manufacturer is required to report to the FDA any adverse reactions that have come to light and to add appropriate notices to the label or withdraw the product from the marketplace. As a result, the label (or package insert) has become one of the most objective and current sources of information on parasiticides.

In the early phases of new product development, the molecule is usually identified by only a code number, S-147 for example. This is to keep the hundreds of thousands of potential products separate and to avoid the trouble of naming each one. Once the product clears the early hurdles of activity and safety, it is given a nonproprietary (generic) name. The nonproprietary name is used in the scientific literature worldwide to identify the molecule. Thus S-147 now becomes milbemycin oxime. As product development proceeds, the marketing staff develops a trade name. This name will be trademarked and applied to a specific formulation. At this point milbemycin oxime becomes Interceptor.

One molecule may have several different trade names that correspond to different formulations or to different countries. For example, milbemycin oxime is marketed and sold as Interceptor for internal parasite control and in combination with lufenuron as Sentinel. These trade names will be used in the advertising and promotion of the product. In this text the nonproprietary name will be used to identify the products, and some of the trade names will be mentioned.

Resistance to Parasiticides

Regular application of antiparasitic drugs to populations of parasites inevitably results in the development of resistant parasite populations through selection of resistant phenotypes. Eventually, the once-effective drug ceases to work and must be replaced by another.

Unfortunately, the replacement also may fail against the resistant strain, especially if it is a chemical congener of the original. This has happened often enough to serve us warning. We need to develop better ways of controlling parasites than to lash away at them crudely and blindly with one chemical after another.

The literature on antiparasitic drugs is enormous. In the interests of both economy and readability, we have tried to list the few references that will guide the veterinarian who needs more specific information about these agents.

It is important to note here whom one calls when potential adverse reactions or problems arise. The American Society for the Prevention of Cruelty to Animals (ASPCA) National Animal Poison Control Center is probably the best staffed and has the largest database available for consultation. They charge a small consultation fee for each case and can be reached at 800-548-2423. The manufacturer of the product also can be consulted and is required by law to notify federal authorities concerning all adverse reactions. The manufacturer may also be prepared to provide assistance in investigating and treating any adverse event.

■ INSECTICIDES

The Federal Environmental Pesticide Control Act (FEPCA) of 1972 is administered by the EPA, which controls the distribution, sale, and use of pesticides within each state and between states. This act even specifies what penalties may be imposed for the misuse of pesticides. State governments may establish even stricter standards than those set by the FEPCA.

Users of pesticides bear a legal responsibility in the United States for knowing which chemicals they are currently permitted to use and for using these chemicals only in strict accordance with the indications and directions on the package labels. Current information on pesticides should be sought from the pesticide coordinator, extension entomologist with livestock responsibility, or extension veterinarian appointed by the state agricultural extension services and land grant colleges.

The diversity of structure, biological activity, and toxicity among insecticides is exceeded only by the number and variety of insects, mites, and ticks that are trying to be controlled. The label of every insecticide container must be read carefully and understood before the contents are applied to the animal. The label is the most up-to-date and authoritative source of information available (Entriken, 2001). In addition, there are several good review texts that discuss the chemistry, mode of action, and toxicity of insecticides (Coats, 1982; Fest and Schmidt, 1982; Hassall, 1982; Ware, 1983; Ware, 1986; Hayes and Laws, 1991; Plapp, 1991).

The treatment of insecticidal overdose or toxicity is a complex subject, which lies outside the scope of this chapter. A few general comments, however, are included about treatment of affected patients.

For more specific up-to-date information, the veterinarian should consult the ASPCA National Animal Poison Control Center at 800-548-2423. They maintain a 24-hour service staffed with veterinary toxicologists to consult about animal poisoning of any type.

Botanicals

The botanical insecticides are derived from plant materials. Ground plant parts (e.g., flowers, leaves, stems, roots) or their extracts may be combined in a variety of formulations. Essential oils from plants are often used as insect attractants or repellents. Botanical insecticides, particularly pyrethrins, have excellent toxic effects against a variety of crop and animal insect pests, very short persistence in the environment, and relatively low toxicity to animals. Pyrethroids are synthetic pyrethrum-like compounds with superior potency and knockdown activity. Rotenone is an insecticidal product obtained from the roots of several plants.

Rotenone

Rotenone was first used by natives in South America to paralyze fish, causing them to surface. In the 1800s it was first used to control leaf-eating caterpillars. Rotenone is the insecticidal component of derris root, cube root, and several other leguminous shrubs. It acts as an inhibitor of mitochondrial respiratory enzymes. Rotenone is insoluble in water but very soluble in alcohols, acetone, carbon tetrachloride, chloroform, and many other organic solvents. It decomposes on exposure to light and air. The oral median lethal dose (LD_{50}) of rotenone for rats is 133 mg/kg and for white mice, 350 mg/kg, but it is toxic to fish. Rotenone, alone or synergized, is the main insecticidal ingredient in Hilo Dip and Good-winol Ointment. It may be applied to cats and dogs as an ointment or dip or in liquid form for the control of a variety of arthropod parasitism including localized demodicosis in dogs and ear mites in cats.

WARNING: Kittens younger than 4 weeks and suckling puppies should not be treated with rotenone products. Rotenone is toxic to swine, fish, and snakes and should not be applied to these animals. Cats and dogs may vomit after licking rotenone from their coats. It may be carcinogenic in rats.

Pyrethrins

The flower head of the pyrethrum plant *Chrysanthemum cinerariaefolium* contains six closely related insecticidal substances (pyrethrin I and II, cinerin I and II, jasmolin I and II) that are known as pyrethrins. Pyrethrins are rapidly degradable in the presence of moisture, air, and light and are also rapidly biodegradable. They are very soluble in kerosene but insoluble in water. The oral LD_{50} of pyrethrum for rats is 200 to 1500 mg/kg, depending on the purity of the product, and the dermal LD_{50} for rats is greater than 1800 mg/kg. Pyrethrins may produce some inhalation problems in rats, but regular aerosol applications should not produce any adverse reactions in domestic animals. Because they are toxic to fish, pyrethrin aerosols should not be used near fish tanks, but regular use has had little impact on game fish and other wildlife.

Pyrethrins rapidly knock down, paralyze, and kill arthropods by disrupting sodium and potassium ion transport in nerve membranes, thus poisoning neurotransmission along the axon and at the synapse. Residues of pyrethrins are sometimes repellent. Pyrethrins are usually combined with a synergist such as piperonyl butoxide or N-octyl bicycloheptene dicarboximide. Synergists increase the insecticidal activity 10 to 20 times (Plapp, 1991). Synergists poison the mixed function oxidases, which detoxify insecticides in the insect.

Because of the safety and rapid knockdown effect of natural pyrethrins, they enjoy widespread use in the home and in agriculture. Natural pyrethrins have more uses approved by the EPA than any other insecticide. Many commercially available insecticides formulated as aerosols, fogs, shampoos, and mists contain a mixture of pyrethrins and a synergist (e.g., Adams Ear Mite Lotion, Aurimite, Buzzoff, Mita-Clear, Mitex, Mycodex Pet Shampoo, Nolvacide, Synerkyl).

Pyrethrin aerosols, fogs, sprays, and powders control face flies, horseflies, houseflies, stable flies, mosquitoes, fleas, lice, and ticks. Pyrethrins are registered for application to beef and lactating dairy cattle and in dairy barns and milk houses. They are not persistent insecticides, so regular and repeated application is necessary. Resistance to pyrethrins has been reported in houseflies and in some cattle ticks.

WARNING: Pyrethrins should not be applied to kittens younger than 4 weeks or to suckling puppies. In case of ingestion, the most toxic component is usually the solvent. Therefore vomiting is contraindicated. Administer activated charcoal and supportive therapy. In case of dermal exposure, the animal should be bathed with a good detergent.

Pyrethroids

Pyrethroids are synthetic pyrethrum-like substances. These new chemicals are more potent and possess greater knockdown effect than do the plant pyrethrins. Pyrethroids are biodegradable but sufficiently stable when exposed to air and light so that weekly or biweekly applications provide excellent control of insects.

Pyrethroids have a greater insecticidal effect when the temperature is lowered. In chemist's language, they have a negative temperature coefficient. Pyrethroids initially stimulate and then depress nerve cell function and eventually cause paralysis. The fast knockdown of flying insects is the result of rapid muscular paralysis. Pyrethroids have low mammalian toxicity, but some pyrethroids provoke sensation of the skin or mucosa. They are toxic to fish.

Research into pyrethroid chemistry has resulted in many new products in recent years. For one to make some sense of this profusion of new products, it is best to divide them by generation. The first generation is represented by allethrin, which is a synthetic duplicate of cinerin I, a component of natural pyrethrin. The second-generation pyrethroids include tetramethrin, resmethrin, bioresmethrin, bioallethrin, and phenothrin. They are more potent than pyrethrum in knockdown potency but decompose rapidly on exposure to air and sunlight. The third-generation pyrethroids are appreciably more potent than earlier generations and are photostable for several days in full sun. They are represented by fenvalerate and permethrin.

The fourth-generation pyrethroids are the newest and most current generation. Many are just now coming to the market. They are photostable and 10 times more potent than the previous generation. The fourth-generation pyrethroids include cypermethrin, flucythrinate, and fluvalinate. The disadvantages of increased potency, and especially increased persistence in the environment, are the development of insect resistance. In fact, insect resistance to synthetic pyrethroids has been documented (Plapp, 1991). Synthetic pyrethroid products commonly used on domestic animals are listed in the following discussion according to generation.

First-Generation Pyrethroids

The first-generation synthetic pyrethroid (allethrin) is a synthetic duplicate of the natural pyrethrin, cinerin I. No more potent or stable than natural pyrethrin, it is rapidly degraded by light and air.

Allethrin

Allethrin, the first-generation pyrethroid, is a mixture of several optical isomers. It has low mammalian toxicity. The LD_{50} of allethrin for rats is greater than 920 mg/kg. Allethrin is formulated in premise sprays with synergists (Farnam Repel X Fly Spray). It is used in the control of flies, mosquitoes, ticks, and fleas in infested animal quarters. Allethrin is also formulated into a flea shampoo (Duocide Shampoo, Mycodex Sensicare Flea and Tick Shampoo) for removing fleas from dogs and cats.

Second-Generation Pyrethroids

The second-generation synthetic pyrethroids were the first step forward from the natural pyrethrins. They increased the knockdown potency 10 to 50 times more than the natural products but were not much more stable in sunlight than the natural pyrethrins.

Resmethrin

Resmethrin, a second-generation synthetic pyrethroid, is not synergized to any appreciable extent by pyrethrum synergists. Of great significance is resmethrin's low mammalian toxicity. Its acute oral LD_{50} for rats is 4240 mg/kg. Resmethrin shows excellent knockdown effect and is cleared for use in sprays and pet shampoo for the control of fleas on dogs and cats.

Tetramethrin

Tetramethrin is a second-generation synthetic pyrethroid, originally developed in Japan. Its acute oral LD_{50} in rats is greater than 2500 mg/kg. Tetramethrin is available in a total release fogger in combination with permethrin to kill cockroaches and fleas (Defend Just for Homes Fogger) in apartments, homes, household storage areas, and pet sleeping areas. As with all foggers, be certain to follow the directions including covering food, avoid contact with pilot lights and open flames, leave the area, and air out the premises thoroughly after treatment. Tetramethrin is also available as an inverted aerosol for control of fleas, ticks, and carpet beetles (Ectokyl Spray, Virbac Knockout, Speer Neoperm, Tetraperm).

Third-Generation Pyrethroids

The third-generation synthetic pyrethroids became available in the 1970s. Photostability is the hallmark of this class. For the first time, increased potency and photostability were fixed in the same molecule.

Permethrin

Permethrin, a third-generation pyrethroid, is an extremely active insecticide with rapid knockdown effect against a variety of insects. Its acute oral LD_{50} for rats is greater than 4000 mg/kg. Like fenvalerate, permethrin is very toxic to fish. It is photostable, with effective residues lasting 4 to 7 days on crop foliage. Permethrin is registered in a variety of formulations as a treatment for residual animal quarters (dairy barns, feedlots, stables, poultry houses, swine, and other animal housing) to control houseflies, stable flies, and other manure-breeding flies.

Permethrin is the most ubiquitous of the pyrethroids approved for use on or around animals. It is available in on-animal sprays (Mycodex), dips (Dermethrin Pet Dip), shampoo (Defend Flea Shampoo), ear tags (Atroban), pour-on (Boss, Expar Pour-On, Permectrin Pour-On), and dust (Permectrin Livestock and Litter Dust), for use on dogs, cats, horses, cattle, and swine. It is also available in a unique concentrated 65% solution for direct application to dogs (Proticall). It then acts systemically to control adult fleas. Permethrin is widely used as a premise spray (Defend, Ectrin, Expar) for use around livestock and pets to control fleas, ticks, and flies.

Fourth-Generation Pyrethroids

The fourth-generation pyrethroids are at the cutting edge of pyrethroid development. They are the most potent and the longest lasting. Currently, they are available only in insecticidal ear tags.

at the rate of 30 to 60 ml per head for the control of face flies, horn flies, stable flies, houseflies, gnats, and mosquitoes. RAVAP, a combination product of dichlorvos and tetrachlorvinphos, is used as a spray or in backrubbers for the control of flies, lice, and ticks, including the spinose ear tick in beef cattle.

DOGS AND CATS. Dichlorvos collars are worn around animals' necks for activity against adult fleas.

PREMISES. Insect control in dairy barns, feedlots, horse barns, and the surrounding resting and breeding areas may be achieved with dichlorvos resin strips, baits, foggers, and regular spraying. Vapona resin strips or bait strips are suitable for fly control in milk rooms.

WARNING: Dichlorvos collars must not be worn by Persian cats, sick cats, greyhounds, or whippet dogs. Exposure to water reduces the effectiveness of dichlorvos collars. The collar must be removed before bathing animals and may be replaced when the animal's haircoat has dried completely. Applications of dichlorvos to animals may be safely repeated every 7 to 14 days. Food animals should not be treated within 1 day of slaughter. For standard precautions to be followed in dealing with organophosphorus insecticides, see earlier discussion.

Ethion

Ethion is an aliphatic organophosphate insecticide with an acute oral LD_{50} for rats of 47 mg/kg. It is formulated into an insecticide ear tag (Commando Insecticide Cattle Ear Tag), which is approved for use on beef and lactating dairy cattle for control of horn flies (including pyrethroids-resistant populations), Gulf Coast ticks, and spinose ear ticks and for help in controlling face flies, lice, stable flies, and houseflies.

Phenyl Derivatives

The phenyl derivatives are structurally more complex organophosphates than the aliphatic derivatives because they have a benzene ring in their structure. They were the second major class of organophosphate to be developed. Because of their structural differences from the aliphatic derivatives, they are longer lasting in the environment. The phenyl derivatives are represented by famphur, fenthion, and tetrachlorvinphos.

Famphur

Famphur is a phenyl derivative organophosphate. Its acute oral LD_{50} for male rats is only 35 mg/kg. It is formulated into a 13.2% pour-on for cattle (Warbex Famphur Pour-On). The product is approved for control of cattle grubs and lice. It should not be used in lactating cattle or dry cattle within 21 days of freshening, nor with sick, weak cattle or calves less than three months old. **Do not use the product**

on Brahman bulls. Do not slaughter cattle within 35 days of treatment.

Fenthion

Fenthion is a potent and a highly persistent insecticide. Its oral LD_{50} for male rats is 255 to 298 mg/kg. Fenthion is very effective when administered topically. It is absorbed systemically to act on external parasites. Fenthion must be handled with care because it readily penetrates human skin.

CATTLE. Fenthion is a ready-to-use 3% pour-on (Tiguvon Pour-On) applied along the back top of beef and nonlactating dairy cattle at the rate of 33 ml/100 kg for the control of flies, lice, and *Hypoderma* grubs. Products containing higher concentrations of fenthion (Lysoff) must be diluted immediately before use. For spot treatment, 3 ml/100 kg of a 20% solution of fenthion in oil (Spotton 20% Solution) may be used. For the control of grubs, fenthion must be applied in the fall immediately after adult fly activity ceases.

One application per season is adequate for the control of *Hypoderma* grubs. Cattle should not be slaughtered within 35 days after a single application. If the drug is applied a second time for the control of cattle lice, usually 35 days after the first application, the cattle should not be slaughtered within 45 days of the second application. Fenthion should not be applied to dairy cows within 28 days of calving and should not be used on lactating dairy cows, on calves younger than 3 months, or on animals under stress.

SWINE. Fenthion is applied to swine as a 3% ready-to-use pour-on (Tiguvon Pour-On) for the control of lice. Apply the solution at the rate of 33 ml/100 kg. Do not apply it to sick, convalescent, or stressed animals. The product should not be applied within 14 days of slaughter.

Tetrachlorvinphos

Tetrachlorvinphos is a phenyl derivative organophosphate with low mammalian toxicity. Its oral LD_{50} of tetrachlorvinphos for rats is 4000 to 5000 mg/kg. Tetrachlorvinphos is available as a wettable powder (Rabon), dust (Rabon Dust Bag), and emulsifiable concentrate with dichlorvos (Ravap EC). These products are approved in dairy cattle for the control of face flies, horn flies, houseflies, stable flies, lice, ticks, and chorioptic mites.

Rabon and Ravap may be applied manually or by dust bag as a ready-to-use 3% dust, by spraying aqueous suspensions, or by backrubber application of concentrates diluted in oil. Rabon prevents the growth of horn fly and face fly larvae when fed to beef and dairy cattle in complete ration (Rabon), mineral supplements, or molasses blocks (Sweetlix Rabon Block) at the rate of 1.54 mg/kg per day.

Regular spraying of barns is recommended for control of flies.

SWINE. Rabon is applied directly to swine for the control of lice. Treatment may be repeated in 2 weeks if necessary.

Heterocyclic Derivatives

The heterocyclic derivatives were the last group of organophosphates to be developed. Chemically they all have a ring structure in which at least one of the atoms in the ring is oxygen, nitrogen, or sulfur. The heterocyclic ring may consist of three, five, or six atoms. The heterocyclic derivatives are the longest lasting of all the organophosphates. They enjoy widespread use on animals and are represented by chlorpyrifos, coumaphos, diazinon, phosmet, and pirimiphos.

Chlorpyrifos

Chlorpyrifos (Dursban) is moderately persistent in the environment and serves well for the control of mosquito and fly larvae, fire ants, and termites. Its acute oral LD_{50} in rats is 163 mg/kg, and its acute dermal LD_{50} in rabbits is 2000 mg/kg.

Chlorpyrifos is available in a wide assortment of premise sprays (Defend, Double Shift), dips, and flea and tick collars, which are indicated for the control of fleas and ticks on dogs only. It is claimed that one application will kill fleas and protect against reinfestation for up to 1 month. For more effective control of fleas, bedding and resting areas should also be sprayed. It is suggested that pregnant bitches and pups younger than 10 weeks should not be treated with chlorpyrifos.

Coumaphos

Coumaphos is a heterocyclic derivative organophosphate of relatively low toxicity for mammals. Mice are very sensitive, however. Their oral LD_{50} is 55 mg/kg, whereas the oral LD_{50} for rats is 90 to 110 mg/kg. Coumaphos hydrolyzes slowly under alkaline conditions, but rapid degradation occurs in the liver of cattle. Coumaphos is available as an emulsifiable concentrate, wettable powder, and 1% dust (Co-Ral) in a variety of formulations for use on animals and premises to control a wide range of parasitic arthropods.

CATTLE. For the control of cattle lice, horn flies, psoroptic mange, screwworms, and ticks, coumaphos is applied as a 1% to 5% dust in self-treatment dust bags, as 1% oil in backrubbers, and as sprays prepared by diluting emulsifiable concentrates with water. Coumaphos may be used on beef and lactating dairy cattle without limitations for slaughter. When concentrated pour-on or dip is applied to cattle, milk should not be used for 14 days after treatment.

SHEEP AND GOATS. Coumaphos 5% ready-to-use dust (Co-Ral) applications are effective against fleeceworms, screwworms, lice, keds, ticks, and chorioptic mites.

SWINE. Coumaphos 0.25% to 3% spray or 1% to 5% ready-to-use dust (Co-Ral) is applied to pigs for the control of lice and screwworm infestations.

HORSES. Coumaphos is sprayed on horses for the control of external parasites, including lice.

Diazinon

Diazinon is a relatively safe heterocyclic organophosphate with a good record of safety. Over several decades it has been used to kill a wide spectrum of insect pests. Its oral LD_{50} for rats is 300 to 400 mg/kg, and its acute dermal LD_{50} in rabbits is 4000 mg/kg.

Diazinon is currently available in a flea collar (Escort) for use on dogs and cats. It is also available in ear tags (Patriot) for use on beef and nonlactating dairy cattle to control horn flies, lice, Gulf Coast ticks, spinose ear ticks, face flies, stable flies, houseflies, and lice. These products can also be used in winter to control lice.

Phosmet

Phosmet is a time-tested heterocyclic organophosphate registered for use on many insect pests. Its oral LD_{50} for male rats is 147 to 316 mg/kg, and its acute dermal LD_{50} for rabbits is 3160 mg/kg.

CATTLE. Phosmet is used as a spray (Del-Phos Emsulsifiable Liquid) for the control of horn flies and ticks. Calves younger than 3 months, dairy animals, and beef animals within 21 days of slaughter should not be treated.

Pirimiphos

Pirimiphos-methyl is a heterocyclic organophosphate. Its acute oral LD_{50} for female rats is 2050 mg/kg. It is formulated into a 20% cattle ear tag (Dominator, Double Barrel), which is approved for use on beef cattle, calves, and nonlactating dairy cattle. Pirimiphos-methyl protects against horn flies (including synthetic pyrethroids-resistant populations) for 5 months.

Chlorinated Hydrocarbons

The first chlorinated hydrocarbon was dichlorodiphenyltrichloroethane (DDT), which is without doubt the pesticide of greatest historical significance. DDT is probably the best known and most notorious chemical of the century. The discovery of its spectacular activity against insects of public health significance in 1939 rapidly spread its use throughout the world. The discovery was so significant that Dr. Paul Muller, the inventor of DDT, was awarded a Nobel Prize. During the war years and for decades after, the primary role of DDT was against mosquitoes for malaria control, against body lice that carry typhus, and against fleas that are vectors for plague.

DDT was responsible for saving millions of lives through prevention of disease and increases in agricultural production. It was widely applied to crops and livestock, but unfortunately, it was soon overused and abused. In later years it was discovered that because of its persistence in body fats, it was accumulating in the food chain and causing disastrous consequences in some wildlife. Of special concern was the effect on eggshell quality in raptors. By the time the effects of bioaccumulation were known, more than 1.8 billion kg had been used worldwide since 1940. The eventual ban by the EPA on January 1, 1973, signaled the end of DDT's spectacular history (Ware, 1983).

Despite its widespread use and historical significance, the mechanism of action for DDT and related chlorinated hydrocarbons has not been completely determined. It is clear that the chlorinated hydrocarbons act as axonic poisons, in similar fashion to the synthetic pyrethroids. The exact mechanism for poisoning neurotransmission along the axon is not entirely clear. The prevailing theory is that the DDT molecule lodges itself like a wedge into the sodium gate. In that way sodium continues to pour across the neuromembrane, which prevents repolarization.

Chlorinated hydrocarbons related to DDT act in much the same way (Ware, 1983), producing neuromuscular hyperexcitability. Poisoning of domestic animals is treated with nervous system depressants such as phenobarbital.

In years past, the shelves of the veterinarian were packed with a wide array of insecticidal products containing chlorinated hydrocarbons. Today the wide spectrum of products has been trimmed down to just one, methoxychlor, for horses, dogs, and cats.

Methoxychlor
Methoxychlor is the methoxy analogue of DDT. Although methoxychlor has prolonged residual insecticidal activity, it shows little tendency to accumulate in animal fat depots. Its oral LD_{50} for rats is 6000 mg/kg. Methoxychlor is used in combination with organophosphate insecticides and synergists (e.g., piperonyl butoxide). Like DDT, methoxychlor presumably interferes with ion movement along the axons. The poisoned insects show tremors, hyperexcitability, and paralysis.

Methoxychlor is available in only two combination products for horses and pets. For horses, a combination product containing 0.5% methoxychlor, pyrethrin, and synergists (Buzz Off) is either sprayed or rubbed on the animal. It may also be sprayed in the adjacent stable areas. The product is effective against stable flies, houseflies, horse flies, horn flies, face flies, deer flies, mosquitoes, and gnats. Avoid contaminating feed or feeding equipment and do not treat overheated or sick animals. Refrain from use on meat or dairy animals.

Methoxychlor is also available in a powder formulation for use on dogs and cats. It is formulated as 0.25% methoxychlor in combination with 12.5% carbaryl (Ritter's Tick and Flea Powder). The powder is labeled for use against fleas, ticks, and lice on dogs and cats. The dust may also be applied to the animals' bedding. Do not use this product on pregnant animals, nursing puppies and kittens, or animals younger than 4 weeks. Wash hands with soap and water after applying.

Formamidines

The formamidines are a promising new group of acaricidal compounds effective against cattle ticks and mange mites of swine and dogs. Formamidines kill by inhibiting monoamine oxidase and are effective against pests that have developed resistance to organophosphates and carbamates. There is also evidence that they act directly on the voltage-sensitive sodium gates in the nerve membrane (Campbell and Rew, 1985). In the United States, amitraz is approved for use in dogs, cattle, and swine.

Amitraz
Amitraz is the only formamidine approved for use on animals in the United States. Its acute oral LD_{50} for rats is 800 mg/kg, and its dermal LD_{50} for rabbits is greater than 200 mg/kg. When applied to the skin of dogs as a 0.025% solution, amitraz produced transient sedation, depression of the rectal temperature, and elevation of blood glucose. Amitraz was well tolerated by dogs when administered orally at 0.25 mg/kg daily for 90 days, but at 1 to 4 mg/kg hyperglycemia was consistently observed. In clinical studies, transient sedation was the most frequently observed untoward effect.

DOGS. Mitaban liquid contains 19.9% amitraz and is diluted to a 0.025% solution for the treatment of generalized demodicosis in dogs. The contents of one 10.6-ml vial are mixed with 2 gallons of warm water for each of three to six treatments spaced 14 days apart. It is suggested that treatment be continued until no viable mites are found in skin scrapings made at two successive treatments, or until six treatments have been applied. The product information leaflet mentions that amitraz should not be used for treatment of localized demodicosis or scabies.

The safety of amitraz has not been evaluated in pregnant bitches or in dogs younger than 4 months. Mitaban concentrate is flammable. Wear rubber gloves when preparing dilutions and applying these to dogs.

Amitraz is also available in a collar for dogs. The product Preventic kills ticks on dogs for 4 months. The collar contains enough amitraz to cause illness if ingested. Therefore the collar must be fitted properly to prevent it from coming loose and being ingested. The amitraz collar must not be used on sick or convalescing animals. It has no effect on fleas, so other means of insect control must be applied.

CATTLE AND SWINE. Amitraz is available in a 12.5% emulsifiable concentrate (Taktic EC) for use against ticks, mange mites, and lice on beef cattle, dairy cattle, and swine. For use against cattle ticks and lice, the product is diluted 760 ml/100 gal of water and applied as a spray or dip. For lice, a second treatment in 10 to 14 days is required. For use against cattle scabies and mange and lice in swine, the product is diluted 760 ml/50 gal of water and used as a spray or dip. For scabies, a second treatment must be applied in 7 to 10 days.

No slaughter withdrawal is required for cattle, and no milk withdrawal for dairy cattle. Swine must not be treated within 3 days of slaughter.

WARNING: Horses must not be treated with amitraz, or fatal colon impaction may result.

Amitraz is also available in a ready-to-use spot-on formulation for use in swine (Point-Guard). It is approved against mange mites and lice in pigs heavier than 20 pounds and in sows and boars. It should not be used in swine within 7 days of slaughter.

Novel Insecticides

Fipronil
Fipronil is a member of a relatively new class of insecticides termed phenylpyrazole. It acts as a potent blocker of the GABA-regulated chloride channel (Gant et al, 1996; Tomlin, 2000). The acute oral LD_{50} of fipronil for rats is 100 mg/kg. A large volume of literature is available to show the mechanism of action, clinical efficacy, and safety when fipronil is used against fleas in dogs and cats. It is approved in a 0.29% spray (Frontline Spray) for use on dogs, cats, puppies, and kittens. This spray is effective against fleas even after bathing (Jeannin et al, 1994; Postal et al, 1994; Tanner et al, 1996). It is also effective against ticks and sarcoptic mange mites (Curtis, 1996; Hunter et al, 1996a; LeNain et al, 1996). The spray should not be used in puppies and kittens younger than 8 weeks.

Fipronil is available in two convenient spot-on formulations for dogs and for cats (Frontline Top Spot). These formulations are effective in spreading the product through the sebum covering the hair and skin with minimal systemic absorption (Birckel et al,

1996; Weil et al, 1997). The product is effective against fleas and ticks for 30 days on cats and dogs and up to 3 months for fleas on dogs (Hunter et al, 1996b; Postal et al, 1996a; Postal et al, 1996b; Cunningham et al, 1997b; Cunningham et al, 1997c). It is also effective after exposure to rain or bathing (Everett et al, 1997). Laboratory and field safety studies reveal no concerns when the product is used according to the label (Consalvi et al, 1996; Arnaud and Consalvi, 1997a; Arnaud and Consalvi, 1997b). Do not use it in puppies younger than 10 weeks or in kittens younger than 12 weeks. Wear rubber gloves when applying the product. Some reports indicate that fipronil is effective against ear mites (Vincenzi and Genchi, 1997).

Fipronil is now available in combination with methoprene, an insect growth regulator. The combination product is sold under the tradename Frontline Plus. For dogs and cats it is effective against fleas and ticks for 30 days. The combination of an adulticide and an insect growth regulator (IGR) provides activity against the immature and adult life stages of the flea, thus breaking the life cycle of the pest.

Imidacloprid
Imidacloprid is the first agent in the class of chloronicotinyl insecticides that irreversibly bind at nicotinic acetylcholine receptor sites. This newly characterized receptor is a subtype that is apparently essential for insect neurofunction, but which is different in pharmacology and tissue distribution from all known mammalian nicotinic receptors (Liu et al, 1995; Londershausen, 1996; Griffin et al, 1997b). Its acute oral LD_{50} in rats is 450 mg/kg. Imidacloprid is available in a 9.1% topical formulation (Advantage) for use in dogs, cats, puppies, and kittens for control of fleas. The product is very effective in laboratory and field use to control fleas (Arthur et al, 1997; Cruthers and Bock, 1997; Cunningham and Everett, 1997; Hopkins, 1997; Hopkins et al, 1997). It apparently is also effective after shampooing (Cunningham et al, 1977a), although the label recommends reapplication after bathing. Safety testing has revealed no concerns when the product is used according to the label (Griffin et al, 1997a). Do not use it in puppies or kittens younger than 4 months or in sick or debilitated animals.

Nitenpyram
Nitenpyram is the first animal health product in the class of neonicotinoids. It has the unique action of rapid oral absorption and low toxicity to dogs and cats. As a result of this action, a single oral dose provides extremely rapid knockdown of flea populations. Studies have shown activity against fleas within 30 minutes. Efficacy was greater than 90% within 4 hours in dogs and within 6 hours in

cats. Nitenpyram has a short half-life and is quickly cleared from th body. Daily dosing in dogs and cats will not result in bioaccumulation.

Nitenpyram is available in tablet form (CAPSTAR). The small tablet contains 11.4 mg and labeled for use in cats and dogs up to 25-lb body weight. The large tablet contains 57 mg and is for use in dogs from 25.1 to 125-lb body weight The wide dosage range is a testament to the favorable margin of safety.

Nitenpyram should not be used in dogs and cats less than 2-lb body weight or less than 4 weeks of age. Pets who are heavily infested with fleas may begin scratching after treatment nitenpyram; this is usually and effect from the dying fleas and not an adverse effect from the product.

Repellents

Repellents are compounds that prevent or discourage pests from approaching a treated area, or induce them to leave soon after approaching. The most intensive research in this area has been to protect humans from flying insects. In general these products are rather volatile and regarded as having little toxicity to the host animal (Hayes and Laws, 1991).

Deet

Deet is the official nonproprietary name for N,N-diethyl-3-methylbenzamide or N,N-diethyl-m-toluamide. Its oral LD_{50} for rats is 2000 mg/kg. Deet is used as a repellent for mosquitoes, gnats, flies, fleas, ticks, and chiggers. For continuing protection, frequent applications are necessary.

Di-N-propyl isocinchomeronate

Dipropyl isocinchomeronate is a relatively safe insect repellent, with an oral LD_{50} for rats of 5.2 to 7.2 g/kg. The chemical is best known by its proprietary name, MGK Repellent 326. It is usually formulated with other insect repellents, insecticides, or synergists for use on pets and livestock.

Insect Growth Regulators

An exciting area of recent advance in the struggle against insects is the advent of IGRs. The sheer number of insecticides covered in this chapter would suggest that insect problems are no longer a threat to the health and welfare of our domestic animals, but anyone who works in the field knows that this is far from the case. The central problem with most insecticides is that they are effective against and directed toward only the adult insect, the one that bites and annoys.

Adulticidal products need to be applied thoroughly and often to control adult insect populations, but this is often unworkable. The applicator trying to stem the flow of adult insects often feels like the Dutch boy with his finger in the dike. The IGRs provide relief from this approach by killing immature insects where they grow and develop, thus breaking the life cycle and providing true relief from insect annoyance. The IGRs typically are juvenile hormone mimics, which bind to juvenile hormone receptors in the immature insect and prevent survival to the next stage of development. Methoprene and pyriproxyfen are the best-known juvenile hormone mimics.

These products are the safest and most effective products available. Their safety lies in the fact that mammalian hosts have no juvenile hormones or juvenile hormone receptors (Londershausen, 1996). Therefore IGR products cannot have any biological effect on the host. The safety of these products has an important side effect. When used properly, they dramatically decrease the use of more toxic adulticides. It follows, then, that insect control programs with IGRs are often safer than programs with adulticides alone.

Cyromazine

Cyromazine is a unique product that has IGR properties limited to the filth flies (e.g., houseflies, lesser houseflies, soldier flies). It has no effect on most of the other orders of beneficial insects. Cyromazine works by blocking the formation of new cuticle in the fly larvae. When it molts from the first to the second instar stage, it does not survive the molt. The product is formulated as a feed premix (Larvadex 1% Premix) and a liquid concentrate (Larvadex 2 SL). The premix is approved for feeding to caged layers and broiler breeders at 1 pound of premix per ton of final feed. Cyromazine passes through the bird and is deposited in the manure where it controls filth flies developing there. The surface spray is used to control fly larvae in other breeding places such as feed spills, dead bird piles, and manure storage areas.

Diflubenzuron

Diflubenzuron is not a true IGR but is included here for simplicity. It does not bind to juvenile hormone receptors. Diflubenzuron is a contact and systemic insecticide that interferes with chitin deposition and thus prevents the shedding of the old skin, leading to the death of larvae or pupae. It also prevents hatching of eggs. In both acute and chronic studies in laboratory animals, diflubenzuron was well tolerated. It is used as a larvacide administered as a bolus (Vigilante) to beef and dairy cattle for the control of horn flies, face flies, stable flies, and houseflies. Diflubenzuron acts by interfering with the growth of larvae in cattle manure. The bolus releases diflubenzuron over a 5-month period. About 80% of diflubenzuron is eliminated in the feces as the unchanged parent compound. Several reports indicate that diflubenzuron and related compounds may provide control of fleas for prolonged periods in household dogs and cats (Henderson and Foil, 1993).

Lufenuron

Lufenuron is actually an insect development inhibitor (IDI) but is included here with the IGRs for simplicity. All IGRs currently available for flea control act by binding to juvenile hormone receptors. Lufenuron acts by a different mechanism, and the term *insect development inhibitor* signifies this difference. Lufenuron is approved for use in dogs and cats for control of fleas (Program) and is approved in combination with milbemycin oxime for control of internal and external parasites of dogs (Sentinel). It is given orally to dogs and cats every 30 days. A new injectable formulation (Program 6-Month Injectable for Cats) has been designed to allow application every 6 months. The drug is very lipophilic, so it resides in the fat tissues of the pet, where it reaches back into the blood stream for at least 30 days. Adult fleas ingest lufenuron when they feed, and the drug is passed transovarially to the flea egg. Most flea eggs exposed to lufenuron fail to hatch, and the few flea larvae that do successfully hatch die during their first molt. The action on the immature flea is thought to be due to disruption of chitin synthesis and deposition. Lufenuron is a convenient and effective agent for flea control in pets. It is known to be safe in pets of all ages, as well as in breeding dogs and cats.

Methoprene

Methoprene is of low toxicity to mammals. Its oral LD_{50} for rats is 34.6 g/kg. Methoprene is an IGR, acting as a juvenile growth hormone mimic that arrests larval development, which in turn results in the death of the larvae. Methoprene is sensitive to ultraviolet (UV) degradation.

Methoprene has enjoyed wide success against fleas. It is available in several preparations, in combination with natural pyrethrin for use on dogs and cats, and formulated into a collar (Ultimate Flea Collar) for extended ovicidal effect in dogs and cats. Methoprene is also formulated in combination with insecticides for control of fleas and other pests. Methoprene is ovicidal and larvacidal against fleas.

Methoprene is formulated into an oral dosage form (Hartz Flea Control Capsules) for use in dogs. When administered weekly (22 mg/kg), they prevent and control flea infestations. In the treatment of active flea infestations, short-term application of flea adulticides may be necessary.

The IGR is also marketed in a topical form for cats (Hartz OneSpot for Cats and Kittens). The product is applied every 30 days to control and prevent flea eggs and larvae. This application is often easier to apply to cats than oral dosage forms.

A combination product containing methoprene and permethrin (Hartz OneSpot for Dogs) is approved for topical application to dogs and puppies every 30 days to provide relief from flea and tick infestation. It is approved for use in dogs older than 6 months. *Do not use in cats.*

Another combination product contains methoprene and phenothrin (Hartz Flea & Tick Drops) and is designed to be used topically in dogs and cats. When used every 30 days it kills fleas and repels ticks with 24 hours of application. It also repels and kills mosquitoes.

Pyriproxyfen

Pyriproxyfen is the newest IGR, sold under the trade name Nylar and included in several flea control sprays, foggers, and collars (Breakthru, Knockout). It is a juvenile hormone mimic. The secretion of juvenile hormone in the immature insect causes it to molt into the next life stage, but the absence of juvenile hormone at the time of the molt allows maturation to occur. The net effect of the juvenile hormone mimic is to interfere with the larval to pupal and pupal to adult molts (Anonymous, 1997b). The acute oral LD_{50} of pyriproxyfen in rats is greater than 5000 mg/kg, which demonstrates the very wide margin of safety. The product is 100% effective against flea reproduction in carpets for more than 6 months after application (Anonymous, 1997b). It represents another important addition to the insecticide arsenal.

Synergists

The synergists are not considered toxic in their own right and have no direct effect in killing insects. They are used with insecticides to enhance insecticidal activity. They are most often used with pyrethrins, in which they can increase the potency twentyfold to fiftyfold. The mode of action is to inhibit mixed-function oxidases, enzymes in the insect that metabolize foreign compounds. When the insect is inhibited from destroying the insecticide, then the agent can kill the pest. The synergists are most commonly listed on the label by their chemical name, which is not designed to be user friendly.

N-Octyl bicycloheptene dicarboximide

N-Octyl bicycloheptene dicarboximide inhibits the microsomal detoxification of insecticides, thus maximizing their toxicity. It is also known by the designation MGK 264. The drug is registered for application to beef and dairy cattle, sheep, goats, horses, swine, dogs, and cats, and to agricultural buildings and animal quarters for the control of annoying insects. It is often formulated with piperonyl butoxide and insecticides as aerosols, pressurized sprays, and free-flowing dusts.

Piperonyl Butoxide

Piperonyl butoxide is a pale yellowish liquid, soluble in alcohols, benzene, Freons, and other organic solvents. It is very safe for animals, with an oral LD_{50} for rats of about 7.5 g/kg. Chlorinated hydrocarbons, carbamates, organophosphates, and particularly pyrethrins and rotenone are synergized by piperonyl butoxide. The insecticidal activity of these compounds is enhanced because piperonyl butoxide inhibits degradation of the insecticide by the insect's microsomal enzymes. Numerous products contain piperonyl butoxide as a synergist formulated with pyrethrins, malathion, carbaryl, or methoxychlor.

Miscellaneous Insecticides

This section discusses miscellaneous insecticides not included in one of the larger classes of chemicals previously discussed. They are often older, more traditional products that have diverse chemistry and different modes of action.

Benzyl benzoate

Benzyl benzoate is an insecticide with an unknown mode of action. It is effective against most ectoparasites, but is used only on dogs infested with sarcoptic, otodectic, or demodectic mites. Benzyl benzoate is marketed as a 36% lotion (Mange Treatment). For spot treatment of localized infestations, apply daily to all lesions for at least 7 days. For the treatment of generalized forms of sarcoptic and demodectic mange, the hair is first clipped from the entire body, and the dog is bathed to remove all crusty materials. Mange lotion is then applied while the dog is still wet. It is recommended that only one third of the body be treated with the acaricide at one time. Benzyl benzoate has no residual effect. Therefore repeated applications are required. Demodectic mange may require prolonged therapy, whereas sarcoptic mange is usually cured with two applications. Benzyl benzoate–containing drugs should not be used on cats. If application is carried out by dipping, protect the patient's eyes with a bland ointment.

Borax

Orthoboric acid is a cellular toxin similar in chemistry to borax. It is applied as a fine powder (Rx for Fleas) in the indoor environment to control fleas. The product is deposited onto carpets at the rate of 1 lb/50 sq ft. The flea larvae ingest the material and are killed. It has no effect on flea eggs, pupae, or adults.

■ ANTIPROTOZOALS

We have tried in this discussion to characterize briefly the biological activities of a few approved and some nonapproved but legally obtainable anti-protozoal drugs. As with any drug, the information on the label or package insert must always be read and directions followed before administering anti-protozoal agents. For more detailed information, the reader should consult detailed review articles (Campbell and Rew, 1985; Schillhorn van Veen, 1986; Snyder et al, 1991; Barr, 1998; Speer, 1999; Lindsday and Blagburn, 2001).

Nonsulfonamides

Albendazole

Albendazole is more completely described later in the section on benzimidazoles. It is included in this section for a discussion of its activity against *Giardia* organisms. Evidence in one study suggests that albendazole is 100% effective in treating giardiasis in dogs (Barr et al, 1993). The dosage given in that study was 25 mg/kg twice a day for four doses. If these results are reliable, then albendazole may prove to be safer and more effective than more traditional therapies.

Albendazole, like other benzimidazoles, is well absorbed (about 50% bioavailable) and converted in the liver to its active metabolites, albendazole sulfoxide and albendazole sulfone. These active metabolites are thought to bind to tubulin molecules; this binding prohibits the formation of microtubules and disrupts cell division. There is also evidence that benzimidazoles can inhibit fumarate reductase, and this blocks mitochondrial function, thus depriving the parasite of energy and resulting in death. In *Giardia* organisms, albendazole causes structural changes in the trophozoite stage, including damage to the adhesive disk and the internal microtubule cytoskeleton, but not the flagella (Lindsay and Blagburn, 2001). The parent drug and its metabolites are excreted primarily in the urine.

Albendazole has proved to be teratogenic, thus limiting its use in pregnant animals. Dogs treated with 50 mg/kg twice daily may have anorexia, and cats treated with 100 mg/kg per day for 14 to 21 days showed weight loss, neutropenia, and mental dullness (Plumb, 1999). Recently, the drug was shown to be toxic in dogs and cats in clinical use (Stokol et al, 1997; Meyer, 1998). Reported toxicities included myelosuppression (anemia, leukopenia, and/or thrombocytopenia), abortion, teratogenicity, anorexia, depression, ataxia, vomiting, and diarrhea. Veterinarians are advised to use caution with this product in dogs. Albendazole is available in an oral suspension and paste (Valbazen) containing 113.6 mg/ml.

Amprolium

The coccidiostatic activity of amprolium is related to its mimicry of thiamine and competition for absorption of thiamine by the parasite. This occurs because of the structural similarity between thiamin and amprolium (USP, 1998). The anticoccidial effect may by reversed by the feeding of excess thiamine. This is most effective against the first-generation schizont stage and thus more effective as a preventative than as a treatment. Amprolium (Amprol, Amprovine) is fed in poultry rations or drinking water to prevent or treat coccidiosis.

BROILERS, LAYERS, AND TURKEYS. Amprolium is given in the water for 2 weeks at 0.0125% (0.025% for severe outbreaks), then given at 0.006% for another 2 weeks.

CATTLE. For treatment of active *Eimeria bovis* and *Eimeria zuernii* infections in cattle, amprolium is formulated as a 9.6% drench solution (Corid Oral Solution), 20% soluble powder (Corid Soluble Powder), or 1.25% feed crumbles (Corid Crumbles). Administration of amprolium is by drench or drinking water, or it is top-dressed on the feed at the approximate dosage of 10 mg/kg for 5 consecutive days. For prevention of coccidiosis caused by *E. bovis* and *E. zuernii* during periods of exposure, a dosage of 5 mg/kg daily for 21 days is recommended. Amprolium premix (Amprovine) is used for beef and dairy calves. Other species of *Eimeria* are also susceptible to amprolium, but the drug label claims efficacy against only *E. bovis* and *E. zuernii*. Cattle dosed with 50 mg/kg of amprolium per day did not have adverse reactions. Animals should not be medicated within 24 hours of slaughter.

SHEEP AND GOATS. Amprolium may protect lambs against coccidia when given at 55 mg/kg twice daily for 19 days (USP, 1998).

PIGS. *Isospora suis* is occasionally a problem in swine. Pigs aged 5 to 10 days die without passing oocysts. Although not approved, amprolium therapy may be beneficial in preventing the disease (USP, 1998).

DOGS. Treatment of dogs and cats requires adapting the approved formulations to small animal use. The target dose for treatment of dogs is 100 to 200 mg/kg by mouth daily in food and water (Plumb, 1999). Dogs may be treated by mixing 30 ml of 9.6% amprolium and 1 gallon (3.8 L) of drinking water and offering it as the sole source of drinking water (Smart, 1971). Alternatively, 1.25 g of 20% amprolium powder can be mixed with enough daily ration for four puppies (USP, 1998). Amprolium should be provided in either the food or water but not both for a period of 7 days. It may be given as a treatment for coccidia or as a preventative for 7 days before shipping puppies or to bitches just before whelping.

CATS. Amprolium may be used at a dose of 60 to 100 mg/kg by mouth, which may be accomplished by direct oral administration (Dubey, 1998). Medication in food or water may be more unreliable in cats than in dogs because of their finicky tastes.

Clindamycin

Clindamycin is currently considered the drug of choice for treating toxoplasmosis. Structurally, clindamycin is a congener of lincomycin. The drug is well absorbed (90%) after oral administration and widely distributed in most tissues, except the central nervous system. It readily crosses the placenta and is extensively bound to plasma proteins. Clindamycin is metabolized in the liver and excreted primarily in the urine and bile. It acts by binding to the 50 S subunit of the bacterial (or parasitic) ribosome and blocking the transpeptidation reaction (Hardman et al, 2001). Gastrointestinal upset is sometimes reported in animals receiving clindamycin. Severe, even fatal, pseudomembranous enterocolitis has been reported in people, caused by overgrowth of *Clostridium difficile.*

Treatment of systemic toxoplasma infection in dogs can be accomplished with oral or intramuscular clindamycin at 10 to 20 mg/kg twice daily for 2 weeks (Greene et al, 1985; Dubey, 1998). Cats can be treated for systemic infections with oral or parenteral clindamycin at 12.5 to 25 mg/kg twice daily for 2 weeks. This regimen is also useful to control the shedding of oocysts (Lappin et al, 1989). The drug should be given with caution in cats with pulmonic toxoplasmosis; parenteral administration to experimentally infected cats resulted in several deaths (Plumb, 1999).

Clindamycin is available in several veterinary formulations (Antirobe): tablets containing 25, 75, or 150 mg and an oral solution containing 25 mg/ml. Similar clindamycin formulations are available for use in people (Cleocin): 75- and 150-mg oral capsules, 15 mg/ml oral pediatric suspension, and an injectable solution containing 150 mg/ml.

Clopidol

Clopidol is a pyrindol coccidiostat that has some activity against ionophore-resistant strains of coccidia. It acts against the sporozoite stage, allowing host cell penetration without development. It is insoluble in water but is available as a feed additive (Coyden 25). The product is fed to chickens at 0.0125% or 0.025%. It should not be fed to laying hens, to chickens older than 16 weeks, or within 5 days of slaughter (Lindsay and Blagburn, 2001).

Decoquinate

Decoquinate is an approved coccidiostatic drug for the control of *Eimeria* infections in chickens, cattle, and goats. This quinolone product kills the sporozoite stage of the life cycle. It disrupts the electron transport in the mitochondrial cytochrome system of the parasite (Plumb, 1999). Decoquinate is primarily indicated for prevention rather than treatment of coccidiosis.

Decoquinate is indicated for prevention of coccidiosis caused by *E. bovis* and *E. zuernii* in ruminating calves and older cattle. It is fed (Deccox) at 0.5 mg/kg per day for at least 28 days during periods of exposure to infective oocysts. In young goats decoquinate is used at the same rate for the prevention of infections caused by *Eimeria christenseni* and *Eimeria ninakohlyakimovae*.

WARNING: Decoquinate should not be fed to breeding animals or lactating dairy cows or goats. Complete feeds containing decoquinate should be consumed within 7 days of manufacture. Bentonite should not be used in decoquinate feeds.

Halofuginone

Halofuginone, a synthetic coccidiostat, is effective against asexual stages. The mechanism of action is unknown. It has been associated with skin tears in chickens and is toxic to fish and aquatic life (Lindsay and Blagburn, 2001). The product is available in a feed additive (Stenorol) for use in broilers and turkeys. It is fed at 2.72 g/ton to chickens and 1.36 to 2.72 g/ton to turkeys. The product should not be fed to layers or within 4 days of slaughter (7 days for turkeys). It should be kept out of lakes, ponds, and streams.

Lasalocid

Lasalocid, an ionophore closely related to monensin, is produced by a streptomycete. Like other ionophores, it forms complexes with sodium and potassium ions. This action renders the parasite membranes permeable to ions, and mitochondrial functions are inhibited. The trophozoite stage is most susceptible to lasalocid (Guyonnet et al, 1990). Lasalocid is the least toxic of the ionophores. It is approved in cattle, sheep, and poultry for the control of coccidia and improvement of feed efficiency.

CATTLE AND SHEEP. The feed additive Bovatec may be mixed into a complete feed for confined cattle or a feed supplement for pasture cattle to deliver a target dose of 1 mg/kg body weight per day. It is effective against *E. bovis* and *E. zuernii* in cattle. Feed continuously during exposure to coccidia. Do not feed to calves to be processed for veal. Sheep are fed to deliver 15 to 70 mg per animal daily depending on body weight. In sheep the product is effective against *Eimeria ovina, Eimeria crandallis, Eimeria ovinoidalis (E. ninakohlyakimovae), Eimeria parva,* and *Eimeria intricata*. Do not feed to horses, or fatal reactions may result. A mineral block containing lasalocid (En-Pro-Al Block Containing Bovatec) is also available for use in pasture cattle only for enhanced rate of gain and not for prevention of coccidia.

POULTRY. Lasalocid is approved in broilers and turkeys to prevent coccidiosis caused by *Eimeria tenella, Eimeria necatrix, Eimeria acervulina,* *Eimeria brunetti, Eimeria mivati,* and *Eimeria maxima*. It is also approved for use in Chukar partridges for prevention of *Emeria legionella*. The product (Avatec) is mixed into a complete ration at a rate of 68 to 113 g/ton. Withdraw product at least 3 days before slaughter.

Maduramicin

Maduramicin, an ionophore coccidiostat, is a fermentation product of *Actinomadura yumaense*. Available as a feed additive (Cygro) for use in broilers, it is fed at 4.54 or 5.45 g/ton of feed. Higher levels may adversely affect growth of the birds. Do not feed to layers or within 5 days of slaughter.

Metronidazole

The nitroimidazoles represent a very useful class of antibiotics that have broad-spectrum activity against trichomonads, amebas, and *Giardia* organisms, as well as anaerobic cocci and bacillus species. The prototypical nitroimidazole is metronidazole, which has become the drug of choice for treatment of *Giardia* organisms. Other drugs in the class (ipronidazole, tinidazole, nimorazole, ornidazole, and benznidazole) have been used to control *Giardia* organisms, although none are currently available in the United States. None of the nitroimidazole drugs are approved for use in animals. The FDA strongly warns against their use in food-producing animals because this class of drug has been shown to produce tumors in laboratory rodents.

Metronidazole (Flagyl) is well absorbed from the gastrointestinal tract. It has low protein binding and is well distributed in the body. After entering the target cell, metronidazole interacts with the protozoal DNA, in which it causes a loss of helical structure and strand breakage (USP, 1998). The liver extensively metabolizes the drug, and in humans hepatic transformation is responsible for 50% of the total elimination. Patients receiving cimetidine or phenobarbital may require adjustment in the dosage because of drug interaction. Metronidazole toxicity may be seen with high doses. Neurologic toxicity includes ataxia, nystagmus, seizures, tremors, or weakness (Dow et al, 1989; USP, 1998).

Numerous studies have demonstrated that metronidazole is an effective treatment for giardiasis (Watson, 1980; Boreham et al, 1984; Kirkpatrick and Farrell, 1984; Zimmer and Burrington, 1986; Zimmer, 1987), although efficacy is rarely 100%. Dogs may be treated orally with 12.5 to 32.5 mg/kg once or twice daily, and therapy should be continued for 8 days. Cats may be treated orally with 17.4 mg/kg once daily, and therapy should be continued for 8 days (USP, 1998). The commercially available product (Flagyl) is formulated in 250- and 500-mg tablets. Parenteral formulations are also available, but their usefulness would seem questionable considering that the giardial trophozoites remain in the lumen of the gastrointestinal tract.

Monensin

Monensin is an antibiotic produced as a fermentation product of *Streptomyces cinnamonensis.* It is used in poultry and cattle for its coccidiostatic and growth-promoting activities. It forms ionophores with sodium and potassium in the host and in the parasite. When the parasite mitochondrial membrane is affected, it is rendered permeable to potassium and sodium ions.

CATTLE. Monensin is available as a feed additive (Rumensin) for cattle for growth promotion and as prevention and control of coccidiosis. For control of coccidiosis due to *E. bovis* and *E. zuernii,* the product should be fed at a rate of 10 to 30 g/ton, or 100 to 360 mg per head per day. It should be fed continuously during periods of exposure to coccidia or when coccidia are likely to be a hazard.

SHEEP AND GOATS. Monensin is approved for use in goats (Rumensin) for the prevention of *E. crandallis, E. christenseni,* and *E. ninakohlyakimovae.* It should be fed at a rate of 20 g/ton of complete ration. Monensin is not approved for use in sheep, but some authorities indicate that it is useful when fed at a rate of 1 mg/kg of body weight per day (Schilhorn van Veen, 1986; McDougald and Roberson, 1988).

POULTRY. Monensin (Conan) is used in broilers and pullets to prevent coccidiosis caused by *E. necatrix, E. tenella, E. acervilina, E. brunetti, E. mivati,* and *E. maxima.* It is fed at a rate of 90 to 110 g/ton of complete feed. It is also approved for use in turkeys to prevent *Eimeria adenoeides, Eimeria meleagrimitis,* and *Eimeria gallopavonis* when fed at 54 to 90 g/ton. Bobwhite quail can be fed monensin at 73 g/ton to prevent coccidiosis caused by *Eimeria dispersa* and *Eimeria lettyae.*

HORSES. Monensin is very toxic to horses, and ingestion is often fatal.

Narasin

Narasin is an ionophore coccidiostat produced by *Streptomyces aureofaciens.* Similar in structure to salinomycin (Lindsay and Blagburn, 2001), it is available as a feed additive (Monteban) for use only in broilers. The product is fed at a rate of 54 to 72 g/ton of feed for prevention of coccidiosis. No withdrawal period is required before slaughter. It should not be fed to layers. Ingestion by adult turkeys, horses, or ponies may be fatal.

Nicarbazine

Nicarbazine is a synthetic coccidiostat effective in preventing cecal and intestinal coccidiosis. The mechanism of action is unknown (Lindsay and Blagburn, 2001). It is available as a 25% feed additive (Nicarb) and approved for use at 0.0125% in the feed of broilers. The product should not be fed to layers or within 4 days of slaughter. It is not effective for treatment of coccidiosis, and it may depress growth in young birds (Lindsay and Blagburn, 2001).

Ponazuril

Ponazuril is a newly developed antiprotozoal product (Marquis) that is approved in the United States for treatment of equine protozoal myeloencephalitis (EPM), which is caused by *Sarcocystis neurona.* This product is unique in the world, in that it is the only product actually approved for this indication (Anonymous, 2001).

The product has been tested at 5 mg/kg and 10 mg/kg. The approved dose is 5 mg/kg orally per day for 28 days. In the pivotal clinical study 54% of the horses with EPM improved at least one grade as judged by the attending veterinarian, and 58% of the horses treated with 10 mg/kg improved at least one grade. In a smaller field study with seven horses, all seven improved when treated with 5 mg/kg. Safety studies demonstrated that administration at doses of 10 mg/kg or greater produced transient episodes of loose feces.

Robenidine

Robenidine is a synthetic coccidiostat chemically similar to guanidine. It is an older drug with a history of developing resistant strains of coccidia, but is now used to treat ionophore-resistant strains. Robenidine is available in a feed additive (Robenz) for use in broilers only. The product is fed at 30 g/ton of feed. It should not be fed to layers or within 5 days of slaughter. Meat and eggs from treated birds have an unpleasant taste if the withdrawal period is not followed (Lindsay and Blagburn, 2001).

Salinomycin

Salinomycin was the third ionophore coccidiostat to enter the market in the United States. A fermentation product of *Streptomyces albus,* it is most active against the sporozoite stage. Salinomycin is available as a feed additive (Bio-Cox, Sacox 60) for use in broilers and quail. It is fed at 40 to 60 g/ton (50 g/ton for quail). No withdrawal period is required before slaughter. The product may be fatal if fed to adult turkeys or horses.

Semduramicin

Semduramicin is an ionophore coccidiostat produced by *Actinomadura roseorufa.* It is available as a feed additive (Aviax) for use in broiler chickens only. The product is fed at 22.7 g/ton for prevention of coccidiosis. It should not be fed to egg-laying chickens or to broilers within 5 days of slaughter.

Sulfonamides

Sulfonamides are the treatments of choice for small-animal coccidia and very useful for the treatment of large-animal coccidiosis. Unfortunately, there is a paucity of research information to support their efficacy. Two pivotal studies with sulfamethoxine and sulfaguanidine against coccidian support their use. However, these two agents are no longer available in the United States (Boch et al, 1981; Correa et al, 1973). Clinicians have empirically substituted more readily available sulfonamides and enjoyed apparent clinical success (Dubey, 1993). Currently there are simple sulfas and potentiated sulfas commonly used in the United States: sulfachlorpyridazine (Vetisulid), sulfadimethoxine (Albon), sulfadimethoxine with ormetoprim (Primor), sulfadiazine with trimethoprim (Di-Trim Tribrissen), sulfamethazine, sulfamethoxazole with rimethoprim (Bactrim, Septra), and sulfaquinoxaline.

The sulfonamides are structural analogues of para-aminobenzoic acid (PABA) that competitively inhibit the dihydropterate synthetase step in the synthesis of folic acid, which is required for synthesis of RNA and DNA. Inhibition by sulfas impairs protein synthesis, metabolism, and growth of the pathogen. A vast array of sulfa agents has been created and described, but most have been lost in the sands of time. The important differences between these agents are their solubility, duration of action, and activity against key pathogens. Fortunately, the sulfas included in this discussion demonstrate acceptable performance in all three categories: solubility is adequate; they are given once or twice daily or in the feed; and they have a reasonably broad spectrum of action. The sulfa drugs are primarily effective against the schizont stages of the coccidia. Thus prolonged treatment may be required for the drug effectively to block the life cycle (USP, 1998).

The diaminopyrimidine potentiators (trimethoprim and ormetoprim) act in concert with sulfonamides by blocking the next step (dihydrofolate reductase) in folic acid synthesis. Chemically, the diaminopyrimidines are related to pyrimethamine, which has antimalarial properties. The agents are highly selective inhibitors of dihydrofolate reductase. This sequential blockade of folic acid synthesis produces significant potentiation of activity. It is a classic case of drug potentiation.

The sulfonamides are weak acids that are well absorbed from the gastrointestinal tract (except for sulfaquinoxaline) and are widely distributed in the body. Sulfadimethoxine and sulfamethoxazole have high serum protein binding, which provides decreased body clearance and long half-lives. They undergo metabolic alteration in the liver and subsequent renal clearance. Trimethoprim and ormeto-prim are also well absorbed from the gut, widely distributed, then hydroxylated and excreted through the urinary tract.

The long history of sulfa use in veterinary medicine has resulted in a wide array of toxic and idiosyncratic reactions in animals. Historically, the most common and most avoidable reactions result from crystallization in the urinary tract with secondary crystalluria, hematuria, and urinary obstruction. Recent reviews in human medicine indicate that the improved solubility of the modern preparations has decreased the risk of crystalluria. Nevertheless, it is still prudent to ensure adequate water intake and proper hydration during sulfa therapy (Cribb et al, 1996). The human literature also suggests that the sulfonamides may be directly nephrotoxic (Cribb et al, 1996). Hematopoietic disorders (thrombocytopenia and leukopenia) have also been reported as a result of sulfa therapy. Sulfaquinoxaline especially has been associated with hypothrombinemia, hemorrhage, and death in puppies receiving therapy for coccidian (Patterson and Grenn, 1975).

Idiosyncratic reactions in animals and people often include immune-mediated phenomena, including hypersensitivity reactions, drug fever, urticaria, nonseptic polyarthritis, focal retinitis, and hepatitis. Fortunately, these reactions occur at very low rates when sulfonamides are used at recommended dose rates and for less than two weeks (USP, 1998).

Four sulfa products are currently available for use in small-animal medicine: sulfadimethoxine, sulfadimethoxine with ormetoprim, sulfadiazine with trimethoprim, and sulfamethoxazole with trimethoprim. Each is available in a variety of formulations.

Sulfadimethoxine

Sulfadimethoxine is a rapidly absorbed, long-acting sulfonamide. It is not acetylated in the dog and is excreted unchanged in the urine. The drug is approved for treatment of coccidiosis in dogs, cats, cattle, chickens, and turkeys, and for treatment of strangles in horses. It has a wide margin of safety. Dogs given multiple oral doses of 160 mg/kg by mouth daily for 13 weeks showed no signs of toxicity. Diarrhea was the only reaction seen in dogs given single oral doses of 16 g/kg (Entriken, 2001).

It is important that all treated animals receive adequate water intake to prevent dehydration and crystalluria, as well as proper nutrition during therapy for coccidiosis. Sulfadimethoxine is available as a 40% injection (Albon), in 125-, 250-, and 500-mg tablets (Albon) and as a pleasant-tasting 5% suspension (Albon), a 12.5% oral solution (Albon), an oral bolus (Albon), a sustained-release bolus (Albon SR), and a soluble powder (Albon).

DOGS AND CATS. The recommended dosage is an initial dose of 55 mg/kg orally or by subcutaneous or intravenous injection for the first day and subsequent doses of 27.5 mg/kg orally once per day for 12 to 21 days. It seems reasonable that since coccidia are enteric pathogens, the oral route would be most effective.

CATTLE AND HORSES. The recommended dosage is an initial dose of 55 mg/kg orally or by subcutaneous or intravenous injection for the first day and subsequent doses of 27.5 mg/kg orally once per day for 4 days. For the sustained-release bolus, give one 12.5-g bolus orally per 200 pounds' body weight. Discard milk for 60 hours (five milkings) after the last treatment. Do not administer drug within 7 days of slaughter. Consult the approved label for accurate dosage and withdrawal information because there is some difference because of dosage form.

POULTRY. Coccidiosis in broilers, pullets, and turkeys can be treated with oral sulfadimethoxine mixed into the drinking water. The usual dosage is 0.05% for chickens and 0.025% for turkeys for 5 days. Do not use drug in chickens older than 16 weeks or in turkeys older than 24 weeks. Do not administer drug within 5 days of slaughter.

Sulfadimethoxine with ormetoprim

Sulfadimethoxine with ormetoprim is the most recently approved potentiated sulfonamide. It constitutes a rational combination that potentiates the action of both drugs by blocking two sequential steps in the synthesis of folic acid. Ormetoprim is a diaminopyrimidine potentiator with very low mammalian toxicity. The available tablets contain 100/20, 200/40, 500/100, or 1000/200 mg of sulfadimethoxine/ormetoprim (Primor). The tablets are designated by the total weight of active ingredient in each tablet. Thus the Primor 120 contains 100 mg of sulfadimethoxine and 20 mg of ormetoprim. The approved starting dosage for dogs is 55 mg/kg orally on the first day of treatment, then 27.5 mg/kg orally once per day for 14 to 21 days. Do not treat beyond 21 days (Entriken, 2001).

It is interesting to note that the only recent controlled study of coccidiosis therapy in dogs was conducted with this drug combination. In that study, 32.5 mg/kg or 66 mg/kg was given continuously in the food for 23 days, subsequent to experimental oocyst infection. The higher dose of 66 mg/kg provided better results and did not produce any adverse reactions (Dunbar and Foreyt, 1985).

Poultry can be treated with the combination in a feed additive (Rofenaid 40). Chickens are fed at 0.0125% sulfa and 0.0075% ormetoprim. Turkeys are treated with 0.00625% sulfa and 0.00375% ormetoprim, and ducks with 0.05% and 0.03%, respectively. Do not feed drug within 5 days of slaughter.

Sulfadiazine with trimethoprim

Sulfadiazine with trimethoprim is the potentiated sulfa with the most years of actual use in veterinary medicine. For many years it was the only potentiated sulfa approved for use in animals. Trimethoprim is a diaminopyrimidine potentiator with very low mammalian toxicity. The available tablets contain 25/5, 100/20, 400/80, or 800/160 mg of sulfadiazine/trimethoprim (Tribrissen, Di-Trim). The tablets are designated by the total weight of active ingredient in each tablet. Thus the Tribrissen 30 contains 25 mg of sulfadiazine and 5 mg of trimethoprim.

The approved dosage is 30 mg/kg orally per day up to 14 days. The preferred dosage for bacterial infections in dogs and cats is 30 mg/kg once or twice daily and may be indicated in severe coccidial infections. The manufacturer recommends that animals with marked hepatic parenchymal damage, blood dyscrasias, or previous sulfonamide sensitivity should not be given this product (Plumb, 1999; Entriken, 2001). Horses may be treated with an oral paste formulation (Tribrissen 400 Oral Paste), which contains 333 mg sulfadiazine and 67 mg trimethoprim per gram. The approved dosage is 5 g of paste per 150 pounds of body weight once daily for 5 to 7 days. The equine injectable formulation contains 400 mg/ml sulfadiazine and 80 mg/ml trimethoprim (Tribrissen 48% injection).

Sulfamethazine

The sodium salt of sulfamethazine may be administered in water (Sulmet) or by oral bolus (Sulfa-Max, Sulfasure, Sulmet) to cattle, sheep, and goats for the control of coccidiosis. The usual dose is 237 mg sulfamethazine per kilogram, which may be administered orally on the first day and followed by 123 mg/kg every day for 4 days (5 days total treatment). A sustained-release bolus (Sustain III) is available, which delivers 32.1 g of sulfamethazine over 3 days. One bolus is given per 200 pounds of body weight. Animals should be provided with plenty of water when they are on sulfonamide medication. Withdrawal recommendations should be followed for food-producing animals.

Sulfamethoxazole with Trimethoprim

Sulfamethoxazole with trimethoprim is a readily available product approved for use in people. It is not currently approved for use in animals. Because of its similarity to veterinary potentiated sulfonamides and because low-cost generics are available, this drug is widely used in veterinary medicine. There is some controversy about the appropriate dosing regimen for this human-labeled product in animals, but many clinicians gain acceptable clinical results using the same dosage as for sulfadiazine.

A 5/1 fixed combination of sulfamethoxazole/trimethoprim is available as tablets and pediatric suspension. The available single-strength tablets contain 400/80 mg, and the double-strength tablets contain 800/160 mg of sulfamethoxazole/trimethoprim, respectively (Bactrim, Septra). The pediatric oral suspension contains 40 mg/ml sulfamethoxazole and 8 mg/ml trimethoprim. The dosage for bacterial infections and coccidiosis in dogs and cats is 30 mg/kg once or twice daily for 14 to 21 days and may be indicated in severe coccidial infections.

Sulfaquinoxaline

Sulfaquinoxaline is a sulfonamide approved for use in poultry, cattle, and sheep for treatment of coccidia. It is not well absorbed from the gastrointestinal tract. Sulfaquinoxaline is available as a water medication (Sul Q Nox). It should be mixed according to the label, which provides cattle with a target dose of 6 mg/lb per day. Chickens should receive 10 to 45 mg/lb per day. Treatment should be administered for 3 to 5 days in cattle and for 2 to 3 days in chickens. Make a fresh solution every day. Do not give drug to lactating dairy cattle. It should not be used within 10 days of slaughter.

■ ANTIHELMINTICS

Several changes have occurred since the last edition of this volume was published (Bowman, 1999), most notably the more widespread use of ivermectin and the emergence of other macrocyclic lactones. Drug manufacturers have discontinued production of many tried and true antihelmintics such as Task Capsules (dichlorvos) and Caparsolate (thiacetarsemide). For simplicity, these drugs do not appear in the current edition. Earlier editions of this text should be consulted for information about discontinued products.

An exhaustive review of the pharmacology, mechanism of action, pharmacokinetics, and efficacy of antihelmintics is outside the scope of this book. We have included a few key references in the text to help the veterinarian. For more exhaustive information on antihelmintics, two excellent works should be consulted (Arundel et al, 1985; Campbell and Rew, 1985). A compendium of products approved by the FDA and commercially available can be found in the *Veterinary Pharmaceuticals and Biologicals* (Entriken, 2001) and the current *Feed Additive Compendium* (Muirhead, 2001).

Gastrointestinal parasites are among the most common infectious agents that veterinarians must manage (Blagburn, 1996). In the landmark parasite prevalence study, Blagburn and colleagues evaluated more than 6000 canine fecal specimens

from all 50 states and the District of Columbia. The results indicate that parasites remain common even in dogs. Nationwide, 36% of the samples tested were positive for roundworm *(Toxocara canis),* hookworm, *(Ancylostoma caninum),* or whipworm *(Trichuris vulpis).* Even more surprising, 52% of the samples from the southwestern United States were positive for at least one of the important nematodes. Although these parasites affect the health of dogs, several are also zoonotic pathogens.

Some research has focused on defining the mechanism of action for antihelmintics. It is hoped that this information will lead eventually to new therapeutic agents. Several reviews discuss this exciting research (Matin, 1993; Londershausen, 1996). The current information has shed new light on mechanisms of drug action and in many cases has changed our opinion on how these drugs work.

Antihelmintics approved by the U.S. FDA and still commercially available are grouped together by class according to their generic names. A few other drugs widely used outside the United States and several nearing approval are also included.

Macrolides

Macrolides (or macrocyclic lactones) have revolutionized the control of parasites in both man and animal. Ivermectin is the best-known agent in this class, which includes avermectins. They are generally regarded as the most effective and least toxic parasiticides yet developed. These products are all similar in that they are antibiotics produced by streptomycete microorganisms, and they have large macrocyclic structures. Although originally thought to act by disturbing GABA-mediated neurotransmission, it is now known that they all bind with high affinity to a glutamate-gated chloride channel (Arena et al, 1991; Martin, 1993; Shoop et al, 1995). The macrocyclic lactones apparently trigger chloride influx, which hyperpolarizes the parasite neuron and prevents initiation or propagation of normal action potentials. The net effect is paralysis and death of the target parasite.

The macrocyclic lactones have revolutionized treatment of parasitic disease. In general, they are highly effective at low doses, are very safe, and provide true broad-spectrum activity against nematodes and arthropods. Commercially, they have crushed the competition. Many conventional drugs that are direct competitors of this class are soon retired from common use and are eventually discontinued by the manufacturer. Many of the old drugs are casualties of the "macrocyclic revolution."

Despite their wonderful activities, macrocyclic lactones have several flaws. They are ineffective against cestodes and trematodes, and they are often expensive. The U.S. patent on ivermectin has now expired; this has allowed generic competitors to enter the market, which may soon change the cost of treatment with ivermectin.

The literature surrounding these products is overwhelming, but there are several good reviews that pare the literature down to comprehendable levels (Bennett, 1986; Campbell, 1989; Shoop et al, 1995).

Doramectin

Doramectin (Dectomax) is the most recent macrocyclic drug to enter the marketplace. It is a fermentation product from a mutant strain of *Streptomyces avermitilis,* and its spectrum of action is similar to avermectin B$_1$, although it has an elimination half-life about twice that of ivermectin (Shoop et al, 1995; Friis and Bjoern, 1997).

CATTLE. Recently approved by the U.S. FDA, doramectin (Dectomax, Dectomax Pour-On) provides broad-spectrum activity against bovine parasites. When injected subcutaneously in cattle at a dose of 200 µg/kg or applied topically at a dose of 500 µg/kg, it is effective against *Ostertagia ostertagi, Ostertagia lyrata, Haemonchus placei, Trichostrongylus axei, Trichostrongylus colubriformis, Cooperia oncophora, Cooperia punctata, Cooperia pectinata, Cooperia surnabada, Bunostomum phlebotomum, Oesophagostomum radiatum, Trichuris* spp., *Dictyocaulus viviparus, Thelazia* spp., *Hypoderma bovis, Hypoderma lineatum, Psoroptes bovis, Sarcoptes scabiei, Hematopinus eurysternus, Linognathus vituli, and Solenopotes capillatus* (Eddi et al, 1993; Gonzales et al, 1993; Goudie et al, 1993; Hendrickx et al, 1993; Jones et al, 1993; Kennedy and Phillips, 1993; Moya-Borja et al, 1993a; Vercruysse et al, 1993; Weatherley et al, 1993; Wicks et al, 1993; Logan et al, 1997; Reinemeyer and Courtney, 2001). Rather surprising is doramectin's activity against the screwworm *Cochliomyia hominivorax,* which is missing from other macrocyclic agents (Moya-Borja et al, 1993b). The injection should not be used within 35 days of slaughter. The pour-on product also has activity against biting lice *Damalinia bovis* and the mange mite *Chorioptes bovis.* It should not be used in cattle within 45 days of slaughter.

SWINE. Doramectin injection (Dectomax) is also approved for use in swine. Injections of 300 µg/kg are effective against *Ascaris suum, Oesophagostomum dentatum, Oesophagostomum quadrispinulatum, Hyostrongylus rubidus, Strongyloides ransomi, Stephanurus dentatus, Sarcoptes scabiei var. suis, Haematopinus suis, and Metastrongylus* spp. (Saeki et al, 1995; Stewart et al, 1996a; Stewart et al, 1996b; Arends et al, 1997a; Arends et al, 1997b; Lichtensteiger et al, 1997; Logan et al, 1997). It should not be used in swine within 24 days of slaughter.

Eprinomectin

Eprinomectin is a true second-generation macrocyclic lactone. It was synthesized from avermectin B$_1$ by the same group that discovered ivermectin. The paper that describes the targeted research effort to find eprinomectin is a beautiful description of targeted research and should be read by any scientist interested in understanding the scope of the pharmaceutical research process (Shoop et al, 1996a). Eprinomectin is synthesized from a fermentation product of *S. avermitilis.* It has extremely broad-spectrum activity, is formulated in an easy-to-apply pour-on formulation, and most surprisingly, has zero time withdrawal for meat and milk. It is the only macrocyclic that can be used in lactating dairy cattle because it partitions away from milk (Shoop et al, 1996b).

CATTLE. Eprinomectin (Eprinex) is approved in a topical formulation, which is applied at 500 µg/kg. It is effective against all common cattle nematodes, including *H. placei, O. ostertagi, O. lyrata, Ostertagia leptospicularis, Cooperia onchophora, C. punctata, C. surnabada, T. axei, T. colubriformis, Nematodirus helvetianus, O. radiatum, D. viviparus,* and *Trichuris* spp. (Cramer et al, 1997; Gogolewski et al, 1997b; Reid et al, 1997; Yazwinski et al, 1997). The efficacy is not affected by coat length or by rain or weather (Gogolewski et al, 1997a). Not surprisingly, it is also effective against several arthropod ectoparasites, including *S. scabiei, Damalinia (Bovicola) bovis,* and *C. bovis* (Eagleson et al, 1997a; Eagleson et al, 1997b; Thompson et al, 1997).

Ivermectin

Ivermectin was the first commercially available macrolide. The avermectins were isolated from the fermentation broth of *S. avermitilis.* The discovery of the antihelmintic activity was made by administering the actinomycetic broth to mice infected with the nematode *N. dubius.* Ivermectin is effective against many nematodes and arthropods. It is very effective against immature *Dirofilaria immitis,* but has minimal effect on adult heartworms. *N. helvetianus* in cattle is one of the least sensitive worms; about 85% efficacy was reported in the literature. The suggested dosage levels are 0.2 mg/kg for cattle, sheep, and horses, and 0.3 mg/kg for swine.

Administration of ivermectin to pregnant rats, mice, and rabbits produced teratism in fetuses only at or near maternotoxic doses. There was no teratogenesis in cattle, sheep, and dogs when ivermectin was administered to pregnant animals at four times the recommended dose. Although toxicity for aquatic animals is high, the binding of ivermectin in soil reduces its concentration to levels that have no impact on the quality of the environment. The acute oral LD$_{50}$ of ivermectin in mice varied from

11.6 to 87.2 mg/kg, and the LD_{50} for rats was 42.8 to 52.8 mg/kg. In a 14-week study with rats, the "no-effect" level was 0.4 mg/kg.

Although originally believed to act by disturbing GABA-mediated neurotransmission, it is now known that ivermectin binds with high affinity to a glutamate-gated chloride channel (Martin, 1993; Shoop et al, 1995). Ivermectin apparently triggers chloride influx, which hyperpolarizes the parasite neuron and prevents initiation or propagation of normal action potentials. The net effect is paralysis and death of the target parasite. In arthropods, ivermectin inhibits transmission of signals at the neuromuscular junctions by the same mechanism. In both cases, death results from paralysis.

HORSES. Ivermectin (Eqvalan paste or liquid) has a broad spectrum of activity against nematodes and arthropod parasites of horses and is administered orally at 0.2 mg/kg of body weight. It is used for the treatment and control of large strongyles: adult *Strongylus equinus;* adult, arterial, and migrating larval stages of *Strongylus vulgaris;* adult and migrating tissue stages of *Strongylus edentatus;* adult *Triodontophorus* spp.; small strongyles, including those resistant to some benzimidazole class compounds (adult and fourth-stage larvae of *Cyathostomum* spp., *Cylicocyclus* spp., *Cylicodontophorus* spp., *Cyclicostephanus* spp.); pinworms; adult and fourth-stage larvae of *Oxyuris equi;* adult and larval stages of *Parascaris equorum;* adult *T. axei;* adult *Habronema muscae;* oral and stomach stages of *Gasterophilus* spp.; adult and fourth-stage larvae of *Dictyocaulus arnfieldi, Strongylus westeri;* summer sores caused by *Habronema* and *Draschia* spp. cutaneous third-stage larvae; and dermatitis caused by microfilariae of *Onchocerca cervicalis.* At times, however, treated horses had edematous reactions caused by a massive release of parasitic antigens.

Oral administration of three times the recommended dose of ivermectin was well tolerated by horses. Pregnant mares treated orally with 0.6 mg/kg of ivermectin throughout the organogenesis period gave birth to normal, healthy foals. Treatment with 0.6 mg/kg of ivermectin did not affect the sexual behavior of stallions, and the quality of semen was not affected. Because safety has not been demonstrated in horses younger than 4 months, ivermectin should not be administered to foals of this age.

CATTLE. Ivermectin (Ivomec) is formulated as a liquid for subcutaneous injection and a paste for oral administration at a dose level of 0.2 mg/kg of body weight. The subcutaneous administration of ivermectin affords excellent efficacy against adult and larval stages of *O. osteragi,* including inhibited fourth-stage larvae of *O. lyrata, H. placei, T. axei, T. columbriformis, C. oncophora, C. punctata, C. pectinata, O. radiatum, B. phlebotomum, D. vivipa-*

rus, and *Strongyloides papillosus* and *Trichuris ovis* (adults only). Its efficacy against the adult *N. helvetianus* and *N. spathiger,* at least with the injectable ivermectin, is about 85%. Ivermectin is highly active against cattle grubs (first, second, and third instars) *H. bovis* and *H. lineatum;* lice *(L. vituli, H. eurysternus, S. capillatus);* and mites *(P ovis, Sarcoptes scabiei var. bovis).* Injectable ivermectin affords consistently good efficacy against sucking lice and mites. The efficacy of ivermectin against biting lice is erratic. Ivermectin is also active against adult *Parafilaria bovicola* and adult and immature conjunctival worm *Thelazia rhodesii.* The drug is absorbed, widely distributed in the tissues, and excreted in the feces as unaltered ivermectin that may prevent the development of coprophilic larvae. Ivermectin is slowly eliminated from the body.

Ivermectin up to 1.2 mg/kg was well tolerated by cattle. Higher doses resulted in transient localized swellings at the injection site. Cattle injected with 8 mg/kg became recumbent within 24 hours after treatment, and three animals died. Ivermectin at a dose of 0.4 mg/kg was administered to pregnant cows 7 to 56 days after insemination. There were no adverse effects on the cows and no teratogenic effects in the calves that were delivered. No adverse effects were observed in the breeding performance or semen quality of bulls treated with ivermectin at 0.4 mg/kg. The only limitation on the label is that animals treated orally should not be sent to slaughter for 24 days, and the withdrawal time for the injectable form is 35 days. The rapid death of cattle grubs after administration of ivermectin may result in acute esophagitis and posterior paresis as a consequence of spinal cord hemorrhages.

Ivermectin is also available in a pour-on formulation for application to cattle. It contains 5 mg/ml of ivermectin and is applied at a rate of 1.0 ml/10 kg. The drug is approved for the removal of *O. ostertagi, H. placei, T. axei, T. colubriformis, Cooperia* spp., *S. papillosus, O. radiatum, Trichuris* spp., *D. viviparus, H. bovis, H. lineatum, S. scabiei var. bovis, L. vituli, H. eurysternus, D. bovis, S. capillatus,* and *Haematobia irritans.* Cattle must not be treated within 48 days of slaughter for human consumption. Because a withdrawal time in milk has not been established, do not use ivermectin in female dairy cattle of breeding age.

Ivermectin is now available in a controlled-release bolus (Ivomec SR Bolus), which is administered orally. Each bolus contains 1.72 g of ivermectin, which is delivered over 135 days. The bolus is given to calves weighing 100 to 200 pounds. The withdrawal period (in Canada) is 184 days (Yazwinski et al, 1995; Ryan et al, 1997).

SHEEP. Ivomec drench at a dose level of 0.2 mg/kg is used for the treatment and control of the adult and fourth-stage larvae of *Haemonchus contortus,* *H. placei* (adults only), *Telordosagia circumcincta,* *T. axei, T. colubriformis, C. oncophora* (adults only), *Cooperia curticei, Oesophagostomum columbianum, Oesophagostomum venulosum* (adults only), *Nematodirus battus, N. spathiger, S. papillosus* (adults only), *Chabertia ovina* (adults only), *T. ovis* (adults only), *Dictyocaulus filaria,* and all the larval stages of the nasal bot *Oestrus ovis.* Overseas, injectable ivermectin is used for the treatment of psoroptic mange. Numerous reports indicate that ivermectin is highly active against benzimidazole-resistant populations of *Haemonchus, Trichostrongylus,* and *Ostertagia* organisms. The dose in sheep and goats is 0.2 mg/kg by subcutaneous injection. There is a label limitation stating that sheep should not be treated within 11 days of slaughter.

SWINE. Ivermectin liquid is administered subcutaneously in the neck area at a dose level of 0.3 mg/kg. It is indicated for the treatment and control of adult and fourth-stage larvae of *A. suum, H. rubidus, Oesophagostomum* spp., *S. ransomi* (including the somatic larvae), the adult lungworm *Metastrongylus* spp., lice *(H. suis),* and mites *(S. scabiei var. suis).* The colostral transmission of *S. ransomi* can be prevented by injecting ivermectin into sows 7 to 14 days before farrowing. Ivermectin was shown to be highly active against the adult and fourth-stage larvae of the swine kidneyworm *S. dentatus.* Swine should not be treated within 18 days of slaughter. In short-term studies, ivermectin was injected into swine up to 30 mg/kg without fatal sequelae, but lethargy, ataxia, labored breathing, and other toxicity signs were noted. No toxic effects were observed in sows treated with 0.6 mg/kg during the first month of gestation, and no teratogenic effects were observed in the litters. Also, no adverse effects were observed in the breeding performance or semen quality of boars treated with 0.6 mg/kg of ivermectin.

Ivermectin is also available in a premix for administration in feed (Ivomec Premix for Swine). It is formulated to provide 0.1 mg of ivermectin per kilogram of body weight daily for a maximum of 7 consecutive days. The drug is indicated for the treatment of *A. suum, Ascarops strongylina, H. rubidus, Oesophagostomum* spp., *Metastrongylus* spp., *H. suis,* and *S. scabiei var. suis.* Medicated feed should be withdrawn 5 days before slaughter.

DOGS. Ivermectin (Heartgard) chewables are administered orally at a dose level of 0.006 mg (6 μg) per kilogram at monthly intervals to prevent the establishment of the *D. immitis.* The initial dose should be given within a month after the first exposure to mosquitoes and throughout the year when mosquitoes are active. The last treatment must be given to dogs within a month after the last exposure to mosquitoes.

Ivermectin has minimal activity against the adult heartworm. It is active only against the third- and fourth-stage larvae and the circulating microfilariae.

A single oral dose of ivermectin administered within 2 months after infection prevents the establishment of the worms in the heart. A single dose of 0.05 mg/kg is adequate to clear the circulating microfilariae when given to dogs 4 weeks after the administration of an adulticide. Ivermectin has not yet been approved as a microfilaricide. When ivermectin (6 μg/kg) is given to heartworm-positive dogs over several months, the circulating microfilariae are eliminated, resulting in an occult infection. Thus dogs on monthly ivermectin should be tested with an occult heartworm test (Bowman et al, 1992; Lok and Knight, 1995).

When replacing diethylcarbamazine in a preventive program, the first dose of Heartgard must be given within a month after stopping diethylcarbamazine. Heartgard should not be given to dogs younger than 6 weeks.

Ivermectin as a single subcutaneous injection at 0.2 mg/kg demonstrated high efficacy against the immature and adult *T. canis, A. caninum, Ancylostoma braziliense, Uncinaria stenocephala,* and *Strongyloides stercoralis.* Its activity against *Toxascaris leonina* and *T. vulpis* is erratic.

Ivermectin is safe in collies at the approved dose of 6 μg/kg. Early studies indicated that when ivermectin was given at a dose of 200 μg/kg (32 times the label dose), some genetic lines of collies could have severe adverse reactions: mydriasis, ataxia, tremors, drooling, paresis, recumbency, excitability, stupor, and coma. A single oral dose of 2 mg/kg and repeated oral doses of 0.5 mg/kg per day for 14 weeks were well tolerated by dogs. Mydriasis, depression, tremors, ataxia, coma, and death have been observed following doses in excess of 20 mg/kg in laboratory dogs (Pulliam et al, 1985). No teratism was observed in fetuses when pregnant bitches received repeated oral doses of ivermectin at 0.5 mg/kg.

A new combination product (Heartguard Plus) containing ivermectin and pyrantel pamoate is available. For more information, see the section on combination products.

CATS. Ivermectin is approved as a heartworm preventive for cats (Heartgard for Cats). Monthly doses of 0.024 mg/kg are effective in preventing the development of *D. immitis* (McTier et al, 1992; Paul et al, 1992a). It is also approved for use against *A. braziliense* and *Ancylostoma tubaeforme* (Nolan et al, 1992; Roberson et al, 1992). A dose of 0.3 mg/kg is required to eliminate *Toxocara cati* (Blagburn et al, 1987; Kirkpatrick and Megella, 1987). Although unapproved in the United States, injectable ivermectin is effective against ear mites *(Otodectes cynotis)* when injected subcutaneously at 0.3 mg/kg every 1 to 2 weeks for two to three doses (Gram et al, 1994).

Acarexx contains 0.01% ivermectin in a liposomal formulation. It is approved for the treatment of ear mites *(O. cynotis)* in cats and kittens 4 weeks of age or older. Recent studies have demonstrated activity against the eggs and immature stages of the ear mite (Bowman et al, 2001; Wexler-Mitchell, 2001).

Milbemycin oxime

Milbemycin oxime was the second macrocyclic lactone to achieve approval by the U.S. FDA. It is a fermentation product of *Streptomyces hygroscopicus aureolacrimosis.* The drug has structural similarities to ivermectin and is believed to work by a similar mechanism of action.

DOGS. Milbemycin oxime tablets (Interceptor) are formulated to deliver 0.5 mg/kg of body weight. When given every 30 days, it is effective in preventing heartworms *(D. immitis)* (Bater, 1989; Bradley, 1989; Grieve et al, 1991). The product also kills *A. caninum* and removes and controls *T. canis* and *T. vulpis* (Bowman et al, 1988; Bowman et al, 1990; Bowman et al, 1991; Blagburn et al, 1992b). Milbemycin oxime has been extensively tested with regard to safety. It is nontoxic to collies at up to 20 times the recommended dose (Blagburn et al, 1989; Sasaki et al, 1990) and can safely be given to pregnant and nursing animals. Although an LD_{50} was never determined in dogs, the drug was well tolerated when given at 200 mg/kg in a single oral dose.

Milbemycin oxime, like ivermectin, is known to kill heartworm microfilariae and inhibit the release of new microfilariae, so all dogs on routine monthly heartworm prophylaxis should be tested with adult antigen tests (Blagburn et al, 1992; Bowman et al, 1992; Lok et al, 1992; Lok and Knight, 1995).

Some work (Garfield and Reedy, 1992; Miller et al, 1993; Miller et al, 1995b) has shown that milbemycin oxime is effective in curing amitraz-resistant *Demodex canis* when given at a dosage of 1 to 2 mg/kg daily for 60 to 90 days. It is also highly effective against *S. scabiei* when given orally at 1 mg/kg every other day for 10 to 14 days (Bourdeau et al, 1997). It is interesting that milbemycin oxime is effective against the nasal mite *Pneumonyssoides caninum* when given at 0.5 to 1.0 mg.kg once a week for 3 weeks (Gunnarsson et al, 1997). These uses are not approved by the FDA.

CATS. Recently approved for use in cats, milbemycin oxime is effective against *D. immitis* at a dose of 0.5 mg/kg every 30 days (Stewart et al, 1992) and against *A. tubaeforme* (Blagburn et al, 1992c) when given at a dose of 1.5 mg/kg.

Milbemite Otic Solution is a 0.1% solution of milbemycin oxime, approved for the treatment of ear mite *(Otodectes cyanotis)* infestations in cats and

kittens 8 weeks of age or older. It is effective against all life stages of the ear mite (Anonymous, 2000).

TURTLES. It is interesting to note that milbemycin oxime is apparently nontoxic in turtles and proved somewhat effective in a small study conducted on red-eared sliders *(Chrysemys scripta elegans)* and Gulf Coast box turtles *(Terrapene carolina major)* (Bodri et al, 1993). It is not approved for this use.

Moxidectin

Moxidectin, the third macrolide to enter the parasite market in the United States, is a chemically altered product of *Streptomyces aureolacrimosus noncyanogenus.* It has the same range of activity and safety margin as ivermectin and milbemycin oxime.

HORSES. Moxidectin (Quest Gel) can be given by oral administration (0.3 mg/kg) against *Cyathostomum* spp., *Cylicocyclus* spp., *Cylicostephanus* spp., *Gyalocephalus capitatus, S. vulgaris, S. edentatus, Triodontophorus brevicauda, Triodontophorus serratus, P equorum, O. equi, T. axei, Habronema muscae,* and *Gasterophilus intestinalis* (Lyons et al, 1992; Bello and Laningham, 1994; Taylor and Kenny, 1995; Anonymous, 1997a; Slocombe and Lake, 1997; Vercruysse et al, 1997b). It seems to be particularly effective against encysted small strongyles. Moxidectin is safe for use in mares during breeding, gestation, and lactation, and for foals older than 4 months.

CATTLE. Moxidectin given orally to calves at 0.2 and 0.4 mg/kg was more than 99% effective against fourth-stage and adult *O. ostertagi, Cooperia* spp., *N. helvetianus,* and adult *Trichostrongylus* spp., *Capillaria* spp., *Trichuris discolor,* and *O. radiatum* (Zimmerman et al, 1992). When given subcutaneously, moxidectin was effective against fourth-stage and adult *O. ostertagi, N. helvetianus B. phlebotomum,* adult *O. lyrata, H. placei, T. axei, T. colubriformis, C. oncophora, C. punctata, Cooperia spatulata, C. pectinata, T. discolor, O. radiatum,* and *D. viviparus* (Eysker and Boersema, 1992; Ranjan et al, 1992; Williams et al, 1992a; Williams et al, 1992b). It was also highly effective against the common cattle grub, *H. bovis,* and *H. lineatum,* when given by injection at 0.1, 0.2, or 0.4 mg/kg (Scholl et al, 1992). A 0.5% pour-on formulation (Cydectin) was approved in the United States to control all the parasites previously mentioned along with mites, lice, and hornflies at a dose of 0.5 mg/kg (Morin et al, 1996; Vercruysse et al, 1997a).

SHEEP. Moxidectin has shown good activity against several strains of ivermectin-resistant strains of *H. contortus* when given at 0.2 and 0.4 mg/kg subcutaneously (Craig et al, 1992).

DOGS. Moxidectin is known to be very active against heartworms *D. immitis* and gastrointestinal nematodes. It is approved by the FDA for prevention of heartworms (Proheart for Dogs) at a dosage of 3 µg/kg orally per month. When moxidectin is administered at 3 µg/kg of body weight monthly, it is 100% effective in preventing the development of adult *D. immitis* (King et al, 1992; McCall et al, 1992; McTier et al, 1992).

At the recommended dose it is safe in rough-coated collies (Paul et al, 1992b), and it produced no adverse effects in collie dogs when given at 20 times the approved dose, although mild toxic signs were seen at 30 times the approved dose (Anonymous, 1997c). Moxidectin showed little effect on circulating microfilariae of *D. immitis* in a short-term study (Hendrix et al, 1992). It also produced no adverse reaction in dogs with patent heartworm infection, although the approved label prohibits use in heartworm-infected dogs (Anonymous, 1997c).

Moxidectin is also effective against gastrointestinal nematodes, although not approved for this use. It was effective against *A. caninum* at 25 µg/kg and *U. stenocephala* at 150 µg/kg. It also demonstrated good activity against *T. canis* and *T. leonina* at the doses tested (25 to 300 µg/kg orally) (Supakorndej et al, 1993).

Proheart 6 is a sustained release formulation that provides therapeutic levels for 6 months after injection. It is approved in the United States for prevention of heartworm *(D. immitis)* and for the treatment of existing larvae and adult hookworm *(A. caninum)* infection (Blagburn et al, 2001; Lok et al, 2001; McCall et al, 2001). It is indicated for use in dogs 6 months of age or older. It is safe for use in collies.

Selamectin

Selamectin is the newest macrocyclic lactone. This novel endectocide is prepared by semi-synthetic modification of doramectin (Bishop et al, 2000). It is the first molecule to provide activity against internal and external parasites of dogs without toxicity in collies.

DOGS AND CATS. Revolution is formulated for topical application in dogs and cats 6 weeks or age or older. The stated dose is 6 mg/kg every 30 days. It is approved for control of external parasites including the elimination and control of fleas *(Ctenocephalides felis)* and ear mites *(O. cynotis)* (Boy et al, 2000; McTier et al, 2001a; McTier et al, 2000b; Shanks et al, 2000b; Shanks et al, 2000c; Six et al, 2000a). In dogs it is approved for the treament and control of sarcoptic mange *(S. scabiei)* and tick infestation *(Dermacentor variabilis)* (Jernigan et al, 2000; Shanks et al, 2001a). It is especially known for the prevention of heartworm *(D. immitis)* in both dogs and cats (Boy et al, 2000). In cats it is also effective in the treatment and control of hookworm *(A. tubaeforme)* and roundworm *(T. cati)* (McTier

et al, 2000c; McTier et al, 2000d; Six et al, 2000b). All this activity is provided in a convenient topical product that demonstrates a good margin of safety in both dogs and cats (Krautmann et al, 2000; Novotny et al, 2000).

Benzimidazoles

The benzimidazoles represent a large family of broad-spectrum agents that have enjoyed widespread use for many years in a wide array of animal species. Excellent review articles (Campbell, 1990; Lacey, 1990; McKellar and Scott, 1990) discuss the history, mode of action, and spectrum of activity of this useful class of anthelmintics.

Thiabendazole was the first benzimidazole discovered, and it represented a major step forward when it became available more than 30 years ago. At the time of its introduction, thiabendazole was a true broad-spectrum product that was very safe to the host animal. Since that time, parasite resistance to the benzimidazoles has been discovered in several species.

Considerable effort has been devoted to determining the mechanism by which the benzimidazoles act on parasites. Conventional wisdom holds that benzimidazoles bind to tubulin molecules, which inhibits the formation of microtubules and disrupts cell division (Frayha et al, 1997; Reinemeyer and Courtney, 2001). It has a much higher affinity for nematode tubulin versus mammalian tubulin, thus providing selective activity against parasites. Evidence also indicates that the benzimidazoles can inhibit fumarate reductase, which blocks mitochondrial function, depriving the parasite of energy and thus resulting in death.

The benzimidazoles are poorly soluble and therefore are generally given by mouth. In general, they are more effective in horses and ruminants because of their slow transit through the cecum and rumen. The dosage is usually more effective when divided, thus prolonging the contact time with the parasite. Three members of the benzimidazole group (albendazole, mebendazole, and oxfendazole) have been found to be teratogenic, thus limiting their use in pregnant animals.

For simplicity the probenzimidazole drug febantel is included in this section. It is a nonbenzimidazole drug that is metabolized to a benzimidazole. It thus shares a similar efficacy and mechanism of action with the other benzimidazoles.

Albendazole

Albendazole, the newest benzimidazole, has potent broad-spectrum antihelmintic activity. It offers a wide margin of safety in cattle when used according to the label specifications.

Albendazole has demonstrated a broad spectrum of antihelmintic activity against gastrointestinal nematodes; lung nematodes, including inhibited larval forms; cestodes; and lung and liver trematodes in farm animals, companion animals, and humans. Albendazole (Zentel) is used overseas for the treatment of intestinal helminth infections, hydatid disease, and cysticercoses of humans.

CATTLE. Albendazole (Valbazen) is administered orally at a dose level of 10 mg/kg for the removal and control of adult and larval stages of *H. contortus, H. placei,* and *O. ostertagi,* including the fourth-stage inhibited larvae, *T. axei, T. colubriformis, N. spathiger, N. helvetianus, C. punctata, C. oncophora, B. phlebotomum, O. radiatum, D. viviparus, Moniezia benedeni, Moniezia expansa,* and adult *Fasciola hepatica* (Bogan and Armour, 1987; Prichard, 1986; Prichard, 1987).

The safety of albendazole in single and repeated treatments was evaluated in healthy and parasitized cattle. A single dose of 75 mg/kg of body weight was well tolerated. Albendazole was embryotoxic when administered to cows at a dosage rate of 25 mg/kg during the first 7 to 17 days of gestation. The conception rate of cows dosed after the twenty-first day of gestation was comparable to that in controls, and all cows gave birth to normal calves.

In the United States, cattle must not be slaughtered within 27 days after treatment. Also, albendazole should not be used in female dairy cattle of breeding age, and the label cautions that the drug should not be given to pregnant cows during the first 45 days of gestation.

SHEEP. Although not approved in the United States, albendazole drench (Valbazen) is administered orally at 3.8 to 5.0 mg/kg for the control of *Haemonchus, Ostertagia,* and *Trichostrongylus* organisms in the abomasum; *Nematodirus, Cooperia, Marshallagia, Bunostomum, Gaigeria, Chabertia, Oesophagostomum, Moniezia,* and *Avitellina* organisms in the intestines; and *Dictyocaulus* organisms in the lungs. For the control of *F. hepatica,* albendazole is administered at 4.75 to 7.5 mg/kg. Outstanding efficacy was observed against *Fascioloides magna* in sheep at a dose of 7.5 mg/kg (McKellar and Scott, 1990). Albendazole at 15 mg/kg is used overseas for the treatment of *Dicrocoelium dendriticum.* The maximum tolerated dose in sheep is reported to be about 37.5 mg/kg.

Albendazole may induce fetal skeletal abnormalities when administered at a dose level of 11 mg/kg or more to ewes during the first 10 to 17 days of pregnancy. No untoward effects have been reported after its use in many thousands of sheep, however.

WARNING: Care should be taken to adhere to recommended dosages, particularly when treating ewes during the first month of pregnancy. Sheep should not be treated within 10 days of slaughter.

DOGS AND CATS. Albendazole is not approved for use in dogs and cats. Dogs treated with 50 mg/kg twice daily may have anorexia, and cats treated with 100 mg/kg daily for 14 to 21 days showed weight loss, neutropenia, and mental dullness (Plumb, 1999). Dogs can be treated for *Filaroides hirthi* at a dosage of 25 to 50 mg/kg twice daily for 5 days (Georgi et al, 1978). *Capillaria plica* can be treated at a dosage of 50 mg/kg twice daily for 10 to 14 days (Brown and Barsanti, 1989) and *Paragonimus kellicotti* at a dosage of 25 mg/kg twice daily for 21 days. The same dosage is effective for *Paragonimus* organisms in cats (Plumb, 1999). Although albendazole is effective against these uncommon parasites, ivermectin and praziquantel are more convenient therapies and likely to be just as effective. More interesting is the use of albendazole against *Giardia* organisms in dogs at 25 mg/kg twice daily for 2 days (Barr et al, 1993).

Febantel

Febantel is a prodrug that is metabolized to fenbendazole and oxfendazole, which are undoubtedly the active parasiticides (McKellar and Scott, 1990). The oral acute toxic dose in mice, rats, and dogs is more than 10 g/kg. At oral doses above 150 mg/kg daily for 6 days, transient salivation, diarrhea, vomiting, and anorexia may be seen in dogs and cats.

Combination products of febantel with praziquantel and pyrantel are discussed in the section on combination products.

Fenbendazole

Fenbendazole is a commercially successful benzimidazole that enjoys wide use in both cattle and dogs. The oral LD_{50} for rats and mice is higher than 10 g/kg. Fenbendazole does not have embryotoxic or teratogenic effects in rats, sheep, and cattle. In the rabbit, fenbendazole was fetotoxic but not teratogenic, and no carcinogenesis was observed in lifetime studies in rats and mice. In a 6-month toxicity study in dogs, no effect was observed at 4 mg/kg or less.

Absorbed fenbendazole is metabolized to at least two active metabolites, oxfendazole sulfoxide and oxfendazole sulfone. In ruminants it is known to undergo enterohepatic cycling, which serves to prolong effective blood levels (USP, 1998).

Fenbendazole is a broad-spectrum anthelmintic with activity against gastrointestinal nematodes and cestodes and lung nematodes in cattle, sheep, goats, and horses. Activity against a variety of helminth parasites in dogs, cats, and many zoo animals also has been reported. In the United States, fenbendazole is approved for control of helminth parasites in horses, cattle, and dogs.

CATTLE. Fenbendazole (Safe-Guard, Panacur; suspension, premix pellets, deworming block, and free-choice mineral supplement) is administered orally or fed to animals at 5 mg/kg for the removal and control of adult and larval stages of *H. contortus, O. ostertagi, T. axei, B. phlebotomum, Nematodirus helvetianus, Cooperia punctata, C. onchophora, Trichostrongylus colubriformis, O. radiatum,* and the lungworm *D. viviparous* (Yazwinski et al, 1985; Yazwinski et al, 1989). For the removal of tapeworms *(Moniezia)* and the inhibited fourth-stage larvae of *Ostertagia,* fenbendazole is used at 10 mg/kg. Overseas, the recommended dose level is 7.5 mg/kg, with additional claims of efficacy against *Trichuris, Strongyloides,* and *Capillaria* species and nematode eggs. The maximum tolerated dose is about 2000 mg/kg. In cattle, fenbendazole is not embryotoxic or teratogenic and does not impair the fertility of bulls (Muser and Paul, 1984).

Fenbendazole has been shown to be effective against *Giardia* organisms in calves when given as a single oral dose at 10 mg/kg (O'Handley et al, 1997).

WARNING: Cattle must not be slaughtered within 8 days of medication with fenbendazole, and dairy cattle of breeding age should not be treated because a suitable milk withdrawal time has not yet been established. In Great Britain, milk from treated cows may be consumed 72 hours after the last administration of fenbendazole.

HORSES. Fenbendazole suspension, granules, or paste (Panacur) is administered orally to horses at 5 mg/kg for the control of *S. vulgaris, S. edentatus, S. equinus, O. equi,* and many species of cyathostomes. For the removal of *P. equorum,* a dose of 10 mg/kg is recommended. Pregnant mares, stallions, and foals may be treated safely with fenbendazole at the recommended dosages. For the control of fourth-stage larvae of *S. vulgaris,* the recommended dosage is 10 mg/kg daily for 5 days (Lyons, et al, 1983; Leneau et al, 1985).

SWINE. Fenbendazole is approved as a feed additive (Safe-Guard) for swine. A total dose of 9 mg/kg is divided and fed over a 3- to 12-day period. This dosage removes the adult and immature forms of *A. suum, H. rubidus, O. dentatum, O. quadrispinulatum, Trichuris suis, S. dentatus, Metastrongylus apri,* and *Metastrongylus pudendotectus* (Biehl, 1986). There is no withdrawal time restriction.

DOGS. Fenbendazole granules (Panacur) at a dose level of 50 mg/kg are mixed in the feed and given to dogs for 3 consecutive days for the removal of *T. canis, T. leonina, A. caninum, U. stenocephala, T. vulpis,* and *Taenia pisiformis* (Burke and Roberson, 1978; Burke and Roberson, 1979; Roberson and Burke, 1982; Cornelius and Roberson, 1986; Bowman, 1992; Reinemeyer, 2000). Higher unap-proved dose levels (50 mg/kg) for several weeks demonstrated excellent activity against the lung fluke *P. kellicotti* (Dubey et al, 1979). Fenbendazole is safe, and there are no known contraindications for its use in dogs with *Giardia* organisms.

CATS. Fenbendazole is not currently approved for use in cats. When given at a dose of 50 mg/kg, it is effective against adult *T. cati, A. tubaeforme, Aelurostrongylus abstrusus,* and *P. kellicotti* (Roberson and Burke, 1980; Bowman, 1992).

SHEEP AND GOATS. Overseas, oral administration of fenbendazole at 5 mg/kg is recommended for removal of adult and immature stages of gastrointestinal nematodes, cestodes, and lung nematodes. Some *Haemonchus* populations apparently have developed resistance to fenbendazole. The FDA has approved the use of fenbendazole for the treatment of lungworms (*Protostrongylus* spp.) in Rocky Mountain bighorn sheep

ZOO ANIMALS. Fenbendazole granules (Panacur) are among the few commercial products actually approved by the FDA for use in zoo animals. The label allows use in lions *(Panthera leo),* tigers *(Panthera tigris),* cheetahs *(Acinonyx jubatus),* pumas *(Felis concolor),* jaguars *(Panthera onca),* leopards *(Panthera pardus),* panthers (*Panthera* spp.), grizzly bears *(Ursus horribilis),* polar bears *(Ursus maritimus),* and black bears *(Ursus americanus).* The label recommends 10 mg/kg orally for 3 consecutive days. It is used to remove ascarids, hookworms, and tapeworms from these species. The actual list is rather complex owing to the large number of host species involved and the common parasites found in each. In summary, the following parasites may be controlled in these zoo animals: ascarids *(T. cati, T. leonina,* and *Baylisascaris transfuga),* hookworms (*Ancylostoma* spp. and *A. caninum),* and tapeworms (*Taenia hydatigena, Taenia krabbei,* and *Taenia taeniaeformis).*

Safety trials in zoo animals dosed at 100 mg/kg (use rate ×10) showed mild signs of anorexia and loose stool. There was no effect on reproduction at this dose.

Fenbendazole is also approved by the FDA for use in large game animals, including ruminants of the subfamily Antiponae, Hippotraginae, and Caprinae, feral swine, and Rocky Mountain bighorn sheep These animals are treated in the feed with 2.5 mg/kg (ruminants), 3.0 mg/kg (swine), or 10.0 mg/kg (bighorn sheep) for 3 consecutive days. The label requires that the drug not be given to game animals 14 days before or during hunting season (Courtney and Roberson, 1995).

Oxfendazole

Oxfendazole is a broad-spectrum benzimidazole approved in the United States for use in horses and cattle. Oxfendazole is metabolized in ruminants to oxfendazole sulfone and fenbendazole, but the primary antihelmintic action is due to the parent drug (Marriner and Bogan, 1981). Its oral LD_{50} is more than 1600 mg/kg for beagle dogs and exceeds 6400 mg/kg for rats and mice.

CATTLE. Oxfendazole suspension (Synathic) is administered at 2.5 mg/kg by oral dosing syringe. The drug is approved for use in beef and nonlactating dairy cattle. It is effective against *D. viviparus, H. contortus, H. placei, T. axei, O. ostertagi, O. radiatum, B. phlebotomum, C. punctata, C. oncophora, Cooperia mcmasteri,* and *M. benedeni* (Todd and Mansfield, 1979).

Cattle must not be slaughtered within 7 days of treatment. Because no milk withdrawal time has been established, do not use oxfendazole in female dairy cattle of breeding age.

HORSES. Oxfendazole is available for horses as a paste (Benzelmin Oral Paste). At a dose of 10 mg/kg, oxfendazole is effective against *S. vulgaris, S. edentatus, S. equinus, P. equorum, O. equi,* and many species of the subfamily Cyathostominae (Lyons et al, 1977; Duncan and Reid, 1978; Colglazier, 1979). Several species of cyathostomes reportedly have developed resistance to oxfendazole (Wescott, 1986; Roberson, 1988).

Oxibendazole

Oxibendazole, a broad-spectrum benzimidazole, apparently is effective against benzimidazole-resistant small strongyles (Drudge et al, 1979). Its acute oral LD_{50} is greater than 10 g/kg in guinea pigs, hamsters, and rabbits, and greater than 32 g/kg in mice. A single dose of 600 mg/kg was well tolerated by cattle, sheep, and ponies, and no adverse reactions were observed in rats and dogs treated with up to 30 mg/kg daily for 3 months. No evidence of teratogenicity or embryotoxicity was observed in rats, mice, sheep, cattle, and horses.

HORSES. Oxibendazole paste or suspension (Anthelcide EQ) is administered orally to horses at 10 mg/kg for the removal and control of *S. vulgaris, S. edentatus,* and *S. equinus;* species of *Triodontophorus, Cyathostomum, Cylicocyclus, Cylicostephanus, Cylicodontophorus, Gyalocephalus,* and *P. equorum;* and adults and larvae of *O. equi* (Drudge et al, 1981a; Drudge et al, 1981b; Drudge et al, 1985). The dose must be increased to 15 mg/kg for treatment of *S. westeri* infection (DiPietro and Todd, 1987). Oxibendazole is not effective against stomach bots, but it is highly effective against benzimidazole-resistant cyathostomes (Drudge et al, 1981a; Drudge et al, 1981b; Drudge et al, 1985).

DOGS. A combination product of oxibendazole and diethylcarbamazine is available for dogs. See the section on broad-spectrum combination products.

Thiabendazole

The discovery of thiabendazole in 1961 marked the beginning of truly broad-spectrum antihelmintics. The first of the benzimidazoles, thiabendazole is a very safe compound. Its acute oral LD_{50} for rats is 3.1 g/kg. Thiabendazole is used as an antihelmintic in sheep, goats, cattle, horses, swine, and other animals in which it is active against the adults and some immature forms of nematodes, and it inhibits embryonation of nematode eggs. It is also active against fungi and mites. Owing to its wide margin of safety, thiabendazole has been used in animals of all ages and in pregnant and debilitated animals. Thiabendazole was available in a variety of pharmaceutical forms (suspension, bolus, paste, feed block, and top-dressing pellets) under various proprietary names. Unfortunately these dosage forms have largely left the market in the United States. Thiabendazole is, however, still readily available as a feed additive for cattle, sheep, goats, swine, and pheasants.

CATTLE. Thiabendazole (TBZ) is administered in a single dose orally to cattle in the feed at 3 g/100 lb of body weight for the control of *Haemonchus* spp., *Ostertagia* spp., *Trichostrongylus* spp., *Nematodirus* spp., and *O. radiatum* (Ames et al, 1966). In severe cases of parasitism or in cases involving *Cooperia,* 5 g/100 lb of body weight is recommended. Thiabendazole is not active against the hypobiotic early fourth-stage larvae of *Ostertagia* organisms (Ames et al, 1963).

WARNING: Milk produced within 96 hours (eight milkings) after thiabendazole medication must not be used for human food. Cattle must not be treated within 3 days of slaughter.

SHEEP AND GOATS. Thiabendazole (TBZ) is indicated for the control of *Haemonchus, Ostertagia, Trichostrongylus, Nematodirus, Cooperia, Bunostomum, Chabertia, Oesophagostomum,* and Strongyloides species at a single dose of 2 g/100 lb body weight (Cairns, 1961; Hebden, 1961; Snijders and Louw, 1966; Lyons et al, 1967; Horak et al, 1970). In heavily parasitized animals (goats only) a dose of 3 g/100 lb body weight should be given. A number of reports indicate that thiabendazole is not as effective against *Haemonchus* and *Trichostrongylus* species as it was when first introduced for general use (Drudge et al, 1964; Hotson et al, 1970; Hall et al, 1979).

WARNING: Do not treat sheep or goats within 30 days of slaughter.

HORSES. Thiabendazole at 44 mg/kg in a drench is effective for the control of *S. vulgaris, S. edentatus, S. equinus, Cyathostomum* spp., *Cylicobrachytus* spp., *Craterostomum* spp., *Oesophagodontus* spp., *Poteriostomum* spp., *O. equi,* and *S. westeri* (Drudge et al, 1962, 1963; Turk et al, 1962). For removal of *P. equorum,* 88 mg/kg must be used (Egerton et al,

1962). For activity against early-migrating larvae of *S. vulgaris* and *S. edentatus,* thiabendazole is administered at 440 mg/kg on 2 consecutive days (Slocombe and McCraw, 1975). Populations of cyathostomes have developed resistance to thiabendazole and other benzimidazole antihelmintics (Drudge et al, 1977; Drudge et al, 1979; Drudge et al, 1984).

SWINE. Thiabendazole is available in a feed premix (TBZ 100, TBZ 200) approved for use in swine. Added to feed, thiabendazole is used to prevent infections with *A. suum.* It is fed at 0.05% to 0.1% of the grain ration for 2 weeks and then continued at 0.005% to 0.02% for 8 to 14 weeks. This practice prevents the appearance of pneumonia because of migrating Ascaris larvae, but has no effect on the larval migrations through the liver. Therefore it does not prevent formation of "milk spot" lesions (Arundel et al, 1985; Biehl, 1986).

WARNING: Pigs are not to be treated within 30 days of slaughter.

PHEASANTS. Thiabendazole (TBZ) is approved for use in pheasant feed for the treatment of gapeworms *(Syngamus trachea).* It is mixed in the feed at 0.05% and fed continuously for 2 weeks. Do not use treated birds for human food within 21 days of last treatment.

Imidazothiazoles

The discovery of tetramisole in 1966 was the first in the development of the imidazothiazoles. Tetramisole was actually a racemic mixture of two optical isomers. Only the L-isomer (levamisole) has antihelmintic activity. The active isomer was subsequently developed as levamisole. In this class of anthelmintic, only levamisole is still readily available.

The imidazothiazoles act as nicotinic agonists that disturb the neuromuscular system, thus causing contraction and subsequent tonic paralysis (Coles et al, 1975; Coles, 1977; Martin, 1993). It seems that the nicotinic acetylcholine receptors of invertebrate parasites are essential for neurofunction but different in physiology and distribution in mammals (Londershausen, 1996). They also are known to interfere with the fumarate reduction system, which plays a key role in mitochondrial energy production (Behm and Bryant, 1979; Arundel et al, 1985).

Levamisole

Levamisole (Levasole, Tramisol, Totalon) is administered orally as a bolus, wettable powder, solution, gel, or feed premix to cattle, sheep, and swine for the control of gastrointestinal and lung nematodes. An aqueous solution of levamisole phosphate (13.6% or 18.2%) is for subcutaneous injection in cattle. A special topical formulation is also available. These preparations are particularly handy for fractious range cattle.

The oral LD_{50} of levamisole for rats is 480 mg/kg and for mice, 210 mg/kg. Some sheep dosed orally with tetramisole at 80 mg/kg died. Subcutaneous injection is more toxic than oral administration. Signs of cholinergic toxicity such as lip licking, salivation, lacrimation, head shaking, ataxia, and muscle tremors may occur at lower dosage levels. At the recommended dosage level, an occasional animal may show transitory muzzle foam and licking of the lips. At twice the therapeutic dosage level, calves may show increased alertness, salivation, head shaking, and muscle tremors.

CATTLE. Levamisole hydrochloride administered orally as a drench, bolus, gel, feed additive, or injectable or topical solution (Tramisol, Levasole, Totalon) is highly effective against *Haemonchus, Ostertagia, Trichostrongylus, Cooperia, Nematodirus, Bunostomum,* and *Oesophagostomum* species in the alimentary tract and *Dictyocaulus* species in the lungs (Baker and Fisk, 1972; Lyons et al, 1972; Lyons et al, 1975a; Curr, 1977; Seibert et al, 1986). The dose for cattle is 8 mg/kg orally, 10 mg/kg topically, and 6 mg/kg by subcutaneous injection of the phosphate salt. Arrested early fourth-stage larvae of *Ostertagia* species are refractory to levamisole.

WARNING: A slight nonpersistent reaction may occur at the site of levamisole phosphate injection. Cattle should not be slaughtered within 9 days of topical medication, 7 days of injection, 6 days of receiving oral gel, or 2 days of oral medication with drench or medicated feed. Levamisole is not to be used in dairy animals of breeding age if one wants to avoid drug residues in milk.

SHEEP. Orally administered levamisole drench or bolus (Levasole, Tramisol) removes *Haemonchus, Ostertagia, Trichostrongylus, Cooperia, Nematodirus, Bunostomum, Oesophagostomum,* and *Chabertia* species from the alimentary tract and *Dictyocaulus* species from the lungs at a dose of 8 mg/kg (Callinan and Barton, 1979; Craig and Shepherd, 1980). Levamisole is also efficacious against the immature stages of *Haemonchus, Nematodirus, Bunostomum, Oesophagostomum, Chabertia,* and *Dictyocaulus* species.

WARNING: Levamisole has an ample therapeutic margin, but an occasional sheep will show side effects (e.g., lip licking, salivation, increased alertness, muscle tremors), even at the recommended dose. Debilitated sheep appear to be more susceptible to toxicity. Sheep should not be slaughtered within 72 hours of treatment.

SWINE. Levamisole administered to swine in water or feed (Levasol, Tramisol) removes *Ascaris* spp., *Oesophagostomum* spp., *S. ransomi, Metastrongylus* spp., and *Hyostrongylus* spp. Levamisole is also effective against the immature forms (including migrating larvae) of *Ascaris* and *Metastrongylus* organisms. The label for levamisole resinate indicates its efficacy against *S. dentatus* when mixed in the feed (Arundel et al, 1985).

WARNING: Levamisole should be administered to pigs of weanling to market age after an overnight fast. Breeding pigs do not need to be fasted before treatment. Pigs should not be treated within 3 days of slaughter. Salivation or muzzle foam is occasionally observed after treatment. Pigs infected with adult lungworms may vomit or cough. These reactions may be caused by the expulsion of paralyzed lungworms from the bronchi.

Tetrahydropyrimidines

The tetrahydropyrimidines include the numerous salts of pyrantel, morantel, and the investigational compound oxantel, which is available outside the United States. They all act as nicotinic agonists, which disturb the neuromuscular system causing contraction and subsequent tonic paralysis (Aubrey et al, 1970; Eyre, 1970; Martin, 1993). In vitro experiments indicate that pyrantel is 100 times more powerful than acetylcholine. It seems that the nicotinic acetylcholine receptors of invertebrate parasites are essential for neurofunction but different in physiology and distribution in mammals (Londershausen, 1996).

In ruminants these products are rapidly metabolized to inactive metabolites. Thus ruminants require higher doses than monogastric animals (Campbell and Rew, 1985).

Pyrantel

Pyrantel is the most widely used of all the tetrahydropyrimidine antihelmintics. The tartrate salt is a white powder, soluble in water, which is used as a powder and pellets in horses and swine. Pyrantel tartrate is well absorbed after oral administration in the rat, dog, and pig. Plasma levels peak within 2 to 3 hours, and the drug is rapidly metabolized and eliminated in the urine.

Pyrantel pamoate is a yellow powder, insoluble in water, which is available as a ready-to-use suspension for dogs and horses and as tablets for dogs. Pyrantel salts are stable in solid form but photodegrade when dissolved or suspended in water, resulting in reduction of potency. Pyrantel pamoate is poorly absorbed from the intestine.

DOGS. Pyrantel pamoate, as a palatable suspension, chewable tablets, or as plain tablets (Nemex), is indicated for the removal of *T. canis, T. leonina, A. caninum,* and *U. stenocephala* from dogs and puppies (Linquist, 1975; Todd et al, 1975; Klein et al, 1978; Jacobs, 1987b; Clark et al, 1991). The recommended dose of 5 mg/kg of Nemex suspension is administered orally or mixed with a small amount of feed. For animals weighing 2.25 kg or less, the dose is increased to 10 mg/kg. Tablets may be administered directly or placed in a small portion of food. Nemex has been shown to be safe in nursing and weanling pups, pregnant bitches, males used for breeding, and dogs infected with *D. immitis.* Its oral LD_{50} is greater than 690 mg/kg in dogs. No significant morphological changes were induced in dogs given 94 mg/kg daily for 90 days. Pyrantel pamoate is compatible with organophosphates and other antiparasitic and antimicrobial agents.

HORSES. Pyrantel pamoate, available for horses as a paste or caramel-flavored suspension (Strongid-Paste, Strongid-T), administered at 6.6 mg of pyrantel base per kilogram eliminates *S. vulgaris, S. edentatus, S. equinus, O. equi, P. equorum,* and several species of the subfamily Cyathostominae, including populations resistant to benzimidazoles (Lyons et al, 1974). Pyrantel pamoate can be administered as a single dose to horses by stomach tube or mixed with the grain ration at 13.2 mg of pyrantel base per kilogram. It was 98% effective against *Anoplocephala perfoliata,* but this is not an approved dose level (Lyons et al, 1986).

Pyrantel tartrate pellets (Strongid C) are fed continuously at a dose of 14.4 mg.kg of body weight daily for the prevention of *S. vulgaris* migration and the control of *S. edentatus, Triodontophorus* spp., *Cyathostomum* spp., *Cylicodontophorus* spp., *Cylicocyclus* spp., *Cylicostephanus* spp., *Poterostomum* spp., *O. equi,* and *P. equorum* (Cornwell and Jones, 1968; Lyons et al, 1975b; Drudge et al, 1982). It is also available in a feed top dressing (Equi-Phar Horse & Colt Wormer) approved for use at 12.5 mg/kg body weight for removal and control of internal parasites. Pyrantel is safe for use in horses and ponies of all ages, including sucklings, weanlings, and pregnant mares. It can be used concurrently with insecticides, carbon disulfide, tranquilizers, muscle relaxants, and central nervous system (CNS) depressants.

SWINE. Pyrantel tartrate (Banminth 48), when fed continuously at 96 g/ton of complete feed as the sole ration, prevents the migration and establishment of *A. suum* and *Oesophagostomum* spp. When fed to pigs for 3 consecutive days, this medicated feed removes the adults and fourth-stage larvae of *A. suum.* Pyrantel tartrate is also mixed with feed at the rate of 800 g/ton of complete feed and fed to pigs for the treatment of *Ascaris* and *Oesophagostomum* species for 1 day at the rate of 1 kg feed per 40 kg body weight (1 pound of feed per 40 pounds body weight) up to 2.3 kg of feed for pigs 91 kg and heavier. Pyrantel is the only approved antihelmintic that will prevent the appearance of "milk spots" on the liver of pigs when administered continuously. It does so by killing the larvae of *A. suum* in the lumen of the gut as they hatch from eggs (Biehl, 1986).

WARNING: Pyrantel should not be given to pigs within 24 hours of slaughter. Because the drug is photodegradable, it should be used immediately after the package is opened. Pyrantel tartrate should not be mixed with rations containing bentonite. Because pyrantel and piperazine appear to be pharmacological antagonists, they probably should not be used concurrently.

CATTLE, SHEEP, AND GOATS. Pyrantel tartrate is not approved by the FDA for use in cattle, sheep, and goats but is effective at 25 mg/kg against *H. contortus, O. ostertagi, Ostertagia (Teladorsagia) circumcincta, T. axei, T. colubriformis, N. battus, N. spathiger, Cooperia* spp., and *Bunostomum* spp. (Arundel et al, 1985; Campbell and Rew, 1985; Reinemeyer and Courtney, 2001).

Morantel Tartrate

Morantel is the 3-methyl analogue of pyrantel. Morantel tartrate (Rumatel) is used for the control of gastrointestinal nematodes in cattle and goats. Its acute oral LD_{50} is 437 mg/kg in male mice and 926 mg/kg in male rats. Morantel tartrate is mixed in a complete feed or top dressed to deliver 9.7 mg/kg of body weight for the removal of adult *Haemonchus* spp., *Ostertagia* spp., *Trichostrongylus* spp., *Cooperia* spp., *Nematodirus* spp., and *O. radiatum* in cattle (Ciordia and McCampbell, 1973; Conway et al, 1973; Anderson and Marais, 1975). The same dose is effective against *H. contortus, O. (Teladorsagia) circumcincta,* and *T. axei* in goats. Activity against larval stages of these nematodes appears to be variable. Morantel may be administered to lactating dairy cows without requiring milk withdrawal. It may be given simultaneously with vaccines, injectable drugs, and external parasiticides without concern. Cattle should not be slaughtered within 14 days after treatment. Goats should not be slaughtered within 30 days of treatment.

Piperazines

Piperazine and the piperazine analogue diethylcarbamazine (DEC) are grouped together because of their central heterocyclic ring. These anthelmintics produce a neuromuscular blockade through disruption of GABA neurotransmission. Most data suggest that the receptors in nematodes and insects resemble the mammalian GABA subtype, but they are clearly different from their vertebrate counterparts (Londershausen, 1996). Piperazine and DEC are quite safe to use in all species but have a narrow spectrum of action (Reinemeyer and Courtney, 2001).

Piperazine

Various salts of piperazine (e.g., madipate, hydrochloride, sulfate, monohydrate, citrate, dihydrochloride) are used as antihelmintics in swine, poultry, horses, dogs, and cats. The amount of piperazine base in each salt varies widely. The adipate, citrate, phosphate, and dihydrochloride salts contain a 37%, 35%, 42%, and 50% piperazine base, respectively (USP, 1998). Antihelmintic activity depends on freeing piperazine base in the gastrointestinal tract. Piperazine is rapidly absorbed from the gastrointestinal tract and quickly cleared by urinary excretion. Elimination is virtually complete within 24 hours. It should be used with caution in animals with hepatic or renal dysfunction. The drug may not be effective in animals with intestinal hypomotility because the paralyzed worms may recover from the effects of the drug before they are passed in the stool. Occasional adverse reactions observed include ataxia, diarrhea, and vomiting.

Piperazine is available as tablets, solution, and soluble powder under several proprietary names (Pipatabs, Tasty Paste). The drug is practically nontoxic. Its oral LD_{50} for rats is 4.9 g/kg and for chickens, 8 g/kg. Piperazine can be administered to animals of all ages.

DOGS AND CATS. Piperazine is administered orally at 45 to 65 mg of piperazine base per kilogram (USP, 1998) although higher doses (100 to 250 mg/kg) have been reported in the literature (English and Sprent, 1965; Sharp et al, 1973; Jacobs, 1987a; Jacobs, 1987b). It is effective against adult *T. canis, T. cati,* and *T. leonina.*

HORSES. Piperazine in an oral drench is effective against *P. equorum* at 110 mg of base per kilogram. Reasonable efficacy was also observed against *S. vulgaris, O. equi,* and many species of small strongyles at 220 to 275 mg/kg (Downing et al, 1955; Poynter, 1955a; Poynter, 1955b; Poynter, 1956; Gibson, 1957). Foals should first be treated when they are 8 weeks old. The treatment may be repeated every 4 weeks if necessary.

CATTLE, GOATS, AND SHEEP. Piperazine is given at 110 mg of base per kilogram orally in a single dose for control of nodular worms (*Oesophagostomum* spp.) and ascarids *(Neoascaris vitulorum)* (USP, 1998; Reinemeyer and Courtney, 2001). It is not often used in ruminants because of its narrow spectrum of action.

SWINE. Piperazine in drinking water is offered to pigs at 110 mg/kg for the removal of *A. suum* and *Oesophagostomum* spp. (Biehl, 1986).

CHICKENS AND TURKEYS. Piperazine is administered in feed or water for 2 days at 32 mg of base per kilogram. It is very effective against *Ascaridia galli* but not against *H. gallinarum* (USP, 1998; Reinemeyer and Courtney, 2001).

Diethylcarbamazine

Diethylcarbamazine citrate is a bitter-tasting heterocyclic compound closely related to piperazine. The drug is readily absorbed from the gastrointestinal tract and distributed to all tissues except for fat. Peak blood levels occur 3 hours after administration. Diethylcarbamazine citrate is rapidly cleared from the body (70% in 24 hours) in the urine. It is eliminated primarily as metabolites with only a small percentage (10% to 25%) as unchanged drug.

Diethylcarbamazine is almost exclusively used in dogs at an oral dose of 6.6 mg/kg to prevent infection with *D. immitis* (Kume et al, 1964; Kume et al, 1967; Warne et al, 1969; Kume, 1974; Hawking, 1979; Knight 1987). It is also somewhat effective as an aid in the treatment of *T. canis, T. cati,* and *T. leonina* infections in dogs and cats at a dose of 55 to 110 mg/kg (Arundel et al, 1985). For the prevention of heartworm infections, diethylcarbamazine is administered orally once a day at 6.6 mg/kg during the mosquito season. Puppies may be started on the prevention program for heartworm at about 2 months of age. It is advisable to begin administration 1 month before the start of the mosquito season and continue until 2 months after the end of the mosquito season. In warm climates, diethylcarbamazine should be given to dogs year round if no other means of *D. immitis* control is available.

Diethylcarbamazine citrate is marketed under several proprietary names (Filaribits, Nemacide) and in many pharmaceutical forms (tablets, chewable tablets, and syrup). Diethylcarbamazine is also available in combination with oxibendazole as Filaribits Plus. For more information, see the section on combination products.

WARNING: Dogs with circulating heartworm microfilariae may develop fatal anaphylactoid reactions if treated with diethylcarbamazine (Palumbo et al, 1977; Furrow et al, 1980; Powers et al, 1980; Atwell and Boreham, 1983; Hamilton et al, 1986). Dogs older than 6 months should be tested for microfilaremia before beginning a regimen of diethylcarbamazine. All those with circulating microfilariae should be freed of adult heartworms and microfilariae before starting the diethylcarbamazine prophylactic regimen. The full therapeutic dose may cause irritation of the gastric mucosa, but a light meal just before medication often reduces gastric irritation and emesis. There are anecdotal reports of sterility in male dogs, but this effect has not been reproduced experimentally (USP, 1998).

Organophosphates

Dichlorvos

Dichlorvos is an organophosphate taken internally to kill parasites. It phosphorylates the acetyl-cholinesterase (AchE) enzyme. Normal AchE eliminates acetylcholine when it is released at the postsynaptic junction. When AchE is inactivated, acetylcholine accumulates at the postsynaptic junction, which results in continued depolarization. The end result is paralysis (Lee and Hodsden, 1963; Hart and Lee, 1966; Fest and Schmidt, 1982). The toxicity of organophosphates is generally related to its ability to inactivate the AchE of the host. Such toxicity is best treated with pralidoxime (2-PAM) and atropine (Woodard, 1957; Nelson et al, 1967; Smith 1986).

Dichlorvos is an organophosphate that is effective against many internal and external parasites. It is rapidly degraded in mammals. The acute oral LD_{50} of dichlorvos for rats is 80 mg/kg. In dogs, the oral LD_{50} of unformulated dichlorvos is 28 to 45 mg/kg, whereas the formulated (resinated) dichlorvos is of low toxicity, with an oral LD_{50} of 387 to 1262 mg/kg. No untoward reactions were observed in pregnant mice, rats, rabbits, sows, mares, bitches, and queens medicated with dichlorvos. Specially formulated dichlorvos is used as an anthelmintic for dogs and cats (Task Tabs) and for swine (Atgard).

DOGS AND CATS. Task Tabs are administered at 11 mg/kg to cats and puppies older than 10 days or weighing more than 0.5 kg. Task Tabs are indicated for the removal of adult *T. canis, T. cati, T. leonina, A. caninum, A. tubaeforme,* and *U. stenocephala* (Batte et al, 1966; Howes, 1972; Olsen et al, 1977). Dichlorvos can be toxic, so check the warning section that follows later. (Please note: Task and Task Capsules contained a slow-release formulation of dichlorvos in nondigestible resin pellets. These products are now unavailable in the United States.)

SWINE. Atgard consists of polyvinyl chloride resin pellets containing dichlorvos. It is mixed into a complete meal type feed (not unground grain or pelleted meal) to deliver 12.5 to 21.6 mg/kg of body weight for the removal of adults and fourth-stage larvae of *A. suum, T. suis,* and *Oesophagostomum* spp., and adult *A. strongylina,* in boars, weaners, fatteners, gilts, and sows (Arundel et al, 1985; Biehl, 1986). For best results, sows and gilts should be medicated shortly before farrowing and again at weaning. It is best to administer the medicated feed to small lots of compatibly sized pigs (e.g., single litters) at one time so they can be watched while feeding to ensure that all eat their share. Preliminary fasting is unnecessary, but alternative sources of feed should be excluded during the medication period. When administered immediately before parturition at 8.8 times the recommended dose, Atgard produced no adverse reactions in sows. There is no preslaughter withdrawal period when the drug is used at the recommended dosage level.

WARNING: Dichlorvos should not be used with other cholinesterase-inhibiting chemicals, taeniacides, antifilarials, muscle relaxants, phenothiazine tranquilizers, or CNS depressants. The drug is contraindicated for dogs and cats showing signs of severe constipation, mechanical blockage of the intestinal tract, liver disease, or circulatory failure. Dogs with *D. immitis* infection should not be treated with dichlorvos. A small number of normal dogs may vomit after treatment, but no other adverse reactions have been reported. Cats are more susceptible to dichlorvos. They may vomit, hypersalivate, appear apprehensive, and pass loose stools after medication. Atropine and pralidoxime (2-PAM) are the recommended antidotes for organophosphate poisoning.

Isoquinolones

The isoquinolones are represented by two closely related cestocides: praziquantel and epsiprantel. This class of cestocide is the safest and most effective yet approved in the United States. They attack the neuromuscular junction and the tegument. The first effect causes an instantaneous contraction and paralysis of the parasite (Andrews et al, 1983). The second effect is a devastating vacuolization and destruction of the protective tegument (Arundel et al, 1985; Frayha et al, 1997). The combined effects of paralysis and tegmental destruction provide excellent activity against cestodes.

Praziquantel

Praziquantel was the first isoquinolone cestocide approved in the United States. It displays marked antihelmintic activity against a wide range of adult and larval cestodes and trematodes of the genus *Schistosoma*. Praziquantel is a very safe antihelmintic. Rats have tolerated daily administration of up to 1000 mg/kg for 4 weeks, and dogs have tolerated up to 180 mg/kg daily for 13 weeks. Adverse reactions in dogs and cats include transient anorexia, diarrhea, incoordination, and lethargy. Vomiting and salivation is typically observed at high dosage rates. The drug has high oral bioavailability, high protein binding, and a marked first-pass effect. It is rapidly metabolized in the kidney and liver, and the half-life for elimination is about 2 hours. About 80% of the dose is eliminated through the urine. The remainder is cleared through the bile and stool. Praziquantel did not induce embryotoxicity, teratogenesis, mutagenesis, or carcinogenesis, nor did it affect the reproductive performance of test animals.

DOGS AND CATS. Praziquantel (Droncit) is administered orally or injected subcutaneously at 2.5 to 7.5 mg/kg for the removal of *D. caninum, Taenia taeniaformis, T. pisiformis, T. hydatigena, T. ovis, Mesocestoides corti, Echinococcus granulosus,* *Echinococcus multilocularis, Spirometra* spp., *Diphyllobothrium latum, Diphyllobothrium erinacei,* and *Joyeuxiella pasquali* (Gemmell et al, 1977; Andersen et al, 1978; Thakur et al, 1978; Thomas and Gonnert, 1978; Andersen et al, 1979; Gemmell et al, 1980; Kruckenberg et al, 1981; USP, 1998). A higher dosage is also highly active when injected subcutaneously or intramuscularly. Praziquantel is not intended for use in puppies or kittens younger than 4 weeks.

SHEEP, GOATS, AND CHICKENS. Although not approved for use in these species, praziquantel may be used for cestode infections from *Avitellina* spp., *Stilesia* spp., *Moniezia* spp., *Choanotaenia infundibulum, Daviainea proglottina,* and *Raillietina cesticellus.* Sheep and goats may be treated with a dose of 10 to 15 mg/kg, and chickens with a dose of 10 mg/kg (Reinemeyer and Courtney, 2001).

Combination products of praziquantel, febantel, and pyrantel are also available. See the section on combination products for more information.

Epsiprantel

Epsiprantel (Cestex) was the second isoquinolone cestocide to be approved in the United States. Acute toxicity studies in mice and rats showed the oral minimum lethal dose of epsiprantel to be more than 5000 mg/kg. Epsiprantel at an oral dosage level of 2.75 mg/kg for cats or 5.5 mg/kg for dogs, as a single oral film-coated tablet, effectively removes *D. caninum, T. taeniaformis, T. pisiformis,* and *T. hydatigena* (Corwin et al, 1989; Manger and Brewer, 1989). Doses as high as 100 mg/kg and 200 mg/kg in cats and dogs were well tolerated. Epsiprantel was given concurrently with diethylcarbamazine, antiinflammatory drugs, insecticides, and other antihelmintic drugs with no incompatibilities observed. Epsiprantel is only slightly absorbed through the digestive tract of cats and dogs. All is eliminated in the feces unchanged.

WARNING: The safety of using epsiprantel in pregnant dogs and cats has not been determined, and it should not be used in puppies and kittens younger than 7 weeks.

Arsenicals

Heavy metals such as arsenic and antimony are well represented in the history of antihelmintics. Today they have been replaced largely by safer and more effective drugs for the most common parasites. Their use is now limited to removal of adult *D. immitis.* The therapeutic effect depends on a reaction between the arsenic salt and sulfhydryl-containing enzymes (Ledbetter, 1984; Gilman et al, 1990). Inactivation of parasite enzyme systems results in death. Arsenic is widely known as a toxin in humans and animals. Due caution is required when using the products.

Thiacetarsemide

Thiacetarsemide (arsenamide sodium) was an organic arsenical solution (Caparsolate) administered intravenously for the treatment of adult *D. immitis* infection in dogs (Otto and Maren, 1947; Courtney et al, 1986). This product is no longer commercially available in the United States. Earlier editons of this text should be consulted for more complete information.

Melarsomine

Melarsomine dihydrochloride (Immiticide) is the only arsenical antihelmintic that is commercially available in the United States. Melarsomine has an efficacy of 92% to 98% for adult *D. immitis* (Dzimianski et al, 1992; Keister et al, 1992; Rawlings et al, 1993; Keister et al, 1995; Miller et al, 1995a). The arsenic content of the product is less than that of thiacetarsemide and is apparently less toxic to the patient. Another novel feature is that the product is administered intramuscularly at a dose of 2.5 mg/kg for two injections given 3 or 24 hours apart. The drug is rapidly absorbed from the injection site with a mean absorption half-life after intramuscular administration of 2.6 minutes, and a peak blood concentration of 8 minutes. The drug is rapidly distributed to most tissues. The parent drug and the arsenoxide metabolite are rapidly eliminated in the feces, probably by biliary excretion. The arsenic acid metabolite is rapidly eliminated in the urine, so there is no significant bioaccumulation (Keister et al, 1995).

Clinical studies indicate that the treatment is well tolerated even in dogs that have clinical signs of heartworm disease (Vezzoni et al, 1992; Case et al, 1995; Miller et al, 1995a). This combination of greater activity and safety has clearly destined melarsomine to become the drug of choice for treatment of heartworm in dogs.

Miscellaneous Antihelmintics

The miscellaneous antihelmintics include a mixture of many different classes of drug. Most are older chemicals that have not yet outlived their usefulness. Some have unique attributes that keep them in use and commercially available.

Clorsulon

Clorsulon, a benzene sulfonamide compound, is very effective in cattle against the immature and mature *F. hepatica*. The product (Curatrem) is given in a drench to cattle and sheep at a dose of 7 mg/kg. A single dose is more than 99% effective in removing *F. hepatica* (Campbell and Rew, 1985; Kilgore et al, 1985; Wallace et al, 1985). The drug should not be given to lactating dairy cattle because no milk withdrawal time has been established. Cattle should not be treated within 7 days before slaughter. Timing for retreatment should be based on risk patterns where the cattle are pastured.

Clorsulon is also available in combination with ivermectin. For more information, see the section on combination drugs.

Dichlorophene

Dichlorophene (Happy Jack Tapeworm Tablets) is a chlorinated analogue of diphenylmethane. It has low toxicity for mammals. The oral LD_{50} of dichlorophene for rats is 2690 mg/kg, and the acute oral LD_{50} for dogs is 1000 mg/kg. Dichlorophene has bacteriostatic, fungicidal, and cestocidal properties. It uncouples electron-transport-linked phosphorylation in the parasite mitochondria. The drug is relatively safe in the host because of its low gastrointestinal absorption (Arundel et al, 1985; Lovell et al, 1990).

Dichlorophene may be used either alone or in combination with other antihelmintic drugs for the removal of *Taenia* and *Dipylidium* tapeworms from dogs and cats (Roberson, 1988). The drug may be administered orally in tablet or capsule form at 220 mg/kg after an overnight fast. The tapeworms are killed, digested, and eliminated in an unrecognizable form. Dichlorophene is most commonly formulated with toluene in over-the-counter preparations. For more information, see the section on combination products. An occasional animal may vomit or have diarrhea after treatment with dichlorophene.

Toluene

Toluene (methylbenzene), a hydrocarbon derived from coal tar, is often used as an industrial solvent. It is quite safe for mammals. The oral LD_{50} of toluene for rats is 7.5 ml/kg. The drug is available in combination with dichlorophene or dichlorvos in over-the-counter antihelmintics sold in grocery stores and pet shops.

DOGS AND CATS. Toluene given orally at 0.22 ml/kg in dogs and cats is 98% effective for the removal of *T. canis, T. cati,* and *T. leonina.* It is 96% effective against *A. caninum* and *A. braziliense* (Courtney and Roberson, 1995). The mechanism of action is postulated to be due either to irritant or depressant effects on the neural cells of the nematode (Lovell et al, 1990). Fasting is suggested for 12 hours before and 4 hours after medication.

WARNING: Toluene is a relatively safe drug, but overdosage produces ataxia, aberrant behavior, mydriasis, vomiting, depression, muscle tremors, and hypersalivation. Treatment should consist of general supportive care, including administration of intravenous fluids, oxygen, and activated charcoal, as well as monitoring for possible renal or hepatic damage (Lovell et al, 1990). Digestible oils, alcohol, and adrenaline should be avoided.

Broad-Spectrum Combinations

The veterinary practitioner is always looking for antihelmintic products that cover ever-increasing spectra of parasites. Broad-spectrum products have two important advantages. First, they obviate dosing with several different products at once when a patient has a mixed parasite infection, which makes administration easier. Second, they provide peace of mind that a parasitized animal will be cleared of parasites missed perhaps in diagnosis. For instance, a puppy from the animal shelter will be better served with a product that is effective in removing both roundworms and hookworms than with a product that is effective only against roundworms.

There are two ways to get broad-spectrum products: either discover a single chemical that has a broad spectrum (not an easy task) or combine several compatible products to build the desired spectrum of activity.

In this section the combination products are discussed. In most cases the formulation may have changed, and the dosing regimen is different than the single-entity drugs discussed in the preceding sections. The toxicity and mechanism of action are covered in the preceding discussion.

Clorsulon and Ivermectin

An injectable product (Ivomec-Plus) containing clorsulon and ivermectin is approved for use in cattle. The product is injected subcutaneously behind the shoulder at a dose of 1 ml/50 kg of body weight. This dose volume delivers 0.2 mg ivermectin and 2 mg clorsulon per kilogram. It is effective against *O. ostertagi, O. lyrata, H. placei, T. axei, T. colubriformis, C. oncophora, C. punctata, C. pectinata, B. phlebotomum, N. helvetianus, N. spathiger, O. radiatum, D. viviparus, F. hepatica, H. bovis, H. lineatum, L. vituli, H. eurysternus, S. capillatus, Psoroptes ovis,* and *S. scabiei var. bovis.* Do not treat cattle within 49 days before slaughter. No milk withholding time has been established, so do not use product in female dairy cattle of breeding age.

Dichlororphene and Toluene

A few small animal proprietary antihelmintic products (Trivermicide Worm Capsules) contain dichlorophene as the cestocidal ingredient and toluene (methylbenzene) as the antinematodal ingredient. Both drugs have low mammalian toxicity.

The dichlorophene and toluene mixture is administered orally in soft capsules to dogs and cats, preferably after a 12-hour fast, at 220 mg dichlorophene and 264 mg (0.22 ml) toluene per kilogram of body weight for the removal of *T. canis, T. leonina, A. caninum, U. stenocephala, T. pisiformis,* and *D. caninum.* The dichlorophene-

toluene mixture is relatively ineffective against *E. granulosus* (Lovell et al, 1990).

WARNING: Toluene is a relatively safe drug, but overdosage produces ataxia, aberrant behavior, mydriasis, vomiting, depression, muscle tremors, and hypersalivation. Treatment should consist of general supportive care, including administration of intravenous fluids, oxygen, and activated charcoal, as well as monitoring for possible renal or hepatic damage (Lovell et al, 1990). Digestible oils, alcohol, and adrenaline should be avoided.

Diethylcarbamazine and Oxibendazole

Filaribits Plus chewable tablets are formulated to deliver 6.6 mg diethylcarbamazine and 5 mg oxibendazole per kilogram of body weight. The medication is administered once a day for the prevention of infections with *D. immitis* and *A. caninum,* and for the removal and control of *T. canis* and *T. vulpis.* Filaribits Plus administration has been associated occasionally with hepatic dysfunction and several fatalities. Signs and symptoms reported as accompanying hepatic dysfunction include anorexia, vomiting, lethargy, jaundice, weight loss, polydipsia, polyuria, ataxia, and dark urine (Vaden et al, 1988). Exhaustive toxicological evaluation by the manufacturer demonstrated that diethylcarbamazine and oxibendazole given individually each showed wide margins of safety. Dogs given a single dose of Filaribits Plus at 640 times the recommended dose levels of the active substances survived without any sequelae. Dogs given 5 times the recommended dose level daily for 2 years had no ill effects and at necropsy showed no drug-related histopathology (Simpson, 1986). One paper (Dickinson and Thornburg, 1988) reported that analysis of a number of cases with hepatotoxic symptoms led them to the conclusion that Filaribits Plus is not an intrinsic hepatotoxin because the incidence of such reactions is low.

Febantel, Praziquantel, and Pyrantel

A three-way combination of febantel, praziquantel, and pyrantel (Drontal Plus) is available in the United States. This product is formulated to deliver 25 to 35 mg of febantel, 5 to 7 mg of praziquantel, and 5 to 7 mg of pyrantel pamoate per kilogram. A single dose is given to dogs to remove *D. caninum, T. pisiformis, E. granulosus, A. caninum, U. stenocephala, T. canis, T. leonina,* and *T. vulpis* (Bowman and Arthur, 1993; Cruthers et al, 1993). This combination is effective against the nematodes when given in a single dose. Febantel alone requires three daily doses to be effective in monogastric animals. This combination should not be used in pregnant dogs, in dogs less than 2 pounds in body weight, or in puppies younger than 3 weeks.

Milbemycin Oxime and Lufenuron

Sentinel is a two-way combination of milbemycin oxime and lufenuron labeled for use in dogs. It is formulated to deliver a minimum dose of 0.5 mg of milbemycin oxime and 10 mg of lufenuron per kilogram of body weight. The product is given once every month to remove or control the important gastrointestinal parasites (heartworm, roundworm, hookworm, and whipworm) and control flea populations.

Praziquantel and Pyrantel

Drontal is a two-way combination of praziquantel and pyrantel labeled for use in cats and kittens. This product is formulated to deliver 5 mg of praziquantel and 20 mg of pyrantel pamoate per kilogram. A single dose is given to cats and kittens to remove *D. caninum, T. taeniaeformis, A. tubaeforme,* and *T. cati.* This combination should not be used in kittens under 1.5 pounds in body weight or younger than 4 weeks.

Ivermectin and Pyrantel Pamoate

Ivermectin combined with pyrantel pamoate is available in a beef-based chewable product (Heartgard-30 Plus). The product is formulated to deliver a target dose of 6 mg of ivermectin and 5 mg of pyrantel pamoate per kilogram of body weight. The product is given orally to dogs every 30 days to prevent *D. immitis* and for the treatment and control of *T. canis, T. leonina, A. caninum,* and *U. stenocephala* (Clark et al, 1992a). The product should be given at monthly intervals during the heartworm season. Recent studies have shown that adult heartworms are not able to maintain detectable levels of microfilariae when exposed to ivermectin, so an antigen test should be used to reveal the presence of adult heartworms (Bowman et al, 1992). Safety tests have revealed that the ivermectin-pyrantel combination is well tolerated (Clark et al, 1992b). Do not give this medication to dogs younger than 6 weeks or to those with existing heartworm infections.

■ REFERENCES

Aiello SE, Mays A: *The Merck veterinary manual,* Whitehouse Station, NJ, 1990, Merck & Co.

Ames ER, Cheney JM, Rubin R: The efficacy of thiabendazole and bephenium etastrongylus hydroxynapthoate against *Ostertagia ostertagi* and *Cooperia oncophora* in experimentally infected calves, *Am J Vet Res* 24:295–299, 1963.

Ames ER, Rubin R, Cheney JM: A critical evaluation of the efficacy of thiabendazole against important heminths of cattle, *Vet Med Small Anim Clin* 61(1):66–70, 1966.

Andersen FL, Conder GA, Marsland WP: Efficacy of injectable and tablet formulations of praziquantel against mature *Echinococcus granulosus, Am J Vet Res* 39(11):1861–1862, 1978.

Andersen FL, Conder GA, Marsland WP: Efficacy of injectable and tablet formulations of praziquantel against immature *Echinococcus granulosus, Am J Vet Res* 40(5):700–701, 1979

Anderson PJS, Marais FS: The control of adult parasitic nematodes of cattle with morantel tartrate, *J S Afr Vet Assoc* 46(4):325–329, 1975.

Andrews P, Thomas H, Pohlke R, et al: Praziquantel, *Med Red Rev* 3(2):147–200, 1983.

Anonymous: New Quest Gel dewormer and boticide, *J Equine Vet Sci* 17(8):406–409, 1997a.

Anonymous: *Nylar technical bulletin,* Minneapolis, 1997b, McLaughlin Gormley King Co.

Anonymous: *ProHeart For Dogs (Moxidectin) heartworm prevention tablets freedom of information summary,* Washington, DC, 1997c, U.S. Food and Drug Administration, Center for Veterinary Medicine.

Anonymous: Milbemite Otic Solution, Freedom of Information Summary for NADA 141-163, http://www.fda.gov/cvm/efoi, 2000.

Anonymous: Freedom of Information Summary for Marquis (NADA 141-188), http://www.fda.gov/cvm/efoi, 2001.

Anonymous: Freedom of Information Summary for Milbemite Otic Solution (NADA 141-163), http://www.fda.gov/cvm/efoi, 2000.

Arena JP, Liu KK, Paress PS, et al: Avermectin-sensitive chloride channels induced by *Caenorhabditis elegans* RNA in *Xenopus oocytes, Mol Pharmacol* 40:368–374, 1991.

Arends JJ, Skogerboe TL, Ritzhaupt LK: *Study one: duration of efficacy of doramectin and ivermectin against* Sarcoptes scabei var. suis, Proceedings of the American Association of Veterinary Parasitologists, Reno, Nev, 1997a.

Arends JJ, Skogerboe TL, Ritzhaupt LK: *Study two: duration of efficacy of doramectin and ivermectin against* Sarcoptes scabei *var.* suis, Proceedings of the American Association of Veterinary Parasitologists, Reno, Nev, 1997b.

Arnaud JP, Consalvi PJ: *Evaluation of acute oral tolerance of fipronil and excipient and the tolerance of Frontline Top Spot in cats and dogs,* Proceedings of the North American Veterinary Conference, Orlando, Fla, 1997a.

Arnaud JP, Consalvi PJ: *Investigative studies to evaluate the safety of Frontline Top Spot treatment for dogs and cats,* Proceedings of the North American Veterinary Conference, Orlando, Fla, 1997b.

Arther RG, Cunningham J, Dorn H, et al: Efficacy of imidacloprid for removal and control of fleas *(Ctenocephalides felis)* on dogs, *Am J Vet Res* 58(8):848–850, 1977.

Arundel JH, Bossche Hvd, Thienpoint D, et al: *Chemotherapy of gastrointestinal helminths,* New York, 1985, Springer-Verlag.

Atwell RB, Boreham PFL: Adverse drug reactions in the treatment of filarial parasites: clinical reactions to diethylcarbamazine therapy in dogs infected with *Dirofilaria immitis* in Australia, *J Small Anim Pract* 24:695–701, 1983.

Aubry ML, Cowell P, Davey MJ, et al: Aspects of the pharmacology of a new anthelmintic: pyrantel, *Br J Pharmacol* 38:332–344, 1970.

Baker NF, Fisk RA: Levamisole as an anthelmintic in calves, *Am J Vet Res* 33:1121–1125, 1972.

Barr SC: Enteric protozoal infections. In Greene CE, editor: *Infectious diseases of the dog and cat,* Philadelphia, 1998, WB Saunders.

Barr SC, Bowman DD, Heller RL, et al: Efficacy of albendazole against giardiasis in dogs, *Am J Vet Res* 54(6):926–928, 1993.

Bater AK: *Efficacy of oral milbemycin against naturally acquired heartworm infection in dogs,* Proceedings of the Heartworm Symposium, Charleston, SC, 1989, pp 107-108.

Batte EG, Moncol DJ, McLamb RD: Critical evaluation of an anthelminitic for dogs, *Vet Med Small Anim Clin* 61:567–570, 1996.

Behm CA, Bryant C: Anthelmintic action: a metabolic approach (a review), *Vet Parasitol* 5:39–49, 1979.

Bello TR, Laningham ET: A controlled trial evaluation of three oral dosages of moxidectin against equine parasites *J Equine Vet Sci* 14(9):483–488, 1994.

Bennett DG: Clinical pharmacology of ivermectin, *J Am Vet Med Assoc* 189(1):100–104, 1986.

Biehl LG: Anthelmintics for swine, *Vet Clin North Am Food Anim Pract* 2(2):481–487, 1986.

Birckel P, Cochet P, Benard P, et al: *Cutaneous distribution of ^{14}C-fipronil in the dog and in the cat following a spot-on administration,* Proceedings of the Third World Congress of Veterinary Dermatology, Edinburgh, 1996.

Bishop BF, Bruce CI, Evans NA, et al: Selamectin: a novel broad-spectrum endectocide for dogs and cats, *Vet Parasitol* 91:163–176, 2000.

Blagburn BL, Hendrix CM, Lindsay DS, et al: Anthelmintic efficacy of ivermectin in naturally parasitized cats, *Am J Vet Res* 48(4):670–672, 1987.

Blagburn BL, Hendrix CM, Lindsay DS, et al: *Post-adulticide milbemycin oxime microfilaricidal activity in dogs naturally infected with* Dirofilaria immitis, Proceedings of the Heartworm Symposium, Austin, Tex, 1992a, pp 159–164.

Blagburn BL, Hendrix CM, Lindsay DS, et al: Efficacy of milbemycin oxime against naturally acquired or experimentally induced *Ancylostoma* spp. and *Trichuris vulpis* infections in dogs, *Am J Vet Res* 53(4):513–516, 1992b.

Blagburn BL, Hendrix CM, Lindsay DS, et al: *Milbemycin: efficacy and toxicity in beagle and collie dogs,* Proceedings of the Heartworm Symposium, Charleston, SC, 1989, pp 109–113.

Blagburn BL, Hendrix CM, Vaughan JL, et al: *Efficacy of milbemycin oxime against Ancylostoma tubaeforme in experimentally infected cats,* Proceedings of the thirty-seventh annual meeting of the American Association of Veterinary Parasitologists, Boston, 1992c.

Blagburn BL, Lindsay DS, Vaughan JL, et al: Prevalence of canine parasites based on fecal floatation, *Comp Cont Educ Pract Vet* 18(5):483–523, 1996.

Blagburn BL, Paul AJ, Butler JM, et al: *Safety of moxidectin canine SR (sustained release) injectable in ivermectin-sensitive collies and in naturally infected mongrel dogs,* Proceedings of the tenth annual meeting of the American Heartworm Society, San Antonio, Tex, 2001.

Boch J, Gobel E, Heine J, et al: Isospora-infektionen bei hund und katze [Isospora infection in the dog and cat], *Berl Munch Tierarztl Wschr* 94:384–391, 1981.

Bodri MS, Nolan TJ, Skeeba SJ: Safety of milbemycin (A3-A4 oxime) in chelonians, *J Zoo Wildl Med* 24(2):171–174, 1993.

Bogan J, Armour J: Anthelmintics for ruminants, *Int J Parasitol* 17(2):483–491, 1987.

Boreham PFL, Phillips RE, Shepherd RW: The sensitivity of *Giardia intestinalis* to drugs in vitro, *J Antimicrob Chemother* 14:449–461, 1984.

Bourdeau P, Blumstein P, Ibisch C: *Treatment of sarcoptic mange in the dog with milbemycin oxime: comparison of four protocols,* Proceedings of the European Society of Veterinary Dermatology, Pisa, Italy, 1997.

Bowman DD: Anthelmintics for dogs and cats effective against nematodes and cestodes, *Comp Cont Educ Pract Vet* 14(5):597–599, 1992.

Bowman DD: *Georgi's parasitology for veterinarians,* Philadelphia, 1999, WB Saunders.

Bowman DD, Arthur RG: *Laboratory evaluation of Drontal plus (febantel/praziquantel/pyrantel) tablets for dogs,* Proceedings of the American Association of Veterinary Parasitologists, Minneapolis, 1993, p 33.

Bowman DD, Johnson RB, Ulrich ME, et al: Effects of long-term administration of ivermectin or milbemycin oxime on circulating microfilariae and parasite antigenemia in dogs with patent heartworm infections, Proceedings of the Heartworm Symposium, Austin, Tex, 1992, pp 151–158.

Bowman DD, Johnson RC, Hepler DI: Effects of milbemycin oxime on adult hookworms in dogs with naturally acquired infections, *Am J Vet Res* 51(3):487–490, 1990.

Bowman DD, Kato S, Fogarty EA: Effects of ivermectin otic suspension on egg hatching of the cat ear mite, Otodectes cynotis in vitro, *Vet Therap* 2(4):311–316, 2001.

Bowman DD, Lin DS, Johnson RC, et al: Effects of milbemycin oxime on adult *Ancylostoma caninum* and *Uncinaria stenocephala* in dogs with experimentally induced infections, *Am J Vet Res* 52(1):64–67, 1991.

Bowman DD, Parsons JJ, Grieve RB, et al: Effects of milbemycin on adult *Toxocara canis* in dogs with experimentally induced infection, *Am J Vet Res* 49(11):1986–1989, 1988.

Boy MG, Six RH, Thomas CA, et al: Efficacy and safety of selamectin against fleas and heartworms in dogs and cats presented as veterinary patients in North America, *Vet Parasitol* 91:233–250, 2000.

Bradley RE: *Dose titration and efficacy of milbemycin oxime for prophylaxis against Dirofilaria immitis infection in dogs,* Proceedings of the Heartworm Symposium, Charleston, SC, 1989, pp 115–120.

Brown SA, Barsanti JA: Diseases of the bladder and urethra. In Ettinger SJ, editor: *Textbook of veterinary internal medicine,* Philadelphia, 1989, WB Saunders.

Buck WB: Toxicity of pesticides in livestock. In Pimental D, Hanson AA, editors: *CRC handbook of pest management in agriculture,* Boca Raton, Fla, 1991, CRC Press.

Burke TM, Roberson EL: Critical studies of fenbendazole suspension (10%) against naturally occuring helminth infections in dogs, *Am J Vet Res* 39(11):1799–1801, 1978.

Burke TM, Roberson EL: Use of fenbendazole suspension (10%) against experimental infections of *Toxocara canis* and *Ancylostoma caninum* in beagle pups, *Am J Vet Res* 40(4):552-554, 1979.

Cairns GC: The efficacy of thiabendazole (MK 360) as an anthelmintic in sheep, *N Z Vet J,* 9:147–152, 1961.

Callinan APL, Barton NJ: Efficacies of thiabendazole and levamisole against sheep nematodes in Western Victoria, *Aust Vet J* 55:255, 1979.

Campbell WC: *Ivermectin and abamectin,* New York, 1989, Springer-Verlag.

Campbell WC: Benzimidazoles; veterinary uses, *Parasitol Today* 6(4):130–133, 1990.

Campbell WC, Rew RS: *Chemotherapy of parasitic diseases,* New York, 1985, Plenum Press.

Case JL, Tanner PA, Keister DM, et al: *A clinical field trial of melarsomine dihydrochloride (RM340) in dogs with severe (Class 3) heartworm disease,* Proceedings of the Heartworm Symposium, Auburn, Ala, 1995, pp 243–250.

Ciordia H, McCampbell HC: Anthelmintic activity of morantel tartrate in calves, *Am J Vet Res* 34:619–620, 1973.

Clark JN, Daurio CP, Barth DW, et al: Evaluation of a beef-based chewable formulation of pyrantel against induced and natural infections of hookworms and ascarids in dogs, *Vet Parasitol* 40:127–133, 1991.

Clark JN, Daurio CP, Plue RE, et al: Efficacy of ivermectin and pyrantel pamoate combined in a chewable formulation against heartworm, hookworm, and ascarid infections in dogs, *Am J Vet Res* 53(4):517–520, 1992a.

Clark JN, Pulliam JD, Daurio CP: Safety study of a beef-based chewable tablet formulation of ivermectin and pyrantel pamoate in growing dogs, pups and breeding adult dogs, *Am J Vet Res* 53(4):608–612, 1992b.

Coats JR: *Insecticide mode of action,* San Diego, 1982, Academic Press.

Coles GC: The biochemical mode of action of some modern anthelmintics, *Pestic Sci* 8:536–543, 1977.

Coles GC, East JM, Jenkins SNL: The mechanism of action of the anthelmintic levamisole, *Gen Pharmacol* 6:309–313, 1975.

Colglazier ML: Critical anthelmintic trials in ponies with oxfendazole and caviphos and concomitant studies on the spontaneous elimination of small strongyles, *Am J Vet Res* 40:384–386, 1979.

Consalvi PJ, Arnaud JP, Jeannin P, et al: *Safety of a 0.25% w/w fipronil solution (Frontline Spray) in dogs and cats, results of a pharmacovigilance survey one year after launch,* Proceedings of the American Association of Veterinary Parasitologists, Louisville, Ky, 1996.

Conway DP, De Goosh C, Arakawa A: Anthelmintic efficacy of morantel tartrate in cattle, *Am J Vet Res* 34:621–622, 1973.

Cornelius LM, Roberson EL: Treatment of gastrointestinal parasitism. In Kirk RW, editor: *Current veterinary therapy IX, small animal practice,* Philadelphia, 1986, WB Saunders.

Cornwell RL, Jones RM: Critical tests in the horse with the anthelmintic pyrantel tartrate, *Vet Rec* 82:483–484, 1968.

Correa WM, Correa CNM, Langoni H, et al: Canine isosporosis, *Canine Pract* 10(1):44–46, 1973.

Corwin RM, Green SP, Keefe TJ: Dose titration and confirmation tests for determination of cestocidal efficacy of epsiprantel in dogs, *Am J Vet Res* 50(7):1076–1077, 1989.

Courtney CH, Roberson EL: Antinematodal drugs. In Adams HR, editor: *Veterinary pharmacology and therapeutics,* Ames, 1995, Iowa State University Press.

Courtney CH, Sundlof SF, Jackson RF: *New dose schedule for the treatment of canine dirofilariasis with thiacetarsemide,* Proceedings of the Heartworm Society, New Orleans, 1986, pp 49–52.

Craig TM, Hatfield TA, Pankavich JA, et al: Efficacy of moxidectin against an ivermectin resistant strain of *Haemonchus contortus* in sheep, *Vet Parasitol* 41:329–333, 1992.

Craig TM, Shepherd E: Efficacy of albendazole and levamisole in sheep against *Thysanosoma actinoides* and *Haemonchus contortus* from the Edwards Plateau, Texas, *Am J Vet Res* 41:425–426, 1980.

Cramer LG, Eagleson JS, Farrington DO: *The use of eprinomectin pour-on formulations against endoparasite infections in cattle,* Proceedings of the 16th International Conference of the World Association for the Advancement of Veterinary Parasitology, Sun City, South Africa, 1997.

Cribb AE, Lee BL, Trepanier LA, et al: Adverse reactions to sulphonamide and sulphonamide-trimethoprim antimicrobials: clinical syndromes and pathogenesis, *Adverse Drug React Toxicol Rev* 15(1):9–50, 1996.

Cruthers L, Bock E: Evaluation of how quickly imidacloprid kills fleas on dogs, *Comp Cont Educ Pract Vet* 19(suppl 5):27, 1997.

Cruthers LR, Slone RL, Arthur RG: *Efficacy of Drontal plus (praziquantel/pyrantel/febantel) tablets for removal of Ancylostoma caninum, Uncinaria stenocephala, and Toxascaris leonina,* Proceedings of the American Association of Veterinary Parasitologists, Minneapolis, 1993, p 34.

Cunningham J, Everett R: Efficacy of imidacloprid on large dogs, *Comp Cont Educ Pract Vet* 19(suppl 5):28, 1997.

Cunningham J, Everett R, Arthur RG: Effects of shampooing or water exposure on the initial and residual efficacy of imidacloprid, *Comp Cont Educ Pract Vet* 19(suppl 5):29-30, 1997a.

Cunningham J, Everett R, Hunter JS, et al: *Residual efficacy of Frontline Top Spot for the control of fleas and ticks in the dog,* Proceedings of the North American Veterinary Conference, Orlando, Fla, 1997b.

Cunningham J, Everett R, Hunter JS, et al: *Residual efficacy of Frontline Top Spot for the control of fleas in the cat,* Proceedings of the North American Veterinary Conference, Orlando, Fla, 1997c.

Curr C: The effect of dermally applied levamisole against the parasitic nematodes of cattle, *Aust Vet J* 53:425–428, 1977.

Curtis CF: Use of 0.25 percent fipronil spray to treat sarcoptic mange in a litter of 5-week-old puppies, *Vet Rec* 139:43–44, 1996.

Dickinson EO, Thornburg LP: Investigating reports of adverse reactions to a DEC-OBZ anthelmintic, *Vet Med Small Anim Clin* 83:1092–1100, 1988.

DiPietro JA, Todd KS: Anthelmintics used in treatment of parasitic infections of horses, *Vet Clin North Am Equine Pract* 3(1):1–14, 1987.

Dow SC, LeCouteur RA, Poss ML, et al: Central nervous system toxicosis associated with metronidazole treatment of dogs: five cases (1984-1987), *J Am Vet Med Assoc* 195(3):365–368, 1989.

Downing W, Kingsbury PA, Sloan JEN: Critical tests with piperazine adipate in horses, *Vet Rec* 67:641–644, 1955.

Drudge JH, Lyons ET, Tolliver BS, et al: Further clinical trials on strongyle control with some contemporary anthelmintics, *Equine Pract* 3(3):27–36, 1981a.

Drudge JH, Lyons ET, Tolliver SC: Resistance of equine strongyles to thiabendazole: critical tests of two strains, *Vet Med Small Anim Clin* 72:433–438, 1977.

Drudge JH, Lyons ET, Tolliver SC: Benzimidazole resistance of equine strongyles: critical tests of six compounds against population B, *Am J Vet Res* 40:590–594, 1979.

Drudge JH, Lyons ET, Tolliver SC: Clinical trials comparing oxfendazole with oxibendazole and pyrantel for strongyl control in thoroughbreds featuring benzimidazole-resistant small strongyles, *Equine Pract* 7(3):23–31, 1985.

Drudge JH, Lyons ET, Tolliver SC, et al: Clinical trials of oxibendazole for control of equine internal parasites, *Modern Vet Pract* 62:679–682, 1981b.

Drudge JH, Lyons ET, Tolliver SC, Kubis JE: Pyrantel in horses, clinical trials with emphasis on a paste formulation and activity on benzimidazole-resistant small strongyles, *Vet Med Small Anim Clin* 77:957–967, 1982.

Drudge JH, Szanto J, Wyant ZN, et al: Critical tests on thiabendazole against parasites of the horse, *J Parasitol* 48(suppl 2, sect 2):28, 1962.

Drudge JH, Szanto J, Wyant ZN, et al: Critical tests of thiabendazole as an anthelmintic in the horse, *Am J Vet Res* 24:1217–1222, 1963.

Drudge JH, Szanto J, Wyant ZN, et al: Field studies on parasite control in sheep: comparison of thiabendazole, ruelene, and phenothiazine, *Am J Vet Res* 25:1512–1518, 1964.

Drudge JH, Tolliver SC, Lyons ET: Benzimidazole resistance of equine strongyles: critical tests of several classes of compounds against population B strongyles from 1977 to 1981, *Am J Vet Res* 45(4):804–809, 1984.

Dubey JP: Intestinal protozoa infections, *Vet Clin North Am Small Anim Pract* 23(1):37–55, 1993.

Dubey JP: Enteric coccidiosis. In Greene CE, editor: *Infectious diseases of the dog and cat,* Philadelphia, 1998, WB Saunders.

Dunbar MR, Foreyt WJ: Prevention of coccidiosis in domestic dogs and captive coyotes *(Canis latrans)* with sulfadimethoxine-ormetoprim combination, *Am J Vet Res* 46(9):1899–1902, 1985.

Duncan JL, Reid JFS: An evaluation of the efficacy of oxfendazole against the common nematode parasites of the horse, *Vet Rec* 103:332–334, 1978.

Dzimianski MT, McCall JW, McTier TL, et al: *Preliminary results of the efficacy of RM 340 administered seasonally to heartworm antigen and microfilaria positive dogs living outdoors in a heartworm endemic area,* Proceedings of the Heartworm Symposium, Austin, Tex, 1992, pp 241–247.

Eagleson JS, Holste JE, Kunklc BN, et al: *The efficacy of topically applied eprinomectin for treatment of Chorioptes bovis infestations,* Proceedings of the 16th International Conference of the World Association for the Advancement of Veterinary Parasitology, Sun City, South Africa, 1997a.

Eagleson JS, Holste JE, Pollmeier M: *Efficacy of topically applied eprinomectin against the biting louse* Damalinia (Bovicola) bovis, Proceedings of the 16th International Conference of the World Association for the Advancement of Veterinary Parasitology, Sun City, South Africa, 1997b.

Eddi C, Bianchin I, Honer MR, et al: Efficacy of doramectin against field nematode infections of cattle in Latin America, *Vet Parasitol* 49:39–44, 1993.

Egerton JR, Cuckler AC, Ames ER, et al: Anthelmintic effect of thiabendazole on intestinal nematodes in horses, *J Parasitol* 48(suppl 2, sect 2):29, 1962.

English PB, Sprent JFA: The large roundworms of dogs and cats: effectiveness of piperazine salts against immature *Toxocara canis* in prenatally infected puppies, *Aust Vet J* 41:50–53, 1965.

Entriken TL: *Veterinary pharmaceuticals and biologicals (VPB),* Lenexa, Kan, 2001, Veterinary Healthcare Communications.

Everett R, Cunningham J, Tanner P, et al: *An investigative study to evaluate the effect of water immersion or shampooing on the efficacy of Frontline Top Spot,* Proceedings of the North American Veterinary Conference, Orlando, Fla, 1997.

Eyre P: Some pharmacodynamic effects of the nematodes: methypyridine, tetramisole, and pyrantel, *J Pharm Pharmacol* 22:26–36, 1970.

Eysker M, Boersema JH: The efficacy of moxidectin against *Dictyocaulus viviparus* in cattle, *Vet Q* 14(2):79–80, 1982.

Fest C, Schmidt KJ: *The chemistry of organophosphorus pesticides,* ed 2, New York, 1982, Springer-Verlag.

Frayha GJ, Smyth JD, Gobert JG, et al: The mechanisms of action of antiprotozoal and anthelmintic drugs in man, *Gen Pharmacol* 28(2):273–299, 1997.

Friis C, Bjoern H: *Pharmacokinetics of doramectin and ivermectin in swine,* Proceedings of the American Association of Veterinary Parasitologists, Reno, Nev, 1997.

Furrow RD, Powers KG, Parbuoni EL: Dirofilaria immitis: II. *Gross and microscopic hepatic changes associated with*

diethylcarbamazine citrate (DEC) therapy in dogs, Proceedings of the Heartworm Symposium, Dallas, Tex, 1980, pp 117–121.

Gant DB, Chalmers AE, Wolff MA, et al: *Mode of action of fipronil,* Proceedings of the American Association of Veterinary Parasitologists, Louisville, Ky, 1996.

Garfield RA, Reedy LM: The use of oral milbemycin oxime (Interceptor) in the treatment of chronic generalized canine demodicosis, *Vet Dermatol* 3:231–234, 1992.

Gemmell MA, Johnstone PD, Oudemans G: The effect of praziquantel on *Echinococcus granulosus, Taenia hydatigena,* and *Taenia ovis* infections in dogs, *Res Vet Sci* 23:121–123, 1977.

Gemmell MA, Johnstone PD, Oudemans G: The effect of route of administration on the efficacy of praziquantel against Echinococcus granulosus infections in dogs, *Res Vet Sci* 29:131–132, 1980.

Georgi JR, Slauson DO, Theorides VJ: Anthelmintic activity of albendazole against *Filaroides hirthi* lungworms in dogs, *Am J Vet Res* 39:803, 1978.

Gibson TE: Critical tests of piperazine adipate as an equine anthelmintic, *Br Vet J* 113:90–92, 1957.

Gilman AG, Rall TW, Nies AS, et al: *Goodman and Gilman's: the pharmacological basis of therapeutics,* New York, 1990, Pergamon Press.

Gogolewski RP, Allerton GR, Pitt SR, et al: Effect of simulated rain, coat length, and exposure to natural climatic conditions on the efficacy of a topical formulation of eprinomectin against endoparasites of cattle, *Vet Parasitol* 69(1/2):95–102, 1997a.

Gogolewski RP, Slacek B, Familton AS, et al: Efficacy of a topical formulation of eprinomectin against endoparasites of cattle in New Zealand, *N Z Vet J* 45:1–3, 1997b.

Gonzales JC, Muniz RA, Farias A, et al: Therapeutic and persistent efficacy of doramectin against Boophilus microplus in cattle, *Vet Parasitol* 49:107–109, 1993.

Goudie AC, Evans NA, Gration KAF, et al: Doramectin: a potent novel endectocide, *Vet Parasitol* 49:5–15, 1993.

Gram D, Payton AJ, Gerig TM, et al: Treating ear mites in cats: a comparison of subcutaneous and topical ivermectin, *Vet Med* 89:1122–1125, 1994.

Greene CE, Cook JR, Mahaffey EA: Clindamycin for treatment of Toxoplasma polymyositis in a dog, *J Am Vet Med Assoc* 187(6):631–634, 1985.

Grieve RB, Frank GR, Stewart VA, et al: Chemoprophylactic effects of milbemycin oxime against larvae of *Dirofilaria immitis* during prepatent development, *Am J Vet Res* 52(12):2040–2042, 1991.

Griffin L, Hopkins TJ, Kerwick C: Imidacloprid: safety of a new insecticidal compound in dogs and cats, *Comp Cont Educ Pract Vet* 19(suppl 5):21–24, 1997a.

Griffin L, Krieger K, Liege P: Imidacloprid: a new compound for control of fleas and flea-initiated dermatitis, *Comp Cont Educ Pract Vet* 19(suppl 5):17–20, 1997b.

Gunnarsson L, Moller L, Einarsson A, et al: *Efficacy of milbemycin oxime in the treatment of nasal mite (Pneumonyssoides caninum) infection in dogs,* Proceedings, European Society of Veterinary Dermatology, Pisa, Italy, 1997.

Guyonnet V, Johnson JK, Long PL: Studies on the stage of action of lasalocid against *Eimeria tenella* and *Eimeria acervulina* in the chicken, *Vet Parasitol* 37:93–100, 1990.

Hall CA, Campbell NJ, Carrol SN: Resistance to thiabendazole in a field population of *Ostertagia circumcincta* from sheep, *Aust Vet J* 55:229–231, 1979.

Hamilton RG, Wagner E, April M, et al: *Dirofilaria immitis:* diethylcarbamazine-induced anaphylactoid reactions in infected dogs, *Exp Parasitol* 61:405–420, 1986.

Hardman JG, Limbird LE, Gilman AG: *Goodman & Gilman's the pharmacological basis of therapeutics,* New York, 2001, McGraw-Hill.

Hassall KA: *The chemistry of pesticides; their metabolism, mode of action, and uses in crop protection,* London, 1982, MacMillan Press.

Hawking F: Diethylcarbamazine and new compounds for the treatment of filariasis, *Adv Pharmacol Chemother* 16:129–194, 1979.

Hayes WJ, Laws ER: *Handbook of pesticide toxicology,* New York, 1991, Academic Press.

Hebden SP: The anthelmintic activity of thiabendazole (MK360), *Aust Vet J* 37:264–269, 1961.

Henderson G, Foil LD: Efficacy of diflubenzuron in simulated household and yard conditions against the cat flea *Ctenocephalides felis* (Bouche') (Siphonoptera: pulicidae), *J Med Entomol* 30(3):619–621, 1993.

Hendrickx MO, Anderson L, Boulard C, et al: Efficacy of doramectin against warble fly larvae *(Hypoderma bovis), Vet Parasitol* 49:75–84, 1993.

Hendrix CM, Blagburn BL, Bowles JV, et al: *The safety of moxidectin in dogs infected with microfilariae and adults of* Dirofilaria immitis, Proceedings of the Heartworm Symposium, Austin, Tex, 1992, pp 183–187.

Hopkins TJ: Imidacloprid: *Ctenocephalides felis* control on dogs under field conditions in Australia, *Comp Cont Educ Pract Vet* 19(suppl 5):25–26, 1997.

Hopkins TJ, Kerwick C, Gyr P, et al: Efficacy of imidacoprid to remove and prevent C*tenocephalides felis* infestations on dogs and cats, *Comp Cont Educ Pract Vet* 19(suppl 5):11–16, 1997.

Horak IG, Louw JP, Raymond SM, et al: The anthelmintic efficacy of feed mash or pellets medicated with thiabendazole, *J S Afr Vet Med Assoc* 41:307–312, 1970.

Hotson IK, Campbell NJ, Smeal MG: Anthelmintic resistance in *Trichostrongylus columbriformis, Aust Vet J* 46:356–360, 1970.

Howes HL: trans-1,4,5,6-Tetrahydro-2-(3-hydroxystyryl)-1-methyl pyrimidine (CP-14,445): a new antiwhipworm agent (36151), *Proc Soc Exp Biol Med* 139:394–401, 1972.

Hunter JS, Keister DM, Jeannin P: *A comparison of the tick control efficacy of Frontline spray treatment against the American dog tick and brown dog tick,* Proceedings of the American Association of Veterinary Parasitologists, Louisville, Ky, 1996a.

Hunter JS, Keister DM, Jeannin P: *The effect of fipronil-treated dog hair on the survival of the immature stages of the cat flea* Ctenocephalides felis, Proceedings of the American College of Veterinary Internal Medicine, San Antonio, Tex, 1996b.

Jacobs DE: Anthelmintics for dogs and cats, *Int J Parasitol* 17(2):511–518, 1987b.

Jacobs DE: Control of *Toxocara canis* in puppies: a comparison of screening techiques and evaluation of a dosing programme, *J Vet Pharmacol Ther* 10:23–29, 1987b.

Jeannin P, Postal JM, Hunter J, et al: *Fipronil: a new insecticide for flea control,* Proceedings of the British Small Animal Veterinary Association, Birmingham, UK, 1994.

Jernigan AD, McTier TL, Chieffo C, et al: Efficacy of selamectin against experimentally induced tick *(Rhipicephalus sanguineus and Dermacentor variabilis)* infestations of dogs, *Vet Parasitol* 91:359–375, 2000.

Jones RM, Logan NB, Weatherly AJ, et al: Activity of doramectin against nematodes endoparasites of cattle, *Vet Parasitol* 49:27-37, 1993.

Keister DM, Dzimianski MT, McTier TL, et al: *Dose selection and confirmation of RM 340, a new filaricide for the treatment of dogs with immature and mature* Dirofilaria immitis, Proceedings of the Heartworm Symposium, Austin, Tex, 1992, pp 225–229.

Keister DM, Tanner PA, Meo NJ: *Immiticide: review of discovery, development, and utility,* Proceedings of the Heartworm Symposium, Auburn, Ala, 1995, pp 201–219.

Kennedy MJ, Phillips FE: Efficacy of doramectin against eyeworms *(Thelazia* spp.) in naturally and experimentally infected cattle, *Vet Parasitol* 49:61–66, 1993.

Kilgore RL, Williams ML, Benz GW, et al: Comparative efficacy of clorsulon and albendazole against Fasciola hepatica in cattle, *Am J Vet Res* 46(7):1553–1555, 1985.

King RR, Courtney CH, Aguilar R: *Heartworm prophylaxis with moxidectin: field trial results from a hyperenzootic area,* Proceedings of the Heartworm Symposium, Austin, Tex, 1992. pp 179–181.

Kirkpatrick CE, Farrell JP: Feline giardiasis: observations on natural and induced infections, *Am J Vet Res* 45(10): 2182–2188, 1984.

Kirkpatrick CE, Megella C: Use of ivermectin in treatment of *Aelurostrongylus abstrusus* and *Toxocara cati* infections in a cat, *J Am Vet Med Assoc* 190(10):1309–1310, 1987.

Klein JB, Bradley RE, Conway DP: Anthelmintic efficacy of pyrantel pamoate against the roundworm, *Toxocara canis,* and the hookworm, *Ancylostoma caninum,* in dogs, *Vet Med Small Anim Clin* 73:1011–1013, 1978.

Knight DH: Heartworm infection, *Vet Clin North Am Small Anim Pract* 17(6):1463–1518, 1987.

Krautmann MJ, Novotny MJ, DeKeulenaer K, et al: Safety of selamectin in cats, *Vet Parasitol* 91:393–403, 2000.

Kruckenberg SM, Meyer AD, Eastman WR: Preliminary studies on the effect of praziquantel against tapeworms in dogs and cats, *Vet Med Small Anim Clin* 76:689–697, 1981.

Kume S: *Supplemental report on diethylcarbamazine as a prophylactic agent,* Proceedings of the Heartworm Symposium, Bonner Springs, Kan, 1974, pp 73–74.

Kume S, Ohishi I, Kobayashi S: Extended studies on prophylactic therapy against the developing stages of *Dirofilaria immitis* in the dog, *Am J Vet Res* 25:1527–1530, 1964.

Kume S, Ohishi I, Kobayashi S: Prophylactic therapy against the developing stages of *Dirofilaria immitis:* supplemental studies, *Am J Vet Res* 28(125):975–978, 1967.

Lacey E: Mode of action of benzimadzoles, *Parasitol Today* 6(4):112–115, 1990.

Lappin MR, Greene CE, Winston S, et al: Clinical feline toxoplasmosis, *J Vet Intern Med* 3:139–143, 1989.

Ledbetter MG: Storage considerations for thiacetarsemide sodium, *J Am Vet Med Assoc* 85(7):753–754, 1984.

LeNain S, Postal JM, Jeannin P, et al: *Efficacy of a 0.25% fipronil spray formulation in the control of a natural tick infestation on dogs,* Birmingham, UK, 1996, British Veterinary Dermatology Group, BSAVA.

Leneau H, Haig M, Ho I: Safety of larvicidal doses of fenbendazole in horses, *Modern Vet Pract* 66:B17–B19, 1985.

Lichtensteiger CA, Dipietro JA, Paul AJ, et al: *Duration of activity of doramectin and ivermectin against Ascaris suum in experimentally infected pigs,* Proceedings of the American Association of Veterinary Parasitologists, Reno, Nev, 1997.

Lindsay DS, Blagburn BL: Antiprotozoan drugs. In Adams HR, editor: *Veterinary pharmacology and therapeutics, Ames,* 2001, Iowa State University Press.

Linquist WD: Drug evaluation of pyrantel pamoate against *Ancylostoma, Toxocara,* and *Toxascaris* in eleven dogs, *Am J Vet Res* 36(9):1387–1389, 1695, 1975.

Liu MY, Latli B, Casida JE: Imidacloprid binding site in *Musca* nicotinic acetylcholine receptor: interactions with physostigmine and a variety of nicotinic agonists with chloropyridyl and chlorothiazolyl substituents, *Pesticide Biochem Physiol* 52:170–181, 1995.

Logan NB, Weatherley AJ, Jones RM: Activity of doramectin against nematode and arthropod parasites of swine, *Vet Parasitol* 66(1/2):87–94, 1997.

Lok JB, Knight DH: *Macrolide effects on reproductive function in male and female heartworms,* Proceedings of the Heartworm Symposium, Auburn, Ala, 1995, pp 165–170.

Lok JB, Knight DH, LaPaugh DA, et al: *Kinetics of microfilaremia suppression in Dirofilaria immitis-infected dogs during and after a prophylactic regimen of milbemycin oxime,* Proceedings of the Heartworm Symposium, Austin, Tex, 1992, pp 143–149.

Lok JB, Knight DH, McCall JW, et al: *Six-month prophylactic efficacy of an injectable, sustained release formulation of moxidectin against Dirofilaria immitis infection,* Proceedings of the tenth annual meeting of the American Heartworm Society, San Antonio, Tex, 2001.

Londershausen M: Approaches to new parasiticides, *Pesticide Science* 48(4):269–292, 1996.

Lovell RA, Trammel HL, Beasley VR, et al: A review of 83 reports of suspected toluene/dichlorophen toxicoses in cats and dogs, *J Am Anim Hosp Assoc* 26:652–658, 1990.

Lyons ET, Drudge JH, Knapp FW: Controlled test of anthelmintic activity of trichlorfon and thiabendazole in lambs with observations on Oestrus ovis, *Am J Vet Res* 28:1111–1116, 1967.

Lyons ET, Drudge JH, La Bore DE, et al: Field and controlled test evaluations of levamisole against natural infections of gastrointestinal nematodes and lungworms in calves, *Am J Vet Res* 33:65–71, 1972.

Lyons ET, Drudge JH, La Bore DE, et al: Controlled test of anthelmintic activity of levamisole administered to calves via drinking water, subcutaneous injection, or alfalfa pellet premix, *Am J Vet Res* 36:777–780, 1975a.

Lyons ET, Drudge JH, Tolliver SC: Critical tests of three salts of pyrantel against internal parasites of the horse, *Am J Vet Res* 35:1515–1522, 1974.

Lyons ET, Drudge JH, Tolliver SC: Field tests of three salts of pyrantel against internal parasites of the horse, *Am J Vet Res* 36:161–166, 1975b.

Lyons ET, Drudge JH, Tolliver SC: Critical tests of oxfendazole against internal parasites of horses, *Am J Vet Res* 38:2049–2053. 1977.

Lyons ET, Drudge JH, Tolliver SC, et al: Pyrantel pamoate: evaluating its activity against equine tapeworms, *Vet Med* 81:280–285, 1986.

Lyons ET, Tolliver SC, Drudge JH: Critical tests in equids with fenbendazole alone of combined with piperazine: particular reference to activity on benzimidazole-resistant small strongyles, *Vet Parasitol* 12:91-98, 1983.

Lyons ET, Tolliver SC, Drudge JH, et al: Critical and controlled tests of activity of moxidectin (CL301,423) against natural infections of internal parasites of equids, *Vet Parasitol* 41:255–284, 1992.

Manger BR, Brewer MD: Epsiprantel, a new tapeworm remedy, preliminary efficacy studies in dogs and cats, *Br Vet J* 145:384–388, 1989.

Marriner SE, Bogan JA: Pharmacokinetics of oxfendazole in sheep, *Am J Vet Res* 42:1143–1145, 1981.

Martin RJ: Neuromuscular transmission in nematode parasites and antinematodal drug action, *Pharmacol Ther* 58(1):13–50, 1983.

McCall JW, McTier TL, Holmes RA, et al: *Prevention of naturally acquired heartworm infection in heartworm-naive beagles by oral administration of moxidectin at an interval of either one or two months,* Proceedings of the Heartworm Symposium, Austin, Tex, 1992, pp 169–177.

McCall JW, Supakorndej P, Dzimianski MT: *Evaluation of retroactive and adulticidal activity of moxidectin SR (sustained release) injectable formulation against Dirofilaria immitis infections in beagles,* Proceedings from the the tenth annual meeting of the American Heartworm Society, San Antonio, Tex, 2001.

McDougald LR, Roberson EL: Antiprotozoan drugs. In Booth NH, McDonald LE, editors: *Veterinary pharmacology and therapeutics, Ames,* 1988, Iowa State University Press.

McKellar QA, Scott EW: The benzimidazole anthelmintics: a review, *J Vet Pharmacol Ther* 13:223–247, 1990.

McTier TL, Jones RL, Holbert MS, et al: Efficacy of selamectin against adult flea infestations *(Ctenocephalides felis felis* and *Ctenocephalides canis)* of dogs and cats, *Vet Parasitol* 91:187–199, 2000a.

McTier TL, McCall JW, Dzimianski MT, et al: *Prevention of experimental heartworm infection in dogs with single, oral doses of moxidectin,* Proceedings of the Heartworm Symposium, Austin, Tex, 1992, pp 165–168.

McTier TL, Shanks DJ, Jernigan AD, et al: Evaluation of the effects of selamectin against adult and immature stages of fleas *(Ctenocephalides felis felis)* on dogs and cats, *Vet Parasitol* 91:201–212, 2000b.

McTier TL, Shanks DJ, Wren JA, et al: Efficacy of selamectin against experimentally induced and naturally acquired infections of *Toxocara cati* and *Ancylostoma tubaeforme* in cats, *Vet Parasitol* 91:311–319, 2000c.

McTier TL, Siedek EM, Clemence RG, et al: Efficacy of selamectin against experimentally induced and naturally acquired ascarid *(Toxocara canis* and *Toxascaris leonina)* infections in dogs, *Vet Parasitol* 91:333–345, 2000d.

Meyer EK: Adverse events associated with albendazole and other products used for treatment of giardiasis, *J Am Vet Med Assoc* 213(1):44–46, 1998.

Miller MW, Keister DM, Tanner PA, et al: *Clinical efficacy and safety trial of melarsomine dihydrochloride (RM 340) and thiacetarsemide in dogs with moderate (Class 2) heartworm disease,* Proceedings of the Heartworm Symposium, Auburn, Ala, 1995, pp 233–241.

Miller WH, Scott DW, Cayatte SM, et al: Clinical efficacy of increased dosages of milbemycin oxime for treatment of generalized demodicosis in adult dogs, *J Am Vet Med Assoc* 207(12):1581–1584, 1995b.

Miller WH, Scott DW, Wellington JR, et al: Clinical efficacy of milbemycin oxime in the treatment of generalized demodicosis in adult dogs, *J Am Vet Med Assoc* 203(10):1426–1429, 1993.

Morin D, Valdez R, Lichtensteiger C, et al: Efficacy of moxidectin 0.5% pour-on against naturally acquired nematode infections in cattle, *Vet Parasitol* 65(1/2):75–81, 1996.

Moya-Borja GE, Muniz RA, Sanavria A, et al: Therapeutic and persistant efficacy of doramectin against *Dermatobia hominis* in cattle, *Vet Parasitol* 49:85–93, 1993.

Moya-Borja GE, Oliveira CMB, Muniz RA, et al: Prophylactic and persistent efficacy of doramectin against *Cochliomyia hominivorax* in cattle, *Vet Parasitol* 49:95–105, 1993.

Muirhead S: *2001 feed additive compendium,* Minnetonka, Minn, 2001, Miller Publishing Co & The Animal Health Institute.

Muser RK, Paul JW: Safety of fenbendazole use in cattle, *Mod Vet Pract* 65:371–374, 1984.

Nelson DL, Allen AD, Mozier JO, et al: Diagnosis and treatment of adverse reactions in cattle treated for grubs with a systemic insecticide, *Vet Med Small Anim Clin* 62:683–684, 1967.

Nolan TJ, Niamatali S, Bhopale V, et al: Efficacy of a chewable formulation of ivermectin against a mixed infection of *Ancylostoma braziliense* and *Ancylostoma tubaeforme* in cats, *Am J Vet Res* 53(8):1411–1413, 1992.

Novotny MJ, Krautmann MJ, Ehrhart JC, et al: Safety of selamectin in dogs, *Vet Parasitol* 91:377–391, 2000.

O'Handley RM, Olson ME, McAllister TA, et al: Efficacy of fenbendazole for treatment of giardiasis in calves, *Am J Vet Res* 58(4):384–388, 1997.

Olsen JL, Rollins LD, Rosenberg MC, et al: Efficacy of dichlorvos administered orally in single and repeated doses for removal of canine whipworms, *J Am Vet Med Assoc* 171:542–544, 1977.

Otto GF, Maren TH: Possible use of an arsenical compound in the treatment of heartworm in dogs, *Vet Med* 42:128, 1947.

Palumbo NE, Perri SF, Desowitz RS, et al: *Preliminary observations on adverse reactions to diethylcarbamazine (DEC) in dogs infected with* Dirofilaria immitis, Proceedings of the Heartworm Symposium, Atlanta, 1977, pp 97–103.

Patterson JM, Grenn HH: Hemorrhage and death in dogs following the administration of sulfaquinoxaline, *Can Vet J* 16(9):265–268, 1975.

Paul AJ, Acre KE, Todd KS, et al: *Efficacy of ivermectin against* Dirofilaria immitis *in cats 30 and 45 days postinfection,* Proceedings of the Heartworm Symposium, 1992, Austin, Tex, pp 117–119.

Paul AJ, Tranquilli WJ, Todd KS, et al: *Evaluation of the safety of moxidectin in collies,* Proceedings of the Heartworm Symposium, Austin, Tex, 1992, pp 179–181.

Plapp FW: The nature, modes of action, and toxicity of insecticides. In Pimentel, editor: *CRC handbook of pest management in agriculture,* Boca Raton, Fla, 1991, CRC Press.

Plumb DC: *Veterinary drug handbook,* Ames, 1999, Iowa State University Press.

Postal JM, Jeannin P, Consalvi PJ, et al: *Efficacy of a 0.25% fipronil pump-spray formulation against cat flea infestations* (Ctenocephalides feils) *in cats,* Proceedings of the World Small Animal Veterinary Association, Durban, South Africa, 1994.

Postal JM, LeNain S, Fillon F, Longo F: *Efficacy of a 10% fipronil spot-on formulation against cat flea infestations* (Ctenocephalides felis) *in cats,* Birmingham, UK, British Veterinary Dermatology Group, BSAVA.

Postal JM, LeNain S, Longo F, et al: *Field efficacy of Frontline Top Spot in the treatment and control of flea infestation,* Proceedings of the World Congress of Veterinary Dermatology, Edinburgh, 1996a.

Powers KG, Parbuoni EL, Furrow RD: Dirofilaria immitis: *I. Adverse reactions associated with diethylcarbamazine therapy in microfilaremic dogs,* Proceedings of the Heartworm Symposium, Dallas, 1980, pp 108–116.

Poynter D: The efficacy of piperazine adipate administered in bran mash to horses, *Vet Rec* 67:625, 1955a.

Poynter D: Piperazine adipate as an equine anthelmintic, *Vet Rec* 67:159–163, 1995b.

Poynter D: A comparative assessment of the anthelmintic activity in horses of four piperazine compounds, *Vet Rec* 68:291–297, 1956.

Prichard RK: Anthelmintics for cattle, *Vet Clin North Am Food Anim Pract* 2(2):489–501, 1986.

Prichard RK: The pharmacology of anthelmintics in livestock, *Int J Parasitol* 17(2):473–482, 1987.

Pulliam JD, Seward RL, Henry RT, et al: Investigating ivermectin toxicity in collies, *Vet Med* 79:33–40, 1985.

Ranjan S, Trudeau C, Prichard RK, et al: Efficacy of moxidectin against naturally acquired nematode infections in cattle, *Vet Parasitol* 41:227–231, 1992.

Rawlings CA, Raynaud JP, Lewis RE, et al: Pulmonary thromboembolism and hypertension after thiacetarsemide vs melarsomine dihydrochloride treatment of *Dirofilaria immitis* infection in dogs, *Am J Vet Res* 54(6):920–925, 1993.

Reid JFS, Eagleson JS, Langholff WK: *Persistent efficacy of eprinomectin pour-on against gastrointestinal and pulmonary nematodes in cattle,* Proceedings of the 16th International Conference of the World Association for the Advancement of Veterinary Parasitology., Sun City, South Africa, 1997.

Reinemeyer CE, Courtney CH: Antinematodal drugs. In Adams HR, editor: *Veterinary pharmacology and therapeutics,* Ames, 2001, Iowa State University Press.

Reinemeyer CR: Treatment of parasites. In Bonogura JD, editor: *Kirk's current veterinary therapy XIII, small animal practice,* Philadelphia, 2000, WB Saunders.

Roberson EL: Chemotherapy of parasitic diseases. In Booth NE, McDonald LE, editors: *Veterinary pharmacology and therapeutics,* Ames, 1988, Iowa State University Press.

Roberson EL, Burke TM: Evaluation of granulated fenbendazole (22.2%) against induced and naturally occuring helminth infections in cats, *Am J Vet Res* 41:1499–1502, 1980.

Roberson EL, Burke TM: Evaluation of granulated fenbendazole as a treatment for helminth infections in dogs, *J Am Vet Med Assoc* 180(1):53–55, 1982.

Roberson EL, Schad GA, Ambrose DL, et al: *Efficacy of ivermectin against hookworm infections in cats,* Proceedings of the Heartworm Symposium, Austin, Tex, 1992.

Ryan WG, Crawford RJ, Gross SJ, et al: Assessment of parasite control and weight gain after use of an ivermectin sustained release bolus in calves, *J Am Vet Med Assoc* 211(6):754-756, 1977.

Saeki H, Ishii T, Ohta M, et al: Evaluation of anthelmintic efficacy of doramectin against gastrointestinal nematodes by fecal examination in cattle in Japan, *J Vet Med Sci* 57:1057–1061, 1995.

Sasaki Y, Kitagawa H, Murase S, et al: Susceptibility of rough-coated collies to milbemycin oxime, *Jpn J Vet Sci* 52(6):1269–1271, 1990.

Schillhorn van Veen TW: Coccidiosis in ruminants, *Comp Cont Educ Pract Vet* 8(10):F52-58, 1986.

Scholl PJ, Guillot FS, Wang GT: Moxidectin: systemic activity against common cattle grubs *(Hypoderma lineatum)* (Diptera:Oestridae) and trichostrongyle nematodes in cattle, *Vet Parasitol* 41:203–209, 1992.

Seibert BP, Guerrero J, Newcomb KM, et al: Seasonal comparisons of anthelmintic activity of levamisole pour-on in cattle in the USA, *Vet Rec* 118:40–42, 1986.

Shanks DJ, McTier TL, Behan S, et al: The efficacy of selamectin in the treatment of naturally acquired infestations of Sarcoptes scabiei on dogs, *Vet Parasitol* 91:269–281, 2001a.

Shanks DJ, McTier TL, Rowan TG, et al: The efficacy of selamectin in the treatment of naturally acquired aural infestations of *Otodectes cynotis* on dogs and cats, *Vet Parasitol* 91:283–290, 2000b.

Shanks DJ, Rowan TG, Jones RL, et al: Efficacy of selamectin in the treatment and prevention of flea *(Ctenocephalides felis felis)* infestations on dogs and cats housed in simulated home environments, *Vet Parasitol* 91:213–222, 2000c.

Sharp ML, Sepesi JP, Collins JA: A comparative critical assay on canine anthelmintics, *Vet Med Small Anim Clin* 68:131–132, 1973.

Shoop WL, Demontigny P, Fink DW, et al: Efficacy in sheep and pharmacokinetics in cattle that led to the selection of eprinomectin as a topical endectocide for cattle, *Int J Parasitol* 26(11):1227–1235, 1996a.

Shoop WL, Egerton JR, Eary CH, et al: Eprinomectin: a novel avermectin for use as a topical endectocide for cattle, *Int J Parasitol* 26(11):1237–1242, 1996b.

Shoop WL, Mrozik H, Fisher MH: Structure and activity of avermectins and milbemycins in animal health, *Vet Parasitol* 59:139–156, 1995.

Simpson J: Toxicity studies of Filaribits plus chewable tablets: acute, subacute, chronic, and reproductive studies conducted, *Norden News* 61(3):16–20, 1986.

Six RH, Clemence RG, Thomas CA, et al: Efficacy and safety of selamectin against *Sarcoptes scabiei* on dogs and *Otodectes cynotis* on dogs and cats presented as veterinary patients, *Vet Parasitol* 91:291–309, 2000a.

Six RH, Sture GH, Thomas CA, et al: Efficacy and safety of selamectin against gastrointestinal nematodes in cats presented as veterinary patients, *Vet Parasitol* 91:321–331, 2000b.

Slocombe JOD, McCraw BM: Suppression of the pathogenic effects of *Strongylus edentatus* larvae with thiabendazole, *Can J Comp Med* 39:256–260, 1975.

Slocombe O, Lake MC: *Dose confirmation trial of moxidectin equine oral gel against Gasterophilus spp. in equines,* proceedings of the American Association of Veterinary Parasitologists, Reno, Nev, 1997.

Smart J: Amprolium for canine coccidiosis, *Mod Vet Pract* 52:41, 1971.

Smith JA: Toxic encephalopathies in cattle. In Howard JL, editor: *Current veterinary therapy: food animal practice 2,* Philadelphia, 1986, WB Saunders.

Snijders AJ, Louw JP: A comparison of anthelmintics administered intraruminally in sheep, *J S Afr Vet Med Assoc* 37:121–131, 1966.

Snyder DE, Floyd JG, DiPietro JA: Use of anthelmintics and anticoccidial compounds in cattle, *Comp Cont Educ Pract Vet* 13(12):1847–1860, 1991.

Speer CA: Coccidiosis. In Howard JL, Smith RA, editors: *Current veterinary therapy 4: food animal practice,* Philadelphia, 1999, WB Saunders.

Stewart TB, Fox MC, Wiles SE: Doramectin efficacy against gastrointestinal nematodes in pigs, *Vet Parasitol* 66(1/2):101–108, 1996a.

Stewart TB, Fox MC, Wiles SE: Doramectin efficacy against the kidney worm *Stephanurus dentatus* in sows, *Vet Parasitol* 66(1/2):95–99, 1996b.

Stewart VA, Hepler DI, Grieve RB: Efficacy of milbemycin oxime in chemoprophylaxis of dirofilariasis in cats, *Am J Vet Res* 53(12):2274–2277, 1992.

Stokol T, Randolph JF, Nachbar S, et al: Development of bone marrow toxicosis after albendazol administration in a dog and cat, *J Am Vet Med Assoc* 210:1753–1756, 1997.

Supakorndej P, McTier TL, McCall JW: *Evaluation of single oral doses of moxidectin against hookworms, ascarids, and whip-worms in dogs,* Proceedings of the American Association of Veterinary Parasitologists, Minneapolis, 1993, p 41.

Tanner PA, Hunter JS, Keister DM: *An investigative study to evaluate the effect of bathing of laboratory dogs on the efficacy of fipronil spray,* Proceedings of the American Association of Veterinary Parasitologists, Louisville, Ky, 1996.

Taylor SM, Kenny J: Comparison of moxidectin with ivermectin and pyrantel embonate for reduction of faecal egg counts in horses, *Vet Rec* 137(20):516–518, 1995.

Thakur SA, Prezioso U, Marchevsky N: Efficacy of droncit against *Echinococcus granulosus* infection in dogs, *Am J Vet Res* 39(5):859–860, 1978.

Thomas H, Gonnert R: The efficacy of praziquantel against cestodes in cats, dogs, and sheep, *Res Vet Sci* 24:20–25, 1978.

Thompson DR, Rehbein S, Loewenstein M, et al: *Efficacy of eprinomectin against Sarcoptes scabei in cattle,* Proceedings of the 16th International Conference of the WorldAssociation for the Advancement of Veterinary Parasitology., Sun City, South Africa, 1997.

Todd AC, Crowley J, Scholl P, et al: Critical tests with pyrantel pamoate against internal parasites in dogs from Wisconsin, *Vet Med Small Anim Clin* 70:936–939, 1975.

Todd KS, Mansfield ME: Evaluation of four forms of oxfendazole against nematodes of cattle, *Am J Vet Res* 40:423–424, 1979.

Tomlin CDS: *The pesticide manual: a world compendium,* Bath, UK, 2000, Farnham, British Crop Protection Council.

Turk RD, Ueckert BW, Bell RR: Observations on thiabendazole as an equine anthelmintic, *J Am Vet Med Assoc* 141:240–242, 1962.

USP: *USP drug information update* (September, pp 1289–1586), Rockville, Md, 1998, United States Pharmacopeial Convention.

Vaden SL, Bunch SE, Duncan DE, et al: Hepatotoxicosis associated with heartworm/hookworm preventative medication in a dog, *J Am Vet Med Assoc* 192(5):651–654, 1988.

Vercruysse J, Claerebout E, Dorny P, et al: Persistence of the efficacy of pour-on and injectable moxidectin against *Ostertagia ostertagi* and *Dictyocaulus viviparus* in experimentally infected cattle, Vet Rec 140(3):64–66, 1997a.

Vercruysse J, Dorny P, Hong C, et al: Efficacy of doramectin in the prevention of gastrointestinal nematode infections in grazing cattle, *Vet Parasitol* 49:51–59, 1993.

Vercruysse J, Eysker M, Demeulenaere D, et al: *Remanent effect of a 2% moxidectin gel on establishment of small strongyles,* Proceedings of the American Association of Veterinary Parasitologists, Reno, Nev, 1997b.

Vezzoni A, Genchi C, Raynaud JP: *Adulticide efficacy of RM 340 in dogs with mild and severe natural infections,* Proceedings of the Heartworm Symposium, Austin, Tex, 1992, pp 231–240.

Vincenzi P, Genchi C: *Efficacy of fipronil (Frontline) against ear mites* (Otodectes cynotis) *in dogs and cats,* Proceedings of the European Society of Veterinary Dermatology, Pisa, Italy, 1997.

Wallace DH, Kilgore RL, Benz GW: Clorsulon: a new fasciolicide, *Mod Vet Pract* 66(11):879–882, 1985.

Ware GW: *Pesticides, theory and application,* San Francisco, 1983, WH Freeman & Co.

Ware GW: *Fundamentals of pesticides: a self instruction guide,* ed 2, Fresno, Calif, 1986, Thompson.

Warne RJ, Tipton VJ, Furusho Y: Canine heartworm disease in Japan: screening of selected drugs against *Dirofilaria immitis* in vivo, *Am J Vet Res* 30:27–32, 1969.

Watson ADJ: Giardiasis and colitis in a dog, *Aust Vet J* 56:444–447, 1980.

Weatherley AJ, Hong C, Harris TJ, et al: Persistent efficacy of doramectin against experimental nematode infections in calves, *Vet Parasitol* 49:45–50, 1993.

Weil A, Birckel P, Bosc F, et al: *Plasma, skin, and hair distribution of fipronil following topical administration to the dog and to the cat,* Proceedings of the North American Veterinary Conference, Orlando, Fla, 1997.

Wescott RB: Anthelmintics and drug resistance, *Vet Clin North Am Equine Pract* 2(2):367–380, 1986.

Wexler-Mitchell E: Ear mites in a 33-cat household, *Vet Forum* 18(10):57–61, 2001.

Wicks SR, Kaye B, Weatherley AJ, et al: Effect of formulation on the pharmacokinetics and efficacy of doramectin, *Vet Parasitol* 49:17–26, 1993.

Williams JC, Barras SA, Wang GT: Efficacy of moxidectin against gastrointestinal nematodes of cattle, *Vet Rec* 131(15):345–347, 1992a.

Williams JC, Nault C, Ramsey RT, et al: Efficacy of Cydectin moxidectin 1% injectable against experimental infections of *Dictyocaulus viviparous* and *Bunostomum phlebotomum* superimposed on natural gastrointestinal infections in calves, *Vet Parasitol* 43:293–299, 1992b.

Woodard GT: The treatment of organic phosphate insecticide poisoning with atropine sulfate and 2-PAM (2-pyridine aldoxime methiodide), *Vet Med* 52:571–578, 1957.

Yazwinski TA, Featherstone H, Tucker C: Effectiveness of the ivermectin sustained release bolus in the control of bovine nematodiasis, *Am J Vet Res* 56(12):1599–1602, 1995.

Yazwinski TA, Greenway TE, Tilley W, et al: Efficacy of fenbendazole against gastrointestinal nematode larvae in cattle, *Vet Med Small Anim Clin* 84:1899–1904, 1989.

Yazwinski TA, Johnson EG, Thompson DR, et al: Nematocidal efficacy of eprinomectin, delivered topically, in naturally infected cattle. *Am J Vet Res* 58(6):612–614, 1997.

Yazwinski TA, Presson BL, Featherstone HE: Comparative anthelmintic efficacies of fenbendazole, levamisole, and thiabendazole in cattle, *Agri-practice* 6(4):4–8, 1985.

Zimmer JF: Treatment of feline giardiasis with metronidazole, *Cornell Vet* 77:383–388, 1987.

Zimmer JF, Burrington DB: Comparison of four protocols for the treatment of canine giardiasis, *J Am Anim Hosp Assoc* 22:168–172, 1986.

Zimmerman GL, Hoberg EP, Pankavich JA: Efficacy of orally administered moxidectin against naturally acquired gastrointestinal nematodes in cattle, *Am J Vet Res* 53(8):1409–1410, 1992.

CHAPTER 5

DIAGNOSTIC PARASITOLOGY

As a busy veterinarian, it is necessary to achieve fairly accurate identification of parasites with a reasonable expenditure of effort. The conventional system is to take advantage of the site and host specificities of parasites and list them according to their customary locations in or on their customary hosts. With the use of this system, it is good to recognize that it must fail in abnormal cases. Whenever doubt arises or the exact identity of a parasite is essential (e.g., as for publication), recourse must be had to detailed morphological study, preferably by a recognized expert.

The diagnostic categories used in the following discussion do not adhere consistently to any particular level of taxonomic nomenclature. This is because the goals of typological taxonomy differ from those of applied parasitology. Taxonomists strive to arrange living organisms into ranks and files in a way that, to their tastes at least, best displays the phylogenetic relationships among them. However, the needs of clinicians and clinical parasitologists are best served by diagnostic categories that do not happen to coincide consistently with any particular level of the taxonomist's classification scheme. Thus we identify an egg from one of several dozens of species of canine tapeworms as a taeniid egg rather than as a *Taenia pisiformis* egg because it is practically impossible to carry the identification of such eggs below the family level. Fortunately, all members of this particular family except *Echinococcus* respond in about the same way to anthelmintic therapy, and the infective larvae of all develop in vertebrate intermediate hosts. Therefore the diagnostic category "taeniid" is adequate to the needs of effective treatment and control. In another instance, the recognition of a worm as a member of its particular phylum may suffice. For example, an acanthocephalan from a pig is almost certain to be *Macracanthorhynchus hirudinaceus*. In still other instances, however, species identification is necessary. For example, the distinction between *Toxocara canis* and *Toxascaris leonina* is important from the standpoints of both animal parasite control and public health.

Unfortunately there are many important practical distinctions that transcend even the lowest levels of conventional systematics. There exist infraspecific races of many nematodes that may differ remarkably in pathogenicity, antigenicity, and response to pharmacological agents yet, on morphological grounds, fall into the same species. Here we must make our way with whatever criterion proves helpful.

■ FECAL EXAMINATION
Qualitative Fecal Examination
Direct Smear

The direct smear made by breaking up a very small particle of feces in a drop of saline is a simple, quick method. When examining outpatients, many small animal practitioners routinely smear the feces adhering to the rectal thermometer directly on a microscope slide. Use of a coverslip improves the optics, subdues eddy currents, and helps prevent soiling of the objective lens of the microscope. The use of saline rather than water prevents the lysis of fragile trophozoites of protozoa that are subject to distortion by osmotic changes. Because the resulting suspension must be thin enough to read through, only a small particle of feces can be examined, but limited efficiency is the only shortcoming of this technique. Negative findings are inconclusive, but positive results are just as valid as those obtained with the more efficient concentration techniques. In fact, the smear presents advantages over concentration techniques in dealing with delicate forms such as nematode larvae and protozoan trophozoites, which are distorted or destroyed by concentration media, and with particularly heavy eggs that fail to float in them. Direct smears of fresh fecal material also allow us to observe motility of amebas, flagellates, nematode larvae, and the like. As a rule, the concentration techniques should supplement rather than supplant the smear, but, in practice, one or the other technique is adopted as a matter of routine.

Detecting Parasite Antigens in Feces

The detection of antigens in feces by various antigen-capture immunoassays is becoming more and more routine, although not necessarily in the field of veterinary medicine. The methods that have been developed in human medicine to detect infections with *Giardia* and *Cryptosporidium* by various enzyme-linked immunosorbent assays (ELISAs) have now been routinely used in veterinary medicine. Such assays are now regularly used in diagnostic laboratories for the examination of the feces of ruminants, dogs, and cats. Other than for these two parasites that are important in people, there are currently no other regularly available assays.

The need to be able to distinguish the eggs of taeniid tapeworms in dogs for the purpose of distinguishing the dangerous eggs of *Echinococcus granulosus* and *Echinococcus multilocularis* from the eggs of *T. pisiformis* and other *Taenia* spp. has led to the development of coproantigen detection ELISAs for these parasites. Thus it is possible to detect the antigens of this parasite in certain laboratories and to distinguish those of *E. granulosus* and *E. multilocularis*, as well as to distinguish them from those of *Taenia* spp. and other intestinal parasites and pathogens (Deplazes et al, 1999). It has also been shown that these types of antigen assays can be used to follow experimental infections with echinococcosis in dogs and to monitor the disappearance from the feces of dogs after treatment (Jenkins et al, 2000). It appears that these assays are now good enough to begin to be used routinely in surveys of canine populations for the presence of these parasites and perhaps to monitor the success of control programs.

Coproantigens are being examined as to their usefulness in the diagnosis of bovine trichostrongylids. This could prove highly useful for prescreening cattle and other ruminants for various drug-testing protocols. In cattle experimentally infected with *Ostertagia ostertagi,* a coproantigen capture ELISA gave very good results in experimentally infected cattle showing a rise over the course of the infection (Agneesens et al, 2001). ELISA values were not really well correlated with worm numbers at necropsy, but some correlation was evident. Cross-reaction with antigens in the feces of cattle with *Cooperia oncophora* did not occur. As more work is done with this system, it appears that these ELISA assays may develop into useful, albeit perhaps often esoteric, tools for the diagnosis of nematode infections in cattle.

Polymerase Chain Reaction (PCR)

The detection of various genetic markers for different parasites found in feces is now being routinely done in the case of several protozoa. The most commonly used are currently various assays for *Cryptosporidium* and *Giardia* (e.g., O'Handley et al, 2000; Xiao et al, 2001). This is being driven mainly by the desire to determine the source of parasites that may have caused zoonotic infections in different waterborne outbreaks. More recently, work has begun on the detection of different trichostrongylid species (Schnieder et al, 1999; Zarlenga et al, 2001). Once such work becomes more standardized and once it is incorporated into a quantitative assay, it may be possible to determine, with DNA extracted from feces, the relative abundance of different worms within the ruminant host. Ultimately this could mean that it might be relatively easy to use a fecal sample from a cow or sheep to identify the worms present within the host without the culture of larvae and in a much shorter period of time than is currently required.

Flotation Concentration of Eggs and Cysts

All flotation techniques take advantage of a difference in the buoyancy of parasites relative to food residues. If some feces are suspended in water, the eggs and solid fecal particles will settle out, allowing the supernatant fats and dissolved pigments to be decanted. If the sediment is then resuspended in a solution intermediate in density between the eggs and fecal debris, the former will float, whereas the latter will sink. In general, techniques based on the flotation principle work well for nematode and cestode eggs and protozoan cysts but fail to float some trematode eggs and distort protozoan trophozoites and certain nematode larvae beyond recognition. Zinc sulfate (specific gravity 1.18) is superior to sucrose of equal density for floating protozoan cysts and nematode larvae because it is slower to shrink and distort them.

Feces puddling is by no means an exact science. The actual procedure followed is less important than a show of respect for the basic principles involved. A workable procedure is outlined as follows:

1. Mix a teaspoonful or so of feces with enough water to make a semisolid suspension. Use a tongue depressor and a paper cup.
2. Place two layers of single-sheet gauze over a second paper cup and empty the fecal suspension into it. Return the gauze with the solid waste to the first cup and discard.
3. Pinch the rim of the second paper cup to form a pouring spout and transfer contents to 15 ml centrifuge tubes.
4. Centrifuge for 3 minutes and decant the supernatant containing fats and dissolved pigments.
5. Add concentrated sucrose solution (specific gravity 1.33) to 1 cm from the top of the tube and resuspend the sediment with an applicator stick.

Insert stopper and mix by four or more inversions. The viscosity of the sugar solution impedes mixing, but the solution must nevertheless be thoroughly mixed with the sediment.

6. Centrifuge for 5 minutes. Without removing the tube from the centrifuge, pick up the surface film containing eggs and cysts by touching it gently with a "glass nail" or wire loop. Transfer the surface film to a microscope slide and add a coverslip. **Variant:** Alternatively, after step 5 has been completed, the centrifuge tube may be filled to the brim with saturated sucrose solution and a coverslip applied to the top. After centrifuging, remove the coverslip by lifting it straight up and place it and its adherent film of sugar solution on a glass slide. This variant will not work with fixed angle-head centrifuges.

7. Scan the slide under ×100 magnification. To avoid omission or overlap of fields, start by scanning along one edge of the coverslip from one corner to the other. Then shift one field width and continue scanning. The shift can be executed precisely by concentrating attention on any object that happens to lie at or near the edge of the field and moving that object to the other edge with the mechanical stage adjustment. As skill in identification is acquired, the scanning may be done under ×50 magnification with considerable saving of time. Very small objects such as *Giardia* cysts and *Cryptosporidium* oocysts must, of course, be hunted with the high dry lens and perhaps studied further under oil immersion.

Gravitational force may be used in lieu of centrifugal force, but it is weaker and therefore takes longer. Several commercially available, disposable fecal analysis kits that work by gravity afford satisfactory results. If sodium nitrate solution (specific gravity 1.20) is used as flotation medium, the preparation is ready for microscopic examination in 10 minutes. Saturated sucrose solution, because of its greater viscosity, requires 15 to 20 minutes to yield equivalent results. A disadvantage of sodium nitrate is that the slide must be examined promptly. Otherwise, osmotic distortion may have rendered the parasites difficult to identify, or crystallization of the medium may have totally obscured the microscopic field.

Fecal Sedimentation Techniques

Sedimentation techniques, like direct fecal smears, demonstrate objects that are too heavy or too delicate to concentrate by the techniques just described. Sedimentation is more sensitive than the direct smear in terms of the number of organisms demonstrated, and the slide is easier to read because much of the fecal debris has been removed. Sedimentation is particularly appropriate for trematode and acanthocephalan eggs, amebas, ciliates, and formalin-fixed *Giardia* cysts. However, sedimentation is far less sensitive than flotation in concentrated sucrose or most nematode eggs and coccidian oocysts including *Cryptosporidium,* less sensitive than flotation in zinc sulfate (specific gravity 1.18) for fresh *Giardia* cysts and *Filaroides* larvae, and less sensitive than the Baermann technique described later for larvae of *Strongyloides, Aelurostrongylus, Dictyocaulus,* and other active nematode larvae. It is unfortunate that there is not one best technique that serves all purposes equally well. However, considering the extreme diversity of the organisms with which we deal, our techniques are remarkably few and simple.

The formalin-ether method should be avoided at all costs because ethyl ether has blown up enough people already. The formalin-ethyl acetate method is safer and probably just as good. Formalin preserves the feces, stops or slows development of most parasites, and reduces the odor of the sample. Ethyl acetate removes fats, pigments, and other substances that interfere with microscopic study. The following outline is freely adapted from Faler and Faler (1984):

1. Mix a teaspoonful or so of feces with 10 ml of water or 10% neutral buffered formalin.
2. Strain the mixture through a tea strainer or two layers of cheesecloth.
3. Transfer strained mixture to a 15-ml centrifuge tube.
4. Centrifuge for 1 to 2 minutes at 1500 to 2000 rpm.
5. Discard the supernatant.
6. Resuspend the sediment in 10 ml of water or formalin and repeat steps 4 and 5 until the supernatant is clear.
7. Resuspend the sediment in 10 ml of water or formalin and add 3 ml reagent grade ethyl acetate.
8. Insert stopper and shake the preparation vigorously for 30 seconds.
9. Remove stopper and centrifuge for 1 minute at 2000 rpm.
10. Decant supernatant, transfer a portion of the sediment to a microscope slide, and examine.

Note: To duplicate the sensitivity of flotation techniques in detecting most nematode eggs and coccidian oocysts, examine at least half of the sediment microscopically.

Concentration of Nematode Larvae by the Baermann Technique

In the Baermann technique, advantage is taken of the inability of most nematode larvae to swim against gravity. The vertical migrations of nematode larvae on vegetation occur in moisture films where surface tension translates their sinusoidal body movements into effective locomotion. By contrast, nematode larvae tend to sink gradually in an appreciable body of water within which there is no surface tension. A typical Baermann apparatus is illustrated in Figure 5-1. Break up a fairly large fecal specimen (5 to 15 g); place it in a tea strainer or wrap it in cheesecloth; and place it in lukewarm water in the funnel. The warmth stimulates larval motility, and many larvae will come to the surface of the fecal mass, fall off, and descend to the pinch clamp. In heavy infections, larvae can be drawn off in a drop of water after an hour or so, but when few larvae are present, it may be necessary to leave the "Baermann" set up overnight. If more than a single drop of water is drawn for examination, it will be necessary to centrifuge, decant, and pipette

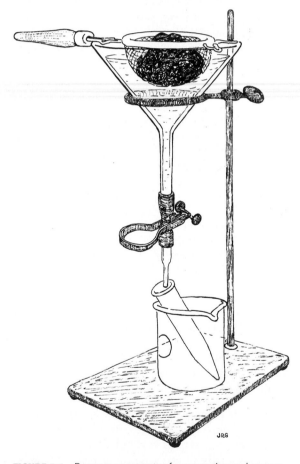

FIGURE 5-1 Baermann apparatus for separating and concentrating nematode larvae from feces, minced tissues, and soil samples. The specimen is placed in the basket of a tea strainer or wrapped in cheesecloth and immersed in lukewarm water in the funnel. Nematode larvae unable to swim against gravity descend to the pinch clamp and may then be recovered in a small volume of water. A few minutes to several hours may be required, depending on the kind of larvae and the degree of infection.

a drop of sediment. There are many refinements and modifications of this technique, but the same simple principle underlies them all.

The infective first-stage larvae of *Filaroides osleri* and *Filaroides hirthi* are lethargic and do not migrate out of the fecal mass. The Baermann technique is therefore an utter failure with respect to *Filaroides* larvae, and it is necessary to resort to the flotation concentration technique with zinc sulfate (specific gravity 1.18) as flotation medium.

Culture of Nematode Larvae

Generic identification of strongylid eggs usually requires rearing infective-stage larvae. Well-formed horse and sheep feces contain just the right amount of water and can usually be successfully cultured merely by placing a few pellets in a covered jar that has been rinsed with 0.1% sodium carbonate solution to inhibit mold growth and by storing the jar in a drawer or dark shelf at room temperature for a week to 10 days. The walls of the jar should always be covered with droplets of condensed moisture. If the culture appears to be drying out, add a few drops of water or sodium carbonate solution. When the jar is returned to the light after incubation, larvae will soon be found squirming about in the condensation droplets on the walls of the jar.

Cattle feces of similar consistency can also be cultured without further preparation, but usually cattle feces are more fluid and require the addition of vermiculite or sand to produce a damp but not wet culture.

All fecal cultural techniques are essentially qualitative because various species of nematodes have differing optimum conditions for hatching, development, and survival. As a result, the relative abundance of species of third-stage larvae harvested from cultures is not a simple function of the relative abundances of species of strongylid eggs that were present at the start. *Haemonchus contortus* or *Strongyloides papillosus* larvae tend to predominate in culture whenever eggs of either of these species are present in the feces, and the possible clinical importance of *Trichostrongylus* or *Cooperia* should not be discounted because they are represented by only a small number of larvae.

Culture of dog feces for the demonstration of *Strongyloides stercoralis* filariform larvae consists of merely storing the specimen in a jar at room temperature. Filariform larvae of the homogonic generation appear by 24 to 48 hours, but, if the isolate under study is principally or entirely heterogonic, substantial numbers of filariform larvae will not appear in less than 96 hours.

When larvae can be seen swimming in droplets of condensed moisture on the walls of the culture jar, rinse the walls of the jar with a small volume of water, collect the rinsings, and concentrate the larvae by centrifugation. Few larvae will be lost with the supernatant if the decanting is done by simply inverting the centrifuge tube in a single motion. Sediment containing the larvae can then be taken up in the small volume of water retained by cohesion and transferred with a bulb pipette to a microscope slide.

Nutrient agar plates provide excellent cultural conditions for certain nematode eggs or larvae that have been separated from feces and concentrated by the techniques already described. For example, rhabditiform larvae that have been concentrated from dog feces by the Baermann technique are deposited on the surface of the agar in a small volume of water and incubated at room temperature. If these are *Strongyloides* larvae, the culture will be found teeming with infective filariform larvae and/or rhabditiform adult worms in less than 2 days.

Identification of larvae often requires that they be killed in an extended posture. This is easily accomplished by judiciously warming the droplet of water before applying the coverslip. Hold a lighted match below the slide and view the cessation of motion and extension of larvae from above. "Relaxation" is the customary euphemism applied to the thermal death of nematodes. Because *Strongyloides* tend to revive, it may be necessary to heat them up again. Avoid overheating the larvae because this distorts them. As an alternative to heating, a drop of Lugol's solution may be added at the edge of the coverslip. This both relaxes and stains the larvae.

Whenever measurements are critical, the coverslip must be supported, or it will press on the larvae and distort them. Ring the coverslip with petroleum jelly to avoid this effect and to retard evaporation. The coverslip may be ringed quickly and conveniently as follows: Spread some petroleum jelly in a thin film on the heel of the left hand. Then, holding a coverslip edgeways between the thumb and forefinger of the right hand, draw each edge of the coverslip in turn through the film to obtain a uniform dam of petroleum jelly all around the perimeter.

Culture of Coccidian Oocysts for Sporulation

Mix a small amount of feces or concentrated suspension of oocysts with 1% potassium dichromate solution and make a shallow pool of this mixture in a Petri dish. Sporulating oocysts need a lot of air, so the pool must be shallow to favor diffusion of oxygen, but do not let the culture dry out; add more dichromate solution if necessary. Sporulation is usually complete after 2 to 4 days incubation at room temperature, but some species require weeks.

Micrometry

Measuring the lengths of parasites with a microscope equipped with a calibrated eyepiece micrometer sometimes provides the most efficient means of reaching a diagnosis. An **object micrometer** is a glass microscope slide etched with a linear scale 1 or 2 mm long and subdivided in units of 10 mm (0.01 mm). An **eyepiece micrometer** is a glass disc etched with a scale of arbitrary units. The disc is inserted into the microscope eyepiece, and the scale may be used to compare linear dimensions of objects in the microscopic field. For example, the ratio of length to width of a particular kind of egg may be determined. To measure absolute lengths, however, one must first calibrate the eyepiece micrometer for each objective magnification against the scale of the object micrometer.

1. Focus the ×10 objective on the scale of the object micrometer.
2. Rotate the eyepiece until the eyepiece scale and objective scale are parallel.
3. Align their zero marks by adjusting the mechanical stage (Figure 5-2).
4. Locate any point past the halfway mark at which the two scales are in perfect register. The ratio of the object length to the number of eyepiece scale divisions up to this point provides a factor for converting all subsequent eyepiece micrometer measurements made with the ×10 objective to absolute units. In Figure 5-2, 40 eyepiece scale divisions correspond exactly to 170 μm of the object micrometer scale, yielding a ratio of 4.25 μm per scale division.
5. Repeat the calibration procedure for all objective magnifications.

Note: Microscopes with variable tube lengths and other sources of variation in secondary magnification must be brought into the same state of adjustment each time measurements are taken or else they must be recalibrated anew. Any variation of the interpupillary distance of certain binocular microscopes alters the tube length and is easily overlooked as a source of error.

Quantitative Fecal Examination
Dilution Egg Counts

The Cornell-McMaster dilution egg counting technique as described in the following paragraphs is based on the work of Stoll (1923 and 1930), Gordon and Whitlock (1939), Whitlock (1941), and Kauzal and Gordon (1941).

Briefly, a sample of feces is weighed and vigorously mixed with water in the proportion of 1 g/15 ml. Aliquots of 0.3 ml are drawn from this suspension

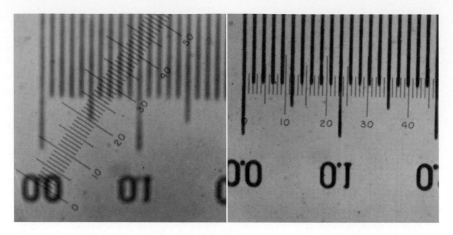

FIGURE 5-2 Eyepiece micrometer calibration. In the left picture, the object micrometer scale is out of focus, and the eyepiece micrometer scale is about one-eighth turn out of alignment. In the right picture, the scales have been made parallel by rotating the eyepiece; the object scale has been brought into focus; and the zero line (0.0) of the object scale has been aligned with the zero (0) line of the eyepiece scale by adjustment of the mechanical stage. Notice that 0.17 mm (170 μm) equals 40 eyepiece divisions (measuring consistently from the right edges of the rather thick object scale lines) so that, at this magnification, each ocular division equals 4.25 μm. An oocyst measuring 9 by 5.5 divisions would thus be 38.2 μm long by 23.4 μm wide.

and mixed with equal parts of saturated sucrose solution in a counting chamber. The parasite eggs float in this medium and come to rest at the undersurface of the chamber cover. In this way, all the eggs in a 0.02-g subsample are brought into the same focal plane of a microscopic field that is relatively free of fecal debris. The number of eggs counted in this aliquot is multiplied by 50 to yield an estimate of the number of eggs per gram of feces.

Materials required
1. Balance sensitive enough to indicate a change of as little as 0.1 g in sample weight.
2. Mixing apparatus (Figure 5-3) consisting of a 250 to 300 ml graduated cylinder with a height-to-diameter ratio of about 2 to 1 (the cylinder of Figure 5-3 was made by sawing off a 500-ml plastic cylinder at the 300-ml mark) and an electric hand drill with a special beater. The beater may be easily fabricated with a brass rod for the shank and a strip of old inner tube for the beater. The beater shank should glide freely through a hole in a rubber stopper that fits the graduated cylinder.
3. Counting chamber (Figure 5-4). Two microscope slides separated by two thicknesses of slide cut into narrow strips and cemented together with aquarium cement. The upper and lower slides should be offset slightly to facilitate filling the chamber. To clean the chamber, rinse under a stream of cold water.
4. Avian tuberculin syringe, 1 ml. The needle hub may be ground off to avoid plugging by coarse debris.

5. Saturated sucrose solution. Add granulated table sugar to boiling water, stirring continuously until no more will dissolve. Cool. Add a few phenol crystals to inhibit mold growth. The specific gravity at room temperature should be at least 1.31.
6. Paper cups, tongue depressors, and dissecting needles.

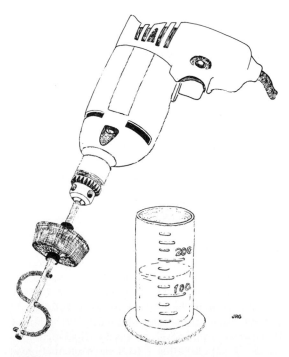

FIGURE 5-3 Mixing apparatus for preparing fecal suspensions.

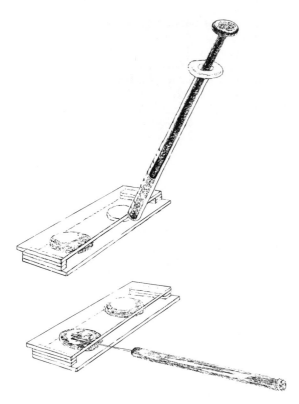

FIGURE 5-4 Loading the counting chamber. Two 0.3-ml volumes of saturated sucrose solution are placed in the counting chamber. Then a 0.3-ml aliquot of fecal suspension is added to each volume of sucrose solution and thoroughly mixed with a dissecting needle.

Procedure

1. Weigh out 10 g of feces in a paper cup (correct for tare) and add to 150 ml water in the graduated cylinder. If less than 10 g of feces is available, reduce the volume of water to preserve the 1:15 proportion.
2. Mix feces and water thoroughly. With the hand drill mixer, only a few seconds are required.
3. (Optional) The suspension may be passed through a tea strainer to remove coarse debris that might interfere with microscopic examination. This is often necessary when examining horse manure but should be avoided if possible because it may yield lower counts.
4. Place 0.3-ml saturated sucrose solution in each half of the counting chamber (Figure 5-4).
5. Stir the fecal suspension, withdraw two 0.3-ml aliquots, and add one to each pool of sucrose solution in the counting chamber.
6. Mix each aliquot-sucrose pool thoroughly with a dissecting needle and allow the preparation to stand for about 15 minutes.
7. Count all the eggs in each pool while scanning with the low power of the microscope. The focal plan containing the eggs may be quickly located

by the presence of air bubbles. Take care to include eggs lying in the optically darkened borders of the pools.

Variations of this technique with the use of calibrated chambers overcome the difficulty of counting eggs in the optically darkened borders of the pools. Unfortunately such chambers often prove difficult to obtain commercially.

An alternative method with an electric stir plate, a magnetic stir bar, a 100-ml beaker, and $MgSO_4$ (Epsom salts) of a specific gravity of 1.2 as the flotation medium is described in the following procedure with a precalibrated counting chamber (Advanced Equine Products, 5004 228th Ave. SE, Issaquah, WA 98029).

1. Place beaker on balance, tare it, and weigh out 4 g of feces into the beaker.
2. Add approximately 10 ml of the $MgSO_4$ solution and *mix well* using applicator sticks or a tongue depressor to break up the fecal matter as much as possible.
3. Bring the volume to 60 ml with additional flotation medium and add a stir bar. Stir for 5 minutes at moderate speed.
4. Using a glass slide to make a score mark, score a pasture pipette halfway between the tip and the barrel and break off the tip to produce a wider bore. (Caution: Pasteur pipettes have caused numerous laboratory accidents; use with care).
5. Load the pipette with the fecal material from the stirring beaker and fill both chambers on the precalibrated counting chamber.
6. Let the preparation stand 5 minutes to allow the eggs to float to the surface and then count all eggs within the grids of both chambers using the ×10 objective.
7. Calculate eggs per gram of feces by multiplying the total number of eggs counted in the two chambers by 50.

Concentration Egg Counts

Dilution egg count procedures are less reliable for quantifying low levels of parasitic infection than are concentration egg counts (see Statistical Considerations, later). Of course, there is a limit to the number of eggs that can be counted conveniently, so one must choose the procedure best suited to the level of infection. A practical solution is proposed as follows:

1. Weigh out 10 g of feces in a paper cup (correct for tare) and add to 150 ml water in the graduated cylinder. If less than 10 g of feces is available, reduce the volume of water to preserve the 1:15 proportion.

2. Mix feces and water thoroughly. With the hand drill mixer, only a few seconds are required.

3. (Optional) The suspension may be passed through a tea strainer to remove coarse debris that might interfere with microscopic examination. This step is often necessary when examining horse manure but should be avoided if possible because it may yield lower counts. *Note:* So far, the procedure is identical to the dilution egg count procedure described before.

4. Draw a 15-ml (1-g) aliquot of well-mixed fecal suspension and transfer it to a 15-ml centrifuge tube.

5. Centrifuge for 3 minutes and decant the supernatant containing fats and dissolved pigments.

6. Add concentrated sucrose solution (specific gravity 1.33) to 1 cm from the top of the tube and resuspend the sediment with an applicator stick. Insert stopper and mix by four or more inversions.

7. Add concentrated sucrose solution to the brim and place a coverslip on top.

8. Centrifuge for 10 minutes. Do not use a fixed-angle centrifuge. The cups must be horizontal during centrifugation.

9. After centrifuging, remove the coverslip by lifting it straight up and place it and its adherent film of sugar solution on a glass slide.

10. Scan the slide under ×50 to ×100 magnification, counting eggs as you go. To avoid omission or overlap of fields, start by scanning along one edge of the coverslip from one corner to the other. Then shift one field width and continue scanning. The shift can be executed precisely by concentrating attention on any object that happens to lie at or near the edge of the field and moving that object to the other edge with the mechanical stage adjustment.

The number of eggs counted by this procedure provides a minimum estimate of the number of eggs per gram of feces. The estimate can be improved by adding another drop of concentrated sucrose solution to the centrifuge tube, placing a second coverslip on top, and repeating steps 7 through 10. If there are too many eggs on the first coverslip to count conveniently, either repeat the procedure with a smaller aliquot or resort to dilution egg counting. Perhaps because the sucrose solution used is twice as concentrated, the concentration procedure is more efficient in detecting *Eimeria* oocysts than is the dilution procedure.

Interpretation of Egg Count Data

Statistical considerations

If it were possible to obtain a **uniform distribution** of parasite eggs in the fecal suspension, we could expect to find the same number of eggs in all aliquots. However, as we mix the suspension, the distribution of eggs does not become uniform but instead becomes a **random distribution** and stays random as long as we continue mixing. Aliquots from a thoroughly mixed suspension thus represent fair samples drawn from a random distribution, and the numbers of eggs counted in replicate aliquots vary in a predictable fashion.

When relatively rare objects are distributed at random in space (or relatively infrequent events are distributed at random in time), the number of objects to be found in each sample volume (or the number of occurrences in each sample time interval) follows a **Poisson distribution.** In a 150-ml fecal suspension there is room for well over a billion eggs, yet even in acute haemonchosis, there rarely will be more than a half million present. This means that for every 2000 volumes the size of one *Haemonchus* egg, no more than one volume will actually contain an egg. Therefore eggs counted in aliquots drawn from a well-mixed fecal suspension meet the specifications for "relatively rare objects distributed at random in space," and we can expect the number counted in each sample volume to follow a Poisson distribution.

The mean and variance of a Poisson distribution are equal. This fact can be turned to practical advantage because it provides a criterion by which we can assess the adequacy of our technique. If the variance of a series of aliquot counts turns out to be much greater than the mean, we may conclude that the mixing, sampling, or counting has been carelessly done. If, on the other hand, the sample variance turns out to be much smaller than the mean, we may conclude that someone has "fudged" the data. Chi-square analysis provides an objective numerical method for testing how well replicate egg counts fit the Poisson distribution (Hunter and Quenouille, 1952), but few practitioners would be tempted to bother with the necessary calculations. A simple alternative is provided by the graph of Figure 5-5. The diagonal lines drawn on this graph enclose a zone within which 95% of all points representing duplicate egg counts should fall, on the average, provided the sampling and counting are adequate. The tolerance bounds on the graph are nearly parallel instead of divergent, as might be expected considering the equality of means and variances inherent in the Poisson distribution, because the axes have square root scales. Square root transformation of a Poisson variate converts the variance to a constant for all but very small values of the variate. In Figure 5-5, of 151 pairs of egg counts, 19 (13%) lie on or outside the boundaries of the 95% zone. This is almost three times too many, and we may conclude that technical performance could be improved.

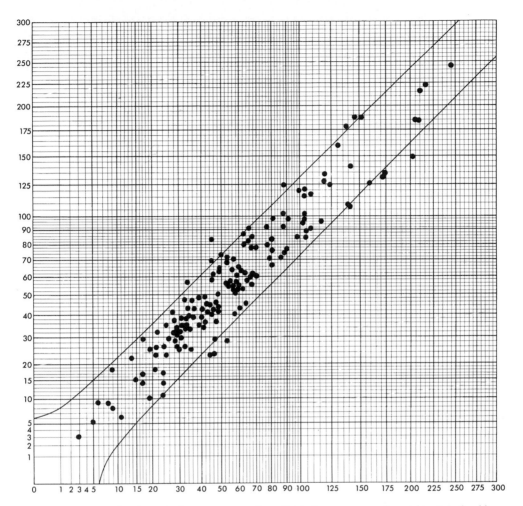

FIGURE 5-5 Plot of 151 duplicate egg counts. According to theory, no more than eight points should have fallen outside the diagonal boundary lines. More careful mixing, sampling, and counting could improve the picture.

Applications

Egg-counting techniques may be applied, in principle, to any patent parasitic infection of any host. For practical purposes, however, they find their greatest utility in estimating levels of strongyle infections in ruminants and horses. Under conditions of ordinary husbandry, these species of domestic animals always shed strongyle eggs in their feces except when they have recently been treated with an effective anthelmintic drug. Therefore the question is not whether these animals are infected with strongyles but, instead, what level of infection is present.

Determining Rates of Environmental contamination

Most contemporary methods for controlling strongyles in grazing livestock depend heavily on periodic medication with anthelmintic drugs to suppress the production of eggs and thereby curtail contamination of the pastures. Unfortunately, when populations of parasites are repeatedly exposed to anthelmintics for several years, they develop resistance to these anthelmintics and their chemical congeners. The more frequently anthelmintic medication is applied, the more rapidly does resistance to them develop. To slow or stop the development of resistance, one should administer anthelmintics only when they are actually needed to reduce a significant rate of pasture contamination. This can be accomplished by performing periodic fecal egg counts on a representative sample of the herd. When egg output is low, treatment may be delayed until it has reached a point deemed significant in relationship to the extent and productivity of pasture, the stocking rate, the species and susceptibility of hosts, and the objectives of the husbandry operation. The **critical number** of eggs per gram at which the herd ought to be treated cannot be specified without taking all of these factors into consideration. For example, 1000 eggs per gram might supposedly be an appropriate **critical number** for clinically normal sheep grazing at low stocking rate under weather conditions favorable to *H. contortus*. However, it would be best not to exceed 100 eggs per gram for brood mares with foals at their sides grazing a small paddock. In both of these cases, the **critical number** would be subject to revision according to the results achieved and any significant modifications of management practices.

Diagnosing Clinical Illness

High egg counts (e.g., more than 5000 eggs per gram for sheep and goats or more than 500 eggs per gram for cattle) are easy to interpret. They indicate that these animals are infected with many reproductively active parasites. However, high counts do not necessarily indicate that the host is suffering from clinical parasitic disease because healthy, well-nourished hosts can often support and compensate for very impressive populations of parasites. Negative egg counts indicate that the host either is uninfected or is infected with nonreproductive worms (e.g., developing or arrested larvae, infertile adults). Negative egg counts are typical of the early stages of winter ostertagiosis in cattle and peracute hookworm disease in newborn pups. Such facts tend to discredit quantitative fecal analysis in the minds of those who require short lists of simple, plausible rules. However, when interpreted by minds familiar with the biology of both host and parasite, egg counts provide one valuable insight into the interaction taking place between them.

■ IDENTIFICATION OF EGGS, CYSTS, AND LARVAE
Parasite vs. Pseudoparasite

One must first learn to distinguish between parasites and superficially similar but unrelated objects such as air bubbles, pollen grains, hair, plant fibers, fat droplets, and corn smut spores. Identification of **pseudoparasites** may occasionally shed light on the host's recent dietary adventures. Suppose, for example, that we find *Moniezia expansa* eggs in a specimen of dog feces. We know then that the dog has recently eaten sheep feces because *M. expansa* is a parasite of sheep and never of dogs. Actually, because *M. expansa* is a true parasite when it is in a sheep, its egg should be called a **spurious parasite** rather than a pseudoparasite when it is found in dog feces, but perhaps that distinction is a bit too pedantic. For practical purposes, if a dog or cat is passing an unidentifiable object in its feces, give the animal an enema, confine it for 24 to 36 hours, and do another fecal examination. If the unidentifiable object is still there, chances are it is a parasite, whereas if it is gone, it was probably a pseudoparasite. It is probably

more efficient to learn to identify the bona fide parasites and to ignore the irrelevant rubbish scattered about them rather than trying to identify all objects in the microscopic field. However, some objects are commonly observed that have regular shapes. Examples of these more common pseudoparasites are shown in Figure 5-6.

In acquiring diagnostic skill, one must not be content with merely comparing general impressions of the microscopic image with a set of pictures in a book. Persons basing their diagnoses on superficial appearances often confuse *Toxascaris* eggs with *Isospora canis* cysts less than half as large. In Figure 5-9, a *T. leonina* egg ×425 and an *I. canis* oocyst ×1000 have been placed side by side to show how easily this mistake could be made. The matter may be resolved with an ocular micrometer or, more simply, through observation of whether a distinct lipid layer (Figure 5-7, *A*) is present *(Toxascaris)* or absent *(Isospora)*.

Fecal specimens for parasitological examination should be fresh and not contaminated with soil or bedding. If feces are allowed to stand, single cells develop into morulae, larvae hatch, and oocysts begin to sporulate. Identification of developmental stages other than those usually encountered is possible but requires greater skill. Contamination with soil or bedding will likely lead to confusion because the specimen may be invaded by free-living nematodes and arthropods. Starting, however, with a fresh, uncontaminated specimen may frequently allow a more specific identification by observation of the subsequent development in fecal culture.

Nematode Eggs

The shell proper of the nematode egg is a smooth, homogeneous, transparent capsule of chitin (Figure 5-7, *A*). Its external surface is covered with a layer of protein that may be smooth (Figure 5-7), rough (*Parascaris;* see Figure 5-41), or uniformly and distinctively patterned (Figure 5-8). An internal lipid layer (vitelline membrane) and a narrow fluid-filled space separate the capsule from its contained embryo.

Nematode eggs representative of the different orders and superfamilies of these parasites have characteristics that typify the group. Thus an egg can usually be identified as that of an oxyurid, ascaridoid, spirurid, rhabditoid, strongylid, or trichinelloid. In general, nematode eggs vary in size from 30 μm to 100 μm in greatest diameter, although a few examples such as *Nematodirus* may be up to 200 μm in length.

The Oxyurid Egg

The eggs of the oxyurid parasites of ruminants, horses, and primates tend to have a rather thick, colorless

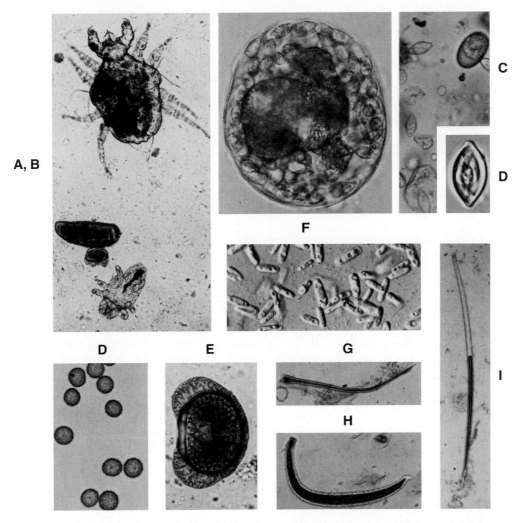

FIGURE 5-6 Pseudoparasites. **A,** *Cheyletiella blakei,* an arachnid parasite of the cat (×108). **B,** *Monocystis,* a protozoan parasite of the earthworm. **C,** *Monocystis* and ruminant *Eimeria* cysts in dog feces (×425). *Inset:* Sporulated *Monocystis* (×1000). **D,** Corn smut spores (×630). **E,** Pine pollen (×425). **F,** *Saccharomycopsis gutulatus,* normal alimentary yeast of rabbits (×425). **G,** Plant hair (×168), **H,** Plant hair (×63), **I,** Plant hair (×63).

shell and to contain a larva when observed. Most of the eggs also appear flattened on one side. The large pinworm of the horse, *Oxyuris equi,* has an egg that appears to have an operculum on one end. Dogs and cats are not hosts to pinworms, so the presence of these eggs in their feces should be considered a spurious finding unless proven otherwise.

The Ascaridoid Egg

The eggs of the ascaridoid parasites of domestic animals are typically thick shelled and oblong to spherical in appearance. When passed in the feces, these eggs tend to contain a single cell. Some eggs, such as those of *Toxocara, Parascaris,* and *Ascaris* are covered with an albuminous coat applied by the

female over the chitinous eggshell. The material may be tanned in the fecal stream giving it a dark-brown color as in *Ascaris* and *Parascaris.* This material may sometimes break off from the eggshell, and the egg will then appear with a clear smooth shell. The eggs of infertile ascaridoids are sometimes found in the feces, and their shape is often less regular than that of the fertilized egg. The eggs of ascaridoids tend to be large overall, around 80 μm to 100 μm in diameter.

The Spirurid Egg

The eggs of the spirurid nematodes found in feces are of at least two basic types. One type of egg, represented by those of *Physaloptera* and *Spirocerca,* is about 30 μm long, covered by a thick colorless shell,

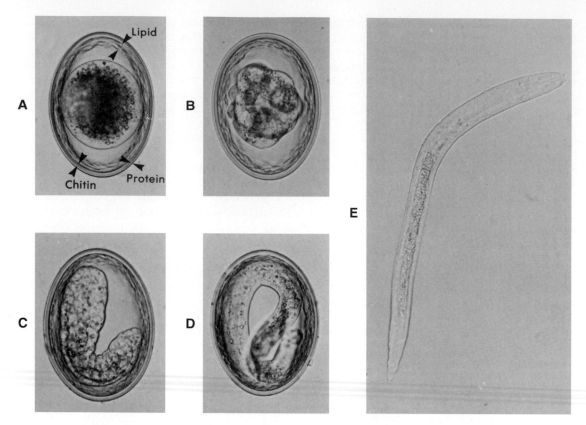

FIGURE 5-7 Development of a *Toxascaris leonina* egg from a tiger. **A,** One-cell stage typically found in fresh fecal specimens with shell layers indicated by opposed arrow heads, **B,** Morula stage. **C,** Early vermiform embryo. **D,** Infective larva in egg shell. **E,** Infective larva artificially hatched in vitro. Hatching of ascarid eggs does not normally occur until they have been ingested by a host (×425).

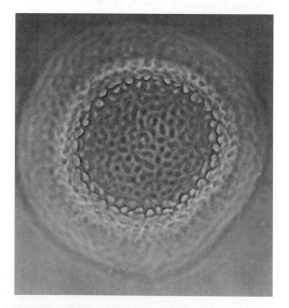

FIGURE 5-8 Surface of a *Toxocara canis* egg cleared in Berlese solution to show the distinctive dimpled pattern of the protein layer (phase contrast ×660).

and contains an embryo. These eggs are typical of those spirurids transmitted by terrestrial coprophagous insects. The other spirurids, such as *Habronema* and *Draschia,* have very thin eggshells that may be distorted by the contained larva. These eggs and the contained larva are typical of those spirurids transmitted by flying insects that obtain their infection through the feeding of maggots on fecal material. Filariids are an ovoviviparous form of spirurid that produce microfilariae rather than eggs.

The Rhabditoid Egg

The rhabditoid eggs found in the feces of domestic animals are of two types. One type represents the spurious eggs of soil nematodes that have been ingested by a host or even laid by free-living coprophagous nematodes that have invaded a fecal pat. The second type of rhabditoid egg represents the eggs of those parthenogenetic females of the *Strongyloides* spp. that produce eggs. In domestic animals in North America, only *S. stercoralis* of the dog and human typically produces larvae. Other *Strongyloides* spp., such as *Strongyloides felis* of cats in Australia and

Southeast Asia and various species in wildlife hosts, also shed larval stages in the feces. The eggs of the *Strongyloides* spp. shed by horses, swine, and ruminants are typically small, with a thin colorless shell, and contain a larva. In feces that are not fresh, size will be one of the best criteria for separating these eggs from those of developed strongylid eggs.

The Strongyle Egg

Females of the superfamilies Strongyloidea, Trichostrongyloidea, and Ancylostomatoidea lay rather thin-walled ellipsoidal eggs containing an embryo in the morula stage of development, and this same stage is found in the host's feces. In this text, such eggs are collectively referred to as "strongyle" eggs because that is what most clinicians and diagnostic parasitologists call them. The eggs of Metastrongyloidea are also thin walled and ellipsoidal, but the developmental stage deposited in the host's tissues by different species of female metastrongyloids varies from a single cell (e.g., *Muellerius*) to a first-stage larva that is ready to hatch (e.g., *Filaroides*). Even those laid in the single-cell stage develop to the first stage and may have hatched by the time they appear in the feces. Therefore either larvated eggs (e.g., *Metastrongylus*) or first-stage larvae are found in the feces of hosts with patent metastrongyloid infections.

A diagnostic dilemma

With few exceptions, the generic identity of individual strongyle eggs cannot be established reliably by microscopic inspection or micrometry (see Figure 5-32). *Nematodirus* eggs stand out because of their large size, and *Bunostomum phlebotomum* eggs have sticky surfaces that accumulate debris, but the rest look very much alike. An ingenious stochastic technique involving the measurement of at least 100 eggs permitted species identification of egg populations or, expressed another way, permitted estimation of the relative abundances of species in mixed infections (Cunliffe and Crofton, 1953). This technique was laborious, limited in application to the eight species of sheep nematodes studied, and strictly valid only on a geographical basis. More recently, Christie and Jackson (1982) combined egg dimensions and information regarding their state of embryonic development after specified times and conditions of incubation. These authors were able to identify more than 90% of *Ostertagia* spp. and *Trichostrongylus vitrinus* eggs but admitted that "for other species supporting information from larval cultures may be needed but this need will vary according to the composition of the sample."

Necropsy of a few animals to establish an accurate diagnosis is justifiable if the unit value of the animal is sufficiently low or the herd sufficiently large.

Owners of valuable animals are understandably reluctant to sacrifice them, however, and recourse must be had to larval identification (see Identification of Strongyle Infective Larvae). Whenever the situation is too urgent to afford the necessary delay of culturing, the clinical signs should be clear enough to suggest a reasonably accurate diagnosis.

Diagnostic morphometry

Electronic image digitizing and analysis systems greatly increase the precision and decrease the labor of identifying objects that cannot be distinguished by qualitative or simple quantitative means. Georgi and McCulloch (1989) used stepwise discriminant analysis of the geometric parameters (length, width, area, perimeter, and areas and arc lengths of both poles) to classify and identify strongylid eggs of sheep and horses. Data were obtained by tracing egg contours on the surface of a digitizing tablet viewed through a drawing tube mounted on a compound microscope. By this means, the image of an egg under the objective lens of the microscope was made to appear to lie at the surface of the digitizing tablet so its perimeter could be conveniently traced by a cursor connected to the digitizing tablet. All coordinates traced by the cursor were automatically fed into a microcomputer and converted by a special program into the 10 geometric parameters. When data representing 12 species of strongylids infecting sheep were analyzed simultaneously, accuracy of classification and identification of individual species ranged from 50% to 100%. "Comparable accuracy of classification was achieved for equine parasites only after pairs of species having morphometrically identical eggs were pooled before analysis and all of the cyathostomin categories except *Gyalocephalus* further pooled after analysis. The final diagnostic categories, 'large strongyle,' *Triodontophorus serratus, T. tenuicollis,* 'small strongyle,' *Gyalocephalus capitatus,* and *Trichostrongylus axei* were correctly classified in 76.6, 74.3, 83.0, 79.1, 100, and 80 per cent of the cases respectively" (Georgi and McCulloch, 1989).

Work continues along the lines of finding easier ways to identify the eggs of cattle and horse by microscopy. This is important not only for the diagnosis of infections but for having better ways to assess infections to verify the efficacy of existing, new, and experimental anthelminthics. Thus this line of inquiry continues. Sommer (1996) produced methods for the morphometric separation of the eggs of different nematodes parasitic in cattle. More recently (Sommer, 1998), work was presented on the ability to separate eggs on the basis of "textures" (i.e., the different shades of gray associated with the egg and its various edges and gray level extremes). With the use of both of these methods, eggs were very consistently identified as to the correct species. As with the work by Georgi and McCulloch, the continued problem is the requirement of time and highly specialized equipment and operators.

The Trichinelloid Egg

The eggs of *Trichuris* and capillarids are typically brown shelled with polar plugs and tend to be elongate or barrel shaped. *Trichuris* is confined to mammalian hosts. Thus when these eggs are found in other vertebrates, the first thought should be that they are capillarid eggs. The eggs of the *Trichuris* spp. tend to have smooth shells, whereas those of capillarids tend to have various forms of delicate surface ornamentation (e.g., pits, roughened areas, small wavy lines). Capillarid eggs, unlike those of *Trichuris* spp., may have polar plugs that are not on the same straight-line axis. However, the eggs of *Trichuris* may become highly distorted after drug therapy that has not removed all female worms. Both *Trichuris* and capillarids tend to have eggs that are single celled or in the early stages of division when passed in the feces. The eggs of *Anatrichosoma* and *Trichosomoides* are different in that they contain a fully formed larva. In the dog, the eggs of the capillarids are smaller than the egg of *Trichuris vulpis,* which is about 80 μm long. Unfortunately, this is not necessarily true for other hosts.

Nematode Larvae

The larvae of nematodes shed in the feces are most readily identified with reference to the host parasitized and are discussed as such for each host as appropriate. The initial goal must be to identify them for what they are and not to confuse them with hairs, threads, or plant fibers. The more common problem is finding an artifact and thinking it a nematode larva. Most individuals will recognize a larva when they see one. The important thing is not to forget to look for them. The nematode larvae found in the feces of domestic animals all tend to be around 300 μm in length. Special attention must be paid to the relative lengths of the buccal capsule and esophagus, the structure of the tail, and the size and position of the genital primordium. If feces are old or collected from the soil, there may be many nematode larvae present that have hatched from eggs of developed parasitic forms or from soil or coprophagous nematodes that have invaded the fecal matter. The process of identification is much more difficult in these situations.

Trematode Eggs

The eggs of trematode parasites of vertebrates tend to have a golden- to dark-brown color and to have an operculum on one end. The eggs can vary in size from 20 μm to 200 μm in maximum length. Some of these eggs contain a fully formed miracidium when passed in the feces, whereas others contain a number of developing cells. In the identification of trematode eggs, attention must be given to the size and shape of the eggs, as well as to whether they contain an embryo, whether the operculum appears as a simple cap or a cap in an indented seat or rim on the eggshell, and whether there are any structures on the shell such as bumps or spines opposite the operculum. The eggs of the schistosomes are not operculate, contain fully developed miracidia when passed with the feces, and often have different types of spines on one end of the eggshell depending on the species involved. Trematode eggs tend to be denser and not to float as well as those of nematodes in many of the lighter flotation media, and in sugar, the eggs often rupture and appear as empty brown shells that may be collapsed on one side. When dealing with the schistosomes, one must take care to wash the feces with saline rather than water because the water induces the miracidium to hatch, making the eggs harder to find and identify.

Cestode Eggs

Some tapeworms commonly shed eggs into the fecal stream (e.g., *Diphyllobothrium*), whereas others more typically shed segments, (e.g., *Taenia*). However, it is not uncommon to find eggs or egg capsules of the latter type in fecal matter from which the segments may have crawled away before collection. The larva that develops in these eggs will have six hooklets (three pairs), but those in the eggs of the Pseudophyllidean tapeworms *Diphyllobothrium* and *Spirometra* will not have developed by the time the eggs are passed in the feces. The eggs of these two species are also operculate and may initially be confused with the egg of a trematode. The confusion may persist even after a good deal of study of the actual eggs and pictures of them. The eggs of the Cyclophyllidean tapeworms will contain six hooklets when passed, which will help to identify the eggs as tapeworm eggs. The "shells" of Cyclophyllidean tapeworms can vary markedly (e.g., the thick, brown surface of a taeniid egg, the thin shells on the individual eggs of *Dipylidium,* and the odd-shaped square to round shells on the various anoplocephalid general). Tapeworm eggs appear to behave erratically in different flotation media and can be hard to demonstrate even when present. Sugar solution works well for taeniid eggs, but not for many of the other egg types that may be encountered.

Acanthocephala Eggs

The eggs of acanthocephala tend to be elongated and have shells composed of three layers. If the larva inside can be seen, the spines present on one end of the larva can often be identified, which clinches the diagnosis. The eggs of some acanthocephala often appear dark brown in the feces (e.g., *Macracanthorhynchus* spp.) and are probably tanned in a manner similar to that of ascaridoid eggs because the eggshells are clear when the eggs leave the female worm. Not all acanthocephalan eggs are brown, and the very clear ones may be difficult to observe, particularly if one is not expecting to find them. There are numerous acanthocephala present in wildlife hosts, and it is there that skill has to be developed in diagnosing infections with different species.

Pentastomid Eggs

In the United States, the eggs of pentastomids will most typically be observed in the feces of snakes or gulls. Elsewhere in the world, they can be observed in the feces of dogs and other hosts. Pentastomid eggs are typically quite large, 100 µm to 200 µm in diameter, with a thin external shell that surrounds what looks like a developing mite. The developing larva is often separated from the eggshell by a rather large area of empty space. The difficulty is in determining whether what is observed is the egg of a pentastomid or the egg of a mite that has been ingested. It is not uncommon to find in feces the eggs of free-living mites and parasitic mites ingested while an animal is grooming. The pentastomid developing within the egg will typically have four or six small claws, which might help distinguish the mite from the pentastomid (see Figure 6-16).

Protozoan Cysts and Oocysts

The cysts and oocysts of protozoa will range from 4 to 30 µm in greatest diameter, with the odd large cysts of *Balantidium* and *Buxtonella* reaching sizes of 40 to 60 µm. The cysts of *Giardia* appear rather clear in both zinc-sulfate and sugar preparations, and their overall appearance is similar to that of amebae that are more round in outline. In many flotation media, cysts of *Giardia* will appear collapsed internally with the ovoid cyst wall remaining intact, whereas collapsed cysts of amebae may appear much like Ping-Pong balls that have been indented various amounts on one side. The oocysts of *Cryptosporidium* are very small and can be found near the surface of the coverslip. They are much easier to see in a sugar flotation where they will appear as a hyaline pink body than in zinc-sulfate where they appear to be clearer. The oocysts of *Isospora* and *Eimeria* do very well in sugar flotation media and present a crisp, clear image of a shell and a central sporoblast. On many species of *Eimeria,* the micropyle and micropylar cap, when present, can be easily discerned. On some *Eimeria* species, it may be difficult to make out the micropyle on all specimens. The oocysts of *Toxoplasma* are similar in size to the cysts of *Giardia*. If the aperture on the condenser diaphragm is not closed and the light coming through the scope is too bright, many of the smaller protozoa will disappear into the background.

■ SKIN SCRAPINGS FOR MANGE DIAGNOSIS

Skin scrapings for mange diagnosis must be obtained in a manner that takes into account both the nature of the lesion and the location of the mite in question.

For lesions with minimal epidermal hyperplasia and lesions caused by deeply burrowing mites (e.g., *Sarcoptes, Demodex*), dip a scalpel blade in mineral oil, pinch a fold of skin firmly between the thumb and forefinger and, holding the blade at right angles to the skin, scrape until blood begins to seep from the abrasion. Most animals do not object to deep scraping, although local anesthesia may occasionally be required. Much of the detritus will adhere to the layer of mineral oil on the scalpel blade and may be transferred to a microscope slide and searched for mites.

For lesions with marked epidermal hyperplasia and exfoliation and lesions caused by lice and superficially dwelling mites (e.g., *Chorioptes*), scrape the detritus into an ointment tin using the cover as a scraper. Examine scrapings under a stereoscopic microscope or with a hand lens to find the lice and mites crawling about. Dip fine-tipped thumb forceps or a dissecting needle into Berlese solution and use this sticky mounting medium to pick up mites and transfer them to a slide for closer study under the compound microscope. Berlese solution is made by mixing 200 g chloral hydrate, 30 g gum arabic, 20 g glycerine, and 50 ml distilled water, by boiling this mixture for 5 to 15 minutes, and by filtering it through cheesecloth. Berlese solution clears the specimen and hardens to produce a permanent preparation. Unfortunately, chloral hydrate is now regulated as a narcotic, and different lots of gum arabic vary considerably in quality so that good Berlese solution is getting hard to come by. Glycerine is a reasonably satisfactory temporary mounting medium. Five percent sodium or potassium hydroxide solution also may be used as a temporary mounting medium that digests epidermis and hair, thus helping to clear the microscopic field of debris.

If the scraping contains much debris and no lice or mites have been found by inspection with the stereoscopic microscope or hand lens, proceed as follows:

1. Add 10 volumes of 5% KOH to 1 volume of skin scrapings in a large (500 to 1000 volumes capac-

ity) beaker, cover with a watch glass or funnel to return condensate, and heat until hair and epidermal scales dissolve. It may be necessary to boil the mixture, but do not allow it to boil dry. **Beware of spattering lye!**

2. Allow to cool.
3. Transfer to a centrifuge tube, centrifuge, decant supernatant, resuspend sediment in water, and centrifuge again. These steps dispose of interfering soaps. Decant the supernatant.
4. Transfer sediment to a Petri dish and search for mites and eggs with a stereomicroscope or ×10 pocket lens, or proceed with step 5.
5. Add saturated sucrose solution to the centrifuge again. Pick mites off the top of the sucrose solution with a wire loop or glass nail and transfer them to a microscope slide for study under the compound microscope.

Ear mites may be removed from the external ear canal with a cotton swab. If the swab is placed on a dark background in sunlight or near an incandescent lamp, white *Otodectes* mites may be seen crawling about within a few minutes.

■ NECROPSY PROCEDURES

Occasionally, severe or fatal parasitosis may escape antemortem diagnosis. For example, pups with peracute hookworm disease may bleed to death before shedding an egg. When disease breaks out in a flock of sheep, postmortem examination of a few sick animals often provides the most efficient and economical means of arriving at a diagnosis. In strongylid infections of sheep, various combinations of primary and secondary pathogens often yield a confusing array of clinical signs that may be resolved by identification and enumeration of the worms.

Necropsy findings must be correlated with the case history and clinical signs to arrive at a definitive diagnosis. This is especially true of parasitic diseases. For example, a diagnosis of acute haemonchosis must rest not only on the demonstration of a sufficient number of *H. contortus* worms in the abomasum, but also on the existence of clinical anemia. If there is no anemia, then there is no haemonchosis. In fact, *H. contortus* worms sometimes desert a moribund host so that, on necropsy examination, pallor and edema of the tissues is found, but no worms. The correct diagnosis is still haemonchosis.

Opening the Cadaver

Arrange a ruminant cadaver on its left side to get the rumen out of the way. Cadavers of other species are about equally accessible from either side, but you should adopt a consistent approach to develop a mental image of the normal appearance and location of the various organs so that any abnormal relationship will be quickly noticed. Incise the skin along the midline from the submaxillary space to the perineum. Reflect the skin from one side, including the superficial thoracic muscles and the pectoral limb with it so as to lay bare the rib cage. Cut the ribs close to the axial muscles and the costal cartilages close to the sternum. Lift away the rib cage, severing attachments to the diaphragm in the process. Incise the abdominal wall along the midline, taking pains to avoid puncturing the viscera. Carry the incision across the brim of the pubis and reflect the abdominal wall. Split the pubic symphysis or incise the ligaments of the hip joint and reflect the pelvic limb.

Thoracic Viscera

Incise the intermandibular muscles, hyoid apparatus, and other attachments and dissect the tongue, larynx, trachea, and esophagus. Removal of the heart and lungs is facilitated by traction on the trachea and esophagus. The points of attachment (aorta, cavae, azygous vein, various ligaments) are easily found and severed. Remove the thoracic viscera from the carcass. Lay open the tracheobronchial tree, heart chambers, cavae, aortic trunk, and ramifications of the pulmonary arteries, and inspect the contents and linings for macroscopic parasites. Very small metastrongylid nematodes (e.g., *Muellerius capillaris, Aelurostrongylus abstrusus, F. hirthi*) are practically invisible grossly. These may be demonstrated in squash preparations of their grayish subpleural nodules. The Baermann technique is useful for demonstrating larvae of lung nematodes (e.g., *Muellerius, Aelurostrongylus*), but usually fails in the case of *F. hirthi* because the larvae of this parasite are too lethargic to migrate out of the lung tissues.

Abdominal Viscera

Examine the peritoneum for cysticerci, tetrathyridia, encysted pentastomid, and acanthocephalan nymphs. *Strongylus edentatus* larvae may often be observed immediately beneath the parietal peritoneum of horses. Examine the surface of the liver for migration racks of ascarid, taeniid, and *Fasciola* larvae, and the kidneys for encysted *Toxocara* larvae. The equine pancreas is a favorite location for *Strongylus equinus* larvae. Place double ligatures around the cardia (or omasoabomasal junction), pylorus, and ileocecal junction, thus isolating the stomach, small intestine, and large intestine. These regions provide differing environments for distinct sets of parasites, and valuable diagnostic information is lost by pooling the collection from the entire gut. Open one region at a time, carefully poking through the ingesta and scanning the mucosa for the smaller forms. Many parasites of dogs, cats, horses, and pigs are large enough to see with the unaided eye, but there are a few very small ones that are important (e.g., *Strongyloides, Trichinella*). Scrape the mucosa of the small intestine and examine the scrapings for small nematodes, coccidia, and the like.

Most of the important nematode parasites of ruminants are very small, and great care must be taken not to overlook them. The population of nematodes sufficient to kill a heifer may pass the notice of a careless prosector completely. The following technique accomplishes the concentration and separation of these worms from much of the ingesta and mucosal debris and, with a bit of extra effort, provides an estimate of the number of worms present.

1. Transfer all ingesta from a particular organ (the abomasum is an easy one with which to begin) to a bucket; scrub or lightly scrape the mucosal surface to ensure complete transfer of worms.
2. Add several quarts of tepid water, mix, and allow to stand for about 5 minutes so that the worms and heavy debris can settle to the bottom; then decant the supernatant. Repeat this process until the sediment consists principally of worms and coarse ingestation.
3. Transfer a *small* amount of sediment to a Petri dish and examine with transillumination, preferably under a magnifying glass or stereoscopic microscope. If the worms have been taken from the cadaver of a recently dead animal, they will become very active in the tepid water and can be easily detected and fished out with a forceps for closer examination.

The small intestine is long, and life is short. Most of the important nematode parasites of the ruminant small intestine can be collected by flushing a liter of water through its first 6 meters. Insert a funnel into the pyloric end of 6 meters of unopened small intestine and pour a beaker of water into it. Massage the water along the length of gut and collect it at the other end; then proceed with steps 2 and 3 above.

A popular alternative to step 2 is to rinse sediment vigorously over a sieve with openings small enough to retain the parasites but large enough to pass water and fine debris. The sieve may then be inverted and back-rinsed to transfer the parasites and coarse debris to a collecting vessel. If time or facilities to examine sediment for parasites is lacking, the sediment can be preserved in 10% formalin and attended to later. Be sure to sieve preserved sediments once again to remove the formalin before attempting to isolate and study the parasites; this may save you a big headache.

Because we are almost certain to find parasites in sheep, young cattle, and horses, it follows that the evaluation of the necropsy findings must rest on the abundance of the parasites as well as on their identity. To obtain an estimate of worm numbers, substitute step 3a for step 3 and proceed as follows:

3a. Transfer the washed sediment to a graduated cylinder and fill with water to 1 liter. We now have all the worms from some particular organ suspended in 1 liter.
4. Stir the suspension thoroughly and withdraw a 50-ml aliquot.
5. Pour a small portion of the 50-ml aliquot into a Petri dish and count all of the worms. Continue until the 50 ml is used up. The number of worms counted times 20 provides an estimate of the total number of worms in the particular organ.

The worm count must be interpreted in the light of other necropsy findings, especially the nutritional status of the cadaver and lesions specifically related to the parasites found. Etiological significance should be attached to *Trichostrongylus* or *Cooperia* only if it is apparent that the animal has suffered severe and protracted diarrhea. The presence of even 10,000 *Trichostrongylus* worms in a well-nourished lamb carcass with formed fecal pellets in the rectum suggests only that we should search further for the cause of death. Etiological significance should be attached to *Haemonchus* only if the carcass shows signs of anemia. Cattle suffering from ostertagiosis can become emaciated on full feed. These animals do not even lose their appetites but suffer from malabsorption that causes them to starve to death in the midst of plenty. It is just as well not to accuse the farmer of starving the animal to death when in fact *Ostertagia* is the culprit.

■ PARASITES OF DOGS
Stages in Feces

The common internal parasitisms of dogs can usually be diagnosed on the basis of the microscopic appearance of eggs, cysts, or larvae found in the feces. Micrometry or fecal culture may be necessary when more specific identification is required than can be accomplished on the basis of microscopic appearance alone.

Nematode Eggs

Eggs of some nematode parasites of dogs are shown in Figures 5-9 and 5-10.

The stage of embryonic development of eggs found in fresh fecal specimens varies among nematode species and thus provides us with diagnostic criterion. In fresh fecal specimens, *Toxocara, Toxascaris, Trichuris,* and the capillarid eggs of

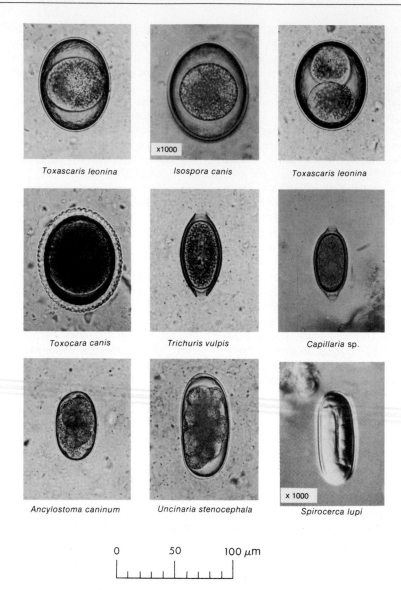

Toxascaris leonina   Isospora canis   Toxascaris leonina

Toxocara canis   Trichuris vulpis   Capillaria sp.

Ancylostoma caninum   Uncinaria stenocephala   Spirocerca lupi

0   50   100 μm

FIGURE 5-9 Eggs of some nematode parasites of dogs (×425, except for *Isospora canis* and *Spirocerca lupi*). *Toxascaris leonina* produces a colorless, subspherical to ellipsoidal egg shell with a smooth shell surface and a prominent lipid layer containing one or sometimes two cells in fresh specimens. *Isospora canis,* a coccidian oocyst and not a nematode egg, is portrayed here ×1000 to illustrate how easily it might be confused with *T. leonina* unless the difference in size or the absence of a lipid layer is noticed. *Toxocara canis* produces a yellowish brown, subspherical egg with a uniformly pitted shell surrounding a single cell in fresh specimens. *Trichuris vulpis* and capillarid eggs are lemon shaped and have bipolar plugs. *T. vulpis* eggs average more than 75 μm, whereas those of Capillarids average less than 75 μm in length. Recovery of *E. aerophilus* eggs from respiratory mucus by tracheal swab requires general anesthesia. The presence of *P. plica* eggs in fresh fecal specimens represents contamination with urine. Urine specimens may also contain eggs of *Dioctophyme renale* (no photomicrograph available), but these have much larger and rougher shells than do the eggs of *P. plica. Ancylostoma* and *Uncinaria* eggs have a smooth, clear, colorless, ellipsoidal shell and contain an embryo in the morula stage of development. *Ancylostoma caninum* eggs average less than 65 μm, whereas *Uncinaria stenocephala* eggs average more than 70 μm in length. Mixed infection with these two common species is easily recognized by the simultaneous presence of eggs of disparate size. De Faria (1910), who first described *A. braziliense,* gave the dimensions of that egg as 65 by 32 μm. *Caution:* the eggs of strongyle parasites of domestic herbivores frequently find their way into dog feces through coprophagy and may be confused with hookworm eggs. Eggs of the order Spirurida are usually smooth walled and contain a larva. The most important of these, *Spirocerca lupi,* produces very small (30 by 12 μm), cylindrical eggs with rounded ends.

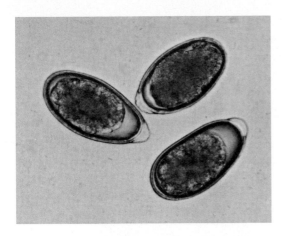

FIGURE 5-10 *Gnathostoma spinigerum* from a dog (×425). This dog belonged to a pet shop owner who occasionally fed it defunct tropical fish. Probably, infection with this exotic parasite was acquired by eating one of these fishes.

Eucoleus aerophilus and *Aonchotheca putorii* contain a single cell. The *Ancylostoma* or *Uncinaria* embryo has already segmented to produce a morula as has the capillarid egg of *Eucoleus böhmi*. Many spirurid eggs contain first-stage larvae, and *Strongyloides* and *Filaroides* have already hatched and appear in the feces as first-stage larvae. The development of a typical nematode egg is portrayed in Figure 5-7.

Unfortunately, the range of sizes of eggs, cysts, and larvae precludes adoption of one standard magnification for all. In the following pages, most of the nematode eggs are represented ×425, most protozoan cysts ×1000, and nematode larvae either ×250 or ×425. The scale at the bottom of Figures 5-9, 5-28, 5-32, and 5-41 corresponds to magnification ×425.

Nematode Larvae

If the canine fecal sample is fresh and not contaminated with soil or extraneous organic material, larvae found swimming about the microscopic field may be either *S. stercoralis* or one of the following metastrongyloids: *F. osleri*, *F. hirthi*, *Crenosoma* sp., or *Angiostrongylus vasorum*. The esophagus of metastrongyloid larvae is longer than the rhabditiform esophagus of the first-stage *Strongyloides* larva, and the tail may have a slight kink as in *Filaroides* or a dorsal spine as in *Angiostrongylus,* whereas the tail of the *Strongyloides* and *Crenosoma* first-stage larva tapers smoothly to a point (Figure 5-11).

If the sample is stale, hookworm larvae may have developed and hatched. These somewhat resemble *Strongyloides* rhabditiform larvae but have a longer buccal capsule and smaller genital rudiment (Figure 5-11). Should doubt remain, culture the

feces for the development of infective stages. The infective sheathed third-stage larvae of hookworms do not begin to appear until after 5 to 7 days' incubation at room temperature, whereas homogonic *Strongyloides* filariform larvae appear as early as 24 to 36 hours, and heterogonic filariform larvae appear in about 4 days. *Strongyloides* filariform larvae are slender, with a very long esophagus, and the tip of their tail appears notched or truncated (Figure 5-12). If the specimen is contaminated with soil or extraneous organic material, free-living nematodes and their larvae may confuse the issue. Under such circumstances, the best course is to obtain a fresh sample directly from the dog's rectum.

Tapeworm Segments

Detached segments of Cyclophyllidean tapeworms are often found crawling about on the perineum or fresh feces of infected dogs (and cats). Hand lens inspection permits identification for practical purposes. Owners sometimes submit for identification shriveled objects that are actually dehydrated tapeworm segments (Figure 5-13, *A*). If these are soaked in water, they will usually regain their familiar appearance (Figure 5-13, *B*). Should doubt remain, the "reconstituted" segment may be squashed between two microscope slides bound together with adhesive tape. The segment may then be identified by the microscopic appearance of its eggs and such organs (e.g., genital pore, uterine diverticula or capsules, parauterine organ) as may persist in gravid segments of various species. Taeniid segments are roughly rectangular with a single, lateral genital pore and contain taeniid eggs (Figures 5-13, 5-14 and 5-17, *A*). *Dipylidium* segments are shaped somewhat like cucumber seeds, have a genital pore on each lateral margin, and contain eggs clustered in packets (uterine capsules) (Figures 5-15 and 5-17, *D*). *Mesocestoides* segments have a dorsal genital pore and eggs massed in a central, thick-walled parauterine organ (Figure 5-16).

Cyclophyllidean Eggs

Taeniid eggs are spherical or subglobular with a radially striated embryophore (a shell-like covering) and contain an embryo (oncosphere or hexacanth embryo) with three pairs of hooks (see Figures 3-34 and 5-17, *A*). If the hooks are not clearly visible, they may sometimes be demonstrated by pressing a needlepoint on the coverslip to break the embryophore (Figures 5-17, *B* and 5-17, *C*). The eggs of *Echinococcus* are a serious menace to human health and cannot be distinguished from those of *Taenia*. In *Echinococcus* endemic areas, therefore, the discovery of taeniid eggs in canine fecal samples demands prompt anthelmintic therapy and caution in the han-

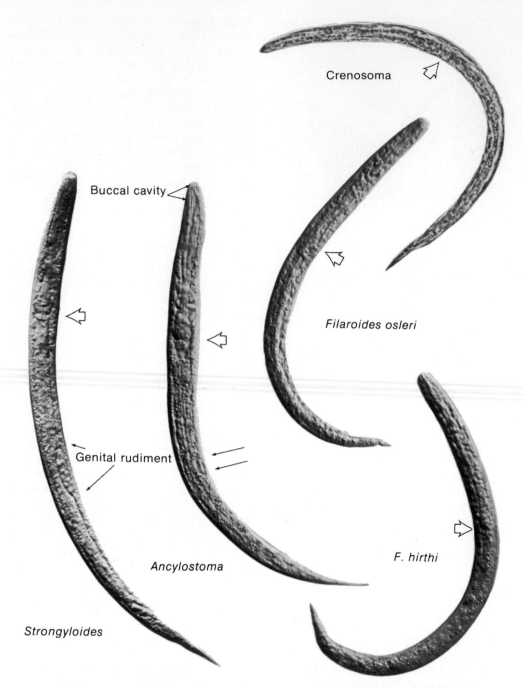

FIGURE 5-11 First-stage larvae of some nematode parasites of dogs. *Crenosoma* and *Filaroides* spp. are metastrongyloid lungworms and usually undergo no development in fecal cultures. *Strongyloides* and *Ancylostoma* first-stage larvae can be distinguished by differences in the relative sizes of their genital rudiments and relative lengths of their buccal cavities. In fecal cultures, both *Strongyloides* and *Ancylostoma* develop to the infective stage (see Figure 5-12).

dling and disposal of feces. The eggs of Dipylidiidae are spherical or subspherical with an unstriated embryophore, contain an oncosphere, and are enveloped in a uterine capsule. In *Dipylidium* there may be up to 29 eggs per capsule (Figure 5-17, *D*). In *Joyeuxiella* and *Diplopylidium* there is only one egg per uterine capsule. The eggs of *Mesocestoides* are oval and thin shelled and contain an oncosphere.

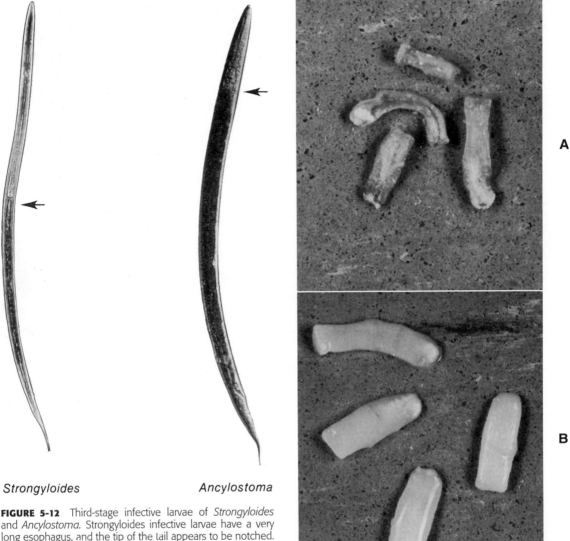

Strongyloides   *Ancylostoma*

FIGURE 5-12 Third-stage infective larvae of *Strongyloides* and *Ancylostoma*. Strongyloides infective larvae have a very long esophagus, and the tip of the tail appears to be notched. (Actually, it is composed of four small projections of the double lateral alae.) *Ancylostoma* infective larvae are usually enclosed in the uncast cuticle (sheath) of the second stage, here seen extending slightly beyond the tail of the third stage.

FIGURE 5-13 A, Dehydrated taeniid segments. **B,** Same segments after an overnight soaking in water (×2).

Diphyllobothriid Eggs

Diphyllobothriid eggs are discharged continuously through the uterine pores of many segments along the body of the worm and hence are passed independently of any detached segment. *Diphyllobothrium* eggs are oval with an operculum at one pole and a small button at the other (Figure 5-18, *A*).

Acanthocephalan Eggs

Acanthocephalan eggs have a thick outer and thinner inner shell enclosing an embryo called an **acanthor**. The external surface of the egg of *Macracanthorhynchus* is elegantly patterned (Figure 5-19).

Trematode Eggs

Eggs of most digenetic trematodes have an operculum at one pole and contain an embryo whose stage of development varies with the species in question (Figure 5-20). Schistosome eggs, on the other hand, lack an operculum and contain a fully developed miracidium that hatches shortly after the egg comes in contact with water. Many, but not all, schistosome eggs have a sharp spine. If a dog has fed recently on trematode-infected tissues such as sheep liver infected with *Dicrocoelium* or *Fasciola* or rabbit entrails infected with *Hasstilesia,* the presence of

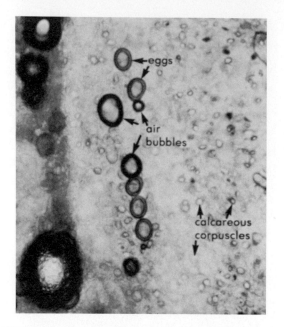

FIGURE 5-14 Taeniid segment in squash preparation (×150).

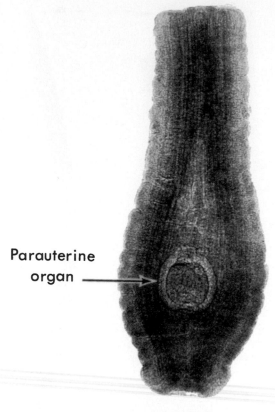

FIGURE 5-16 *Mesocestoides* sp. gravid segment; fresh, unrelaxed, and viewed with transmitted light (×35).

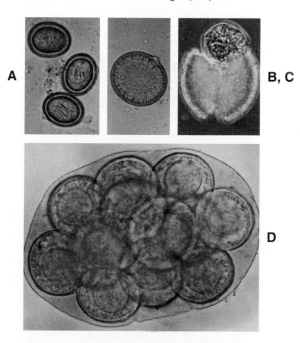

FIGURE 5-17 Tapeworm eggs. **A,** Three taeniid eggs. **B,** Taeniid egg, hooks not visible. **C,** Oncosphere emerging from the broken embryophore of the taeniid egg at left. **D,** *Dipylidium* egg capsule (×380).

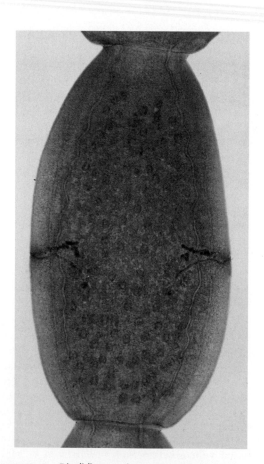

FIGURE 5-15 *Dipylidium caninum* segments (×2).

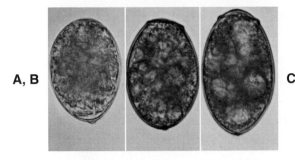

FIGURE 5-18 Operculate eggs (×425). **A,** *Diphyllobothrium* egg. **B** and **C,** Unidentified eggs; their prominent opercula suggest that, except for their small size, these might be *Paragonimus* eggs (see Figure 5-20, *B*). This figure illustrates the difficulty of distinguishing *Diphyllobothrium* eggs from those of certain trematodes.

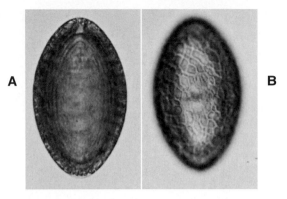

FIGURE 5-19 *Macracanthorhynchus ingens* (Acanthocephala) egg (×425). **A,** Acanthor in focus. **B,** Surface of shell in focus.

myriad trematode eggs in its fecal specimen may lead to misdiagnosis.

Coccidian Oocysts and Sporocysts

Isospora

Isospora spp., *Hammondia,* and *Neospora* oocysts have colorless, ovoid or ellipsoidal, smooth-surfaced walls without micropyle or polar cap and contain a single sporont when passed in the feces of the host (see Figure 5-9). Sporulation occurs in 2 to 4 days at room temperature. The fully sporulated *Isospora* oocyst then contains two sporocysts, each of which contains four sporozoites (Figure 5-21, *A*). Because dogs tend to be coprophagic, oocysts of various other coccidia, especially *Eimeria* spp. of herbivores, are very common pseudoparasites in dog feces. If the *Eimeria* spp. in question have micropyles, polar caps, or other distinguishing features, they present no diagnostic problem (Figure 5-21, *B*), but many species are

difficult to differentiate from *Isospora* spp. Differentiation of *Eimeria* and *Isospora* may be accomplished by fecal culture for oocyst sporulation. Sporulated *Eimeria* oocysts contain four sporocysts, each of which contains two sporozoites (Figure 5-21, *C*).

Identification of species of *Isospora, Hammondia,* and *Neospora* requires micrometry. Oocyst dimensions in micrometers for species infecting dogs are as follows: *I. canis,* 32-42 × 27-33; *Isospora ohioensis,* 19-27 × 18-23; *Isospora burrowsi,* 17-22 × 16-19; *Hammondia heydorni,* 10-13 × 10-13 (Trayser and Todd, 1978); *Neospora caninum* 11.7 × 11.3 (Lindsay et al., 1999).

Sarcocystis

Sarcocystis spp. sporulate within the host, and the fragile oocyst wall often breaks so that the sporocyst containing four sporozoites is the form usually found in the feces (see Figure 5-30, *D*). Sporocysts measure 11-28 × 7-13 μm, but it is not possible to

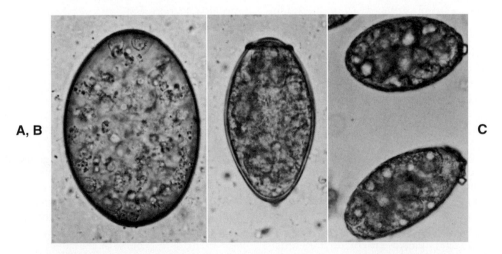

FIGURE 5-20 Trematode eggs (×425). **A,** *Alaria* sp. **B,** *Paragonimus kellicotti.* **C,** *Nanophyetus salmincola.*

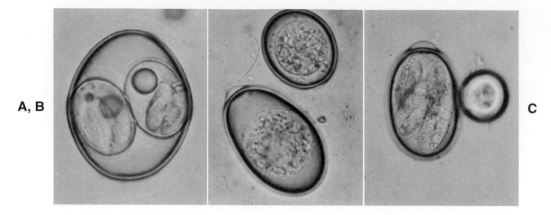

FIGURE 5-21   Coccidian oocysts (×1000). **A,** *Isospora canis,* sporulated. **B,** *Eimeria* spp., one-cell stage. **C,** *Eimeria* sp., sporulated. *Isospora* spp. sporulated oocysts contain two sporocysts, each of which contains four sporozoites. *Eimeria* spp. sporulated oocysts contain four sporocysts, each of which contains two sporozoites. See Figure 5-9 for *I. canis* one-cell stage.

distinguish species of *Sarcocystis* by micrometry of sporocysts (Dubey, 1976). The host relationships of common species of *Sarcocystis* are presented in Table 2-1.

Amebas

Entamoeba histolytica, a serious human pathogen, may appear in canine fecal specimens as either trophozoite or cyst. The trophozoites are more likely to be encountered in diarrheal feces and the cysts in formed fecal specimens. Trophozoites of the large race of *E. histolytica* are 10 to 30 μm across, and their nuclei have marginated chromatin and a small central endosome. *E. histolytica* trophozoites display ameboid movement and often ingest erythrocytes. The mature cysts are 10 to 20 μm in diameter and contain four nuclei.

Entamoeba coli trophozoites are 20 to 30 μm in diameter. Their nuclei have a relatively large eccentric endosome. Erythrocytes are not found in *E. coli* trophozoites. As many as eight nuclei may be counted in *E. coli* cysts.

Entamoeba gingivalis, a parasite of the oral cavity, infects both man and dog. Only trophozoites, ranging in size from 5 to 35 μm, are found in oral scrapings.

Flagellates

Giardia sp. trophozoites are less than 21 μm long, bilaterally symmetrical, and pear shaped. Two nuclei with large central endosomes look like a pair of eyes (see Figure 5-60). *Giardia* cysts are less than 12 μm long, are ellipsoidal, and contain four nuclei.

Trichomonas and related genera do not form cysts and occur in feces (usually diarrheal) only as mononucleated trophozoites.

Ciliates
Balantidium coli

Balantidium coli trophozoites are ovoid with a cytostome at one end; measure 25 to 150 μm in diameter; contain one macronucleus and one micronucleus, two contractile vacuoles, and inclusions; and are covered with rows of cilia (see Figure 2-7). Cysts are spherical or ovoid, measure 40 to 60 μm in diameter, and have a wall consisting of two membranes (see Figure 2-7).

Diagnosis of Heartworm Infection in Dogs

The diagnosis of heartworm infection in dogs is complicated by the fact that circulating microfilariae will not be found in the blood of infected dogs that either have occult infections or have been on preventive therapy. Similarly, if infected dogs have been placed on macrolide preventatives, there will be no circulating microfilariae present in the blood. In these dogs, the diagnostic method of choice is an antigen detection test. However, when a dog has not been on preventive therapy, when the treatment history is not known, or when the dog has been on preventive therapy for only part of the year, especially when the preventive is daily diethylcarbamazine, it is important to determine whether circulating microfilariae are present in the blood. Although the antigen detection tests typically identify infected dogs with circulating microfilariae, there appear to be rare cases in which dogs with high numbers of microfilariae in circulation have negative test results for circulating antigen. For whatever reason, if these test results are negative, the safest course of action—before starting or restarting one of the dogs in this latter group on a preventive regimen—is to examine the blood with a method that will identify microfilariae. To confirm the negative status of the dog or to rule out occult infection, one can also perform an antigen detection test.

Fixation and Identification of Microfilariae in Blood

The simplest procedure for diagnosing the presence of microfilariae in the blood of dogs is to place a drop of heparinized venous blood on a slide, add a coverslip, and examine the preparation under low and high dry magnification. Microfilariae reveal their presence by agitating the erythrocytes in their immediate vicinity. In general, if more than 5 or 10 microfilariae are observed per drop of blood, they are probably *Dirofilaria immitis*. If a smaller number are observed, they may represent either heartworm or another filariid parasite infection. In North America, the only other filariid recognized in dogs is *Dipetalonema reconditum* (Newton and Wright, 1956, 1957), but in certain other parts of the world, there are still other species to withstand. The following procedure is about 15 times as sensitive as the direct smear and permits more accurate differentiation of microfilariae of *D. immitis* and *D. reconditum*.

Technique of Knott (1939) Modified

1. Draw a sample of venous blood into a syringe containing a suitable anticoagulant such as EDTA or heparin.
2. Draw 1 to 2 ml of air into the syringe and mix the blood and anticoagulant by rocking the syringe so as to run the air bubble back and forth along the length of the barrel. Prolonged delay and thermal extremes are to be avoided. Remix blood immediately before proceeding with step 3.
3. Place 1 ml of blood in a 15-ml centrifuge tube. Add 10 ml of 2% formalin, stopper, and mix by inversion and shaking. *Note:* When submitting blood samples to a laboratory for identification of microfilariae, complete only steps 1, 2, and 3 to prepare them for shipment.
4. Wait 2 or 3 minutes.
5. Centrifuge for about 5 minutes and pour off the supernatant by inverting the centrifuge tube only once. Remove the drop that clings to the rim of the tube with absorbent paper.
6. Add one drop of 0.1% methylene blue to the sediment, mix, and transfer some stained sediment to a slide for microscopic examination.

There are other microfilarial concentration techniques, but the Knott test is preferred because it is standard, inexpensive, and includes the best preparative technique for specimens submitted to the

laboratory. The quality and concentration of the formalin solution are critical. Two percent formalin is 2 ml of stock 37% formaldehyde solution (i.e., formalin) and 98 ml of distilled water. This reagent tends to deteriorate in storage and should be made up fresh periodically.

Differentiation of Microfilariae

Microfilariae of *D. immitis* are 6.0 to 7.0 µm wide, whereas those of *D. reconditum* are less than 5.6 µm wide. Length measurement is a more tedious and less reliable differential criterion. When fixed by the preceding technique, the tails of *D. reconditum* microfilariae tend to be curved like an ovariectomy hook. The anterior end of the *D. immitis* microfilaria tapers gently, whereas that of *D. reconditum* maintains about the same diameter throughout. The **cephalic hook** of *D. reconditum* (Figure 5-22) is demonstrable with the ×40 objective of any modern, standard, compound microscope in samples prepared by the Knott technique described earlier. It is not necessary to resort to thick smears or special stains to demonstrate the cephalic hook. Patience is required at first but, with practice, the cephalic hook proves the quickest, easiest, and most reliable differential criterion.

Annotated Host-Organ Listing of Parasites of Dogs

Toxoplasma gondii may occur in any tissue of any host as extracellular or intracellular tachyzoites or as bradyzoites in cysts (see Figures 6-36 and 6-37). *N. caninum* may occur in similar locations.

Alimentary System

Mouth
PROTOZOAN
Trichomonas canistomae (Mastigophora). Found around gum margins; nonpathogenic.

Esophagus and stomach
Nematodes
Spirocerca lupi (Spirurida). Found in fibrous nodules in the wall of the esophagus and sometimes the stomach (see Figures 6-91 to 6-93).

Physaloptera rara and *Physaloptera preputialis* (Spirurida) (see Figures 3-123 and 3-124).

Gnathostoma spinigerum (Spirurida). Relatively rare in North America (see Figure 3-122).

Small Intestine
NEMATODES
T. canis and *T. leonina* (Ascaridoidea). *Toxocara* has a ventriculus intercalated between the esophagus and the intestine (Figure 5-23), whereas *Toxascaris*

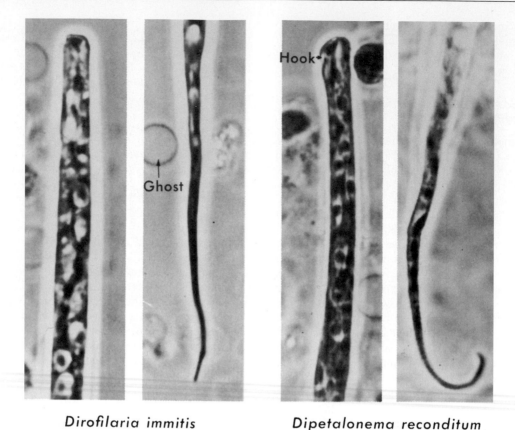

Dirofilaria immitis   *Dipetalonema reconditum*

FIGURE 5-22   Microfilariae of *Dirofilaria immitis* and *Dipetalonema reconditum* (×2000). See text for exposition of differential characters.

has none (Figure 5-24). The ventriculus is visible in transilluminated fresh specimens under the stereoscopic microscope and in fixed, cleared specimens under the compound microscope. Large, fixed specimens may be dissected to determine the presence or absence of a ventriculus. The tail of male *Toxocara* is fingerlike (Figure 5-25), whereas the tail of male *Toxascaris* tapers to a point (Figure 5-26). Female *Toxocara* and *Toxascaris* may be distinguished by comparing their eggs (see Figure 5-9).

The canine roundworm, *Baylisasaris procyonis,* is showing up in dogs as adult worms. This is a dangerous parasite because the zoonotic disease produced by the ingestion of embryonated eggs can be devastating and life threatening. Although a rather rare condition, cases are regularly occurring. When fully mature, the worms tend to be larger than *T. canis* or *T. leonina,* and the eggs can be differentiated by the facts that they are smaller, have a rough external shell (see Figure 3-119), and appear browner than the eggs of the two common dog ascaridoids.

Ancylostoma caninum, Ancylostoma braziliense, and *Uncinaria stenocephala* (Ancylostomatoidea). Mature hookworms are found anchored to the mucosa

by their buccal capsules unless the cadaver has cooled out or the host has died of an overdose of barbiturate, in which case many specimens will be found

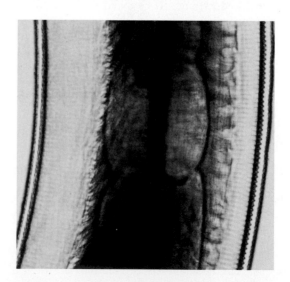

FIGURE 5-23   *Toxocara.* A ventriculus is intercalated between the esophagus and the intestine (×108).

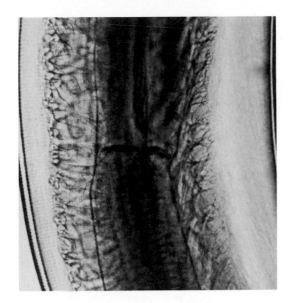

FIGURE 5-24 *Toxascaris.* There is no ventriculus between the esophagus and the intestine (×108).

unattached. Preadult *A. caninum* burrow deeply and destructively in the mucosa, and the mesenteric lymph nodes may be hemorrhagic as a result during the prepatent phase of severe infections. An adult *A. caninum* is colored red, whereas *A. braziliense* and

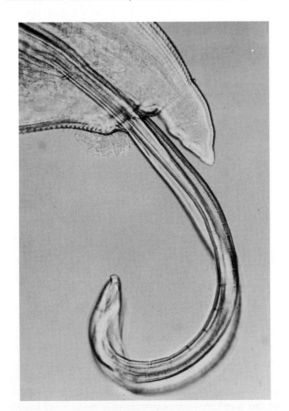

FIGURE 5-25 *Toxocara.* The tail of the male is fingerlike (×108).

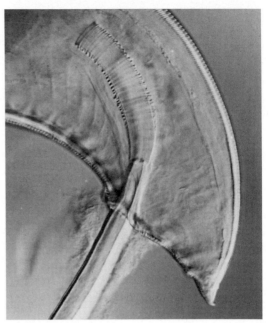

FIGURE 5-26 *Toxascaris.* The tail of the male tapers gradually (×168).

U. stenocephala are grayish white. The red color of *A. caninum* quickly fades on fixation, however. Specimens may be differentiated by microscopic examination of their buccal structures: *A. caninum* has three pairs of pointed teeth on the ventral border of the buccal capsule. *A. braziliense* has one pair of pointed teeth, and *U. stenocephala* has a pair of rounded plates instead of teeth (see Figure 3-94).

S. stercoralis (Rhabditoidea) (see Figure 3-108). The tiny (2.2 mm) parthenogenetic parasitic female worms may be found in scrapings of the mucous membrane.

Trichinella spiralis (Trichinelloidea) (see Figure 3-137). The small adults are found threaded through the mucosa of the duodenum.

CESTODES

T. pisiformis, Taenia hydatigena, Taenia ovis, Taenia multiceps, Taenia serialis (Taeniidae) (see Figures 3-33, 3-34, 3-35, 3-37).

E. granulosus and *E. multilocularis* (Taeniidae) (see Figure 3-43).

Dipylidium caninum, Diplopylidium, and *Joyeuxiella* (Dipylidiidae) (see Figures 3-54, 5-15, and 5-17).

Mesocestoides spp. (Mesocestoididae) (see Figures 3-57 and 5-16).

Diphyllobothrium latum (Diphyllobothriidae) (see Figures 3-25, 3-26, and 5-18, A).

TREMATODES

Alaria americana (5 mm), *Alaria arisaemoides* (10 mm), *Alaria canis* (3.2 mm), and *Alaria michiganensis* (1.9 mm) (Diplostomatidae) (see Figure 3-22).

Mesostephanus appendiculatum (1.8 mm), *Mesostephanus longisaccus* (1 mm) (Cyathocotylidae). These cyathocotylids resemble *Alaria* in having a bulbous tribocytic organ but differ in not being divided into distinct fore- and hind-body regions.

Echinochasmus schwartzi (2.1 mm) (Echinostomatidae) is a slender echinostomatid with a collar of spines surrounding the oral sucker.

Apophallus venustus (1.4 mm), *Cryptocotyle lingua* (2.2 mm) and *Phagicola longa* (1.2 mm) (Heterophyidae).

Plagiorchis sp. This small (1.2 mm) plagiorchiid has a spindle-shaped, spinous body with well-developed suckers; the genital pore is anterior to the ventral sucker.

Nanophyetus salmincola (1.1 mm; see Figure 3-13) and *Sellacotyle mustelae* (0.4 mm) are ovoid and pear shaped, respectively, and have spinous bodies and well-developed suckers.

ACANTHOCEPHALANS

Oncicola canis is small (14 mm) and spindle-shaped (see Figure 3-148). *Macracanthorhynchus ingens* is very large (see Figures 3-143 and 5-19).

PROTOZOANS

FLAGELLATE. *Giardia lamblia* (Flagellate) (see Figure 5-60).

COCCIDIA. *Isopora canis, I. ohioensis, I. burrowsi, H. heydorni,* and *N. caninum.* Oocysts contain a single poront when shed in the feces (see Figure 5-9). Schizonts, gamonts, and oocysts may also be found in istosections or mucosal scrapings.

Sarcystis cruzi, Sarcocystis ovicanis, Sarcocystis miescheriana, Sarcystis bertrami, Sarcystis fayeri, Sarcystis hemionilatrantis (see Table 2-1 and Figure 5-30).

Cryptosporidium spp.

Cecum and colon

NEMATODE

T. vulpis (Trichuroidea) (see Figures 3-140, 3-141, and 5-9).

PROTOZOANS

E. histolytica and *E. coli* are cyst-forming amebas. Trophozoites of *E. histolytica* may contain phagocytosed erythrocytes.

Trichomonas spp. and *Pentatrichomonas hominis* are non–cyst-forming mucosoflagellates.

B. coli (see Figure 2-7).

Liver and Pancreas

NEMATODES

T. canis and *T. leonina* sometimes erratically invade the common bile duct.

Calodium (= Capillaria) hepaticum (see Figure 6-105).

NEMATODE LARVAE

T. canis.

Filaroides spp.

TREMATODES

Opisthorchis tenuicollis, Opisthorchis viverini, Clonorchis sinensis, Metorchis albidus, and *Metorchis conjunctus* (Opisthorchiidae) in bile ducts (see Figure 3-10). Eggs of *Heterobilharzia americana* in tissues surrounded by granulomatous reaction.

Peritoneum and Peritoneal Cavity

CESTODE LARVA

Mesocestoides tetrathyridium (see Figures 6-63 and 6-64).

NEMATODE

Dioctophyme renale (up to 1 meter! Trichinelloidea). A giant red worm in the peritoneal cavity or renal pelvis (see Figure 3-135).

Respiratory System

Nasal passages

NEMATODES

E. (= Capillaria) böhmi (Trichinelloidea).

ARTHROPODS

Pneumonyssoides caninum (Mesostigmata) (see Figure 6-9).

Linguatula serrata (130 mm, Pentastomida). Bloodsucking, wormlike parasite of the nasal cavity and paranasal sinuses.

Trachea and bronchi

NEMATODES

F. osleri (Metastrongyloidea) (see Figures 3-104 and 5-11). In nodules near the bifurcation of the trachea.

Crenosoma vulpis (Metastrongyloidea) (see Figures 3-101 and 5-11). Small worms (16 mm) found on bronchial and bronchiolar mucosa.

E. (= Capillaria) aerophilus (Trichinelloidea).

Lung parenchyma

NEMATODES

F. hirthi and *Filaroides milksi* (Andersonstrongylus milksi) (Metastrongyloidea) (Georgi, 1975, and see Figures 3-102, 5-11, 6-82, and 6-83).

D. immitis (Filarioidea) (see Figures 3-129 and 5-22). Large (30 cm) worms in pulmonary infarcts.

NEMATODE LARVAE

Petechial hemorrhages, areas of focal necrosis, and nodular inflammation of lung tissue may be caused by migrating nematode larvae. Such lesions should be investigated by preparing squashes and by the Baermann technique. Identification of nematode larvae in histological preparations is considered below.

A. vasorum eggs and larvae.

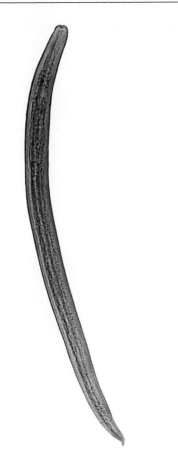

FIGURE 5-27 *Toxocara* larva from a rabbit's liver (×250).

S. stercoralis (Rhabditoidea) filariform larvae (see Figure 5-12).

A. caninum, A. braziliense, and *U. stenocephala* (Ancylostomatoidea) (see Figure 5-12)

T. canis (Ascaridoidea) (Figure 5-27).

Microfilariae of *D. immitis.*

TREMATODE

Paragonimus kellicotti (Troglotrematidae) (see Figures 3-14, 3-15, and 5-20, *B*).

Vascular System
Pulmonary artery, right heart, and venae cavae

PROTOZOANS

T. gondii, cardiac muscle.

Trypanosoma cruzi, cardiac muscle.

NEMATODES

D. immitis (300 mm, Filarioidea) in right ventricle, right atrium, pulmonary arteries, and rarely venae cavae (see Figures 3-129 and 5-22).

A. vasorum (25 mm, Metastrongyloidea). Much smaller than *D. immitis* and located in the pulmonary arterial branches. First-stage larvae resembling those of *Aelurostrongylus* (Figure 5-28) are shed in the host's feces.

T. canis larvae in cardiac muscle.

Mesenteric and portal veins

TREMATODE

H. americana (Schistosomatidae) (see Figures 3-24 and 6-50).

Blood

NEMATODE MICROFILARIAE

D. immitis and *D. reconditum* (Filarioidea) (see Figure 5-22).

PROTOZOANS

Babesia canis (piroplasm) (see Figure 2-26).

T. cruzi (hemoflagellate). Trypomastigotes of this flagellate may be scarce in blood films. Examine heart muscle histologically for amastigotes (see Figure 6-17).

Skeletal Muscles

PROTOZOANS

N. caninum (see Figure 2-20).

NEMATODE LARVAE

T. spiralis (Trichinelloidea) (see Figures 3-139, 5-59, and 6-103).

A. caninum (Ancylostomatoidea). Larvae in vacuoles in muscle fibers with little or no evidence of host reaction (see Fig. 6-79).

Connective Tissues

NEMATODES

D. reconditum (32 mm, Filarioidea) (see Figure 3-134).

D. immitis (300 mm, Filarioidea) (see Figure 3-127).

D. insignis (360 mm, Spirurida) (see Figures 3-120, 3-121, and 6-96).

INSECT LARVAE

Cuterebra (30 mm, Cuterebridae) (see Figures 1-26, 1-27, 6-1, and 6-3).

Cochliomyia hominivorax (17 mm, Calliphoridae) (see Figures 1-12 and 1-19).

Phaenicia sericata, Phormia regina, Protophormia terraenovae (17 mm, Calliphoridae) (see Figures 1-12 and 1-19).

Wohlfahrtia vigil and *Wohlfahrtia opaca* (Sarcophagidae) (see Figure 1-19).

Urogenital System
Kidney

NEMATODE

D. renale (up to 1 meter! Trichinelloidea). A giant red worm in the renal pelvis or peritoneal cavity (see Figure 3-135).

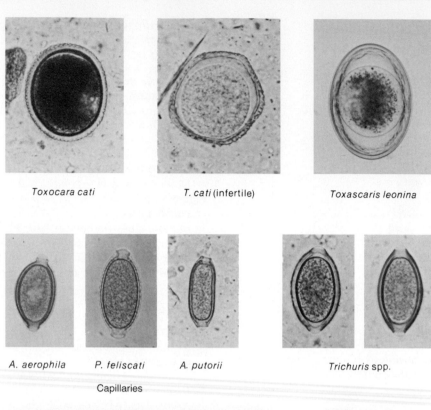

Toxocara cati   T. cati (infertile)   Toxascaris leonina

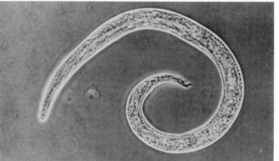

A. aerophila   P. feliscati   A. putorii   Trichuris spp.

Capillaries

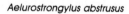

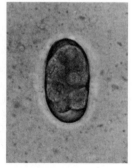

Aelurostrongylus abstrusus   Ancylostoma tubaeforme

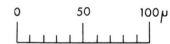

0   50   100 μ

FIGURE 5-28 Nematode parasites of cats. *Toxocara cati* eggs are smaller and more delicate than *T. canis* eggs (Figure 5-9). *Toxascaris leonina* is a parasite of both cats and dogs. The egg in this figure came from a tiger. Capillarid eggs may be those of *E. aerophilus* in the lungs, *P. feliscati* or *P. plica* in the urinary bladder, or *A. putorii* in the stomach and small intestine. Recovery of eggs from respiratory mucus or urine therefore aids in identification. *Calodium (=Capillaria) hepaticum* (Figure 6-105) is a common pseudoparasite of cats when this parasite is endemic in the local rodent population. *Trichuris* spp. are rare parasites of North American cats. The *Trichuris* egg at left was observed in the feces of a cat from Puerto Rico that was found during necropsy to contain three female *Trichuris* sp. worms. The egg at right, from a New York State cat, was presumptively identified as *Trichuris* sp. because of its close resemblance (except for smaller size) to *Trichuris vulpis* (Figure 5-9). *Aelurostrongylus abstrusus* larvae may be identified by their curiously shaped tail. *Ancylostoma tubaeforme*, *A. braziliense*, and *Uncinaria stenocephala* all produce typical strongyle eggs. *Strongyloides* spp. rhabditiform larvae (Figure 5-11) and *Trichinella spiralis* prelarvae and defunct adults are sometimes found in the feces of cats.

NEMATODE LARVAE
T. canis (see Figure 5-27).

A. caninum.

Urinary Bladder
NEMATODE
Pearsonema (=Capillaria) plica (60 mm, Trichinelloidea).

Nervous System
Brain and spinal cord
PROTOZOAN
N. caninum (see Figure 2-20).

NEMATODES
Baylisascaris sp. (Thomas, 1988).

Eye
NEMATODES
T. canis in retina (Hughes et al, 1987).

D. immitis (Filarioidea) (see Figures. 3-129 and 5-22). In the anterior chamber of the eye, or epidural space, erratically.

Thelazia californiensis (19 mm, Spirurida) (see Figure 3-125). In the conjunctival sac and ducts of the lacrimal gland.

Skin and Hair

INSECTS
Adult dipterans.

Linognathus setosus (Anoplura) (see Figure 1-33).

Trichodectes canis (Mallophaga) (see Figures 1-41 and 1-42).

Heterodoxus spiniger (Mallophaga) has club-shaped antennae that lie in cephalic grooves, and the anterior margin of the head is pointed; restricted to warm climates.

Ctenocephalides canis, Ctenocephalides felis, Pulex irritans, Echidnophaga gallinacea (Siphonaptera) (see Figures 1-47, 1-48, and 1-50).

ARACHNIDS
Rhipicephalus sanguineus, Dermacentor variabilis, Dermacentor andersoni, Amblyomma americanum, Amblyomma maculatum, Ixodes spp., and others (Ixodidae) (see Figures 1-66 to 1-75).

Sarcoptes scabiei (Sarcoptidae) (see Figures 1-84 and 6-4).

Otodectes cynotis (Psoroptidae) (see Figure 1-91).

Demodex canis (Demodicidae) (see Figures 1-95 and 6-7).

Cheyletiella yasguri (Cheyletidae) (see Figures 1-96 and 6-6).

NEMATODE LARVA
Rhabditis strongyloides (Rhabditida) (see Figures 3-106, 6-69, and 6-70).

■ PARASITES OF CATS
Stages in Feces

Cats share a few parasites (e.g., *T. leonina, E. (=Capillaria) aerophilus, D. caninum, P. kellicotti*) with dogs, and cross-infections with others may occur on rare occasions. However, the most common cat parasites (Figures 5-28, 5-29, and 5-30) are different species of the genera found in dogs (e.g., *Toxocara cati, Ancylostoma tubaeforme, Isospora felis*). Pseudoparasitism in cats is usually the result of predation rather than coprophagy. For example, the eggs of *Capillaria hepatica* accumulate in infected rodent livers and may be found in the feces of a cat that has eaten such a rodent (see Figure 6-105). Feline *Trichuris* infection often excites lively debate because its rare appearances in North American cats violate a time-honored belief that it does not exist at all. In any case, it is certainly of little practical importance aside from its tendency to complicate the differential diagnosis of pulmonary and vesical capillariasis.

Isospora, Hammondia, Besnoitia, and Toxoplasma

The species of *Isospora* infecting cats are entirely distinct from those infecting dogs. The largest oocyst is that of *I. felis*. A midsize oocyst is *Isospora rivolta*. There are several species and genera producing smaller oocysts, including *Besnoitia besnoiti, Besnoitia darlingi, Besnoitia wallacei,* and *Besnoitia jellisoni,* along with *T. gondii* and *Hammondia hammondi*. Careful micrometry affords differentiation of the larger species of oocysts, but, unfortunately, the most important species, *Toxoplasma*, remains confounded with *Hammondia*. Until this dilemma is resolved, oocysts smaller than 14 μm should be regarded as *Toxoplasma*, just to be on the safe side (see Figure 5-30).

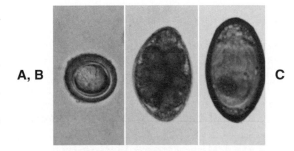

FIGURE 5-29 Eggs of cat platyhelminths. **A,** *Taenia taeniaeformis.* This taeniid cestode egg has a radially striated embryophore and contains a fully developed oncosphere. **B,** *Spirometra mansonoides.* This diphyllobothriid cestode egg has an operculate capsule and contains an undeveloped embryo. **C,** *Platynosomum fastosum.* This dicrocoeliid trematode egg also has an operculate capsule but contains a fully developed

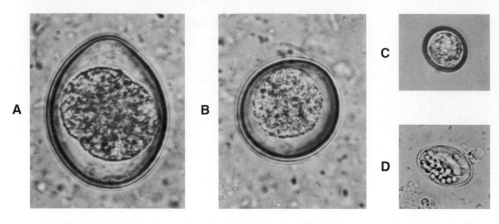

FIGURE 5-30 Coccidian cysts of cats (×1000). **A,** *Isospora felis.* **B,** *I. rivolta.* **C,** *Toxoplasma gondii.* **D,** *Sarcocystis* sp. *Sarcocystis* sporocysts released by rupture of the oocyst wall are only slightly larger than *T. gondii* but are ovoid rather than subspherical and contain four sporozoites. (*Sarcocystis* sp. photomicrograph from Dubey JP: *J Am Vet Med Assoc* 162[10]:876, 1973.)

Species	Oocyst Dimensions (μm)
I. felis	38-51 × 27-39
I. rivolta	21-28 × 18-23
B. besnoiti	14-16 × 5-14
B. darlingi	11-13 × 11-13
B. wallacei	16-19 × 10-13
T. gondii	11-13 × 9-11
H. hammondi	11-13 × 10-12

Sarcocystis

Sarcocystis sporulates within the host, and the fragile oocyst wall often breaks. Therefore the sporocyst measuring 9-12 × 7-12 μm and containing four sporozoites is the form usually found in the feces (see Figure 5-30). It is not possible to distinguish species of *Sarcocystis* by micrometry.

Cryptosporidium

The oocysts of *Cryptosporidium felis* are best floated in saturated sucrose solution. Because they are a mere 5 μm in diameter, slides must be scanned at high dry magnification. *Cryptosporidium* oocysts tend to lie in the focal plane immediately below the coverslip (i.e., at the top of the air bubbles) (see Figure 2-16).

Annotated Host-Organ Listing of Parasites of Cats

T. gondii may occur in any tissue of any host as extracellular or intracellular tachyzoites or as bradyzoites in cysts (see Figures 2-19, 6-36, and 6-37). Sexual reproduction with formation of oocysts (see Figure 5-30) occurs only in the intestinal mucosae of members of the cat family (Felidae).

Alimentary System
Mouth
PROTOZOAN
Trichomonas felistomae (flagellate). Found around the gum margins; nonpathogenic.

Stomach and Esophagus
NEMATODES
Gnathostoma spinigerum (Spirurida) (see Figure 3-122).

Physaloptera spp. (Spirurida) (see Figures 3-123 and 3-124).

Ollulanus tricuspis (1 mm Trichostrongyloidea) (see Figure 3-79).

Aonchotheca (=Capillaria) putorii (Trichinelloidea) (see Figure 5-28).

Small intestine
NEMATODES
T. cati and *T. leonina* (Ascaridoidea) (see Figures 3-117, 5-23 to 5-26, and 5-28).

A. tubaeforme, A. braziliense, U. stenocephala (Ancylostomatoidea) (see Figures 3-94, 3-97, 5-28, and 5-31).

S. stercoralis (2.2 mm, Rhabditida) (see Figures 3-108).

T. spiralis (Trichinelloidea) (see Figure 3-137).

A. (=Capillaria) putorii (Trichinelloidea) (see Figures 5-28).

CESTODES
Taenia taeniaeformis (Taeniidae) (see Figures 3-34, 3-36, 6-52, and 6-53).

E. multilocularis (Taeniidae) (see Figure 3-43).

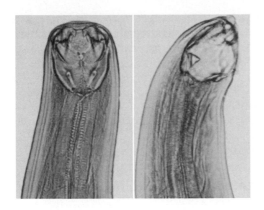

FIGURE 5-31 *Ancylostoma tubaeforme. Left,* the dorsoventral aspect of the stoma, and *right,* its lateral aspect (×78).

D. caninum (Dipylidiidae) (see Figures 3-53, 5-5, and 5-17).

Mesocestoides latus and *Mesocestoides variabilis* (Mesocestoididae) (see Figures 3-57 and 5-16).

Spirometra mansonoides (Diphyllobothriidae) (see Figures 3-27 and 3-29).

TREMATODES
Alaria spp. (5 mm, Diplostomatidae) (see Figures 3-20 to 3-22).

A. venustus (1.4 mm.) and *P. longa* (1.2 mm). (Heterophyidae).

Mesotephanus spp. (1.8 mm, Cyathocotylidae).

ACANTHOCEPHALAN
Oncicola spp. (see Figure 3-148).

PROTOZOANS
I. felis, I. rivolta, Besnoitia spp., *H. hammondi, T. gondii* (coccidia) (see Figure 5-30).

Sarcocystis hirsuta, Sarcocystis tenella, Sarcocystis porcifelis, Sarcocystis leporum (coccidia) (see Table 2-1 and Figure 5-30).

Giardia sp.
C. felis.

Large intestine
NEMATODES
Strongyloides tumefaciens and *S. felis* (common in Australia; Speare and Tinsley, 1987) (5 mm, Rhabditida) (see Figure 3-108).

Trichuris campanula and *Trichuris serrata* (Exotic, South America: Trichinolloidea) (see Figures 3-140 and 5-28).

Liver, Bile Ducts, and Gallbladder; Pancreatic Duct
NEMATODES
C. (=Capillaria) hepaticum (see Figure 6-105).
T. canis larvae, granulomas (Parsons et al, 1988).

TREMATODES
O. tenuicollis, M. albidus (4.6 mm), *M. conjunctus* (6.6 mm), *Amphimerus pseudofelineus* (22 mm), *Parametorchis complexus* (10 mm), *C. sinensis* (Asia) (Opisthorchiidae) (see Figures 3-10 and 3-17).

Platynosomum fastosum (8 mm), *Eurytrema procyonis* (3.3 mm) (Dicrocoeliidae) (Figures 3-19 and 5-29).

Respiratory System
Nasal Cavity, Trachea, and Bronchi
NEMATODES
E. (= Capillaria) aerophilus (Trichinelloidea) (see Figure 5-28).

Mammomonogamus spp. (Syngamidae) (see Figure 3-91).

Lung Parenchyma
NEMATODES
A. abstrusus (9 mm, Metastrongyloidea) (see Figures 5-28 and 6-81).

TREMATODE
P. kellicotti (Troglotrematidae) (see Figures 3-14, 3-15, and 5-20, B).

Vascular System
Heart
NEMATODES
D. immitis (Filarioidea) (see Figures 3-130 and 6-97).

A. vasorum.

T. canis larvae, granulomas (Parsons et al, 1988).

Blood
PROTOZOAN
Cytauxzoon felis (Piroplasm) (see Figure 2-27).
NEMATODE MICROFILARIA
D. immitis (see Fig. 5-22).

Skeletal Muscles
NEMATODE LARVA
T. spiralis (Trichinelloidea) (see Figures 3-139, 5-59, and 6-104).

Connective Tissues
INSECT LARVA
Cuterebra spp. (30 mm) (see Figures 1-27, 6-1, and 6-3).

Urogenital System
Kidneys
NEMATODE
T. canis larvae, granulomas (Parsons et al, 1988).

Urinary Bladder

NEMATODES

P. (=Capillaria) plica (60 mm), *Pearsonema feliscati* (32 mm) (Trichinelloidea) (see Figure 5-28).

Nervous System

NEMATODE

D. immitis adults migrating erratically in meninges and ventricles (see Figure 3-130).

INSECT LARVA

Cuterebra spp. (30 mm) (see Figures 1-27, 6-1, and 6-3).

Skin and Hair

INSECTS

Adult dipterans.
Felicola subrostratus (Mallophaga) (Fig. 1-43).
C. canis, C. felis, Echidnophaga gallinacea (Siphonaptera) (see Figures 1-47 and 1-48).

ARACHNIDS

Dermacentor spp., *Haemaphysalis leporispalustris, Ixodes* spp. (Ixodidae) (see Figures 1-66 to 1-76).
Notoedres cati, S. scabiei (Sarcoptidae) (see Figures 1-84 to 1-86).
O. cynotis (Psoroptidae) (see Figure 1-91).
Lynxacarus radovskyi (Listrophoroidea) (see Figure 1-94).
Cheyletiella blakei (Cheyletidae) (see Figures 1-96 and 6-6).
Demodex cati (Demodicidae) (see Figure 1-95).
Neotrombicula whartoni, Walchia americana (Trombiculidae) (see Figures 1-98 and 1-99). *N. whartoni,* a bright red chigger, has been found in the external ear canal of cats. *W. americana,* normally a parasite of the gray squirrel *Sciurus carolinensis,* is capable of causing a severe and generalized dermatitis in cats (Lowenstine et al, 1979).

■ PARASITES OF RUMINANTS
Stages in Feces
Nematode Eggs

Other than the numerous eggs of various strongylid parasites that will be present in the feces, one commonly finds the eggs of *Strongyloides, Trichuris,* and capillarids (Figure 5-32). The strongylid eggs present in ruminant feces cannot be readily identified to genus or species with the exception of certain types (e.g., *Nematodirus battus*). When a more specific diagnosis is required, it is necessary to culture the stages present in the feces to the infective stage.

Other Nematodes

Eggs of the following ruminant nematodes are not illustrated in Figure 5-32. *Toxocara vitulorum* (parasite of cattle) eggs are subglobular with a uniformly pitted surface and one cell. *Note:* Patent *Ascaris suum* infections are occasionally reported from sheep and cattle. *A. suum* eggs (see Figure 5-58) are easy to distinguish from those of *T. vitulorum.* *Gongylonema* eggs are thick walled, have bipolar opercula, and contain vermiform embryos. *Skrjabinema ovis* eggs are typical pinworm eggs with one side slightly flattened.

Identification of Strongyle Infective Larvae

Identification of third-stage infective larvae in cultured ruminant feces is challenging but not formidable. Usually, two or more genera are present, and one can best determine just how many there are by scanning the slide at low power and mentally grouping those of similar appearance. Certain species stand out from the crowd. For example, *Strongyloides* larvae are more slender than any of the others, lack a sheath, and have a long cylindrical esophagus and truncated tail. Two sizes, of which the larger is "standard," are portrayed in Figure 5-33. Dr. Georgi has encountered both sizes in a single culture. Similarly, *Bunostomum* spp. are distinguished from other sheathed strongyle larvae by their smaller size. Other genera of sheathed larvae may be grouped according to the length of their caudal sheath extension (the extension of the sheath beyond the tip of the larva's tail): short, *Trichostrongylus* and *Ostertagia;* medium, *Haemonchus* and *Cooperia;* and long, *Oesophagostomum* and *Chabertia,* as illustrated in Figures 5-33 and 5-34. Within these groupings, further identification depends on micrometry and observation of such morphological details as the caudal tubercles of *Trichostrongylus,* the "oval bodies" of *Cooperia,* and the number and shape of the intestinal cells of *Oesophagostomum* and *Chabertia.* The odd larva may defy identification, but accurate diagnosis of the predominating genera in a culture is not a difficult task. Proceed as follows:

Place a drop of larval suspension on a microscope slide. Relax the larvae by gentle warming or by adding a drop of Lugol's solution (5 g iodine crystals and 10 g potassium iodide in 100 ml distilled water). Ring the coverslip with petroleum jelly for support and thus prevent distortion of the larvae. Avoid higher magnifications at first but instead scan the slide under low power to get an impression of how many different kinds of larva are present. Then seek representatives of each kind; examine these under higher power; and take whatever measurements may be necessary for generic or specific diagnosis. The data of Table 5-1 are taken from the works of Dikmans and Andrews (1933, sheep) and Keith

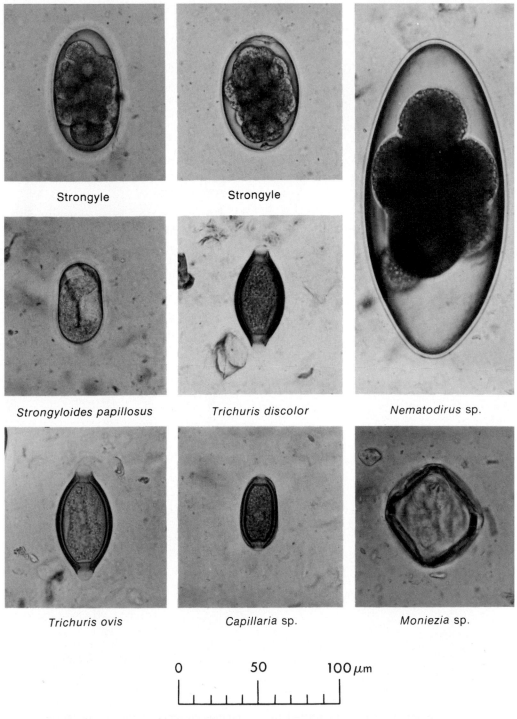

Strongyle

Strongyle

Strongyloides papillosus   *Trichuris discolor*   *Nematodirus* sp.

Trichuris ovis   *Capillaria* sp.   *Moniezia* sp.

0   50   100 µm

FIGURE 5-32 Eggs of common ruminant parasites. Strongyle eggs are ellipsoidal, are smooth walled, and contain a morula. Although *Nematodirus* spp. eggs are very large, some species are considerably smaller than the one shown here. *Marshallagia marshalli* eggs (not shown) are also very large but differ from *Nematodirus* eggs in having more parallel sides and less pointed poles. *Strongyloides papillosus* eggs are slightly smaller than strongyle eggs and contain a rhabditiform larva in fresh fecal specimens. On incubation, the larvae soon hatch and develop into infective filariform larvae (Figure 3-62) or free-living adult males and females, predominantly the latter. *Trichuris* spp. eggs of ruminants are more than 60 µm long; those of *Capillaria* spp. are less than 60 µm long. *Moniezia* spp. eggs contain a pear-shaped embryophore containing an oncosphere. *Thysanosoma* spp. eggs (not shown here) are grouped in uterine capsules.

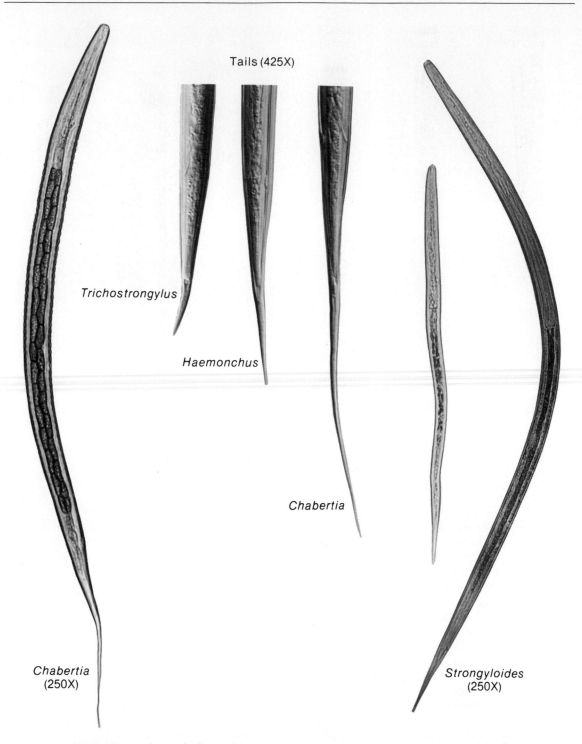

Tails (425X)

Trichostrongylus

Haemonchus

Chabertia

Chabertia
(250X)

Strongyloides
(250X)

FIGURE 5-33   Infective third stage larvae of nematode parasites of sheep. Both large and small *Strongyloides* infective larvae are represented at the same magnification.

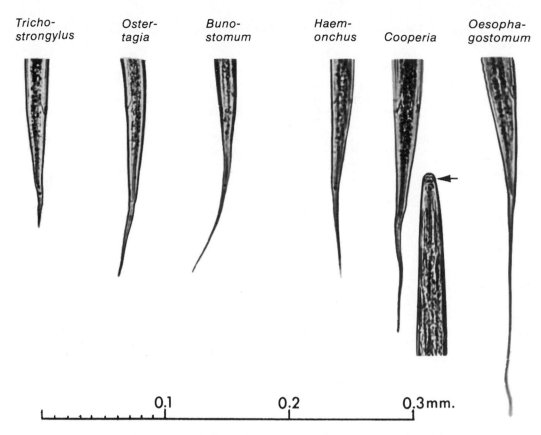

Tricho-strongylus Oster-tagia Buno-stomum Haem-onchus Cooperia Oesopha-gostomum

0.1   0.2   0.3 mm.

FIGURE 5-34 Tails of infective third stage larvae of nematode parasites of cattle and the anterior end of a *Cooperia* larvae showing the conspicuous oval bodies *(arrow)*, which represent optical cross sections of a bundle of fibers surrounding the buccal capsule (×350). (From Whitlock JH: *The diagnosis of veterinary parasitisms,* Philadelphia, 1960, Lea & Febiger.)

(1953, cattle). The number of intestinal cells is 16, except as otherwise noted. Taxa grouped with braces are similar in appearance and require more care for their differentiation than comparisons among groups.

Work continues to develop some means by which to automate the identification of the different nematode parasites of ruminants. Toward the identification of trichostrongylid larvae, as with eggs, automated imaging analysis has been tried for the differentiation of larvae from culture (Theodoropoulos et al, 2000). The process seems to work if the system is appropriately "taught," but again, the problem is that such identification methods would be restricted to well-equipped laboratories because of the high cost and specialization of the equipment that is required.

Lungworm Larvae

Dictyocaulus viviparus is the only lung nematode of cattle. *Dictyocaulus filaria, Protostrongylus rufescens,* and *M. capillaris* are common lung nematodes of sheep and goats in North America. Differential diagnosis is based on morphological features of the first-stage larvae found in the host's feces (Figure 5-35). *Dictyocaulus* spp. larvae are tough enough to be countable by the Cornell-McMaster egg-counting technique, but the counting should be done promptly to avoid osmotic shriveling of the larvae. For sensitive qualitative diagnosis of lungworm infections, the Baermann is the technique of choice.

Trematode Eggs

Trematode eggs may fail to float in the concentrations of sugar solutions ordinarily used. They are best concentrated by washing feces through sieves to remove coarse debris, then centrifuging the washings. The eggs will be found in the sediment. The formalin-ethyl acetate sedimentation technique is also appropriate. The operculum of trematode eggs is sometimes difficult to see. When in doubt, press the coverslip with a pencil point. Usually, the type of operculum found on trematode eggs will pop open under such pressure (Figure 5-36, *B*).

Fasciola hepatica eggs are large (up to 150 μm) and operculate, and contain a cluster of yolk cells

TABLE 5-1 ■ Table of Measurements of Infective Third-Stage Larvae of Strongyles Infecting Sheep and Cattle

Genus (sensu latu)*	Measurements (microns)			Special morphological features
	Overall	Tail of sheath†	Extension of sheath‡	
Strongyloides				Length of esophagus at least $\frac{1}{3}$ length of body caudal
Sheep	574–710		Sheath	extremity of larva truncated (Fig. 5-33)
Cattle	524–678		Absent	
Trichostrongylus				
Sheep	622–796	76–118	21–40	Tiny tubercles on tip of tail
Cattle	619-762	83–107	25–39	
Ostertagia				
Sheep	797–910	92–130	30–60	
Cattle	784–928	126–170	55–75	
Haemonchus				
Sheep	650–751	119–146	65–78	Sheath kinked at tip of tail; anterior end tapers
Cattle	749–866	158–193	87–119	
Cooperia oncophora				
Sheep	804–924	124–150	62–82	Two conspicuous oval bodies at anterior end of
Cattle	809–976	146–190	79–111	esophagus
Cooperia spp.				
Sheep	711–850	97–122	35–52	Two conspicuous oval bodies at anterior end of
Cattle	666–866	109–142	47–71	esophagus
Nematodirus				
Sheep	922–1118	310–350	250–290	Unlikely to be encountered in cultures less than 2 weeks
Cattle	1095–1142	296–347	207–266	old; forked tail with rodlike process; intestine has 8 cells.
Bunostomum				
Sheep	514–678	153–183	85–115	Small size, long tail sheath
Cattle	500–583	129–158	59–83	
Oesophagotomum				
Sheep	771–923	193–235	125–160	16-24 triangular intestinal cells
Cattle	726–857	209–257	134–182	
Chabertia				
Sheep	710–789	175–220	110–150	24-32 rectangular intestinal cells

*Taxa grouped with braces are similar in appearance and require more care for differentiation than other groups.
†Anus to tip of sheath.
‡Tip of larva to tip of sheath.

(Figure 5-36, *A*). *Fasciola gigantica* (Africa, Hawaii, Philippines, and India) are like those of *F. hepatica* but larger (more than 150 μm). Eggs of *Fascioloides magna,* normally a parasite of deer, resemble those of *F. hepatica* but are infrequently found in the feces of infected domestic ruminants because the eggs are trapped in the hepatic cysts containing the adult worms in cattle and because the flukes fail to mature in sheep and goats. Paramphistomatid (rumen fluke) eggs are large and easily confused with those of *Fasciola* spp. (Figure 5-36). *Dicrocoelium dendriticum* eggs are small (50 μm), lopsided, and yellowish brown, and contain a miracidium (Figure

5-36, *C*). *Eurytrema pancreaticum* (Far East) eggs resemble those of *D. dendriticum.* Schistosome eggs lack an operculum, contain a fully developed miracidium, and are armed with a spine.

Coccidia of Ruminants

Oocysts of *Eimeria* spp. are often found in considerable numbers in the feces of healthy ruminants. Even experimental lambs raised on wire become infected with coccidia. Despite their frequent occurrence in healthy animals, coccidia are quite capable of causing serious disease in cattle, sheep, and goats. At

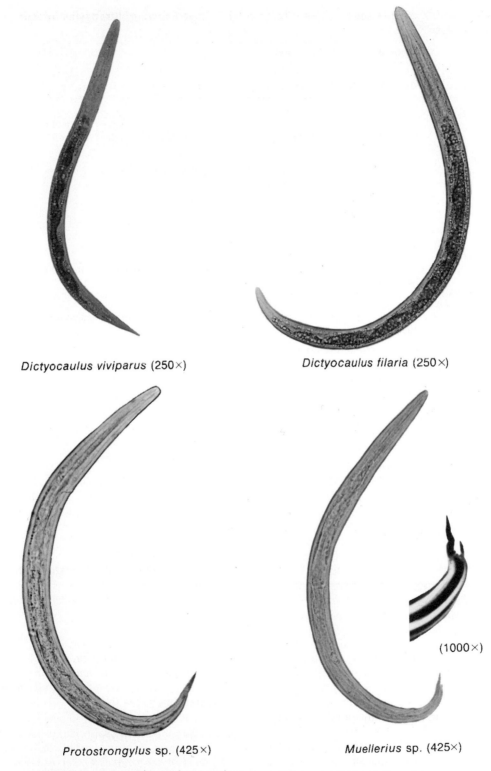

Dictyocaulus viviparus (250×)

Dictyocaulus filaria (250×)

(1000×)

Protostrongylus sp. (425×)

Muellerius sp. (425×)

FIGURE 5-35 First-stage larvae of ruminant lungworms. *Dictyocaulus viviparus* is the only lungworm of cattle, and *D. viviparus* first stage larvae are the only larvae of parasitic nematodes found in fresh cattle dung. Notice the prominent granules. *Dictyocaulus filaria* first stage larvae from sheep are large and have bluntly rounded tails and a "button" at the mouth, and likewise have prominent granules. *Protostrongylus rufescens* larvae are rather stout and have conically tapering tails without spines. *Muellerius capillaris* larvae have a curiously shaped tail with a dorsal spine *(inset)*.

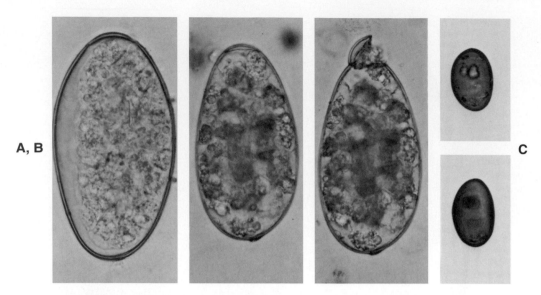

FIGURE 5-36 Eggs of some trematode parasites of ruminants (×425). **A,** *Fasciola hepatica.* **B,** *Paramphistominae.* **C,** *Dicrocoelium dendriticum.*

times, severe disease signs appear before oocysts are shed in the feces. Diagnosis of clinical coccidiosis must be based not only on identification of the oocysts in the feces (Figures 5-37 and 5-38), but also on consideration of the case history and clinical signs.

Figure 5-37 presents the unsporulated and sporulated oocysts of nine species of *Eimeria* from sheep. Goats have a closely similar set, which do not, however, cross-infect and are probably all distinct species. Corresponding species of *Eimeria* of sheep and goat are listed in Table 5-2. The species listed for sheep are those illustrated in Figure 5-37. *Eimeria ahsata, Eimeria bakuensis,* and *Eimeria crandallis* differ mainly in size and the ranges overlap, so differentiating these three species is problematical. Therefore these three species are listed in Table 5-2 under "Ahsata Group," and their counterpart goat parasites are listed under "Arloingi Group." Oocysts of *Eimeria caprovina, Eimeria absheronae,* and *Eimeria caprina* resemble those of *Eimeria faurei* very closely, so we have also assigned these species to an unofficial composite group. (In the table, asterisks indicate those species most likely to be responsible for clinical signs of coccidiosis.)

Cryptosporidium

The oocysts are best concentrated by flotation in saturated sucrose solution. Because the oocysts of *Cryptosporidium parvum* are a mere 5 μm in diameter, the slide must be scanned under high dry magnification. *Cryptosporidium* oocysts tend to lie in the focal plane immediately below the coverslip (i.e., at the top of the air bubbles) (see Figure 2-15). Cattle

are hosts of two species of *Cryptosporidium, C. parvum* of the small intestine and *Cryptosporidium andersoni* of the abomasum. The oocysts of *C. andersoni* are larger than those of *C. parvum* being about 7 mm in diameter (see Figure 2-16).

Annotated Host-Organ Listing of Parasites of Ruminants

T. gondii may occur in any tissue of any host as extracellular or intracellular tachyzoites or as bradyzoites in cysts (see Figures 6-36 and 6-37).

Alimentary System
Mouth, esophagus, and forestomachs
PROTOZOANS
Sarcocystis sarcocysts in muscles of tongue and esophagus (see Figures 6-35).
CESTODE LARVAE
Taenia spp. cysticerci in muscles of tongue (see Figures 3-39, 6-56, and 6-57).
INSECT LARVA
Hypoderma lineatum in wall of esophagus.
NEMATODES
Gongylonema pulchrum (150 mm), *Gongylonema verrucosum* (100 mm) (Spirurida) (see Figure 5-68). Woven in a neat, sinusoidal pattern in the esophageal *(G. pulchrum)* or ruminal *(G. verrucosum)* mucosa.
TREMATODES
Cotylophoron cotylophoron, Paramphistomum cervi, Paramphistomum liorchis, Paramphistomum microbothroides (Paramphistomatidae) (see Figure 3-12).

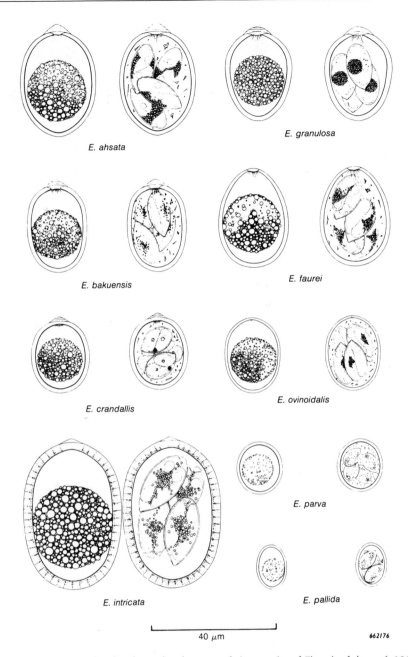

E. ahsata

E. granulosa

E. bakuensis

E. faurei

E. crandallis

E. ovinoidalis

E. intricata

E. parva

E. pallida

40 μm

662176

FIGURE 5-37 Unsporulated and sporulated oocysts of nine species of *Eimeria* of sheep (×1000). (From Joyner, et al: *Parasitology* 56:533, 1966. Crown copyright. Reproduced by permission of the Controller of Her Britannic Majesty's Stationery Office.)

Abomasum

PROTOZOAN

Eimeria gilruthi megaschizonts (see Figure 6-29).

NEMATODES

H. contortus, Haemonchus placei, Haemonchus similis, Mecistocirrus digitatus, O. ostertagi, Ostertagia bisonis, Ostertagia (Telodorsagia) circumcincta, Ostertagia orloffi, Ostertagia trifurcata, Ostertagia (Grosspiculagia) lyrata, Ostertagia (Grosspiculagia) occidentalis, Ostertagia (Telodorsagia) davtiani, Ostertagia (Pseudostertagia) bullosa, Marshallagia marshalli, and *T. axei (Trichostrongyloidea).*

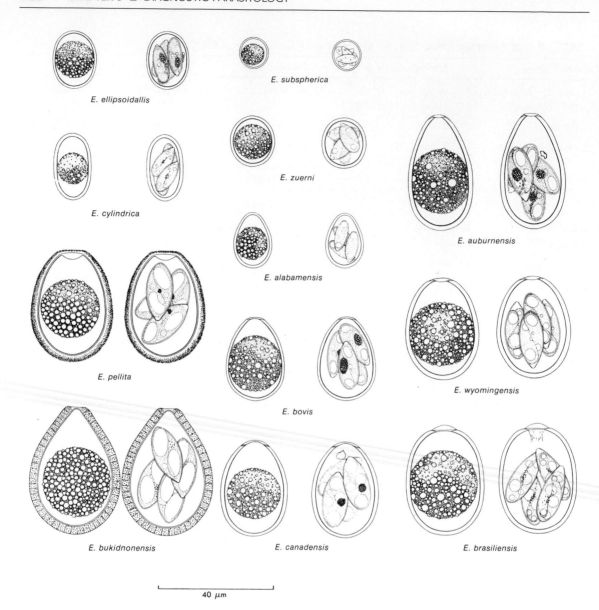

E. ellipsoidallis

E. subspherica

E. cylindrica

E. zuerni

E. auburnensis

E. alabamensis

E. pellita

E. bovis

E. wyomingensis

E. bukidnonensis

E. canadensis

E. brasiliensis

40 μm

FIGURE 5-38 Unsporulated and sporulated oocysts of 12 species of *Eimeria* of cattle (×1000). (From Joyner, et al: *Parasitology* 56:536, 1966. Crown copyright. Reproduced with permission from the Controller of Her Britannic Majesty's Stationery Office.)

Genus	Length (mm)	Figure(s)
Haemonchus	14 to 30	3-71, 3-74
Mecistocirrus	43	3-76
Ostertagia (s.I.)	7 to 9	3-65, 3-71
T. axei	7	3-69, 3-71, 6-72

Small Intestine

NEMATODES

T. vitulorum (30 cm, Ascaridoidea). This exotic parasite of cattle is only rarely seen in the United States, has an esophageal ventriculus, and produces subspherical eggs with a pitted shell surface. *A. suum,* an occasional parasite of ruminants, lacks a ventriculus and produces ellipsoidal eggs with a mammillated shell surface

Cooperia curticei, Cooperia bisonis, C. oncophora, Cooperia pectinata, Cooperia punctata, Cooperia spatulata, Cooperia occidentalis, Trichostrongylus colubriformis, Trichostrongylus longispicularis, Trichostrongylus capricola, Trichostrongylus vitrinus, Nematodirus helvetianus, Nematodirus spathiger, Nematodirus filicollis, Nematodirus abnormalis, Nematodirus lanceolatus, N. battus (Strongylida: Trichostrongyloidea).

TABLE 5-2 ■ Corresponding Species of Eimeria of Sheep and of Goats

Ahsata group	Arloingi group	Faurei group	Absheronae group
(E. ahsata,* E. bakuensis,* and E. crandallis)	*(E. arloingi,* E. hirci, and E. christenseni*)*	*(E. faurei and E. caprovina)*	*(E. absheronae,* E. caprina, and E. caprovina)*
E. intricata	*E. kocharii*	*E. ovinoidalis**	*E. ninakohlyakimovae**
E. granulosa	*E. jolchijevi*	*E. parva*	*E. alijevi**
		E. pallida	*E. pallida*

*Those species most likely to be responsible for clinical signs of coccidiosis.

Genus	Length (mm)	Figure(s)
Cooperia	6 to 16	3-71, 3-77
Trichostrongylus	6 to 7	3-69, 3-71
Nematodirus	20 to 25	3-71, 3-75

B. phlebotomum (cattle), *Bunostomum trigonocephalum* (sheep) (25 mm, Ancylostomatoidea) (see Figure 3-92).

S. papillosus (6 mm, Rhabditida) (see Figure 3-108).

Aonchotheca (= *Capillaria*) *bovis, Aonchotheca* (=*Capillaria*) *brevipes* (Trichinelloidea) (see Figure 5-32).

Oesophagostomum spp. third- and fourth-stage larvae (Strongyloidea) (see Figure 3-89).

CESTODES
M. expansa, Moniezia benedeni (Anoplocephalidae) (see Figures 3-49, 3-50, and 5-32).

Thysanosoma actinoides, Wyominia tetoni (Anoplocephalidae).

Thysaniezia, Stilesia, Avitellina (Anoplocephalidae). Exotic anoplocephalids of ruminants.

PROTOZOANS
Eimeria spp. (coccidia) (see Figures 5-37, 5-38, and 6-29).

Cryptosporidium spp.

G. lamblia (flagellate) (see Figure 5-60).

Cecum and Colon

NEMATODES
Oesophagostomum radiatum (cattle), *Oesophagostomum columbianum* (sheep and goats), *Oesophagostomum venulosum* (sheep and goats), *Chabertia ovina* (sheep and goats) (18 to 22 mm, Strongyloidea) (see Figures 3-87 to 3-89). The fourth-stage larvae of *O. radiatum* in cattle and *O. columbianum* in sheep may be found in abscesses in the gut wall (see Figure 3-89).

Trichuris discolor (52 mm, cattle), *Trichuris ovis* (70 mm, sheep and goats) (Trichinelloidea) (see Figure 5-32).

S. ovis, Skrjabinema caprae (8 to 10 mm, Oxyurida).

PROTOZOANS
Eimeria spp. (coccidia) (see Figures 5-37, 5-38, and 6-29).

Entamoeba bovis (ameba).

Buxtonella sulcata (ciliate).

Liver

NEMATODES
A. suum (Ascaridida). This swine ascarid sometimes matures in the bile ducts of sheep and cattle.

Stephanurus dentatus (Strongyloidea) (see Figure 3-90). Immature *S. dentatus* worms migrate through the bovine liver and cause severe trauma.

CESTODES
T. actinoides, W. tetonis (Anoplocephalidae).

CESTODE LARVAE
E. granulosus, E. multilocularis hydatids (Taeniidae) (see Figures 3-44 to 3-47, 6-55, and 6-62).

T. hydatigena cysticerci (Taeniidae) (see Figure 3-36).

TREMATODES
F. hepatica, F. gigantica, F. magna (Fasciolidae) (see Figures 3-2, 3-11, and 5-36, *A*). *F. hepatica* (30 mm) is endemic in western and Gulf states of the United States and in Hawaii, Puerto Rico, British Columbia, and eastern provinces of Canada. *F. gigantica* (75 mm) is endemic in Hawaii and Africa. *F. magna* (100 mm) occurs in foci throughout North America.

D. dendriticum (Europe, Asia, Africa, South America, and central New York State), *E. pancreaticum* (Asia and Brazil) (Dicrocoeliidae) (see Figures 3-18 and 5-36, *C*).

Peritoneum and Peritoneal Cavity

NEMATODE
Setaria labiatopapillosa (Filarioidea) (see Figure 3-132).

CESTODE LARVA
T. hydatigena larva (Taeniidae) (see Figure 3-38).

PENTASTOMID NYMPH
L. serrata (see Figure 1-100).

Respiratory System
Nasal cavity and paranasal sinuses
INSECT LARVA
Oestrus ovis larva in sheep and goats (Oestridae) (see Figure 1-21).

Trachea and bronchi
NEMATODES
D. viviparus (80 mm; cattle), *D. filaria* (100 mm; sheep and goats) (Trichostrongyloidea) (see Figures 3-71, 3-80, and 5-35).

P. rufescens (50 mm; sheep) (Metastrongyloidea) (see Figures 3-99 and 5-35).

Mammomonogamus laryngeus (Syngamidae) (see Figure 3-91). Male and female worms are fused in copula; endemic in Puerto Rico.

Lung parenchyma
NEMATODES
M. capillaris (Metastrongyloidea) (see Figures 3-100 and 5-35).

O. columbianum larvae (erratic migration) (see Figure 3-89).

CESTODE LARVA
E. granulosus (Taeniidae) (see Figures 3-44, 3-45, and 6-61).

Vascular System
Heart
CESTODE LARVAE
T. ovis, Taenia saginata (Taeniidae).

Arteries
NEMATODES
Elaephora schneideri (sheep; Filarioidea).
Elaeophora poeli (cattle; Filarioidea).
Onchocerca armillata (cattle; Filarioidea).

Veins
TREMATODES
Schistosoma mattheei in sheep, *Schistosoma mansoni* in South American cattle (Schistosomatidae) and other species worldwide (see Figure 3-24).

Lymph nodes
PENTASTOMID
L. serrata (see Figures 1-100 and 6-11 to 6-16).

Blood
NEMATODE MICROFILARIA
S. labiatopapillosa.
PROTOZOANS
Babesia bigemina, Babesia bovis, Babesia divergens, Babesia argentina, Theileria parva, Theileria annulata, Theileria mutans (piroplasms) (see Figure 2-27).

Trypanosoma theileri (cattle), *Trypanosoma melophagium* (sheep) (hemoflagellates) (see Figure 2-1). Rarely seen in blood films; readily demonstrable by blood culture.
RICKETTSIAS
Anaplasma marginale, Eperythrozoon wenyoni.

Skeletal Muscles and Connective Tissues
CESTODE LARVAE
T. saginata (Taeniidae). Cysticerci found most frequently in the muscles of mastication, tongue, heart, and muscular portion of the diaphragm of cattle; scolex with four suckers but no hooks.

T. ovis (Taeniidae). Pea-sized vesicles are found in the heart and esophagus and beneath the epicardium and diaphragmatic pleura of sheep and goats.

T. hydatigena (Taeniidae) (see Figure 3-38). Sometimes found in skeletal muscles but more commonly in liver or on peritoneal membranes.
INSECT LARVAE
Hypoderma bovis, H. lineatum (Hypodermatidae) (see Figure 1-21).
NEMATODES
Onchocerca gutterosa, Onchocerca lienalis, Onchocerca bovis, Onchocerca gibsoni (Filarioidea). Adult *Onchocerca* worms are found in deep connective tissues, microfilariae in the dermis. In Australian cattle, *O. gibsoni* produces nodules in the brisket that require extensive trimming. We have seen *O. gibsoni* in corned beef purchased in a local supermarket.
PROTOZOANS
Sarcocystis spp. sarcocysts in muscles (coccidia) (see Table 2-1 and Fig. 6-35).

Urogenital System
PROTOZOANS
Trichomonas foetus (flagellate) (see Figure 2-4).
T. gondii, placentas of aborting sheep.

Nervous System
Brain, spinal cord, and meninges
PROTOZOAN
Sarcocystis-like organism, brain of cattle (Dubey et al, 1987).
NEMATODE
Parelaphostrongylus tenuis (Metastrongylidae) (see Figures 6-85 and 6-86).
CESTODE LARVA
T. multiceps (Taeniidae) in brain of sheep and goats (see Figures 3-41 and 6-59).
INSECT LARVA
H. bovis (Hypodermatidae).

Eye

NEMATODES

T. californiensis (sheep), *Thelazia gulosa* (cattle), *Thelazia skrjabini* (cattle) (Spirurida), in conjunctival sac and lacrimal duct (see Figure 3-125).

Skin and Hair

INSECTS

Dipteran Adults. *Musca autumnalis, Stomoxys calcitrans, Haematobia irritans* (muscidae) (see Figures 1-13, 1-14, and 1-15).

Glossina spp. (Africa) (see Figure 1-16).

Melophagus ovinus (Hippoboscidae) (see Figure 1-17).

H. bovis, H. lineatum (Hypodermatidae).

Tabanidae (see Figures 1-10 and 1-11).

Dipteran Larvae. *H. bovis, H. lineatum* (30 mm, Hypodermatidae) (see Figure 1-21).

Calliphoridae, Sarcophagidae (see Figures 1-12, 1-18, and 1-19).

Anoplurans. *Haematopinus eurysternus, Haematopinus quadripertussus, Haematopinus tuberculatus, Linognathus vituli, Solenopotes capillatus* (cattle), *Linognathus ovillus, Linognathus pedalis, Linognathus oviformes* (sheep), *L. oviformes, Linognathus stenopsis* (goat) (see Figures. 1-30, 1-32, and 1-34).

Mallophagans. *Damalinia bovis* (cattle), *Damalinia ovis* (sheep). *Damalinia caprae, Damalinia limbatus, Damalinia* (Holokartikos) *crassipes* (goats) (see Figure 1-39).

Siphonapterans. *E. gallinacea* (see Figure 1-48).

Ctenocephalides felis can cause severe distress in calves.

ARACHNIDS

Metastigmata: Ixodidae. *Amblyomma americanum, Amblyomma cajennense, Amblyomma imitator, Amblyomma inornatum, Amblyomma maculatum, Amblyomma oblongoguttatum* (see Figure 1-61).

Boophilus annulatus, Boophilus microplus (see Figure 1-74).

D. andersoni, Dermacentor albipictus, Dermacentor occidentalis, Dermacentor nigrolineatus, D. variabilis, Dermacentor *(=Otocentor)* nitens (see Figures 1-75 and 1-76).

Ixodes cookei, Ixodes pacificus, Ixodes scapularis (see Figures 1-62, 1-68, and 1-69).

Metastigmata: Argasidae. *Otobius megnini* ("spinose ear tick") (see Figure 1-65).

Ornithodorus coriaceus, Ornithodorus turicata (see Figure 1-64).

Astigmata. *S. scabiei* (see Figure 1-84).

Chorioptes bovis (see Figures 1-89 and 1-90).

Psoroptes communis, Psoroptes cuniculi (see Figure 1-88).

Prostigmata. *Demodex bovis, Demodex ovis, Demodex caprae* (see Figures 1-95 and 6-8).

Psorobia ovis.

Trombiculidae (see Figures 1-98 and 1-99).

Mesostigmata. *Raillietia auris* (cattle), *Raillietia caprae* (goats). Ear mites (see Figure 1-81).

PROTOZOAN

B. besnoiti (coccidian).

NEMATODES

Stephanofilaria stilesi (6 mm, Filarioidea). Very small adult filariids in skin of ventral abdomen.

Parafilaria bovicola (Filarioidea). Adults in subcutaneous tissues cause "summer bleeding" in cattle.

O. gutterosa, O. lienalis, O. bovis (Filarioidea). Microfilariae found in dermis of cattle.

E. schneideri (Filarioidea).

R. strongyloides (Rhabditida) (see Figures 3-106, 6-69, and 6-70).

■ PARASITES OF HORSES
Stages in Feces

The intestinal parasites of horses form a unique group. Horses host only two coccidian species, *C. parvum* and *Eimeria leukarti* (Figure 5-39), and only three species of tapeworms, all of which belong to the family Anoplocephalidae (Figure 5-40). Nematodes form the largest group (Figure 5-41), which includes one ascarid, two pinworms, one species of *Strongyloides,* three habronematid spirurids, and many strongylids. The horse hosts no hookworms or whipworm but 54 species of strongylids more than make up for these deficiencies. The strongylids are cosmopolitan in distribution, and naturally infected horses tend to harbor a dozen or more species simultaneously. The diagnostic dilemma associated with strongylid eggs is thus accentuated in the case of the horse. However, the major diagnostic categories can be identified by egg morphometry, as explained previously under the section Diagnostic Morphometry, or by fecal culture and reference to Figure 5-42.

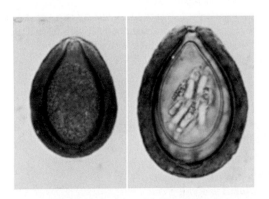

FIGURE 5-39 *Eimeria leuckarti* unsporulated *(left)* and sporulated *(right)* oocysts (×425).

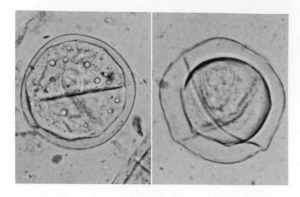

FIGURE 5-40 *Anoplocephala magna (left)* and *A. perfoliata (right)* eggs (×425). The oncospheres are enclosed by pear-shaped embryophores. The egg of *Paranoplocephala mamillana* is only three fourths as large as these.

Identification of Equine Microfilariae

Equine microfilariae are portrayed diagrammatically in Figure 5-43.

The sheathed microfilariae of *Setaria equina* may be demonstrated in blood samples by the techniques described for detecting the microfilarias of the canine heartworm.

Parafilaria multipapillosa microfilariae may be found in blood discharged from "summer bleeding" nodules caused by the adult female worms. They are less than 200 μm long, are unsheathed, and have a rounded posterior extremity (Supperer, 1953).

Microfilariae of *Onchocerca cervicalis, Onchocerca reticulata,* and *Elaeophora böhmi* may be demonstrated by excising a small piece of skin from near the linea alba and placing it in physiological saline solution. The microfilariae of these three species will soon be observed migrating out of the dermis into the saline solution. Leave the preparation set up overnight to detect low levels of microfiladerma.

O. cervicalis microfilariae are slender, delicate, and 207 to 240 μm long.

O. reticulata microfilariae are 330 to 370 μm long and have a long, whiplike tail ending in a fine point.

E. böhmi microfilariae are 300 to 330 μm long and may be distinguished from *O. reticulata* by a difference in the distance from the genital cell to the tip of the tail, which is greater than 140 mm for *O. reticulata* and less than 120 μm for *E. böhmi.*

Annotated Host-Organ Listing of Parasites of Horses
Alimentary System
Mouth
INSECT LARVAE
Gasterophilus intestinalis, Gasterophilus nasalis, Gasterophilus hemorrhoidalis.

PROTOZOAN
Trichomonas equibuccalis (mucosoflagellate). Found around gum margins of cheek teeth.

Stomach
NEMATODES
Draschia megastoma, Habronema muscae, Habronema microstoma (Spirurida) (see Figure 3-128).

T. axei (Trichostrongyloidea) (see Figures 3-69 and 3-71). May cause hypertrophic gastritis with mucosal proliferations.
INSECT LARVAE
G. intestinalis (see Figures 1-23 and 1-24).

Small intestine
NEMATODES
Parascaris equorum (Ascaridoidea) (see Figure 5-41).

Strongyloides westeri (Rhabditida) (see Figures 3-108, 5-41, and 6-71).
CESTODES
Anoplocephala magna, Paranoplocephala mamillana (see Figures 3-51, 3-52 and 5-40).
PROTOZOANS
Cryptosporidium spp.

E. leukarti (see Figures 5-39 and 6-30).

Giardia sp. (see Figure 5-60)
INSECTS
G. nasalis, G. hemorrhoidalis larvae, in duodenum.

Large intestine
NEMATODES
O. equi (150 mm), *Probstmayria vivipara* (3 mm) (Oxyurida) (see Figures 3-110 to 3-112, and 5-41).

FAMILY STRONGYLIDAE. The horse is host to about 60 species belonging to the family Strongylidae, and as many as 20 different species are often found in the same horse. Subfamily *Strongylinae. Strongylus vulgaris, S. edentatus, S. equinus, T. serratus, Triodontophorus brevicauda, T. tenuicollis, Triodontophorus nipponicus, Oesophagodontus robustus, Craterostomum acuticaudatum* (see Figures 3-62, 5-44, and 5-47, bottom row).

Subfamily Cyathostominae. Genera: *Cyathostomum, Cylicocyclus, Cylicostephanus, Cylicodontophorus, Poteriostomum, Paraposteriostomum, Petrovinema, Coronocyclus, Gyalocephalus* (Figures 5-45 to 5-55).

Each series can be identified by careful study of the stomal region alone. With fresh specimens, detail sufficient for identification can be seen without recourse to clearing agents. Simply mount the specimen under a coverslip in a drop of water. With this simple preparation it is usually possible to roll the specimen so that both dorsal and lateral aspects may be studied. Even preserved specimens may be

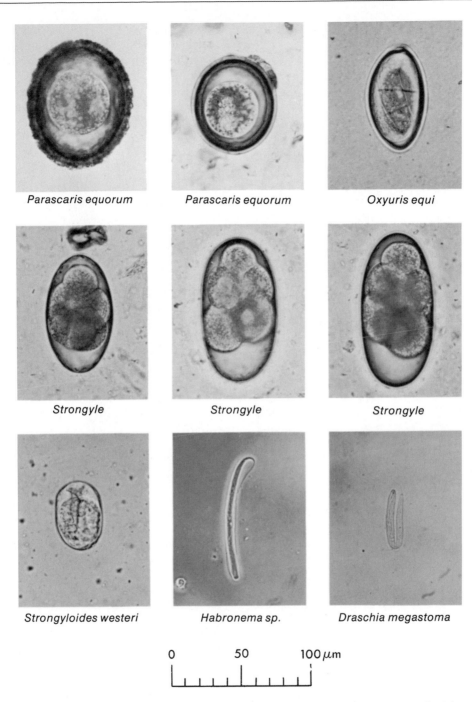

Parascaris equorum   *Parascaris equorum*   *Oxyuris equi*

Strongyle   *Strongyle*   *Strongyle*

Strongyloides westeri   *Habronema sp.*   *Draschia megastoma*

0   50   100 μm

FIGURE 5-41 Eggs of some nematode parasites of horses. *Parascaris equorum* eggs are yellowish brown with thick, subspherical, rough-surfaced shell walls and contain one cell. Eggs are often found with their external protein layer partially or completely detached. The exposed portions of such shells are smooth and clear. *Oxyuris equi* eggs are more likely to be recovered from anal scrapings than from fecal specimens. The egg shown here was collected by momentarily pressing the adhesive side of a piece of Scotch tape against a horse's anus and then was mounted by sticking the tape to a microscope slide. Strongyle eggs present the usual differential diagnostic problem. Recourse may be had to fecal culture and identification of infective third stage larvae (Figure 5-42). *Strongyloides westeri* eggs are smaller than strongyle eggs and contain a rhabditiform larva in fresh specimens. *Draschia* and *Habronema* eggs are cigar shaped and contain a vermiform embryo. Such eggs are difficult to demonstrate in feces. If a technique for antemortem diagnosis of gastric habrone-miasis is essential, resort to xenodiagnosis using *Musca domestica* larvae for *D. megastoma* and *H. muscae,* and *Stomoxys calcitrans* larvae for *H. microstoma.*

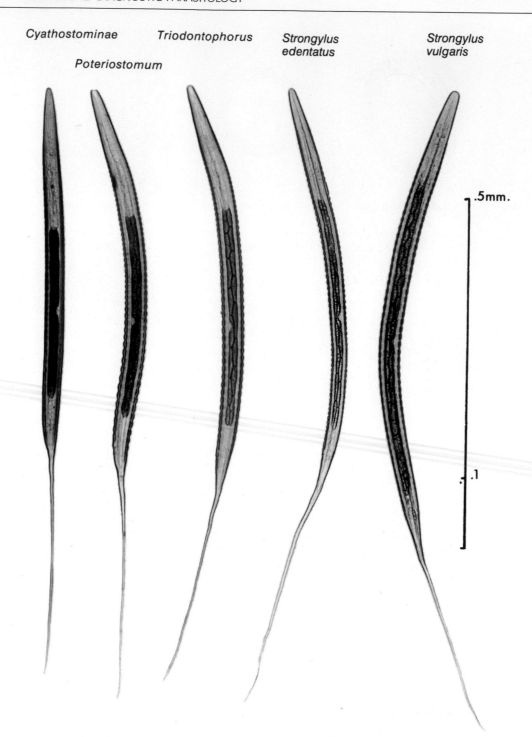

FIGURE 5-42 Infective third-stage larvae of some horse strongylids. Larvae of the subfamily Cyathostominae, represented here by *Cyathostomum catinatum,* have 8 intestinal cells. *Gyalocephalus capitatus* (not shown) has 12, *Poteriostomum* has 16, *Triodontophorus* has 18 (but the *T. serratus* larvae shown here have only 16), *Strongylus edentatus* has 18 to 20, and *Strongylus vulgaris* has 32 intestinal cells. *S. vulgaris* is easily distinguished from all the rest by its large size and long column of intestinal cells.

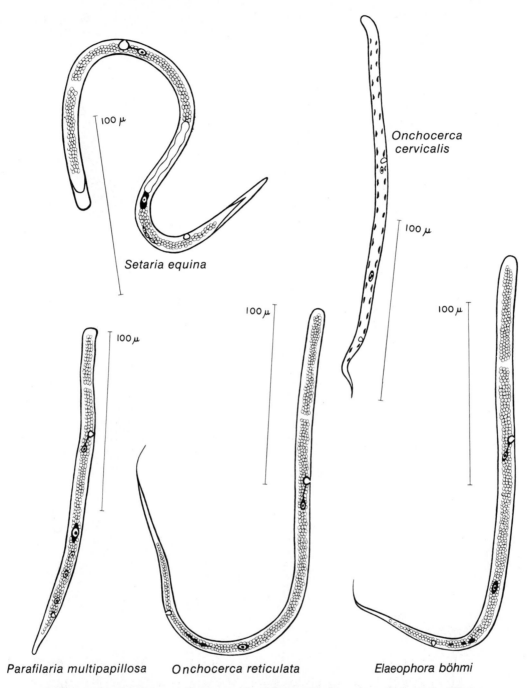

Onchocerca cervicalis

100 μ

Setaria equina

100 μ

100 μ

100 μ

100 μ

Parafilaria multipapillosa   *Onchocerca reticulata*   *Elaeophora böhmi*

FIGURE 5-43 Microfilariae of filariid parasites of horses. (Redrawn from Supperer R.: *Wiener Tierärztliche Monatschr* 40:214–216, 1953.)

studied in this manner but tend to be considerably less transparent than fresh specimens. For comparisons to be made easily, illustrations of the species that bear the greatest resemblance to one another have been grouped together. The nomenclature of J. Ralph Lichtenfel's excellent monograph *Helminths of Domestic Equids* (Proc Helminth Soc Wash, 42, 1975) along with a recent update on the taxonomy of the group (Lichtenfels et al, 1998) is the system that has been applied in the following pictorial key.

CESTODE

Anoplocephala perfoliata (see Figures 3-52 and 5-40). Found mainly in the cecum, this tapeworm tends also to cluster in the ileum near the ileocecal valve, where it is associated with ulceration and chronic inflammation of the ileal wall.

Text continued on p. 345

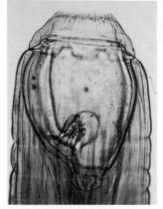

Strongylus vulgaris

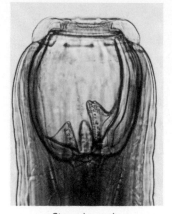

Strongylus equinus

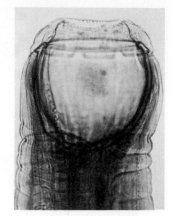

Strongylus edentatus

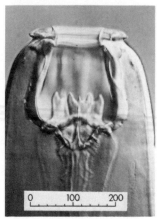

Triodontophorus brevicauda

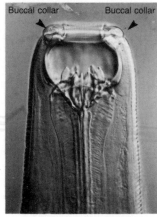

Buccal collar   Buccal collar

Triodontophorus serratus

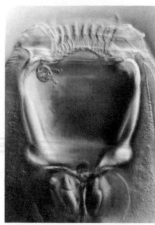

Oesophagodontus robustus

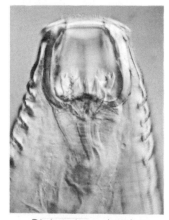

Triodontophorus nipponicus

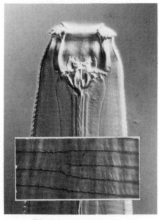

Triodontophorus tenuicollis

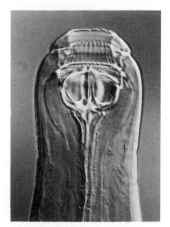

Gyalocephalus capitatus

FIGURE 5-44 Members of the subfamily Strongylinae (large strongyles) and *Gyalocephalus capitatus* (subfamily Cyathostominae). *Strongylus vulgaris* and *Oesophagodontus robustus* (×72); *Strongylus equinus* (×40); *Strongylus edentatus* (×33); *Triodontophorus* spp. and *Gyalocephalus capitatus* (×112).
(*Strongylus* spp. cleared and mounted by the glycol methacrylate method of Pijanowski, et al: *Cornell Vet* 62:333–336, 1972).

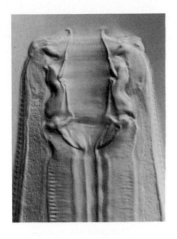
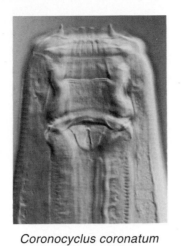
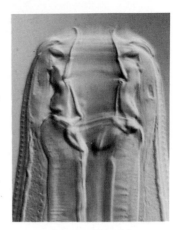

Coronocyclus coronatum

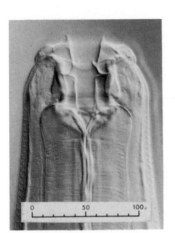
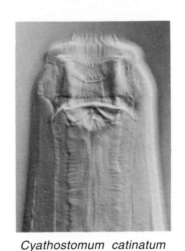
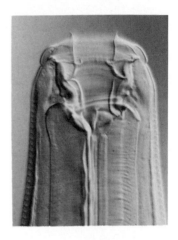

Cyathostomum catinatum

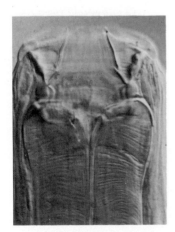
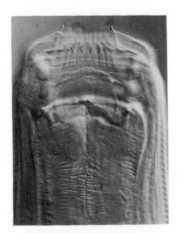
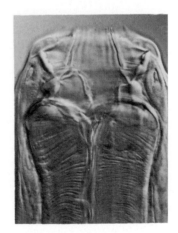

Cyathostomum tetracanthum

FIGURE 5-45   Members of the subfamily Cyathostominae. Dorsoventral *(left)*, dorsal surface *(center)*, and lateral *(right)* views of the heads of *Coronocyclus coronatus (top row)*, *C. catinatum (middle row)*, and *Cyathostomum tetracanthum (bottom row)*. (All ×283.)

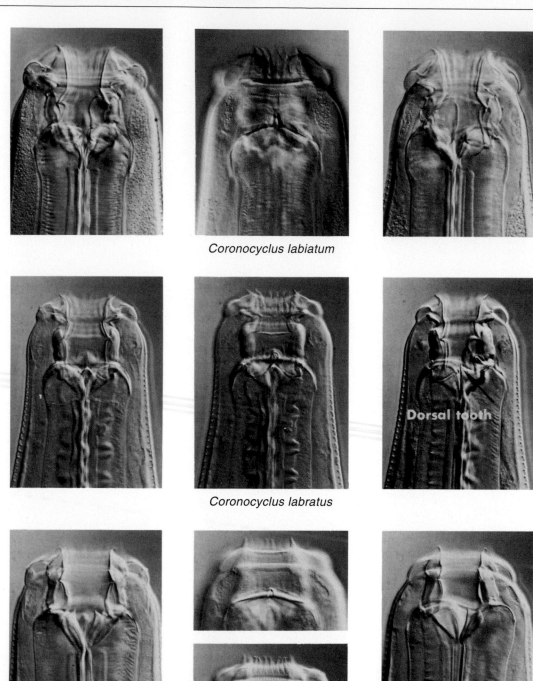

Coronocyclus labiatum

Coronocyclus labratus

Dorsal tooth

Cylicostephanus goldi

FIGURE 5-46 Members of the subfamily Cyathostominae. Dorsoventral *(left)*, dorsal surface *(center)*, and lateral *(right)* of the heads of *Coronocyclus labiatus (top row)*, *C. labratus (middle row)*, and *Cylicostephanus goldi (bottom row)*. (All ×283.)

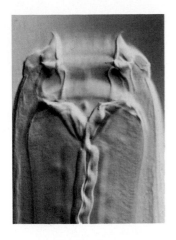
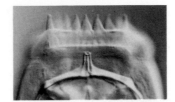
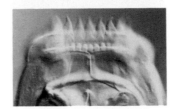
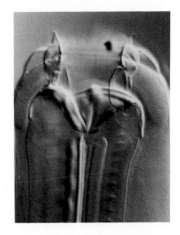

Cylicostephanus asymetricus

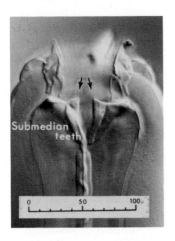
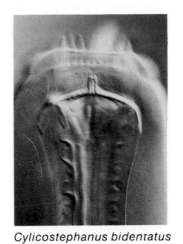

Cylicostephanus bidentatus

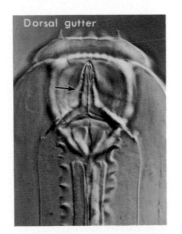
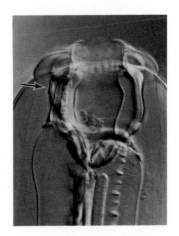

Craterostomum acuticaudatum

FIGURE 5-47 Members of the subfamily Cyathostominae and *Craterostomum acuticaudatum* (subfamily Strongylinae). Dorsoventral *(left)*, dorsal surface *(center)*, and lateral *(right)* views of the heads of *Cylicostephanus asymetricus (top row)*, *C. bidentatus (middle row)*, and *Craterostomum acuticaudatum (bottom row)*. (All ×283.)

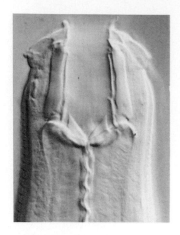
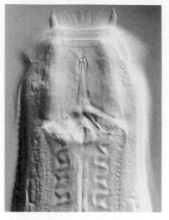
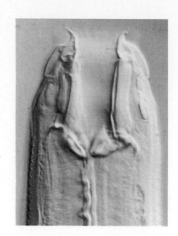

Cylicostephanus calicatus

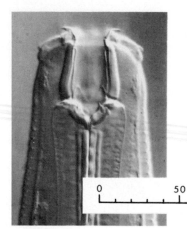
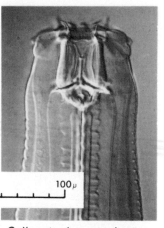
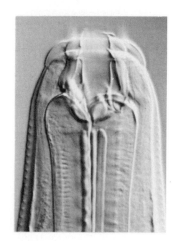

0   50   100 μ

Cylicostephanus minutus

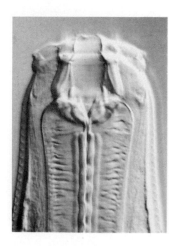
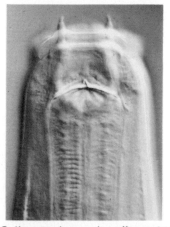
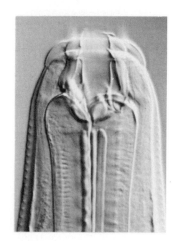

Cylicostephanus longibursatus

FIGURE 5-48 Members of the subfamily Cyathostominae. Dorsoventral *(left)*, dorsal surface *(center)*, and lateral *(right)* views of the heads of *Cylicostephanus calicatus (top row)*, *C. minutus (middle row)*, and *C. longibursatus (bottom row)*. (All ×425.)

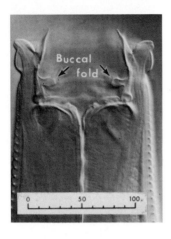
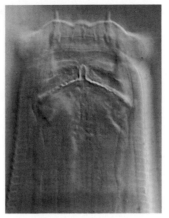
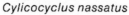
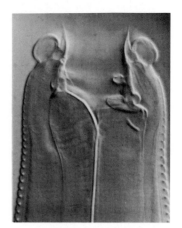

Cylicocyclus nassatus

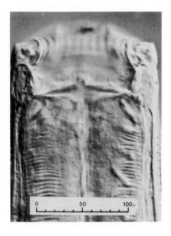
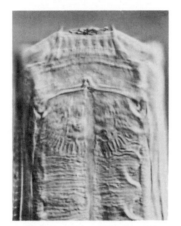
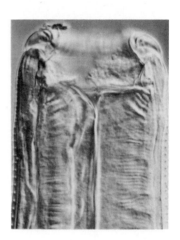

Cylicocyclus ashworthi

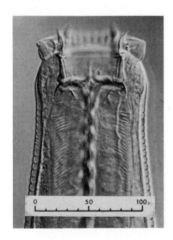
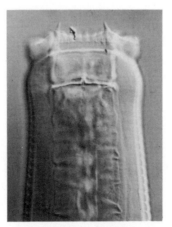
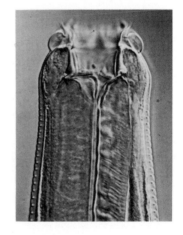

Cylicocyclus leptostomus

FIGURE 5-49 Members of the subfamily Cyathostominae. Dorsoventral *(left)*, dorsal surface *(center)*, and lateral *(right)* views of the heads of *Cylicocyclus nassatus (top row)*, *C. ashworthi (middle row)*, and *C. leptostomus (bottom row)*. (*C. nassatus* and *C. leptostomus* ×283, *C. ashworthi* ×242.)

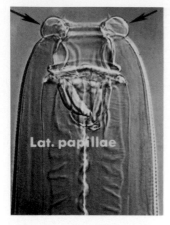
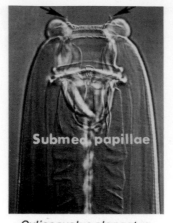
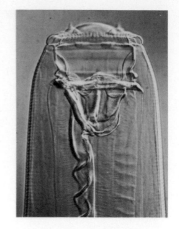

Cylicocyclus elongatus

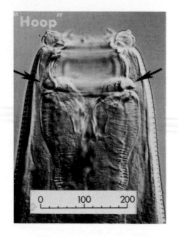
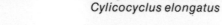
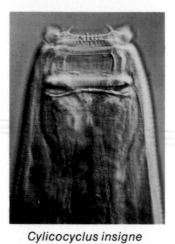
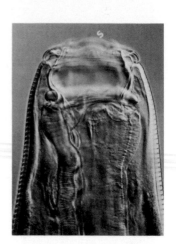

Cylicocyclus insigne

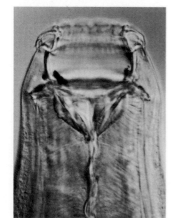
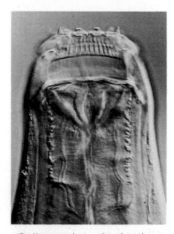
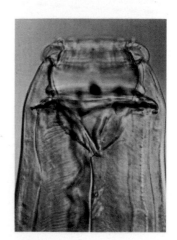

Cylicocyclus ultrajectinus

FIGURE 5-50 Members of the subfamily Cyathostominae. Dorsoventral *(left)*, dorsal surface *(center)*, and lateral *(right)* views of the heads of *Cylicocyclus elongatus (top row)*, *C. insigne (middle row)*, and *C. ultrajectinus (bottom row)*. (All ×112.)

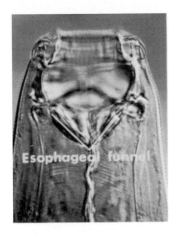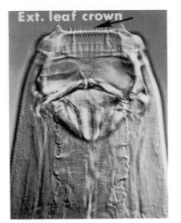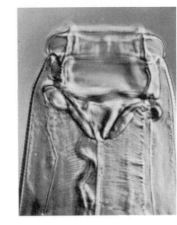

Poteriostomum imparidentatum

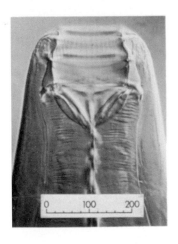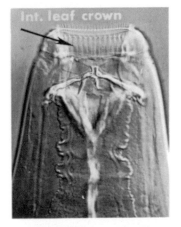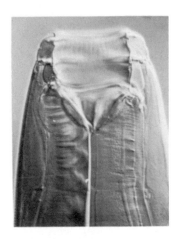

Poteriostomum ratzii

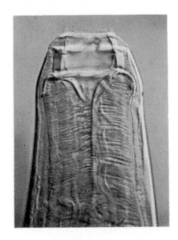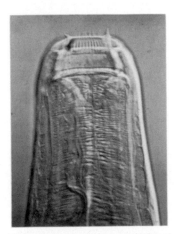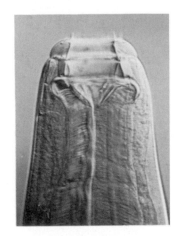

Paraposteriostomum mettami

FIGURE 5-51 Members of the subfamily Cyathostominae. Dorsoventral *(left)*, dorsal surface *(center)*, and lateral *(right)* views of the heads of *Poteriostomum imparidentatum (top row)*, *Poteriostomum ratzii (middle row)*, and *Paraposteriostomum mettami (bottom row)*. (All ×112.)

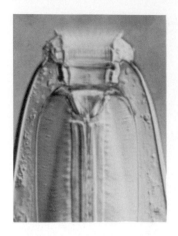
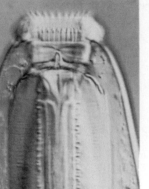
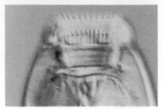
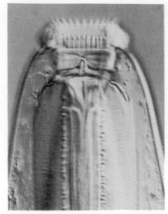

Cylicodontophorus bicoronatus

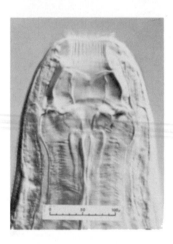
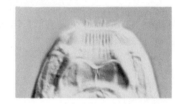
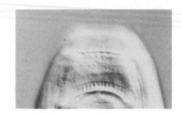
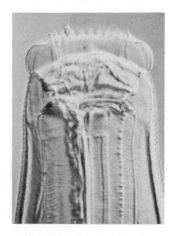

Paraposteriostomum euproctus

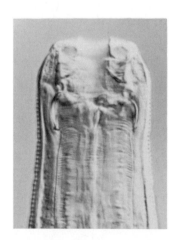
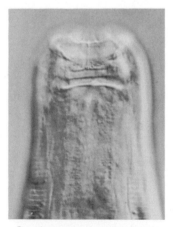

Cyathostomum pateratum

FIGURE 5-52 Members of the subfamily Cyathostominae. Dorsoventral *(left)*, dorsal surface *(center)*, and lateral *(right)* views of the heads of *Cylicodontophorus bicoronatus (top row)*, *Paraposteriostomum euproctus (middle row)*, and *Cyathostomum pateratum (bottom row)*. (All ×170.)

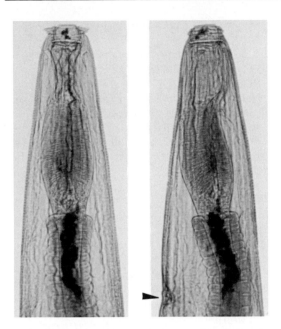

FIGURE 5-53 *Cylicocyclus auriculatus* (subfamily Cyathostominae) (×50). Note prominent lateral head papillae. Arrow indicates position of excretory pore.

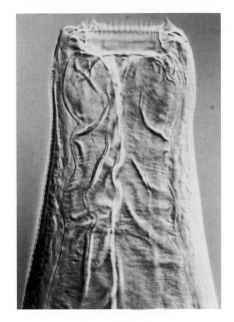

FIGURE 5-55 *Cylicocyclus brevicapsulatus,* the only homely member of the subfamily Cyathostominae (×168).

INSECT

G. hemorrhoidalis larvae.

Liver

NEMATODE LARVAE

P. equorum (Ascaridoidea).
S. edentatus, S. equinus (see Figures 6-75 to 6-79).

CESTODE LARVA

E. granulosus (Taeniidae) (see Figures 3-44 to 3-46 and 6-61).

Pancreas

NEMATODE

S. equinus (see Figure 6-78).

Peritoneum and Peritoneal Cavity

NEMATODES

S. equina (150 mm; Filarioidea) (see Figures 3-133 and 5-43).

S. edentatus (44 mm; Strongylinae) (see Figures 6-75 to 6-79).

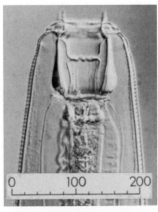

Petrovinema poculatum

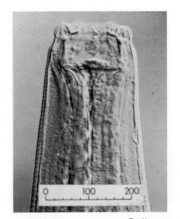

Cylicocyclus radiatus

FIGURE 5-54 Members of the subfamily Cyathostominae.

Respiratory System
Paranasal sinuses
INSECT LARVA
Rhinoestrus purpureus (Oestridae; exotic).

Bronchi and bronchioles
NEMATODE
Dictyocaulus arnfieldi (65 mm; Trichostrongyloidea) (see Figures 3-71 and 3-80).

Lung parenchyma
NEMATODE
S. edentatus (aberrant migration) (see Figure 6-75).
PNEUMOCYSTIS
Pneumocystis carinii (uncertain classification) (see Figure 6-39) are small protozoan-like fungi causing acute pneumonia in immunosuppressed hosts

Vascular System
Arteries
NEMATODES
S. vulgaris (Figure 5-56)
E. böhmi (Filarioidea) (see Figure 5-43). Found in intimal nodules of the wall of the aorta and other vessels. Exotic.

Blood
NEMATODE MICROFILARIA
S. equina (Filarioidea) (see Figure 5-43).
PROTOZOAN
Babesia caballi (piroplasm) (see Figure 2-27).

Skeletal Muscles and Connective Tissues

NEMATODES
T. spiralis first-stage larvae, found in Europe in horses fattened for human consumption.

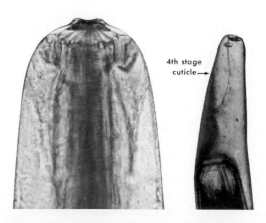

4th stage
cuticle→

FIGURE 5-56 *Strongylus vulgaris* fourth stage (*left*, ×108) and immature fifth stage (*right*, ×38) from a mural thrombus of the cranial mesenteric artery of a horse.

O. cervicalis adults in nuchal ligament.
PROTOZOAN CYSTS
S. bertrami, S. fayeri (coccidians) (see Table 2-1 and Figures 6-34 and 6-35).
INSECT LARVAE
H. bovis, H. lineatum (see Figure 1-21). In dorsal subcutaneous tissues of horses, erratically.
NEMATODE MICROFILARIAE
O. cervicalis, O. reticulata (Filarioidea) (see Figures 6-99 and 6-100). Microfilariae in dermis.

Urogenital System
Kidneys
NEMATODE
Halicephalobus (= Micronema) deletrix.
PROTOZOAN
Klossiella equi (coccidian) (Fig. 6-33).

Testes
NEMATODE
S. edentatus (see Figures 6-75 to 6-79). Immature fifth stage in vaginal tunics.

Nervous System
Brain and spinal cord
NEMATODES
S. vulgaris (see Figures 5-44 and 5-56). Fourth or fifth stages migrating erratically; even one worm can cause fatal neurological disease.
Setaria spp. (Filarioidea) (see Figures 3-32, 3-33, and 5-43). Erratic migration with neurological disease.
H. (Micronema) deletrix (Rhabditoidea).
D. megastoma (Spirurida) (Mayhew et al, 1983).
INSECTS
H. bovis, H. lineatum (Diptera). Erratic migration in atypical host. One larva can cause fatal neurological disease.
PROTOZOAN
Equine protozoan myelitis (EPM) organism, *Sarcocystis neurona.*

Eye
NEMATODES
Thelazia lacrymalis (Spirurida) (see Figure 3-125). Found in conjunctival sac and lacrimal ducts.
D. megastoma and *Habronema* spp. Larvae may cause habronemic conjunctivitis.
Onchocerca spp. microfilariae (see Figure 5-43).

Skin and Hair

INSECTS
M. autumnalis, S. calcitrans (Diptera: Muscidae) (see Figures 1-13 and 1-14).

Hippobosca equina, Lipoptena cervi (Diptera: Hippoboscidae) (see Figure 1-17).

G. intestinalis, G. nasalis, G. hemorrhoidalis (Diptera).

Tabanus spp., *Chrysops* spp. (Diptera: Tabanidae) (see Figures 1-10 and 1-11).

Haematopinus asini (Anoplura).

Damalinia equi (Mallophaga: Ischnocera).

Echidnophaga gallinacea (Siphonaptera) (see Figure 1-48).

Triatoma sanguisuga (Hemiptera: Triatominae) (see Figure 1-56).

INSECT LARVAE

H. bovis, H. lineatum (Diptera) (see Figure 1-21). In subcutis of the saddle area.

ARACHNIDS

Amblyomma, Anocentor, Boophilus, Dermacentor, Haemaphysalis, Hyalomma, Ixodes, Rhipicephalus (Metastigmata: Ixodidae) (see Figures 1-66 to 1-75).

S. scabiei (Sarcoptidae; Astigmata) (see Figure 1-84).

P. communis, P. cuniculi, C. bovis (Psoroptidae; Astigmata) (see Figures 1-88, 1-89, and 1-90).

Trombiculidae (Prostigmata) (see Figures 1-98 and 1-99).

Demodex equi (Prostigmata) (see Figure 1-95).

NEMATODE MICROFILARIAE AND LARVAE

P. multipapillosa (Filarioidea) (see Figure 5-43). Microfilariae in serosanguineous discharge from ulcerated nodules.

O. cervicalis, O. reticulata (Filarioidea) (see Figures 5-43, 6-99, and 6-100). Microfilariae of *Onchocerca* are almost universally present in the dermis of horses, especially the dermis of the ventrum.

R. strongyloides (Rhabditida) (see Figure 3-106).

D. megastoma, H. muscae, H. microstoma (Spirurida). Larvae of these species excite exuberant granulomatous reactions in skin wounds, areas of skin subject to frequent wetting, and ocular conjunctiva.

■ PARASITES OF SWINE
Stages in Feces

Intestinal protozoa include eight species of *Eimeria* and *Isospora suis* (Figure 5-57), *Entamoeba* spp., *Iodamoeba buetschlii, Endolimax nana, Giardia* spp., other flagellates, and the very common ciliate *B. coli* (see Figure 2-7).

The following nematodes are not represented in Figure 5-58: *S. dentatus* eggs are large and morulated and are found in urine specimens from infected swine. The last urine voided contains the highest concentration of eggs. *Strongyloides ransomi* eggs resemble those of *S. papillosus* (see Figure 5-32). *Ascarops* and *Physocephalus* produce thick-walled, larvated eggs.

Examination for Trichinae
Squash Preparation

Moderate to heavy *T. spiralis* infections can be diagnosed by simply squashing bits of muscle tissue between two glass slides and scanning under low power. The diaphragm and masseter muscles are especially likely to yield positive findings.

1. Detach a small scrap of meat and place it on a microscope slide.
2. Cover with a second microscope slide and press the two slides together with the thumb and forefinger, thus squashing the scrap of meat.
3. While maintaining pressure, bind the slides firmly together by wrapping each end with adhesive tape.
4. Trim off any meat protruding from between the slides to avoid contaminating the microscope stage.
5. Scan the entire field under low power. Larvae, if present, are easily visible (Figure 5-59). *Note:* This procedure is also applicable to the other tissue-dwelling parasites such as the smaller lungworms of sheep and carnivorans, encysted Toxocara larvae, and the like.

Tissue Digestion

Peptic digestion is used to detect light infection with *T. spiralis* and other nematodes in tissues. Gastric juice digests the muscle tissue but not the larvae of *T. spiralis*. Pepsin-acid solution consists of 0.2 g granular pepsin and 1.0 ml concentrated hydrochloric acid in 100 ml distilled water.

1. Weigh out 4 g of tissue and mince it with a scalpel.
2. Add 100 ml of pepsin-acid solution and allow to stand for about 1 to 6 hours at 37 °C.
3. Decant excess supernatant carefully, suspend sediment, and transfer to a Petri plate.
4. Count larvae under a dissecting microscope. Larvae may be retrieved with a Pasteur pipette for closer study under the compound microscope.

Annotated Host-Organ List of Parasites of Swine
Alimentary System
Mouth and Esophagus

NEMATODES

G. pulchrum (150 mm; Spirurida) (see Figure 5-68).

Eucoleus (=*Capillaria*) *garfiai* found in the epithelia of the tongue of wild pigs (Trichinelloidea).

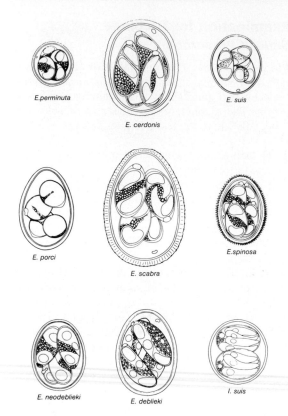

FIGURE 5-57 Sporulated oocysts of eight species of *Eimeria* and one species of *Isospora* from swine. (From Vetterling JM: *J Parasitol* 51:909, 1965.)

Stomach

NEMATODES
Physocephalus sexalatus (see Figure 3-127), *Ascarops strongylina*, *Gnathostoma hispidum* (see Figure 3-122), and *Simondsia paradoxum* (Spirurida).

Hyostrongylus rubidus (9 mm) and *Ollulanus tricuspis* (1 mm) (Trichostrongyloidea) (see Figures 3-71 and 3-77).

Aonchotheca (= Capillaria) gastrosuis (Trichinelloidea) (see Figure 5-28).

Small intestine

NEMATODES
A. suum (410 mm; Ascaridoidea) (see Figures 3-113 and 5-58).

Globocephalus urosubulatus (6 mm; Ancylostomatoidea) (see Figure 3-93).

S. ransomi (5 mm; Rhabditida) (see Figure 3-108).

T. spiralis (4 mm; Trichinelloidea) (see Figure 3-137).

ACANTHOCEPHALAN
M. hirudinaceus (470 mm.) (see Figure 3-143).

PROTOZOANS
Eimeria debliecki and about 10 other species of Eimeria, I. suis (coccidians).

G. lamblia (mucosoflagellate) (see Figure 5-60).

Cecum and colon

NEMATODES
Oesophagostomum dentatum, Oesophagostomum brevicaudum, Oesophagostomum georgianum, Oesophagostomum quadrispinulatum (Strongyloidea) (see Figure 3-87).

T. suis (Trichinelloidea) (see Figures 3-140 and 5-58).

PROTOZOANS
E. histolytica, E. coli, Entamoeba suis, E. nana, I. buetschlii (amebas).

Chilomastix mesnili, Tetratrichomonas buttreyi, Trichomitus rotunda, T. suis (mucosoflagellates).

B. coli (ciliate) (see Figures 2-7).

Liver, Pancreas, and Peritoneal Cavity

NEMATODE LARVAE
A. suum (Ascaridoidea) (see Fig. 3-114). Migrating larvae cause "milk spot" lesions on the liver surface.

S. dentatus (Strongyloidea) migrating larvae in liver and pancreas (see Figure 3-90).

TREMATODES
F. hepatica, F. gigantica (see Figures 3-2 and 3-11).

CESTODE LARVAE
E. granulosus (Taeniidae) (see Figures 3-44 to 3-46 and 6-60).

T. hydatigena (Taeniidae) (see Figure 3-38).

Respiratory System

Bronchi and bronchioles

NEMATODES
Metastrongylus apri, Metastrongylus salmi, Metastrongylus pudendotectus (Strongylida) (see Figure 3-98).

Lung parenchyma

NEMATODE LARVA
A. suum (see Figure 3-114).

CESTODE LARVA
E. granulosus (Taeniidae) (see Figures 3-44 to 3-46 and 6-61).

TREMATODE
P. kellicotti (Troglotrematidae) (see Figures 3-14, 3-15, and 5-20, *B*).

Skeletal Muscles and Connective Tissues

NEMATODE LARVA
T. spiralis (Trichinelloidea) (see Figures 5-59 and 6-104).

CESTODE LARVAE
Taenia solium (Taeniidae) (see Figures 6-56 and 6-56). *S. mansonoides* (Diphyllobothriidae) (see Figures 3-31 and 6-64).

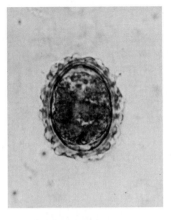

Ascaris suum

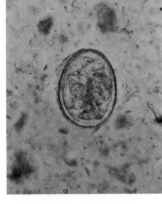

A. suum (infertile)

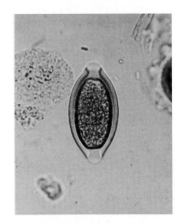

Trichuris suis

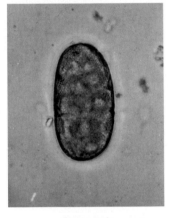

Strongyle

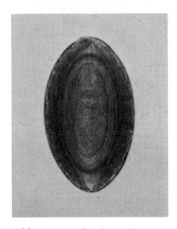

Metastrongylus sp.

Macracanthorhynchus hirudinaceus

FIGURE 5-58 Eggs of some parasites of swine (×425). *Ascaris suum* eggs have a rough, bile-stained, external protein layer. Infertile *A. suum* eggs are common. Strongyle eggs may represent infection with *Hyostrongylus rubidus, Oesophagostomum* spp., *Globocephalus urosubulatus,* or *Necator americanus,* but, most commonly, with only the first two. *Trichuris suis* are typical of the genus. *Trichuris suis* and *T. trichiura* (human whipworm) are possibly nonspecific. *Metastrongylus* spp. eggs are small and subglobular and contain a larva. *Macracanthorhynchus hirudinaceus* (Acanthocephala) eggs have three concentric, ellipsoidal shells surrounding the acanthor embryo.

TREMATODE LARVA

Alaria (mesocercaria, Diplostomatidae).

PROTOZOAN CYSTS

S. miescheriana, S. porcifelis, Sarcocystis suihominis (coccidians) (see Table 2-1 and Figures 6-34 and 6-35).

Urogenital System

NEMATODE

S. dentatus (45 mm; Strongylida) (see Figure 3-90). Stout, white worms in the kidneys, ureters, urinary bladder, perirenal fat, pork chops, spinal canal, and elsewhere as a result of erratic migrations.

Skin and Hair

INSECTS

Musca, Stomoxys (Diptera) (see Figures 1-13 and 1-14).

Haematopinus suis (Anoplura) (see Figure 1-31).

P. irritans, E. gallinacea, Tunga penetrans (Siphonaptera) (see Figures 1-48 and 1-50).

ARACHNIDS

Metastigmata (ticks) (see Figures 1-66 to 1-77).

S. scabiei (Astigmata) (see Figure1-84).

Demodex phylloides (Prostigmata).

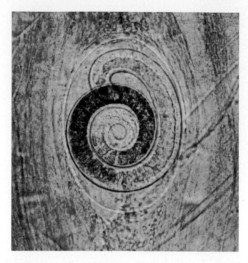

FIGURE 5-59   *Trichinella spiralis* cyst in a fresh squash preparation of pork muscle (×160).

■ PARASITES OF LABORATORY RABBITS AND RODENTS

Many parasites lose all opportunity to complete their life histories the day their host becomes a member of a laboratory animal colony. Although they may limit the usefulness of their immediate hosts as experimental subjects, such parasites present no continuing problem of control. Heartworm infection, for example, renders a dog unfit for experiments involving the circulatory or respiratory system but, in the absence of mosquitoes, must remain confined to the host in which it arrived. On the other hand, a surprising variety of arthropod, protozoan, and helminth parasites do succeed in maintaining impressive populations even in reasonably hygienic laboratory animal colonies. Hair-clasping mites, mucosoflagellates, coccidians, *Hymenolepis* tapeworms, and pinworms are particularly common. The following incomplete outline includes only the common parasites of laboratory rabbits, rats, mice, guinea pigs, monkeys, and apes.

Stages in Feces

A few of the more common parasites of rodents and rabbits are represented in Figure 5-60.

Annotated Host-Organ Listing of Common Parasites of Rabbits
Alimentary System
Stomach
NEMATODES
Obeliscoides cuniculi, Graphidium strigosum (18 to 20 mm; Trichostrongyloidea) (Figure 5-61).

Spicules of *O. cuniculi* 0.54 mm; of *G. strigosum* 2.4 mm.

Intestine
NEMATODES
Trichostrongylus retortaeformis, Nematodirus leporis (Trichostrongyloidea) (see Figures 3-69 and 3-71).
   S. papillosus (6 mm; Rhabditida).
   Passalurus ambiguus (11 mm; Oxyurida) (see Figure 3-109).
   Trichuris leporis (Trichinelloidea).
CESTODE
   Cittotaenia ctenoides (Anoplocephalidae) (see Figure 5-60).
PROTOZOANS
   Eimeria spp. (coccidian) (see Figure 5-60). Ten species of *Eimeria* parasitize the intestinal epithelium and cause diarrhea and emaciation.
   Entamoeba cuniculi (ameba). Nonpathogenic.

Liver and Peritoneal Cavity
PROTOZOAN
Eimeria stiedae causes biliary coccidiosis.
CESTODE LARVA
T. pisiformis (Taeniidae) (Figure 5-62).

Skin and Hair
ARACHNIDS
P. cuniculi (Astigmata) (see Figure 1-88).
   Sarcoptes, Chorioptes (Astigmata) (see Figures 1-84, 1-89, and 1-90).
   Leporacarus gibbus (Figure 5-63).
   Cheyletiella parasitovorax (Prostigmata) (see Figure 1-96).

Annotated Host-Organ Listing of Common Parasites of Rats
Alimentary System
Stomach and intestines
NEMATODES
Nippostrongylus brasiliensis (6 mm; Trichostrongyloidea) (see Figure 5-64).
   Strongyloides ratti (Rhabditida) (see Figure 3-108).
   Gongylonema neoplasticum (Spirurida).
   Syphacia muris, Aspiculuris ratti (Oxyurida) (see Figure 5-65).
   Heterakis spumosa (16 mm; Ascaridida).
   T. spiralis (Trichinelloidea) (see Figure 3-137).
   Trichuris muris (Trichinelloidea).
CESTODE
Hymenolepis diminuta (Hymenolopidae) (see Figure 5-35). Scolex without hooks.

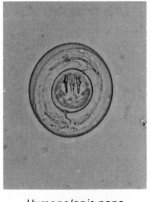
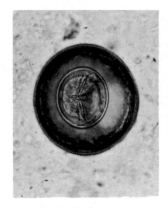
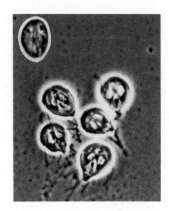

Hymenolepis nana   *H. diminuta*   *Giardia*

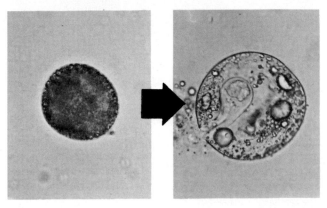
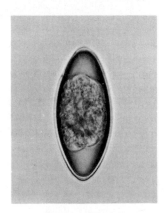

Cittotaenia ctenoides   *Aspiculuris*

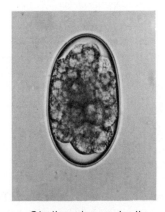
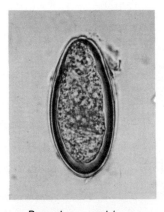
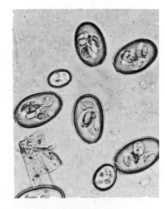

Obeliscodes cuniculi   *Passalurus ambiguus*   *Eimeria*

FIGURE 5-60 Common parasites of laboratory mice, rats, and rabbits. For a more comprehensive listing of laboratory animal parasites by host and organ, see text. MOUSE AND RAT: *Hymenolepis nana* and *H. diminuta* (Hymenolepidae) are also parasites of man. *Hymenolepis nana* infection in rodent colonies is directly infective to human beings; no intermediate host is required by this tapeworm. Various beetles and cockroaches serve as intermediate hosts for *H. diminuta* and, facultatively, for *H. nana*. *Giardia* (Mastigophora) trophozoites *(group of five, center)* and cysts *(inset, upper left)* are common parasites of mice. RABBIT: *Cittotaenia ctenoides* (Anoplocephalidae) eggs appear as amorphous spheres *(left of arrow)* until crushed by pressure on the coverslip *(right of arrow)*, whereupon the oncosphere and pear-shaped embryophore become visible. *Obeliscoides cuniculi* eggs are typical strongyle eggs. *Passalurus ambiguus* (Oxyuridae) are somewhat asymmetrical and have a cap at one end. *Eimeria,* sporulated oocysts. Avoid mistaking *Saccharomycopsis gutulatus* (see Figure 5-6) for a bona fide parasite of the rabbit. All ×425 except Giardia (×1000).

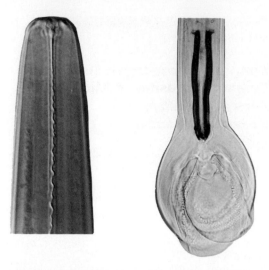

FIGURE 5-61 *Obeliscoides cuniculi,* stomal end *(left)* and bursa and spicules of male *(right)* (×120).

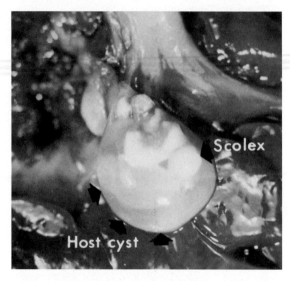

FIGURE 5-62 Cysticercus of *Taenia pisiformis* on the surface of the liver of a domestic rabbit (about ×3).

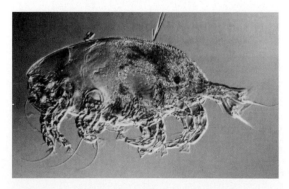

FIGURE 5-63 *Leporacarus gibbus,* a hair-clasping mite of rabbits (×100).
(Specimen courtesy of Dr. Stephen Weisbroth.)

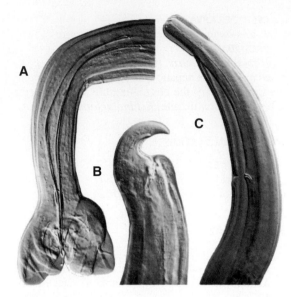

FIGURE 5-64 *Nippostrongylus brasiliensis.* **A,** Bursa and spicules of male (×125). **B,** Caudal end of female (×150). **C,** Esophageal region (×150).

PROTOZOANS

Eimeria nieschultzi and other species (coccidians) (see Figure 5-35).

Giardia (mucosoflagellate) (see Figure 5-60).

Liver

NEMATODE

C. (=Capillaria) hepaticum (Trichinelloidea) (see Fig. 6-105).

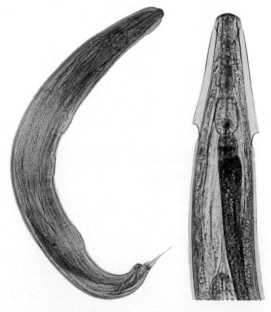

FIGURE 5-65 Pinworms of mice: *Syphacia obvelata* male *(left)* and *Aspiculuris tetraptera* anterior end *(right)* (×80).

CESTODE LARVA

T. taeniaeformis (Taeniidae) (see Figure 6-58).

PROTOZOAN

Hepatozoon muris (plasmodium). Schizogony takes place in the hepatic cells; gamonts are found in the monocytes of the circulating blood. The vector is a mesostigmatid mite, *Echinolaelaps echidninus*.

Urogenital System

NEMATODES

Capillarid spp., *Trichosomoides crassicauda* (Trichinelloidea) (see Figure 3-142).

Skin and Hair

INSECTS

Polyplax spinulosa (Anoplura) (Figure 5-66).
Xenopsylla cheopis (Siphonaptera) (see Figure 1-49).

ARACHNIDS

Ornithonyssus bacoti (Mesostigmata).
Radfordia ensifera (Prostigmata).

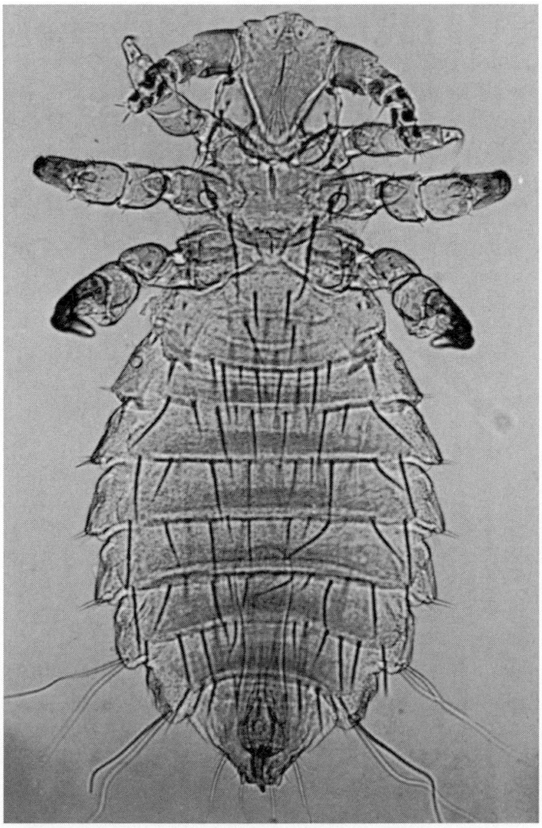

FIGURE 5-66 *Polyplax spinulosa* male (×108).

Notoedres muris (Astigmata) (see Figures 1-85 and 1-86).

Annotated Host-Organ Listing of Common Parasites of Mice

Alimentary System

Stomach and intestines

PROTOZOANS

Cryptosporidium muris (stomach) and *C. parvum* (small intestine).

NEMATODES

Heligmosomoides polygyrus (syn. *Nematospiroides dubius;* Trichostrongyloidea). Reddish, tightly coiled.
N. brasiliensis (6 mm; Trichostrongyloidea) (see Figure 5-64).
Syphacia obvelata, Aspiculuris tetraptera (Oxyuroidea) (see Figure 5-65).
H. spumosa (Ascaridida).
T. muris (Trichinelloidea).

CESTODES

Hymenolepis nana, H. diminuta (Hymenolepididae) (see Figure 5-60). The scolex of *H. nana* is armed with hooks; that of *H. diminuta* is unarmed.

Urogenital System

Kidneys

PROTOZOAN

Klossiella muris (coccidian).

Skin and Hair

INSECTS

Polyplax serrata (Anoplura) (see Figure 1-35).

ARACHNIDS

Myobia musculi, Radfordia affinis (Prostigmata) (see Figure 1-97). Myobiids do not migrate away from a dead host; the carcass must be scanned carefully with a stereoscopic microscope to find them.
Myocoptes musculinus (Astigmata) (see Figure 1-93).
O. bacoti, Allodermanyssus sanguineus (Mesostigmata).

Annotated Host-Organ Listing of Common Parasites of Guinea Pigs

Alimentary System

NEMATODE

Paraspidodera uncinata (Oxyurida).

CESTODE

H. nana (see Figure 5-60).

PROTOZOANS

Eimeria caviae (coccidian).
Balantidium sp. (ciliate) (see Figure 2-7).
Cryptosporidium wrairi.

Skin and Hair

INSECTS

Gliricola porcelli, Gyropus ovalis, Trimenopon hispidum (Mallophaga) (see Figure 1-45).

ARACHNIDS

Chirodiscoides caviae (Astigmata) (see Figure 1-92).

Trixacarus caviae.

■ PARASITES OF MONKEYS AND APES

The kinds of parasites to be found depends on the species and geographical origin of the monkey and on the duration and environmental conditions of its captivity. Certain parasites (e.g., *Strongyloides* and *Oesophagostomum*) flourish in captive monkeys. Others, especially those whose natural intermediate hosts are no longer available, tend to fade away. In mixed colonies, parasites that are not discriminating in their selection of hosts may spread to species of monkeys that, for geographical or ecological reasons, rarely or never infect in the wild. Such cross-infections are more likely to cause disease because of the lack of mutual adaptation of host and parasite. The following therefore represents a composite listing of the more common parasites of monkeys and apes without particular regard to natural host species' preferences or geographical origins.

Stages in Feces

Some eggs of primate parasites are shown in Figure 5-67. Many of the parasites are shared with humans, and a text such as *Atlas of Human Parasitology* (Ash

and Oribel, 1990) can be consulted for the identification of the many shared parasites.

Alimentary System

NEMATODES

Cephalobus parasiticus (Rhabditida). These harmless parasites of the stomach and intestines of *Macaca iris mordax* (and probably others) resemble the free-living generation of *Strongyloides*. Their rhabditiform larvae may be confused with those of *Strongyloides* on fecal examination. They do not, however, develop into filariform larvae, so the dilemma may be resolved by culturing the fecal specimen.

Strongyloides fuelleborni, S. stercoralis (Rhabditida) (see Figure 3-108). Simian strongyloidosis is a human health hazard.

Nochtia nochti (Trichostrongyloidea). Bright red worms lying within or protruding from gastric papillomata in the prepyloric region of the stomach. Cross sections of *N. nochti* in histological preparations display 16 distinct longitudinal cuticular ridges and channeled lateral alae.

Trichostrongylus, Molineus, Nematodirus (Trichostrongyloidea) (see Figure 3-71).

Oesophagostomum (Conoweberia) apiostomum, Oesophagostomum stephanostomum, Ternidens deminutus (Strongyloidea) (see Figures 3-62 and 5-68). Stout-bodied "nodular worms" with leaf crowns and transverse ventral cervical groove.

Necator, Ancylostoma, Globocephalus (Ancylostomatoidea) (see Figures. 3-93 and 3-94).

Ascaris lumbricoides (Ascaridoidea) (Figure 3-112). Trichuris spp. (Trichinelloidea).

Enterobius spp. (Oxyurida) (Figure 5-68). Pinworms are quite host specific. Generally speaking,

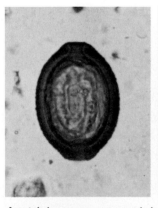 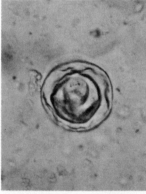 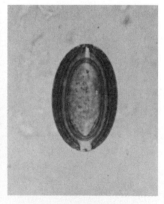

Anatrichosoma cynomolgi   *Anoplocephalidae*   *Prosthenorchis elegans*

FIGURE 5-67 Three parasites of primates. For a more complete listing of simian parasites by host and organ, see text. *Anatrichosoma cynomolgi* adult worms tunnel in the nasal mucosa. Anoplocephalid eggs have a pear-shaped embryophore surrounding the oncosphere. *Prosthenorchis elegans* (Acanthocephala) eggs have a thick outer shell and thin inner shells enclosing the embryo (acanthor).

a species of pinworm infects a genus of monkeys. *Enterobius vermicularis* and *Enterobius anthropopitheci* occur in chimpanzees. *Enterobius* spp. are usually considered nonpathogenic, but sometimes they invade the wall of the intestine and produce serious or even fatal disease.

Streptopharagus, Gongylonema, Protospirura, Physocephalus, Rictularia, Physaloptera (Spirurida) (see Figures 3-123, 3-124, 3-126, and 5-68). *Protospirura muricola,* a parasite of rodents that uses the cockroach *Leucophaea maderae* as intermediate host, has been observed to cause perforation of the stomach in captive monkeys (Foster and Johnson, 1939).

CESTODES
Bertiella studeri (Anoplocephalidae). Large, four suckers, no hooks.

H. nana (Hymenolepidae) (see Figure 5-60). Very small, four suckers, hooks.

ACANTHOCEPHALANS
Prosthenorchis, Moniliformis (see Figure 5-61).
TREMATODE
Gastrodiscoides hominis (Paramphistomatidae).
PROTOZOANS
B. coli (ciliate) (see Figure 2-7). Acute enteritis (Teare and Loomis, 1982).

E. histolytica, pathogenic as in humans.

G. lamblia (flagellate) (see Figure 5-60).

Liver and Pancreas

PROTOZOANS
Hepatocystis kochi schizonts.
E. histolytica, hepatic abscess.
NEMATODES
C. (=Capillaria) hepaticum (Trichinelloidea) (see Figure 6-105). Worms and eggs in hepatic parenchyma.

Trichospirura leptostoma. A 10- to 20-mm worm with a long capillary pharynx; associated with varying degrees of fibrosing pancreatitis. Found in pancreatic duct of American primates.

Respiratory System
Nose and throat
NEMATODE
Anatrichosoma (Trichinelloidea) (see Figure 5-61).
ANNELIDS
The leeches that attack the pharyngeal mucosa of monkeys are large, black annelids with a large cup-shaped caudal sucker. The presence of this bloodsucking parasite is suggested by chronic epistaxis in a recently captured monkey. When the host drinks infested water, the young leeches enter the mouth, nose, pharynx, or larynx and attach to the mucous membrane. They remain in these locations for several weeks unless removed.

ARACHNID
Rhinophaga spp.

Lungs
NEMATODES
Filaroides (Metastrongyloidea).
Metathelazia (Spirurida).
CESTODE LARVA
E. granulosus (Taeniidae) (see Figures 3-44 to 3-46 and 6-61).
ARACHNID
Pneumonyssus simicola (Mesostigmata).

Serous Cavities

NEMATODE
Dipetalonema spp. (Filarioidea) (see Figure 3-134).
CESTODE LARVAE
T. hydatigena (cysticercus) (see Figure 3-38).
Mesocestoides (tetrathyridium) (see Figures 6-63 and 6-63).
S. mansonoides (plerocercoid) (see Figures 3-31 and 6-64).
PENTASTOMID NYMPHS
Porocephalus, Armillifer, Linguatula.
ACANTHOCEPHALANS
Prosthenorchis spp.

Blood

NEMATODE MICROFILARIAE
Dirofilaria, Dipetalonema, Tetrapetalonema, Loa, Brugia (Filarioidea). Differentiation of the many kinds of microfilariae found in monkeys from all parts of the tropics is a task for the specialist. Many species remain to be described.
PROTOZOANS
Simian malaria organisms, *Plasmodium, Hepatocystis.*

Muscles and Connective Tissues

NEMATODES
Onchocerca, Dirofilaria, Dipetalonema, Tetrapetalonema, Loa, Brugia (Filarioidea) (see Figures 3-129 and 3-134). *Onchocerca* microfilariae are found in the dermis.
CESTODE LARVAE
Taenia (cysticercus).
Mesocestoides (tetrathyridium) (see Figures 6-63 and 6-64).
Spirometra (plerocercoid) (see Figures 3-31 and 6-65).

Skin and Hair

INSECTS
Pedicinus, Pthirus (Anoplura) (see Figure 1-37).

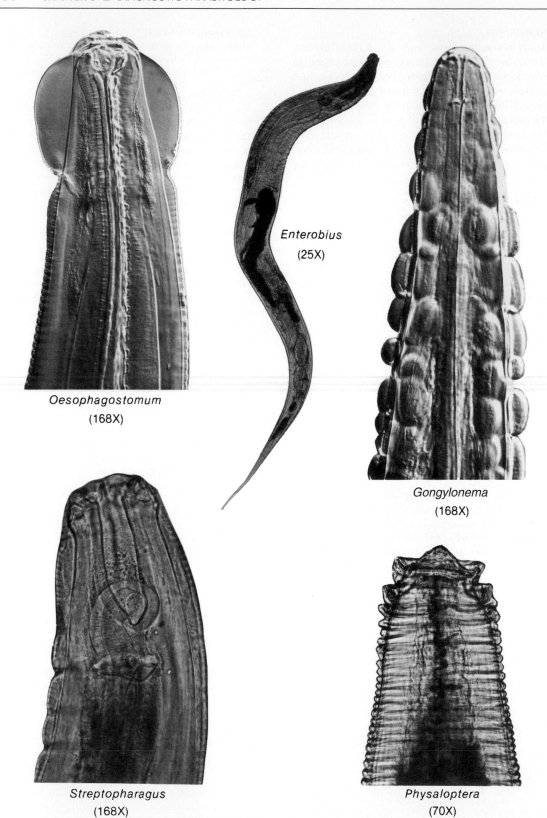

Oesophagostomum
(168X)

Enterobius
(25X)

Gongylonema
(168X)

Streptopharagus
(168X)

Physaloptera
(70X)

FIGURE 5-68 Some nematode parasites of monkeys and apes.
(Specimens courtesy of Dr. M.M. Rabstein.)

NEMATODES

Anatrichosoma cutaneum (Trichinelloidea). Very slender (25 by 0.2 mm) worms give rise to subcutaneous nodules, edema about the joints, and elongated, serpiginous blisters of the palms and soles. Adult females burrow in the epidermis of the palms and soles.

Onchocerca microfilariae.

Dracunculus (Spirurida) (see Figures 3-120 and 3-121).

■ REFERENCES

Agneessens J, Claerebout E, Vercruysse J: Development of a copro-antigen capture ELISA for detecting *Ostertagia ostertagi* infections in cattle, *Vet Parasitol* 97:227–238, 2001.

Ash LR, Orihel TC: *Atlas of human parasitology,* Chicago, 1990, ASCP Press.

Becklund WW: Revised check list of internal and external parasites of domestic animals in the United States and possessions and in Canada, *Am J Vet Res* 25:1380–1416, 1964.

Benbrook EA: *Outline of parasites reported for domesticated animals in North America,* ed 6, Ames, 1963, Iowa State University Press.

Binford CH, Connor DH: *Pathology of tropical and extraordinary diseases,* vols 1 and 2, Washington, D.C., 1976, A.F.I.P.

Chitwood MB, Lichtenfels JR: Identification of parasitic metazoa in tissue sections, *Exp Parasitol* 32:407–519, 1972.

Christie M, Jackson F: Specific identification of strongyle eggs in small samples of sheep feces, *Res Vet Sci* 32:113–117, 1982.

Craig TM, Barton CL, Mercer SH, et al: Dermal leishmaniasis in a Texas cat, *Am J Trop Med Hyg* 35:1110–1102, 1986.

Cunliffe G, Crofton DH: Egg sizes and differential egg counts in relation to sheep nematodes, *Parasitology* 43:275–286, 1953.

Cushion MT, Walzer PD, Smulian AG, et al: Terminology for the life cycle of *Pneumocystis carinii, Inf Immun* 65:43–65, 1997.

Deplazes P, Alther P, Tanner I, et al: *Echinococcus multilocularis* coproantigen detection by enzyme-linked immunosorbent assay in fox, dog, and cat populations, *J Parasitol* 85:115–121, 1999.

Dikmans G, Andrews JS: A comparative morphological study of the infective larvae of the common nematodes parasitic in the alimentary tract of sheep, *Trans Am Micros Soc* 52:1–25, 1933.

Dubey JP: A review of *Sarcocystis* of domestic animals and of other coccidia of cats and dogs, *J Am Vet Med Assoc* 169:1061–1078, 1976.

Dubey JP, Perry A, Kennedy MJ: Encephalitis caused by a *Sarcocystis*-like organism in a steer, *J Am Vet Med Assoc* 191:231–232, 1987.

Faler K, Faler K: Improved detection of intestinal parasites, *Mod Vet Pract* April:273–276, 1984.

Foster AO, Johnson CM: A preliminary note on the identity, life cycle, and pathogenicity of an important nematode parasite of captive monkeys, *Am J Trop Med* 19:265–277, 1939.

Gardiner CH, Fayer R, Dubey JR: *An atlas of protozoan parasites in animal tissues,* Washington, D.C., 1998, AFIP, American Registry of Pathology.

Georgi JR: Differential characters of *Filaroides milksi* Whitlock, 1956 and *Filaroides hirthi* Georgi and Anderson, *Proc Helminthol Soc Wash* 46:142–145, 1975.

Georgi JR, McCulloch CE: Diagnostic morphometry: Identification of helminth eggs by discriminant analysis of morphometric data. *Proc Helminthol Soc Wash* 56: 44–57, 1989.

Gordon HMcL, Whitlock HV: A new technique for counting nematode eggs in sheep faeces, *J Counc Sci Industr Res (Australia)* 12:50–52, 1939.

Hughes PL, Dubielzig RR, Kazacos KR: Multifocal retinitis in New Zealand sheep dogs, *Vet Pathol* 24:22–27, 1987.

Hunter GC, Quenouille MH: A statistical examination of the worm egg count sampling technique for sheep, *J Helminthol* 26:157–170, 1952.

Jenkins DJ, Fraser A, Bradshaw H, et al: Detection of *Echinococcus granulosus* coproantigens in Australian canids with natural or experimental infection, *J Parasitol* 86:140–145, 2000.

Kauzal GP, Gordon HMcL: A useful mixing apparatus for the preparation of suspensions of faeces for helminthological examinations, *J Counc Sci Industr Res* (Australia) 14:304–305, 1941.

Kazacos KR: Raccoon roundworms *(Baylisascaris procyonis):* a cause of animal and human disease. Station Bulletin No. 422. Agr. Expt. Sta., 1983, Purdue University.

Keith RK: Infective larvae of cattle nematodes, *Australian J Zool* 1:223–235, 1953.

Knott J: A method for making microfilarial surveys on day blood, *Trans Roy Soc Trop Med Hyg* 33:191–196, 1939.

Lichtenfels JR: Helminths of domestic equids, *Proc Helminthol Soc Wash* (Special Issue) 42:1–92, 1975.

Lichtenfels JR, Kharchenko VA, Krecek RC, et al: An annotated checklist by genus and species of 93 species level names for 51 recognized species of small strongyles (Nematoda: Strongyloidea: Cyathostominea) of horses, asses, and zebras of the world, *Vet Parasitol* 79:65–79, 1988.

Lindsay DS, Upton SJ, Dubey JP: A structural study of the *Neospora caninum* oocyst, *Int J Parasitol* 29:1521–1523, 1999.

Lowenstine LJ, Carpenter JL, O'Connor BM: Trombiculosis in a cat, *J Am Vet Med Assoc* 175:289–291, 1979.

Mayhew IG, Lichtenfels JR, Greiner EC, et al: Migration of a spirurid nematode through the brain of a horse, *J Am Vet Med Assoc* 180:1306–1311, 1983.

Newton WL, Wright WH: The occurrence of a dog filariid other than *Dirofilaria immitis* in the United States, *J Parasitol* 42:246–258, 1956.

Newton WL, Wright WH: A reevaluation of the canine filariasis problem in the United States, *Vet Med* 52:75–78, 1957.

Nichols RL: The etiology of visceral larva migrans, I: diagnostic morphology of infective second-stage *Toxocara* larvae, *J Parasitol* 42:349–362, 1956.

Nichols RL: The etiology of visceral larva migrans, II: comparative larval morphology of *Ascaris lumbricoides, Necator americanus, Strongyloides stercoralis,* and *Ancylostoma caninum, J Parasitol* 42:363–399, 1956.

O'Handley RMO, Olson ME, Fraser D, et al: Prevalence and genotypic characterisation of Giardia in dairy calves from Western Australia and Western Canada, *Vet Parasitol* 90:193–200, 2000.

Parsons JC, Bowman DD, Gillette DM, et al: Disseminated granulomatous disease in a cat caused by larvae of *Toxocara canis, J Comp Pathol* 99:343–346, 1988.

Schell SC: *How to know the Trematodes,* Dubuque, 1970, Wm. C. Brown Company.

Schnieder T, Heise M, Epe C: Genus-specific PCR for the differentiation of eggs or larvae from gastrointestinal nematodes of ruminants, *Parasitol Res* 85:895–898, 1999.

Sommer C: Digital image analysis and identification of eggs from bovine parasitic nematodes, *J Helminthol* 70:143–151, 1996.

Sommer C: Quantitative characterization of texture used for identification of eggs of bovine parasitic nematodes, *J Helminthol* 72:179–182, 1998.

Speare R, Tinsley DJ: Survey of cats for *Strongyloides felis, Austral Vet J* 64:191–192, 1987.

Stoll NR: Investigations on the control of hookworm disease, XV: an effective method of counting hookworm eggs in human feces, *Am J Hyg* 3:59–70, 1923.

Stoll NR: On methods of counting nematode ova in sheep dung, *Parasitology* 22:116–136, 1930.

Supperer R: Filariosen der Pferde in Österreich, *Wiener Tierärztliche Monatschr* 40:214–216, 1953.

Swenson CL, Silverman J, Stromberg PC, et al: Visceral leishmaniasis in an English Foxhound from an Ohio research colony, *J Am Vet Med Assoc* 193:1089–1092, 1988.

Teare JA, Loomis MR: Epizootic of balantidiasis in lowland gorillas, *J Am Vet Med Assoc* 181(11):1345–1347, 1982.

Theodoropoulos G, Loumos V, Anagnostopouos C, et al: A digital image analysis and neural network based system for identification of third-stage parastic strongyle larvae from domestic animals, *Comp Meth Prog Biomed* 62:69–76, 2000.

Thomas JS: Encephalomyelitis in a dog caused by *Baylisascaris* infection, *Vet Pathol* 25:94–95, 1988.

Toft JD, Eberhard ML: Parasitic diseases. In: Taylor BT, Abee CR, Henrickson R, editors: *Nonhuman primates in biomedical research: diseases,* San Diego, 1998, Academic Press, pp. 111–206.

Trayser CV, Todd KS: Life cycle of *Isospora burrowsi* n. sp. (Protozoa: Eimeriidae) from the dog *Canis familiaris, Am J Vet Res* 39:95–98, 1978.

Verster A: A taxonomic revision of the genus Taenia Linnaeus, 1758. *Onderstepoort J Vet Res* 36:3–58, 1969.

Whitlock JH: A practical dilution egg count procedure *J Am Vet Med Assoc* 98:466–469, 1941.

Whitlock JH: *The diagnosis of veterinary parasitisms,* Philadelphia, 1960, Lea & Febiger.

Xiao L, Bern C, Kimor J, et al: Identification of 5 types of Cryptosporidium parasites in children in Lima, Peru, *J Inf Dis* 183:492–497, 2001.

Zarlenga DS, Chute MB, Gasbarre LC, et al: A multiplex PCR assay for differentiating economically important gastrointestinal nemaatodes of cattle, *Vet Parasitol* 97:199–209, 2001.

CHAPTER 6

HISTOPATHOLOGICAL DIAGNOSIS

MARK L. EBERHARD

The microscopic identification of parasites in tissue sections is an interesting challenge. Often a diagnostician is provided with a single slide that shows only pieces of the parasite. In an attempt to identify an object believed to be a parasite, one should gather as much information about the patient as possible, including life history and clinical signs. It is also important to be familiar with the kind of parasites most likely to be found in the particular host and tissue under study, as well as in the specific geographical area. The host-organ listing of parasites in the preceding chapter should be considered as a checklist of possibilities. The main objective of this section is to emphasize some of the major microscopic anatomical features of parasites that can be helpful in their identification in histologic sections. For the arthropods and metazoan parasites, several defining characteristics can be listed for each group of parasites, but the presence or absence of a body cavity and digestive tract, and the type and distribution of muscle fibers are important criteria to be considered in making an initial placement into a major group. Table 6-1 includes the main microscopic characteristics of arthropods (including pentastomes), trematodes, cestodes, nematodes, and acanthocephalans as a quick reference.

For further reading and assistance with diagnosis of parasites in tissues, the following sources are helpful. A monograph dealing with the present subject is *Identification of Parasitic Metazoa in Tissue Sections* by MayBelle Chitwood and J. Ralph Lichtenfels, first published in *Experimental Parasitology* 32:407-519, 1972, and later reprinted by the U.S. Department of Agriculture. Texts dealing with the subject include *Pathology of Tropical and Extraordinary Diseases,* vol. 1 and 2, by C.H. Binford and D.H. Connor, Washington, D.C., 1976, Armed Forces Institute of Pathology; *Pathology of Infectious Diseases,* vol. 1 and 2, by D.H Connor, F.W. Chandler, D.A. Schwartz, H.J. Manz, and E.E. Lack, Stamford, Conn., 1997, Appleton & Lange; *An Atlas of Proto-*

zoan Parasites in Animal Tissues, by C.H. Gardiner, R. Fayer, and J.P. Dubey, USDA Agriculture Handbook No. 651, U.S. Government Printing Office, Washington, D.C., 1988 and ed. 2, published by AFIP, American Registry of Pathology, Washington, D.C.; *Diagnostic Pathology of Parasitic Infections with Clinical Correlations,* ed. 2, by Y. Gutierrez, Philadelphia, 1990, Lea & Febiger; *Parasites in Human Tissues* by T. C. Orihel and L. R. Ash, Chicago, 1995, American Society of Clinical Pathology Press; and *Pathology of Infectious Diseases,* vol. 1, Helminthiases, by W.M. Meyers, R.C. Neafie, A.M. Marty, and D.J. Wear, AFIP, 2000, American Registry of Pathology, Washington, D.C.

Arthropods

Arthropods, composed of hundreds of thousands of species, have such diverse features that attempting to describe them succinctly is nearly impossible. However, there are several morphologic features that can be seen in sections that are typical of the group. Arthropods have a chitinous exoskeleton, usually thick and dark, although often the exoskeleton itself does not take up stain. In certain areas of the body, the exoskeleton is jointed, and in these areas the cuticle is thin. Arthropods have striated muscle, which is diagnostic. Arthropods also have a tracheal system that in section appears as variously sized tubes coursing throughout the body. The large tracheal tubes have chitinous reinforcing rings. Often seen in sections of arthropods are darkly staining fat bodies. Frequently, arthropods have rounded to elongated bodies in tissue section, and, on occasion, paired jointed legs can be observed. Together or alone, these features serve to distinguish the arthropods.

The three major groups of arthropods that are encountered in tissue sections are (1) the insects (subphylum Mandibulata, class Insecta), which include fly larvae (maggots) that cause myiasis; (2) mites and, rarely, ticks (subphylum Chelicerata, class

TABLE 6-1 ■ Main Microscopic Characteristics of the Arthropods and Metazoan Parasites

	Body cavity	Muscle layer	Digestive tract	Special features
Arthropods	Present	Striated	Present	Chitinized or sclerotized cuticle Segmented body Jointed appendices
Pentastomids	Present	Striated	Present	Chitinized cuticle with sclerotized openings Acidophilic glands
Trematodes	Absent (parenchymatous body)	Unstriated Subtegumental Inconspicuous	Present	Tegument Spines Suckers Hermaphrodites
Cestodes	Absent (parenchymatous body)	Outer layer (subtegumental) Inner layer sparse (parenchymal and sparse)	Absent	Tegument Calcareous corpuscles Scolex Suckers Segmented body (adult stage)
Nematodes	Present (pseudocoelom)	Unstriated Prominent Polymyarian (coelomyarian) Meromyarian (platymyarian)	Present	Cuticle Thin hypodermis Characteristic esophagus and intestine in cross section
Acanthocephalans	Present (pseudocoelom)	Unstriated Prominent	Absent	Thick hypodermis with lacunar system Proboscis

Arachnida); and (3) the pentastomes (subphylum Pentastomida).

Maggots

Fly larvae in tissue sections display a body cavity (Figure 6-1), segmentation, striated muscles attached at various points to the chitinous exoskeleton (Figure 6-2), and tracheae, often with cuticular rings. Some species have prominent spines (Figure 6-3). *Cuterebra* larvae are obligate endoparasites of rodents and lagomorphs. These larvae frequently invade dogs, cats, and occasionally man, where they are usually found in the cervical subcutaneous tissues but have been reported to migrate through the central nervous system with disastrous results (Figures 6-1 and 6-3). First-stage *Hypoderma* larvae migrate extensively in cattle, and erratic migration through the brain of horses has been reported. The spiracular plate is important in identification of fly larvae and may need to be retrieved from the wet tissues or paraffin block (see Figure 1-20).

Mites

Parasitic mites seen in tissues have segmented legs, spines, and hairs externally, and striated muscles, reproductive organs, intestine, yolk glands, and developing eggs internally; all or some of these may be seen in section. Species such as *Sarcoptes, Notoedres,* and *Trixacarus* have spines on their dorsum (see Figures 1-82 and 1-83) and feed at the stratum germinativum and dermis (Figure 6-4). In some hosts such as the red fox, *Vulpes fulva,* sarcoptic mange is characterized by extraordinary hyperkeratosis (Figure 6-5). Hyperkeratosis is also typical of mange caused by *Chorioptes* and *Cheylietiella* organisms, but the mites lie more superficially in the stratum corneum (Figure 6-6).

Demodex spp. are cigar-shaped mites found in the hair follicles or associated sebaceous glands (Figure 6-7). In severe demodectic mange in dogs, *Demodex canis* may be found in the lymph nodes. Demodectic mange in cattle and swine tends to be nodular (Figure 6-8).

Mites of the respiratory tract (e.g., *Pneumonyssus* and *Sternostoma*) have more delicate exoskeletons than their ectoparasitic relatives. *pneumonyssoides caninum* (Figure 6-9) of the canine nasal passages may be compared with *Sarcoptes scabiei* (see Figure 6-4).

Trombiculid larvae (chiggers) feed through a stylostome or feeding tube extending into the dermis (Figure 6-10).

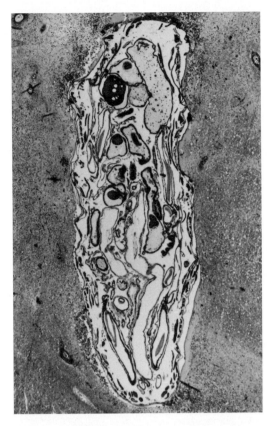

FIGURE 6-1 *Cuterebra* in the brain of a cat (×22). The internal organs lie in a body cavity rather than in a parenchymatous matrix.

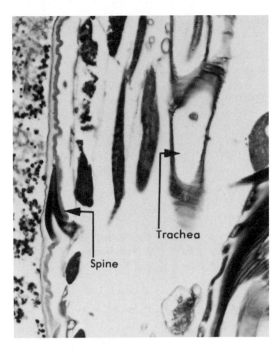

FIGURE 6-3 *Cuterebra* organisms in the brain of a cat (×220).

Pentastomids

Pentastomids, although commonly known as *tongue worms,* derived their name from the early belief that they had five mouths. In reality, they possess one mouth surrounded by four hooks (see Figure 1-100). Pentastomid adults are worm-like parasites in the

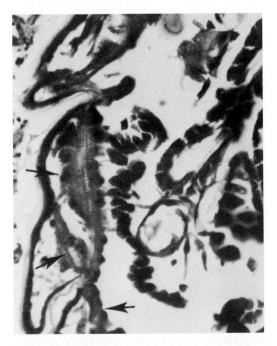

FIGURE 6-2 Dipteran larva in the brain of a calf (×250). The body is segmented and striated muscles *(arrows)* attach at various points to the exoskeleton.

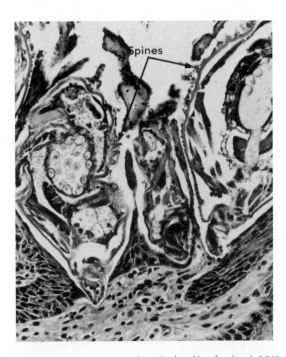

FIGURE 6-4 *Sarcoptes* organisms in the skin of a dog (×230).

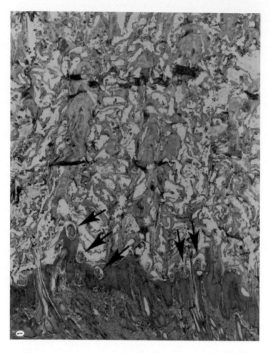

FIGURE 6-5 Hyperkeratosis caused by *Sarcoptes scabiei* in the fox (×22). The mites *(arrows)* are found in the deeper layers of the greatly thickened epidermis.

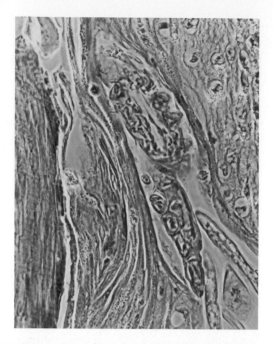

FIGURE 6-7 *Demodex canis* in the hair follicle of a dog (×430).

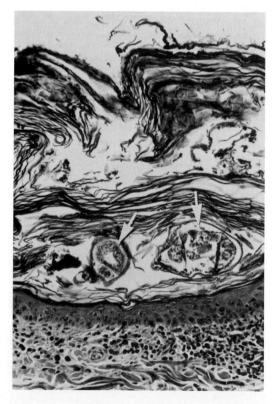

FIGURE 6-6 *Cheyletiella yasguri* in the skin of a dog (×150). These mites *(arrows)* lie in the stratum corneum.

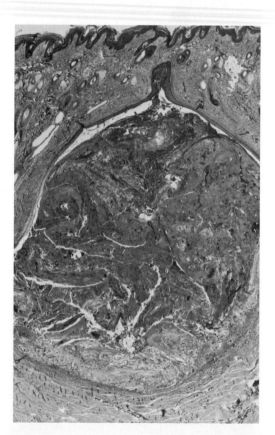

FIGURE 6-8 Demodectic mange in a bull (×16). Demodectic mange in cattle takes the form of nodular accumulations of myriads of mites and cellular debris in proportions depending on the age of the lesion.

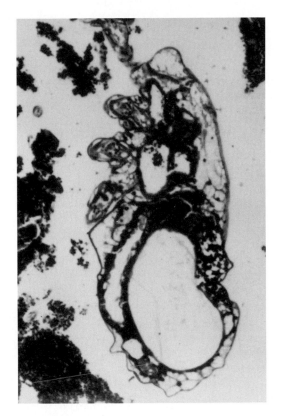

FIGURE 6-9 *Pneumonyssoides caninum* in the nasal sinus of a dog (×92).

respiratory passages of predaceous reptiles, birds, and mammals that become infected when they ingest nymphs encysted in the tissue of their prey. The pentastome nymph is the form usually seen in tissue sections. The nymphs have a spherical to oval shape and a pseudosegmented annulated body covered by a thick cuticle with sclerotized openings called stomata (Figures 6-11 and 6-12). Pentastomids have a digestive system and large acidophilic glands alongside the intestine. These acidophilic glands are characteristic, staining bright pink with prominent blue nuclei in hematoxylin and eosin (H&E) stain sections (Figures 6-13 to 6-15). Although the musculature is striated and located within the subcuticular region, these muscles are not arranged for moving appendages, which are lacking in all but the embryonic and larval stages The intermediate host becomes infected by ingesting the eggs (Figure 6-16); each egg contains a larva with four or six appendages, depending on the species.

Protozoans

At the light microscope level, protozoa are characterized as single-celled (unicellular) organisms with a nucleus and various other organelles. However, it is often difficult to distinguish even distantly related intracellular protozoans purely on the basis of

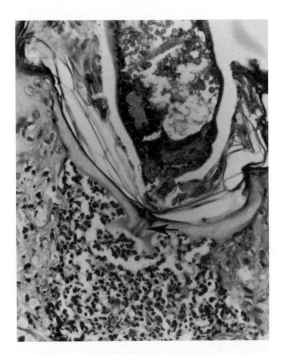

FIGURE 6-10 *Walchia americana* in the skin of a cat (×225). The *stylostome* or feeding tube extends to an area of dermis infiltrated with inflammatory cells.

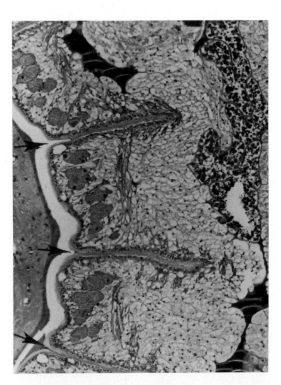

FIGURE 6-11 Pentastomid in a lymph node of a South American otter (×94). The cuticle is marked by deep annulations *(arrows)*.

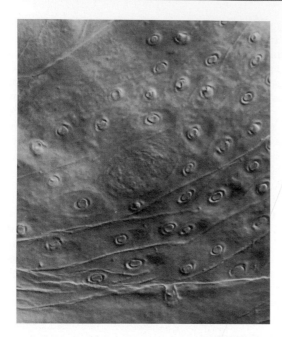

FIGURE 6-12 Surface view of the cuticle of a pentastomid showing the pores (×440).

structure, especially in tissue sections. It is one matter to start out with a known experimental infection and recognize the salient features of a particular organism, but it is quite another to be able to identify the same organism in material

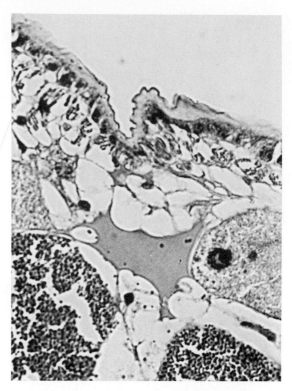

FIGURE 6-14 Pentastomid tissue in a racoon liver showing acidophilic glands and a cuticular sclerotized opening (×666). (Specimen provided by Dr. Ori Brener.)

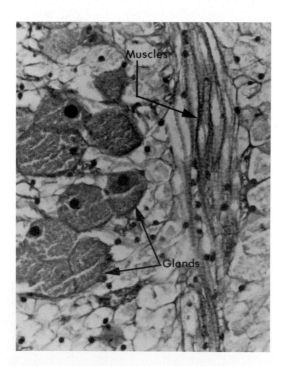

FIGURE 6-13 Pentastomid tissue showing striated muscle and acidophilic glands (×460).

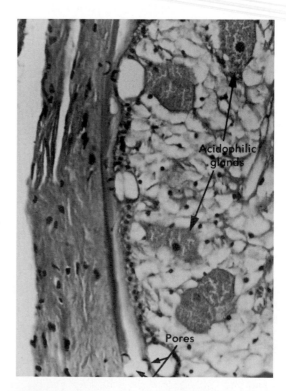

FIGURE 6-15 Pentastome larva in histological section showing cuticular pores (×290).

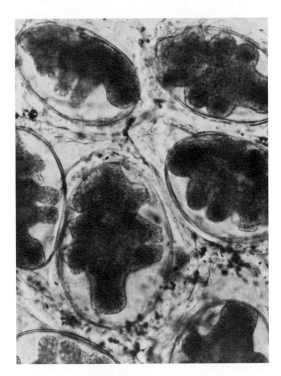

FIGURE 6-16 Pentastomid eggs with developing embryos (×160).

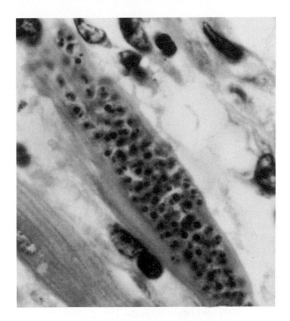

FIGURE 6-17 *Trypanosoma cruzi* amastigotes in cardiac muscle (×1300). Both nucleus and kinetoplast can be seen in individual organisms.

submitted for diagnosis. For example, *Trypanosoma cruzi* amastigotes should be easy to distinguish from *Toxoplasma gondii* bradyzoites because the former have a kinetoplast and the latter do not. However, the kinetoplast may be visible in only a small proportion of the amastigotes and might be overlooked. It is usually necessary to take into account the history, clinical signs, and pathological changes in reaching a diagnosis. Molecular biology can provide more definitive diagnosis but can be expensive and frequently is not feasible.

Flagellates

Both trypomastigotes and amastigote stages of *T. cruzi* occur in the vertebrate host, but generally, only the amastigotes are seen in tissue sections. *T. cruzi* amastigotes are generally found in muscle cells of the esophagus, colon, and heart, where they may be responsible for megaesophagus, megacolon, and myocarditis, respectively. Amastigotes are small, round to oval bodies, measuring 1.5 to 4 μm in diameter (often smaller after tissue processing) and contain a nucleus and a rod-shaped kinetoplast. They do not store PAS-positive material (Figure 6-17).

In *Leishmania* infections, only the amastigote stage is present in the vertebrate host. *Leishmania* amastigotes, similar in morphology to *T. cruzi* amastigotes, can be found in skin, bone marrow,

and visceral organs such as the spleen, often in macrophages or in other cells of the reticuloendothelial system (Figure 6-18). Often present in small numbers, but even when present in large numbers, diagnosing *Leishmania* in tissue sections can be challenging, because of the difficulty in seeing both the nucleus and kinetoplast. Differentiating *Leishmania* from *Histoplasma* organisms is the most common source of confusion. Exudate or impression touch preps from cutaneous lesions or lymph node (Figure 6-19) and bone marrow aspirates (Figure 6-20) may be prepared and stained with Wright-Giemsa solution. These are especially helpful because the full structure of the organism, including both the nucleus and kinetoplast, is generally more clearly visible.

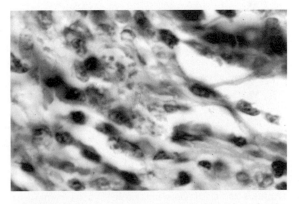

FIGURE 6-18 *Leishmania* amastigotes in a lymph node of a dog (×690).

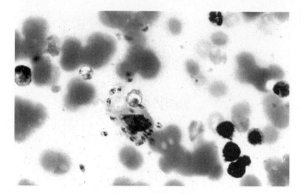

FIGURE 6-19 *Leishmania* amastigotes in a touch prep of an axillary lymph node from the same dog as seen in Figure 6-18 (×690). The nucleus and kinetoplast are clearly evident in several of the organisms.

Ciliates

Balantidium coli trophozoites may secondarily invade the wall of the large intestine of swine that have various forms of enteritis. They are characterized by their large size and the presence of a macronucleus and a micronucleus and cilia (Figures 2-5 and 6-21). Rumen ciliates may be found in the lung as a result of terminal inhalation of rumen contents (Figure 6-22), in which case there is no evidence of inflammatory reaction. Rumen ciliates may also be found in hepatic vessels in cases of very severe enteritis (Figure 6-23). In horses with severe enteritis, the extravagantly shaped ciliates normally present in the large intestine may secondarily penetrate the submucosa. These ciliates have large, often polymorphic macronuclei, and some have tufts of long cilia.

Coccidians

The coccidia are members of the phylum Apicomplexa, which includes not only the coccidia, but such

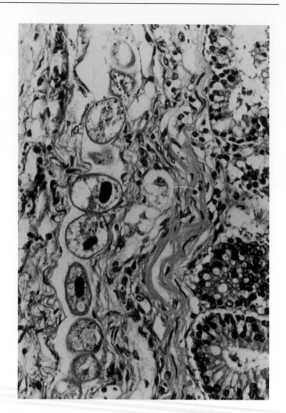

FIGURE 6-21 *Balantidium coli* in the submucosa of the large intestine of a pig (×280).

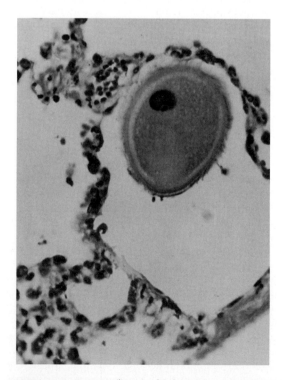

FIGURE 6-22 Rumen ciliate in the lung of a cow (×360). Agonal inhalation of ruminal contents accounts for the atypical location of this ciliate.

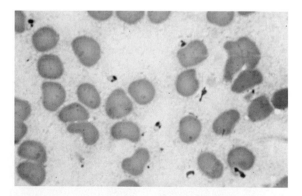

FIGURE 6-20 *Leishmania* amastogotes in bone marrow aspirate of the same dog as seen in Figures 6-18 and 6-19 (×690). Readily evident are the nucleus and kinetoplast.

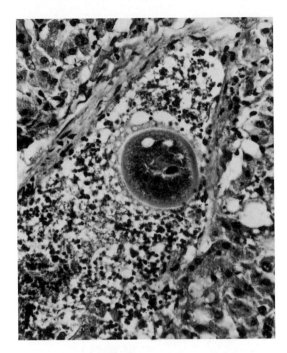

FIGURE 6-23 Ciliate in vein in the liver of a bull with severe enteritis (×250).

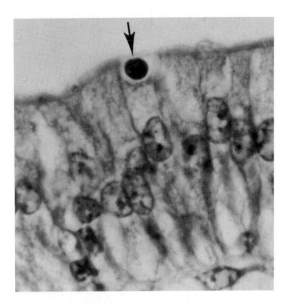

FIGURE 6-24 *Eimeria* trophozoite *(arrow)* in an intestinal epithelial cell of a chicken (×1300).

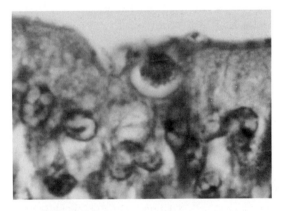

FIGURE 6-25 *Eimeria* schizont in an intestinal epithelial cell of a chicken (×1400).

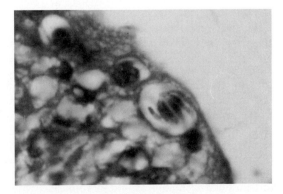

FIGURE 6-26 Another *Eimeria* schizont in an intestinal epithelial cell of a chicken (×1400).

seemingly diverse parasites as *Plasmodium, Theileria,* and *Babesia.* The life history and development of the major genera of coccidians are described in Chapter 2. A description of the histological appearance of the various stages follows, but host specificity, site specificity, life cycle, and details of development characteristic of the genera and species of coccidia must also be taken into consideration in arriving at a diagnosis.

Asexual stages
The infective stage contained in the oocyst is the sporozoite (= zoite). When a sporozoite enters a cell, it rounds up as a trophozoite in a membrane-lined parasitophorous vacuole (Figure 6-24). Trophozoites undergo nuclear division and initiate a cycle of asexual multiplication resulting in production of merozoites. Meronts (= schizonts) develop from trophozoites by a process called *merogony* (= schizogony, endopolygony). Depending on the species, meronts may be found in enterocytes (Figures 6-25 through 6-27), biliary epithelial cells (e.g., *Eimeria stiedae*/rabbit), endothelial cells (Figures 6-28 and 6-29), renal epithelial cells (e.g., *Klossiella equi*), or even uterine epithelial cells. Ordinary meronts contain from less than ten to hundreds of merozoites; some meronts (megaschizonts) (Figure 6-29) may contain over 100,000 merozoites. At some point, merozoites produced by asexual reproduction form sexual stages called *microgametes* (= male) and *macrogametes* (= female).

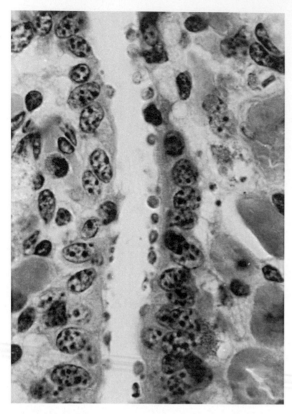

FIGURE 6-27   *Cryptosporidium* organisms projecting from the luminal surface of intestinal epithelial cells of a calf (×1050).

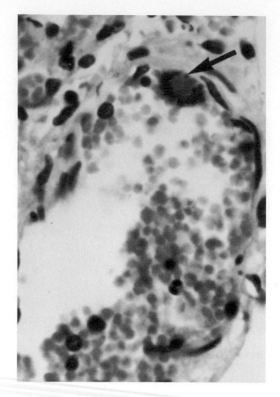

FIGURE 6-28   *Sarcocystis cruzi* schizont *(arrow)* in endothelium of a small artery of a calf with a fatal, naturally acquired infection (×812).
(Specimen provided by Dr. Paul Frelier.)

Sexual stages

A merozoite produced by the final merogonic generation enters a fresh host cell and develops into either a male or a female gametocyte. The female gametocyte enlarges, stores food materials, and induces a hypertrophy of both the cytoplasm and the nucleus of its host cell. When mature, the female gametocyte is called a macrogamete. The male gametocyte also induces hypertrophy of the cytoplasm and the nucleus of its host cell (Figures 6-30 and 6-31) as it undergoes repeated nuclear division and becomes multinucleate. Each nucleus is finally incorporated into a flagellated microgamete. When a macrogamete is penetrated and fertilized by a microgamete, it becomes a zygote. Currently, wall-forming bodies, already present in the macrogamete, become clearly visible as large, spherical, eosinophilic granules in the cytoplasm of the zygote. These later coalesce to form the oocyst wall (Figures 6-31 and 6-32). In *K. equi,* the sexual (as well as asexual) stages occur in the glomerular endothelium and in the proximal convoluted tubules of the kidneys. The distinctive sporonts (Figure 6-33) in the renal tubular epithelium produce as many as 40 sporoblasts, which develop into sporocysts, each of which may contain 8 to 15 sporozoites.

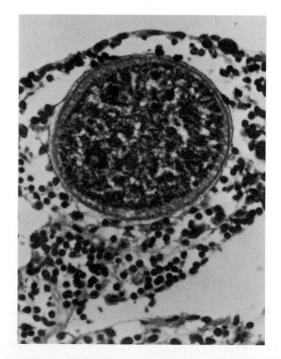

FIGURE 6-29   *Eimeria bovis* developing megaschizont in central lacteal of an intestinal villus (×425).

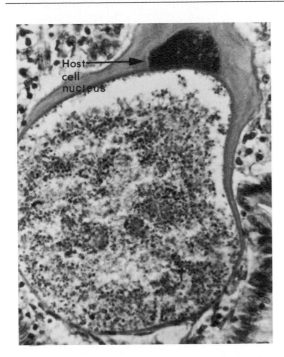

FIGURE 6-30 Male gamont of *Eimeria leuckarti* in the submucosa of the small intestine of a horse (×350). The cytoplasm and nucleus of the host cell *(arrow)* are greatly hypertrophied, and enormous numbers of flagellated microgametes have developed.

The life cycle just mentioned is the general pattern for those organisms that have a one-host life cycle, such as *Cryptosporidium* and *Eimeria*. For those parasites that have a two-host life cycle, such as *Sarcocystis, Toxoplasma, Hammondia* and *Neospora*, the sexual cycle typically occurs in the definitive (predator) host, and the asexual cycle typically occurs in

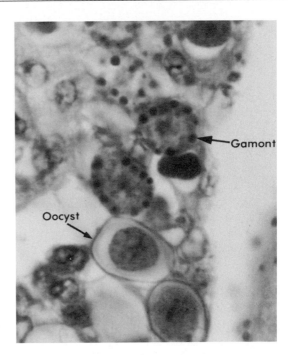

FIGURE 6-32 Female gamonts and oocysts of *Eimeria* organisms in an intestinal epithelial cell of a chicken (×1400). The female gamonts contain wall-forming bodies.

the intermediate (prey) host. In the two-host cycle, the sporulated oocyst is ingested by the intermediate host and excysts in the gut; sporozoites (= zoites) migrate to extraintestinal tissue sites, where several types of tissue cysts are produced. In *Sarcocystis*

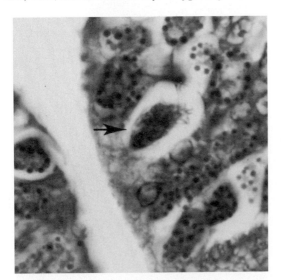

FIGURE 6-31 Male gamont *(arrow)* of *Eimeria* organisms in an intestinal epithelial cell of a chicken (×1400). The surrounding female gamonts contain wall-forming bodies.

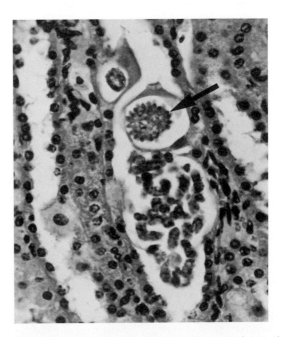

FIGURE 6-33 Sporont of *Klossiella equi (arrow)* in the renal tubular epithelium of a horse (×425).

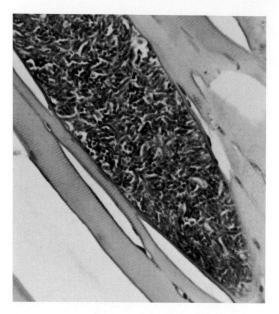

FIGURE 6-34 Sarcocyst of *Sarcocystis muris* in skeletal muscle of a mouse (×1300).
(Specimen provided by Dr. Marguerite Frongillo.)

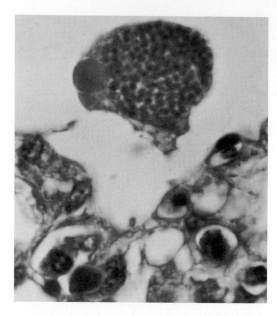

FIGURE 6-36 *Toxoplasma gondii* in the lung of a fatally infected cat (×1200). A macrophage has engulfed many *T. gondii* tachyzoites and two erythrocytes.

organisms, the cysts, called *sarcocysts,* are found in skeletal and cardiac muscle fibers (Figures 6-34 and 6-35). These sarcocysts vary in size from a few micrometers in diameter to macroscopically visible cysts and stain intensely with hematoxylin. After merogony, the sarcocysts are packed full of stages called *bradyzoites;* bradyzoites are the infective stage for the definitive host. Septa subdivide the interior of the sarcocyst but may escape notice because they stain poorly or not at all with H&E. In *Toxoplasma* organisms, ingested oocysts release sporozoites (or zoites) that enter host tissues and multiply as tachyzoites. Tachyzoites are 4 to 6 μm long, crescent-shaped, rapidly multiplying stages

that spread throughout the host tissues (Figure 6-36) and eventually encyst. Cysts persist in tissues such as brain, muscle, and retina, and are round to oblong in shape, thin walled, and contain few to hundreds of bradyzoites (Figure 6-37). Cysts containing bradyzoites, when found in striated muscle fibers, might be confused with either sarcocysts or accumulations of *T. cruzi* amastigotes.

Some of the Apicomplexa have moved away entirely from the gut and incorporated an arthropod

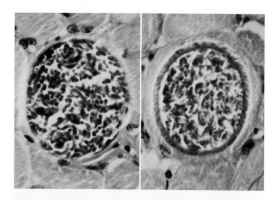

FIGURE 6-35 Sarcocysts of *Sarcocystis cruzi (left)* and *Sarcocystis bovifelis (right)* in skeletal muscle of the calf in Figure 5-23 (×300). The cyst wall of *S. bovifelis* is thicker and appears striated.

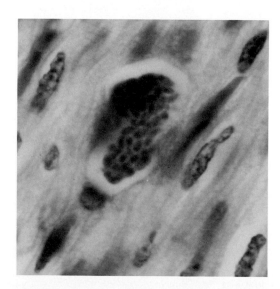

FIGURE 6-37 *Toxoplasma gondii* bradyzoites in a cyst in cardiac muscle of a puppy (×1200).

intermediate host in their life cycle. *Cytauxzoon felis,* considered by some to be *Theileria felis,* is a hemosporidian parasite of domestic cats (and possibly wild cats as well) and is one such parasite. Histologically the most striking feature is the presence of schizonts in cells of the mononuclear phagocytic system. The affected monocytes become enlarged, engorged, and occlude the lumen of small- and medium-size vessels of the lungs, liver, spleen, and lymph nodes (Figure 6-38).

Parasites of Uncertain Classification

Pneumocystis

The taxonomic position of *Pneumocystis* has been controversial for decades. It was considered by many to be a protozoan, but recently, molecular studies have shown that it is a fungus, class Ascomycota. *Pneumocystis* infections cause interstitial pneumonia, especially in horses with immune deficiencies. These organisms stain brownish black with Gomori's methenamine silver stain (Figure 6-39).

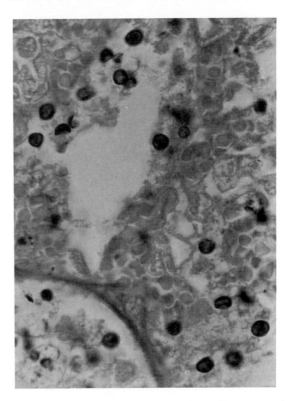

FIGURE 6-39 *Pneumocystis carinii* in horse lung; Gomori methenamine silver stain (×1000). (Specimen provided by Dr. J.M. King.)

Microsporidia

Much like *Pneumocystis,* microsporidia organisms have been considered parasites until recently; molecular study has indicated a closer relationship to fungi. When seen in tissues, microsporidia are typically very small, oblong structures, 1 to 4 μm

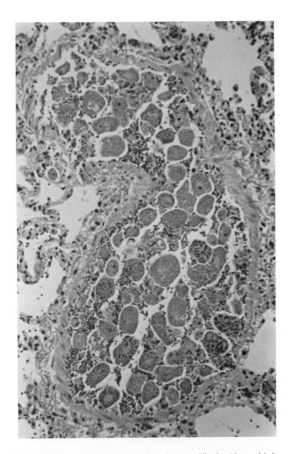

FIGURE 6-38 A pulmonary vein of a cat filled with multiple, enlarged, mononuclear cells containing schizonts of *Cytauxzoon felis* (×200).

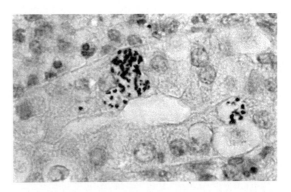

FIGURE 6-40 Gram stain of kidney from a rhesus monkey *(Macaca mulatta)* infected with SIV and *Encephalitozoon hellum* (×860). Clusters of Gram-positive *E. hellem* organisms are seen within the cytoplasmic vacuoles of renal tubular epithelium. The adjacent interstitium is infiltrated with neutrophils and macrophages. (Specimen provided by Dr. P.J. Didier.)

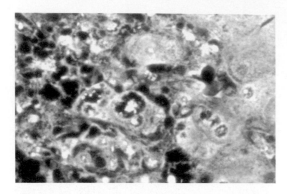

FIGURE 6-41 Calcofluor white M2R stain of liver from a rhesus monkey *(Macaca mulatta)* infected with SIV and *Encephalitozoon cuniculi* (×825). Individual and clusters of blue-white fluorescing *E. cuniculi* are apparent within vacuoles of hepatocytes near necrotic zones.
(Specimen provided by Dr. P.J. Didier.)

in length by 1 to 2 μm in diameter. They are best visualized after staining with Gram (Figure 6-40), Gram-chromotrope, or optical brighteners such as Calcofluor White (Figure 6-41). Biopsy or autopsy material may show organisms in most any tissue, including eye, muscle, digestive tract, respiratory tract, liver, gallbladder, kidney, bone, or brain.

■ METAZOA
Trematodes

Most trematodes are parasites of the digestive tract, but a number are found in the lumen of various ducts or organs (e.g., bile or pancreatic ducts, lungs, ureters, blood vessels, and sometimes brain tissue). Sometimes larval forms may also be encountered in sections. Except for the schistosomes, trematodes are hermaphrodites and generally have dorsoventrally flattened bodies. Trematodes are solid bodied and thus lack a body cavity; their organs are embedded in a loosely arranged parenchymatous matrix (Figures 6-42 and 6-43). Unlike cestodes, trematodes have a digestive tract (although often not a prominent structure in histologic sections), no calcareous corpuscles, and a spongy parenchyma that is not subdivided by muscular bands into a cortical and medullary region (Figures 6-43 and 6-44). Trematodes have vitelline glands composed of large clusters of eosinophilic cells with abundant cytoplasm (Figure 6-45).

Trematodes also are characterized by a thick outer homogeneous body surface called the *tegument* (Figure 6-46). The trematode tegument is an organized continuous syncytial epithelium that forms a seemingly thick multilaminated membrane. The tegumental membrane of trematodes is composed of a homogeneous prominent outer layer, which may contain external spines known as *tegumental spines* (Figure 6-46). Not only the presence, but also the

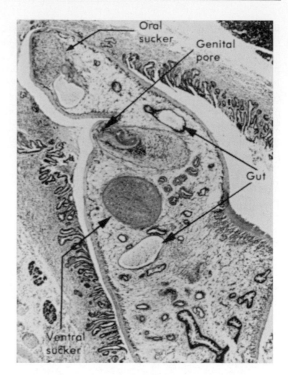

FIGURE 6-42 *Fasciola hepatica* in a bile duct of a rat (×27). (Specimen provided by Dr. Helen Han Hsu.)

number, size, and location of these spines can be of taxonomic value. Lying underneath the outer tegumental layer are a thinner pale intermediate layer and an inner layer of scattered sparse nuclei (Figures 6-46 and 6-47). Immediately beneath the tegument is a poorly developed, nonstriated muscle layer with a circular and longitudinal arrangement. Although both trematodes and cestodes have suckers, the oral sucker of trematodes is connected to a rudimentary gut (Figure 6-47), a feature that does not exist in cestodes. Sections through the uterus may contain eggs, which by their size, shape, and state of embryonic development can provide valuable clues to the identity of the specimen (Figure 6-48). Additionally, schistosome eggs tend to form granulomatous inflammatory reactions in tissues (Figure 6-49). The arrangement of the sex organs and distribution of vitelline glands in the trematode body are much-used taxonomic characteristics. For example, vitelline glands lie in positions both dorsal and ventral to the gut in *Fasciola* organisms, but all are ventral to the gut in *Fascioloides* organisms. Occasionally the position of such structures can be ascertained in tissue sections and is helpful in making a diagnosis.

The body size and form of some trematodes is quite distinctive. For example, *Fasciola* and *Fascioloides* organisms are relatively large worms, whereas others such as the heterophyids are quite small. Also,

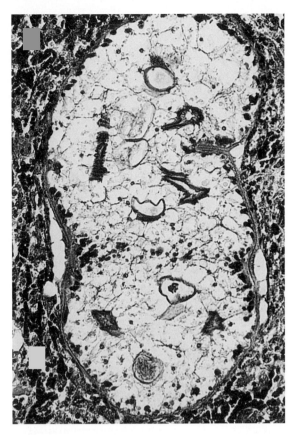

FIGURE 6-43 Trematode in the liver of a lizard. Trematodes have flat-shaped bodies without a body cavity, so that their organs are embedded in a loosely arranged parenchymatous matrix. Trematodes have a digestive tract, but lack calcareous corpuscles. Their spongy parenchyma is not subdivided by muscular bands (×100).
(Specimen provided by Dr. O. Brener.)

diplostomatids have a flattened forebody and a cylindrical hindbody (Figure 6-50; see also Figure 3-20), whereas in the dioecious schistosomes, the slender female is enclosed in the gynecophoral groove of the male worm (Figure 6-51).

Cestodes

Cestodes, like trematodes, have a solid spongy body with no body cavity, but lack a digestive system (Figure 6-52). They are covered by a tegument formed by the cytoplasmic projections of epidermal cells, which appears in histological sections as a thick, homogeneous noncellular external layer supported by a basal membrane. The internal organs of cestodes are embedded in a loose matrix. This parenchymal meshwork is divided into a distinct outer cortical and inner medullary portions by a system of longitudinal and transverse muscle fibers (Figures 6-53 and 6-54). The outer cortical region contains the subtegumental muscle layer and

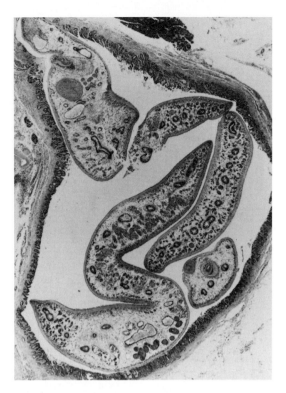

FIGURE 6-44 *Fasciola hepatica* in a bile duct of a rat (×13). (Specimen provided by Dr. Helen Han Hsu.)

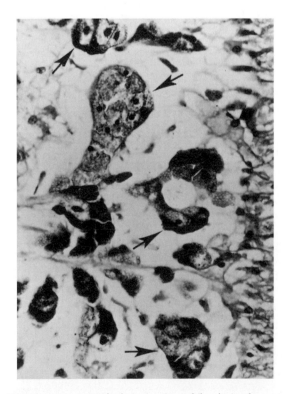

FIGURE 6-45 *Fasciola hepatica* in a bile duct of a rat. Vitelline glands *(arrows)* filled with secretion granules (×250). (Specimen provided by Dr. Helen Han Hsu.)

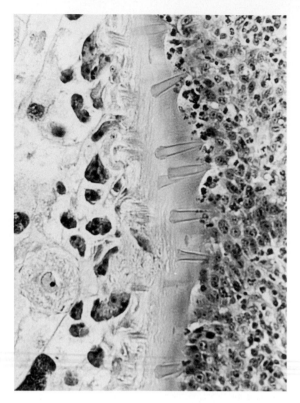

FIGURE 6-46 *Paragonimus westermani* in the lung of a macaque. The tegumental membrane of trematodes is composed of a homogenous prominent outer layer, which may project external spines known as tegumental spines (×170). (Specimen provided by the Armed Forces Institute of Pathology.)

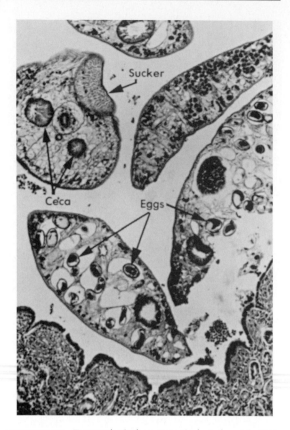

FIGURE 6-48 Trematodes in the pancreatic duct of a cat (×100).

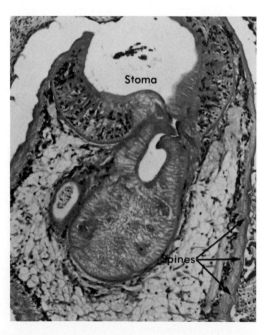

FIGURE 6-47 *Fasciola hepatica* in a bile duct of a rat (×90). (Specimen provided by Dr. Helen Han Hsu.)

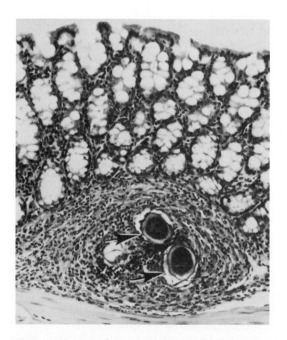

FIGURE 6-49 Granuloma containing eggs *(arrows)* of *Schistosoma mansoni* (×120). (Specimen provided by Dr. Helen Han Hsu.)

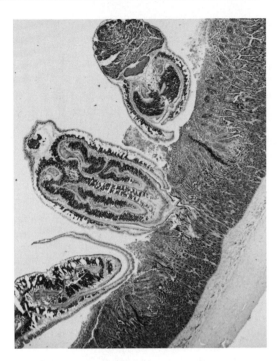

FIGURE 6-50 *Alaria* organisms in the small intestine of a dog (×10). *Alaria,* typical of the family Diplostomatidae, is divided into forebody and hindbody.

scattered epidermal cells. The parenchymal muscles, reproductive structures, and osmoregulatory ducts are found within the inner medullar portion of the body (Figure 6-53).

Scattered throughout the matrix of the body are calcareous corpuscles. These round- to oval-shaped bodies are unique to the parenchyma of cestodes and are especially prominent in larval stages, and serve as key diagnostic features. These solid bodies frequently have a concentric appearance in tissue

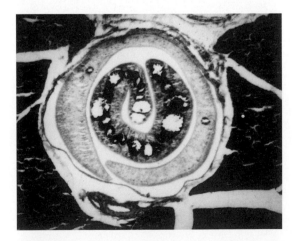

FIGURE 6-51 *Heterobilharzia americana* in a pancreatic vein of a beagle (×80). The smaller female is seen being held in the gynecophorous canal of the male.

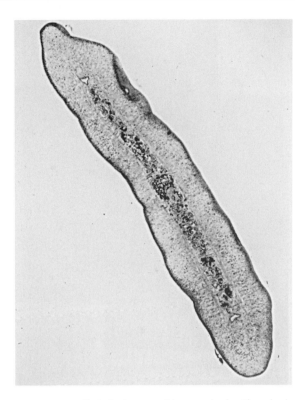

FIGURE 6-52 Cestodes have a solid spongy body with no body cavity and no digestive system. The internal organs of cestodes are embedded in a loose matrix, a parenchymal meshwork of loosely arranged cells divided into distinct outer and inner portions by a system of longitudinal subtegumental and transverse parenchymal muscle fibers (×30).

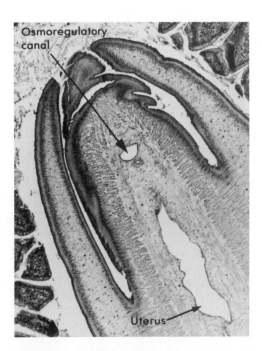

FIGURE 6-53 *Taenia taeniaeformis* in the small intestine of a cat (×50).

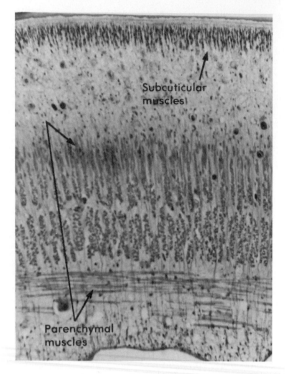

FIGURE 6-54 *Taenia taeniaeformis* of Figure 5-70 at higher power showing the subtegumental and parenchymal muscle layers (×140).

section and a complex chemical composition that includes calcium carbonate (Figure 6-55; see also Figure 6-64). Adult cestodes have holdfast structures such as bothria, suckers, and hooklets on the anterior end for attachment to the host. Rarely, these structures are seen in histological sections, but they can be useful in identification if present.

Almost all adult tapeworms are parasites of the digestive tract. Thus the stages typically observed in tissue sections are larvae. The larva consists of a head, which is similar to that of the adult, and associated tissue such as a bladder or elongated solid body (see Figure 3-38). Larval tapeworms do not possess reproductive organs or eggs. Pleurocercoid (spargana), tetrathyridium, and cysticercus, including simple, coenurus, strobilicercus, and unilocular or multilocular, hydatid cysts are the most common and important larval stages of cestodes found in tissues of domestic animals (see Figures 3-39 and 3-44). If the histological section includes only the bladder wall of the larva stage, the calcareous corpuscles might be the only unique feature identifying the parasite as a cestode. A section through the scolex that includes the hooks identifies the specimen as a member of the family Taeniidae (Figures 6-56 and 6-57), although *Taenia saginata,* the beef tapeworm of man, is an exception because it has no rostellar hooks, even in the larval cysticercus stage. Additionally, the length measurements of the hooks may provide further information for the identification of the cestode if both long and short hooks happen to

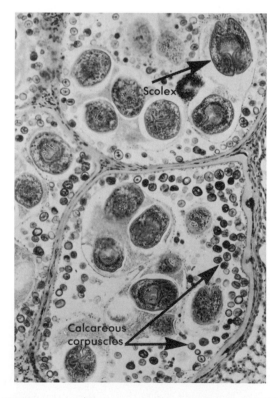

FIGURE 6-55 *Echinococcus multilocularis* alveolar hydatid (×108).

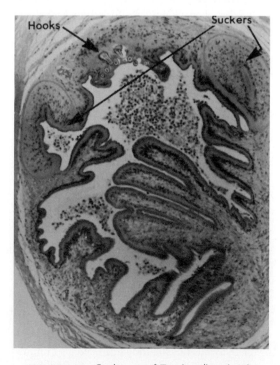

FIGURE 6-56 Cysticercus of *Taenia solium* (×96).

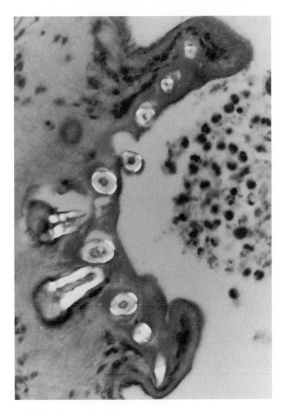

FIGURE 6-57 Cysticercus of Figure 6-56 showing birefringence of hooks in polarized light (×425).

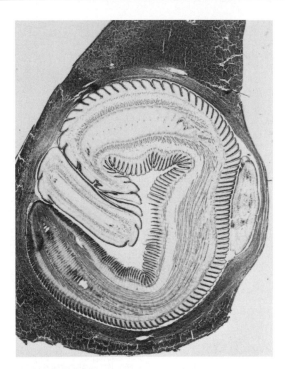

FIGURE 6-58 Strobilocercus of *Taenia taeniaeformis* encysted in the liver of a muskrat *(Ondatra zibethica)* (×12).

be present in the section or if they can be isolated from wet tissue.

Tentative identification of taeniid larvae also may be based on their host and site specificity. For example, a cysticercus attached to the peritoneal membrane of a cottontail rabbit is probably the larva of *Taenia pisiformis,* whereas a cysticercus on the same tissue of a ruminant or a pig is most likely the larva of *Taenia hydatigena.* Strobilocerci of *Taenia taeniaeformis* are cysticerci that have precociously begun to elongate the segment as larvae and are found in the liver of rodents (Figure 6-58; see also Figure 3-40).

A cysticercus-type cyst with more than one scolex connected to the same bladder wall is called a *coenurus* (Figure 6-59). *Taenia crassiceps* presents a source of confusion in this regard because it forms many cysticerci by budding, and these all lie within the same host cyst but are not attached to a common bladder wall (Figure 6-60).

Hydatid cysts exhibit expansive growth and have thick laminated membranes separating the germinative layer, with its sessile scolices or brood capsules, from the surrounding host connective tissue capsule (Figure 6-61; see also Figures 3-44, 3-45, and 3-46). In sterile hydatid cysts, the laminated membrane is the only diagnostic feature available. Alveolar hydatid

cysts have much thinner laminated membranes, and their manner of growth is invasive instead of expansive (Figure 6-62).

Tetrathyridia of *Mesocestoides* organisms differ from taeniid larvae in lacking a bladder (Figure 6-63) and in possessing four suckers with no hooks. Their calcareous corpuscles are large but not as dense as those of other larvae (Figure 6-64).

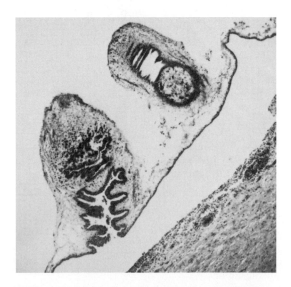

FIGURE 6-59 Coenurus in the brain of a cat showing two scolices on a thin bladder wall (×45).

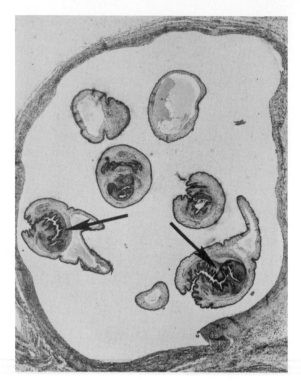

FIGURE 6-60 Cysticerci of *Taenia crassiceps* in a subcutaneous cyst of a gray squirrel (×16). Note inversion of scolices *(arrows)*. This is an unusual cysticercus in that it proliferates by budding and may be found widely disseminated in various tissues of rodents.

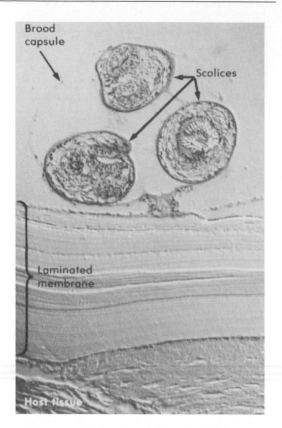

FIGURE 6-61 *Echinococcus granulosus* hydatid cyst (×202).

Plerocercoids of *Spirometra* organisms (Figure 6-65), also called spargana in the medical literature, are solid bodied, ribbon-like larvae that are unsegmented and undifferentiated. They have no bladder, and the scolex is not yet developed, so no suckers or hooks are present. Observation of calcareous corpuscles in a parenchymatous matrix without evidence of other structures may be the only feature on which to identify a plerocercoid.

Nematodes

Nematodes are also called *roundworms,* in part because of their appearance in cross section (Figure 6-66). Adult nematodes have a distinct body cavity containing tubular organs that include a digestive tract and male or female reproductive organs (Figure 6-66; see also Figure 6-91). The body cavity is described as a pseudocavity or pseudocoelom because it is not a true peritoneum lined by mesodermal tissue. The body wall of nematodes consists of three layers: an outer cuticle, an intermediate hypodermal layer, and an inner muscle layer.

The cuticle is an acellular layer that varies in thickness between different groups of nematodes. The

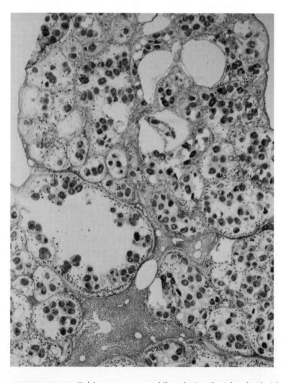

FIGURE 6-62 *Echinococcus multilocularis* alveolar hydatid (×24).

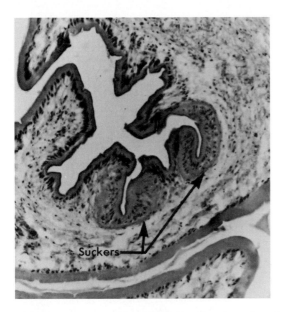

FIGURE 6-63 *Mesocestoides* tetrathyridium from the peritoneal cavity of a baboon (*Papio* sp.); region of scolex showing two suckers (×200).

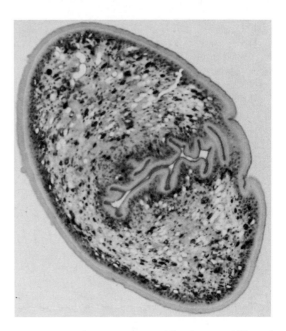

FIGURE 6-65 *Spirometra mansonoides* plerocercoid from the subcutaneous tissues of a mouse (×108).

cuticle is generally thought of as being composed of three layers, which are readily seen in some groups but not in others. Prominent cuticular modifications include lateral or sublateral alae, which are winglike flanges of the cuticle running longitudinally along the body (Figure 6-67), or spines, bosses (see Figure 6-95), striations, or ridges (see Figures 6-98 and 6-99). All of these can have significant taxonomic and identification value.

The hypodermis, which lies just beneath and secretes the cuticle, is thin but projects into the body

cavity at the lateral, ventral, and dorsal margins of the worm. These are called the lateral dorsal, and ventral chords, respectively. The lateral chords are generally prominent, whereas the dorsal and ventral chords are often inconspicuous. The lateral chords divide the muscle layer into dorsal and ventral fields (see Figure 6-66).

The muscle cells run longitudinally and form a layer between the hypodermis and the body cavity. Muscle cells in nematodes are composed of a basal

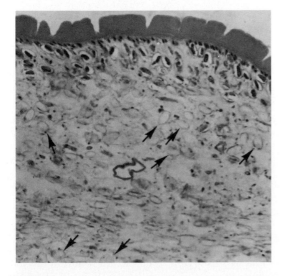

FIGURE 6-64 *Mesocestoides* tetrathyridium of Figure 6-63 parenchyma with large, "empty" calcareous corpuscles *(arrows)* (×250).

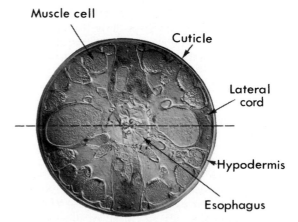

FIGURE 6-66 Cross section through the esophageal region of *Strongylus vulgaris* showing the division of somatic musculature into dorsal and ventral fields by the lateral cords. In this particular body region of *S. vulgaris,* the dorsal and ventral cords are exceptionally well developed, and these anatomically separate their respective muscle fields into halves. However, functional separation, expressed in terms of coordinated muscular activity, remains predominantly dorsoventral (×62).

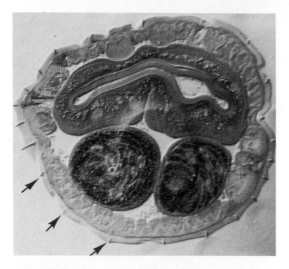

FIGURE 6-67 Cross section through *Haemonchus contortus* (×140). The entire circumference of the cuticle is marked by longitudinal ridges *(arrows)*, and the prominent brush border on the luminal surface of the gut is evident.

contractile and a cytoplasmic section that connects to the dorsal or ventral chord. In transverse sections of a particular parasite, the muscle cells can be numerous (polymyarian) (Figure 6-68; see also Figure 6-97), or few in number (meromyarian) (see Figures 6-66 and 6-77). This anatomic disposition is one of the important keys used in nematode identification. On the basis of muscle cell numbers, nematode musculature can be classified as either polymyarian or meromyarian.

Muscle cells can also be classified according to their shape, in addition to being classified by number. Coelomyarian muscle cells have a darkly staining contractile portion extending up the lateral sides of the muscle cell, which gives the cell a cylindrical appearance and an abundant, noncontractile cytoplasmic portion that looks empty with most stains (see Figure 6-68). The coelomyarian muscles are invariably polymyarian, which means that there are more than 12 columnar muscle cells lining the pseudocoelom. Platymyarian muscle cells appear flat because the fibrillar contractile portion is localized only on the broad base of the muscle cells and oriented perpendicularly to the cuticle. Platymyarian muscles have less than 12 fibers and are called meromyarian (see Figures 6-66 and 6-97). Most of the nematodes have coelomyarian muscle. However, platymyarian muscles are found in three groups: the rhabditids, the oxyurids, and the strongyles (see Figure 6-66).

The anatomy of the digestive tract of nematodes also gives additional details for correct parasite identification. In cross section, the lumen of the esophagus is cuticle lined and typically triradiate and may be muscular throughout or have a posterior section

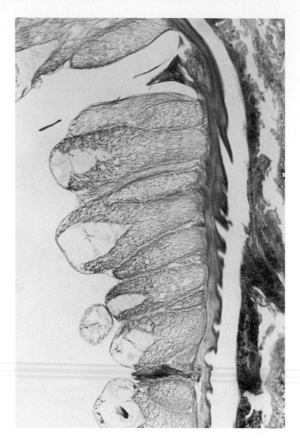

FIGURE 6-68 Muscle cell of *Eustrongyloides* spp. from a great blue heron. Each somatic muscle cell is composed of a basement membrane adjacent to the hypodermis, contractile muscle fibers, and a delicate sarcoplasmic portion containing the nucleus. The coelomyarian muscle cells have a darkly staining contractile portion extending up the lateral sides of the muscle cell, which gives the cell a cylindrical appearance and an abundant, noncontractile cytoplasmic portion that appears to be empty with most stains (×170).

that is glandular in nature. In the Adenophorea (=Aphasmidia), order Enoplida, the esophagus is a thin tube embedded in a structure called the *stichosome,* and in the anterior region of the worm, the cuticle and hypodermis form a single or double bacillary band. Both of these structures are unique to this group. The intestine is lined by a single layer of epithelial cells that may be columnar or cuboidal and may consist of few to many cells. On occasion the cells may be multinucleated, and a distinct brush border may or may not be present (see Figures 6-67, 6-86, and 6-93).

Rhabditida

Pelodera strongyloides larvae are found in the hair follicles of dogs, swine, and cattle (Figure 6-69). They have double lateral alae (Figure 6-70), and their musculature is platymyarian.

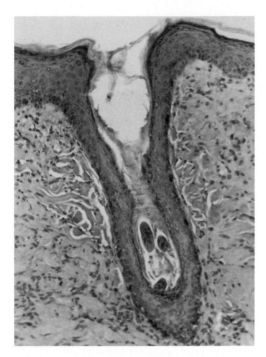

FIGURE 6-69 *Rhabditis (Pelodera) strongyloides* in a hair follicle of a dog (×130).

Halicephalus deletrix is another normal saprophytic nematode that has been reported to invade mammalian tissue and disseminate to various sites, most notably the brain, with fatal outcome. The infection has been reported widely in horses. These worms are small (adult females are 250 to 450 μm

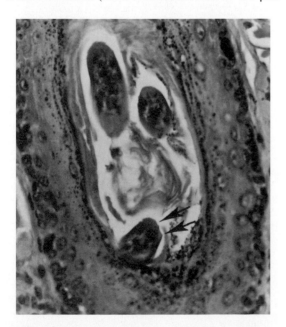

FIGURE 6-70 Same as Figure 6-69, enlarged to show double lateral alae *(arrows)* (×400).

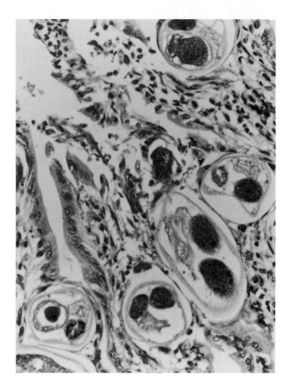

FIGURE 6-71 *Strongyloides westeri* in the mucosa of the small intestine of a horse (×250).

in length by no more than about 25 μm in diameter, and only females and larvae have been reported in tissues, suggesting that they are parthogenetic. Distinctive features in section, in addition to the small size and location, include the presence of a rhabditoid esophagus, a single genital tube, and a thin body wall in which the cuticle, hypodermis, and muscle layers cannot be distinctly separated.

This genus is also parthogenetic, and only female worms and larvae are found in the tissues. The adult parasitic female worms of this species are found deep in the mucous membrane of the small intestine (Figure 6-71) and are characterized by meromyarian/platymyarian muscles, a simple intestine composed of only two cells, and the eggs in utero, which are few in number, lined up in single rows, and often with developing larvae. *Strongyloides* larvae (see Figure 5-12) have double lateral alae.

Strongylida

Strongyles are divided into four superfamilies: Trichostrongyloidea, Strongyloidea, Ancylostomatoidea, and Metastrongyloidea. All except metastrongyles have platymyarian muscles.

Trichostrongyloidea

The adults of this group tend to be small worms that typically inhabit the stomach or small intestine. In

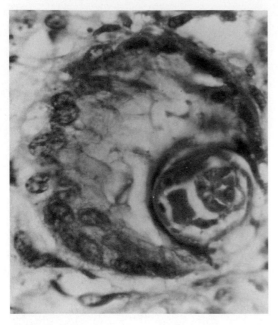

FIGURE 6-72 *Trichostrongylus axei* in the abomasal mucosa of a heifer (×1000).

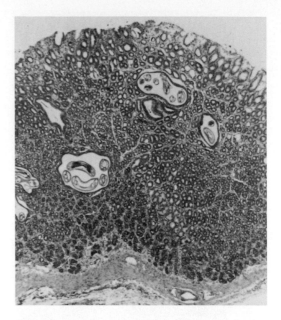

FIGURE 6-73 *Ostertagia ostertagi* in the abomasal mucosa of a heifer (×25).
(Specimen provided by Dr. Lois Roth.)

cross section, they are characterized by the small number of platymyarian muscle cells and an intestine composed of few cells, often with prominent nuclei and a microvillus border. Most trichostrongyles, with the exception of *Trichostrongylus* organisms, have marked longitudinal ridges on the surface of the cuticle (see Figure 6-67). Fourth-stage larvae are found throughout the mucosa of the stomach and intestine of ruminants and a wide range of other hosts. For example, *Trichostrongylus axei* fourth-stage larvae and juvenile adults are found between the basement membrane and epithelial cells of the abomasal mucosa (Figure 6-72). Fourth-stage larvae and juvenile adults of *Ostertagia* organisms are found in dilated gastric glands of the abomasum (Figures 6-73 and 6-74).

Strongyloidea

Most adult strongyles inhabit the intestinal tract and are larger than the trichostrongyles. In section, they exhibit characteristic features, including platymyarian muscles and the typical strongyle intestine. The cuticle is not adorned with ridges. In the strongyles, the presence of a large buccal capsule and specialized mouthparts are of great taxonomic value but are often not seen in tissue sections. Some of the larval stages of strongyles are spent in tissues other than the gut, whereas some form nodules in the intestinal wall. *Strongylus vulgaris, Strongylus edentatus,* and *Strongylus equinus* migrate extensively and sometimes erratically in the horse. *S. edentatus* tends to migrate retroperitoneally, and it is characterized by

a thick, multilayered cuticle (Figure 6-75). *S. equinus* immature adults are frequently found in the pancreas; sections through the buccal capsule reveal the presence of teeth at their base (Figure 6-76 to 6-79).

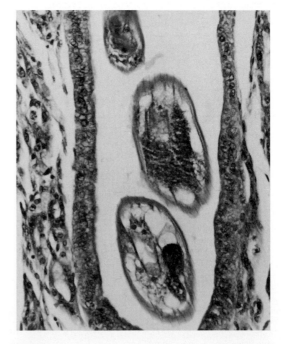

FIGURE 6-74 *Ostertagia ostertagi* in the abomasal mucosa (×370). Higher magnification of Figure 6-73 shows longitudinal cuticular ridges typical of the superfamily Trichostrongyloidea.

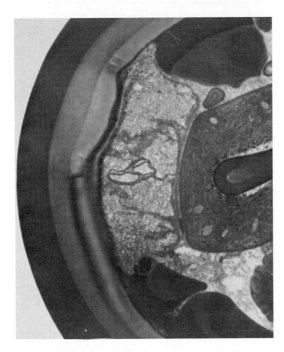

FIGURE 6-75 Cross section of *Strongylus edentatus* showing the thick, multilayered cuticle of this species (×220).

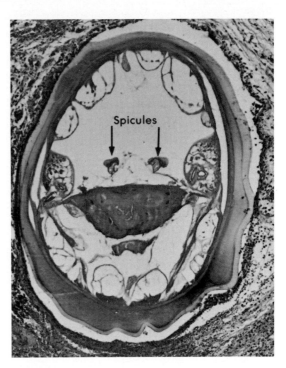

FIGURE 6-77 Higher magnification of Figure 6-76, showing a section through the caudal end of the worm (×100). Note the thick, multilayered cuticle, spicules, and prominent lateral cords. The cytoplasm of the meromyarian-platymyarian muscle cells was lost in histological processing (see also Figure 6-75).

Ancylostomatoidea

This group of worms, typically referred to as *hookworms*, inhabits the gut as adults and have typical strongyle features in section. The larvae of hookworms are relatively small, usually only 14 to 16 µm in diameter and have double lateral alae (Figure 6-80).

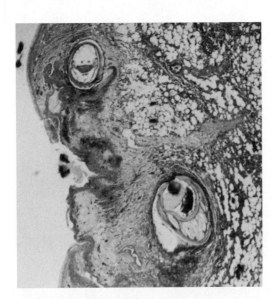

FIGURE 6-76 *Strongylus edentatus* immature male in the lung of a horse (×15). Two sections of worm are visible. The upper is a cross section near the caudal end of the worm (see also Figure 6-77), and the lower is an oblique section through the buccal capsule (see also Figure 6-78).

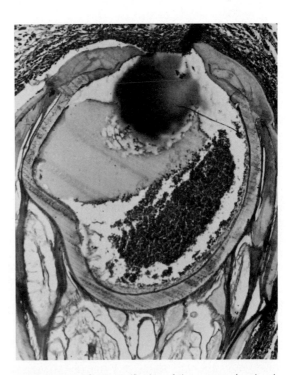

FIGURE 6-78 Higher magnification of Figure 6-76, showing the buccal capsule (×100).

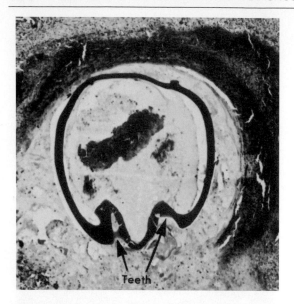

FIGURE 6-79 *Strongylus equinus* immature adult worm in the pancreas of a horse (×100). Although moribund, the teeth in the base of the buccal capsule are still readily visible and distinguish this species from *S. edentatus.*

Metastrongyloidea

Adult metastrongyles, often referred to as *lungworms,* typically parasitize the lungs or airways, but some may invade blood vessels or the central nervous system. In section, the body wall tends to be thin, the musculature is often polymyarian/coelomyarian in nature, and the gut is typical strongyle type, although the microvilli are less prominent than in other strongyles. Many metastrongyles contain embryonated eggs or larvae in utero and shed these stages into the surrounding tissues.

Aelurostrongylus abstrusus is the most common nematode parasite of the lungs of the domestic cat. Adults, eggs in varying stages of development, and larvae are found in nests in the lung parenchyma (Figure 6-81). *Angiostrongylus vasorum* adults may be found in the right side of the heart and pulmonary vessels of dogs, whereas the eggs and larvae are found in the lung parenchyma.

Filaroides hirthi adults are found in the lung parenchyma of the dog surrounded either by normal lung tissue (Figure 6-82) or by cellular inflammatory reaction (Figure 6-83). Eggs contain first-stage larvae when laid, and the eggs do not accumulate in the lung tissue. Autoinfection by *F. hirthi* may lead

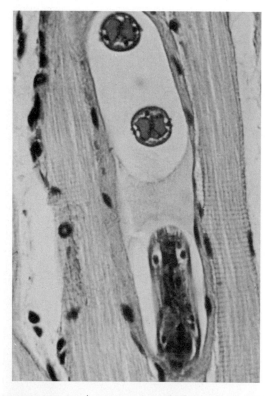

FIGURE 6-80 *Ancylostoma caninum* third stage larvae within skeletal muscle fibers (×650). Note the double lateral alae. (From Lee KT, Little MD, Beaver PC: *J Parasitol* 61:589-598, 1975.)

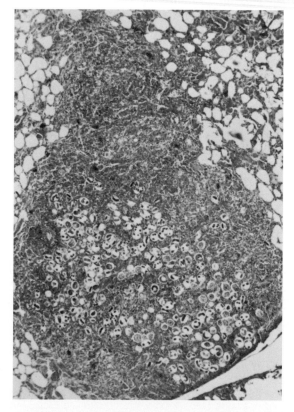

FIGURE 6-81 Eggs and larvae of *Aelurostrongylus abstrusus* in a nodule in the lung of a cat (×32).

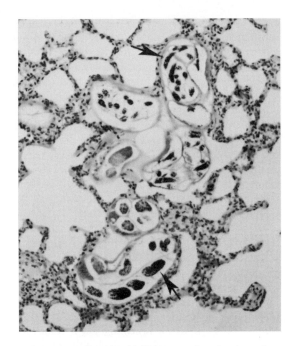

FIGURE 6-82 *Filaroides hirthi* in normal canine lung tissue (×108). The dark objects are eggs and larvae *(arrows)* in the uterus of female worms.

to a state of hyperinfection in which lung tissue is almost completely replaced by adult worms and larvae may be found widely scattered in lymph nodes, pancreas, intestinal tract, liver, and brain. *Filaroides osleri* adults are found in fibrous nodules projecting into the lumen of the trachea and principal bronchi (Figure 6-84; see also Figure 3-104).

Muellerius capillaris of sheep and goats, like *A. abstrusus* of cats, is found in nodules in the lung parenchyma. These nodules contain adult worms, eggs in varying stages of development, and larvae. If the tails of larvae can be located in the tissue section, *Muellerius* organisms can be distinguished from *Protostrongylus* organisms (see Figure 5-35). *Protostrongylus* spp. adults may be found in either parenchymal nodules or airways. *Dictyocaulus* spp. adults are found in airways. *Parelaphostrongylus tenuis* adults are found in the meninges and nervous tissue of the spinal cord and brain of sheep and goats (Figures 6-85 and 6-86), but their eggs and larvae, indistinguishable from those of *Muellerius* organisms, are found widely scattered in the lung parenchyma rather than concentrated in nests.

Ascaridida

The ascarids comprise a diverse group of worms, and as adults, some, such as *Ascaris* and *Parascaris* organisms, are the largest of the intestinal nematodes. In tissue section, in addition to their large size, the ascarids characteristically have a thick, multilayered

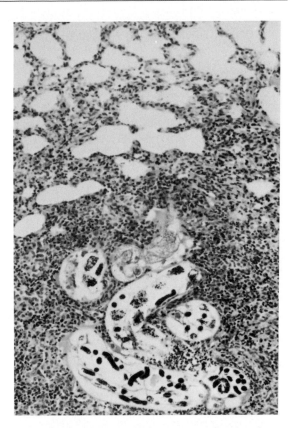

FIGURE 6-83 *Filaroides hirthi* worm surrounded by a cellular inflammatory reaction (×108).

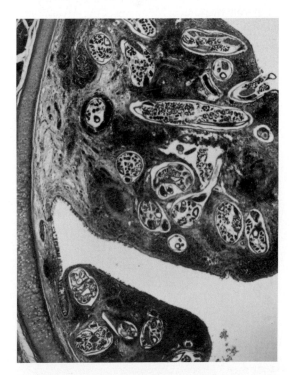

FIGURE 6-84 *Filaroides osleri* in fibrous nodules in the trachea of a dog (×2).

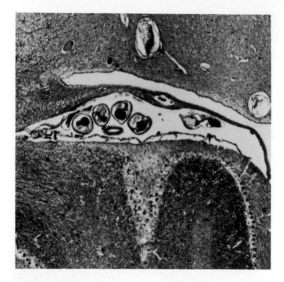

FIGURE 6-85 *Parelaphostrongylus tenuis* in the meninges of a goat (×25).

cuticle, polymyarian/coelomyarian muscles (often with cytoplasmic processes that extend into the body cavity), an intestine with numerous columnar epithelial cells and short microvilli, and large lateral cords. The Ascaridida are often divided into two large groups or superfamilies. One, the Ascaridoidea, parasitize land-dwelling vertebrates, whereas the second group, the Heterocheiloidea, parasitize birds, fish, and marine mammals. Members of the Ascaridoidea, including the genera *Ascaris, Parascaris, Toxocara, Toxascaris,* and *Baylisascaris,* have three simple

lips on the anterior end; thick, multilayered cuticle; a club-shaped esophagus; columnar epithelial gut cells with a single nucleus near the base of each cell; prominent coelomyarian/polymyarian muscle; and typical eggs in the uterus that have a thick shell, often wrinkled or sculptured on the surface (Figures 6-87 to 6-89). Genera in Heterocheiloidea, such as *Anisakis, Terranova, Contracaecum* and *Porrocaecum,* have much the same features in section, except all in this group also have a caecum (anteriorly directed), a ventriculus (posteriorly directed), or both. These may be obvious if sections are cut through the level of the esophageal-intestinal junction.

Those ascarids that parasitize mammals often have larvae that are capable of tissue migration, and larvae of genera such as *Ascaris, Toxocara,* and *Baylisascaris* cause "larval migrans" syndrome. Ascarid larvae have single lateral cuticular alae. They also have a single excretory cell with H-shaped anterior and posterior projections called *excretory columns.* The presence of single lateral alae and paired excretory columns makes ascarid larvae relatively easy to distinguish in tissue sections (Figure 6-90). *Toxocara* larvae migrating or arrested in somatic tissues tend not to exceed 26 μm in diameter, but *Baylisascaris* larvae continue to grow as they migrate and may reach 55 to 69 μm.

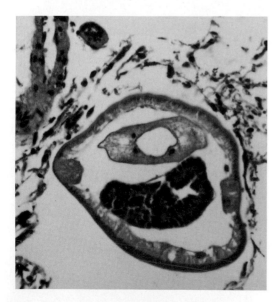

FIGURE 6-86 Section of *Parelaphostrongylus tenuis* (×290) illustrating the nature of the syncitial intestine with multinucleate cells.

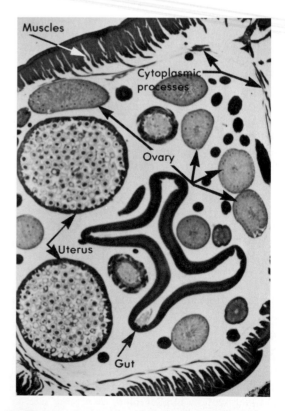

FIGURE 6-87 Cross section of *Parascaris equorum* (×25).

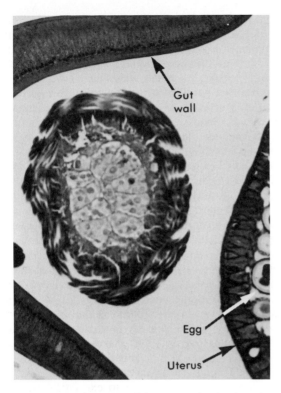

FIGURE 6-88 Enlargement of Figure 6-87, showing the columnar intestinal cells with one nucleus near the base of each cell (×140).

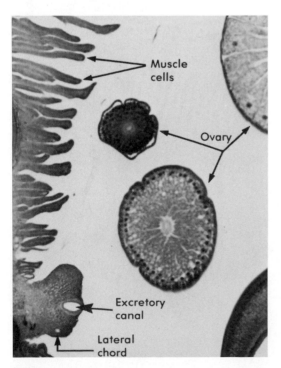

FIGURE 6-89 Enlargement of Figure 6-87, showing other details (×120).

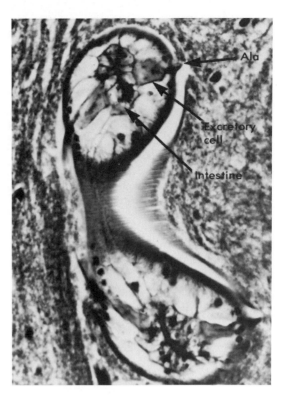

FIGURE 6-90 *Baylisascaris procyonis* in the brain of a Chukar partridge showing relationship of the intestine and excretory cells to the single lateral ala (×530).
(Specimen provided by Dr. Malcolm Peckham.)

Spirurida

The order Spirurida consists of the superfamilies Gnathostomatoidea, Physalopteroidea, Rictularioidea, Thelazioidea, Spiruroidea, Dracunculoidea, and Filarioidea. The spirurids represent an extremely diverse group of nematodes that parasitize a wide range of hosts and anatomic locations in those hosts. As adults, spirurids range in size from thin and threadlike in the case of *Gongylonema*, to stout, robust worms such as *Gnathostoma*, to incredibly long in the case of *Dracunculus*. Some species localize in the lumen of the gut, others are associated with the wall of the gut, and others have moved away from the gut entirely. Despite this variability, there are a number of similarities in both biological and morphological aspects. As a group, the spirurids use insects as intermediate hosts. In many, small, thick-shelled eggs containing a well-developed larva are passed in the feces and ingested by an insect intermediate host. In the Dracunculoidea, female worms migrate to the surface and release first-stage larvae into water where they are ingested by copepods. In the Filarioidea, not only have the adult worms moved away from the gut, but the female worms release motile larvae called *microfilariae* that either circulate in the blood or reside in the skin and are picked up by blood-sucking insects that serve as intermediate hosts. Features of spirurids in tissues include a cuticle that often has some ornamentation, including spines, bosses, transverse striations, or longitudinal ridges. The esophagus tends to be long and divided into an anterior muscular and posterior glandular portion; the glandular portion is very cellular and stains much more intensely. The general spirurid intestine is often large and folded on itself, and is composed of many cells, often with the nuclei arranged in a row, a prominent brush border but rather weak basement membrane. The lateral cords are prominent, and the musculature is polymyarian/coelomyarian in nature. In most spirurids, female worms contain small, thick-shelled eggs containing a larva. In the case of the Dracunculoidea and Filarioidea, large numbers of larvae or microfilariae, respectively, are contained in utero. This combination of features makes the spirurids relatively distinctive in sections.

Spirocerca lupi (Figure 6-91) provides an example of the superfamily Spiruroidea. The adults typically are found in nodules in the wall of the esophagus and stomach, and sometimes in the wall of the aorta or rectum. In cross section, they are characterized by large lateral cords that project into the body cavity, an intensely stained glandular esophagus (Figure 6-92), an intestine with a prominent brush border and many cells with the nuclei lined up in a row that gives the appearance of three layers, a uterus filled with small eggs containing intensely stained larva, and coelomyarian/polymyarian muscle cells (Figures 6-92 and 6-93). The larvae have hooks and combs associated with the stoma, although these structures require oil immersion microscopy to be seen properly (Figure 6-94).

The genus *Gongylonema,* another member of the Spiruroidea group, is encountered in the tissues of animals with some frequency and has several distinctive morphologic features. Typically found threaded in the mucosa of the mouth, esophagus or stomach, the members of *Gongylonema* have characteristic spirurid features in section, including a divided esophagus, a polymyarian/coelomyarian musculature, and the presence of small, thick-shelled, embryonated eggs. *Gongylonema* organisms are distinctive, however, in that the anterior end has large

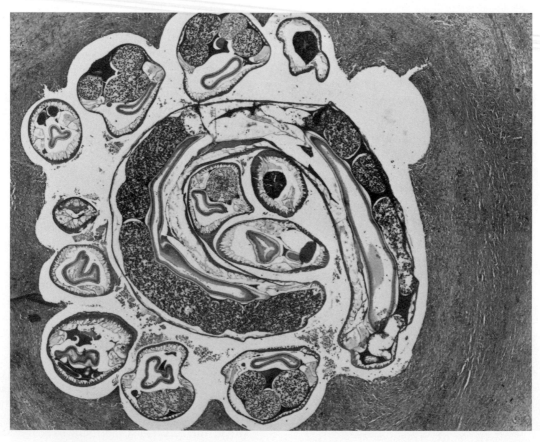

FIGURE 6-91 *Spirocerca lupi* (×22).
(From Georgi ME, Han H, Hartrick DW: Cornell Vet 70:43-49, 1980.)

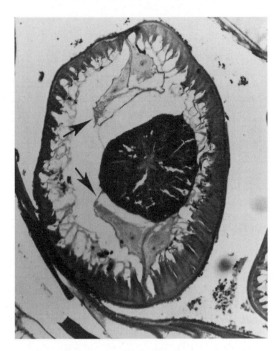

FIGURE 6-92 Cross section of *Spirocerca lupi* in the region of the glandular esophagus showing the lateral cords *(arrows)* projecting into the pseudocoelom (×95).

cervical alae and is covered with cuticular plaques or bosses on the anterior end, and the lateral cords are asymmetrical (Figure 6-95).

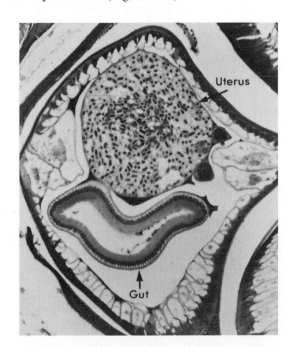

FIGURE 6-93 Cross section of *Spirocerca lupi* showing the nature of the intestine with a prominent brush border and many cells with nuclei lined up in a row and uterus filled with tiny eggs (×95).

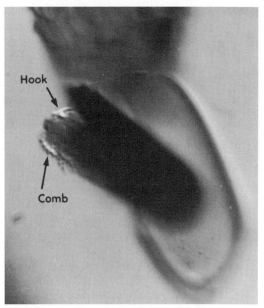

FIGURE 6-94 *Spirocerca lupi* egg with broken shell from which the larva projects (×1800).

Dracunculus insignis, of the superfamily Dracunculoidea, is characterized by flat lateral cords separating semilunar dorsal and ventral muscle fields composed of coelomyarian/polymyarian muscles, a very reduced intestine, and a large uterus filled with larvae (Fig. 6-96).

Members of the superfamily Filarioidea, although having many typical spirurid features in section, are relatively distinct. Most distinctive is their location, as adults, in virtually all tissues except the gut. Filarids range greatly in size, from some that are only 1 or 2 cm in length to others such as *Dirofilaria immitis,* where the female worm may reach 30 cm

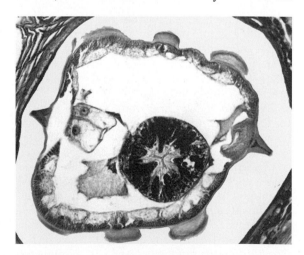

FIGURE 6-95 Cross section through the esophageal region of *Gongylonema* in a rat (×335). The dissimilar lateral cords, glandular esophagus, lateral cuticular alae, and cuticular bosses are all evident.

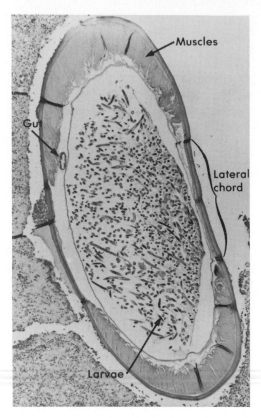

FIGURE 6-96   Cross section of *Dracunculus insignis* in a subcutaneous granuloma in a dog (×39).
(Specimen provided by Dr. S. Neuenschwander.)

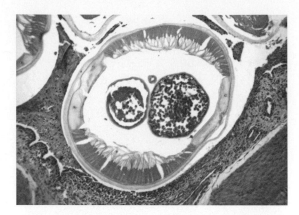

FIGURE 6-97   *Dirofilaria immitis* in heart of a dog (×65). The thick, smooth cuticle, large coelomyarian/polymyarian muscles, small intestine, and paired uteri are evident.

in length by 1 mm in diameter; however, all tend to be slender. The cuticle may be thin or thick and in some groups contains distinctive ridges or striations. The musculature is coelomyarian/polymyarian, the esophagus may be divided but is generally not as prominent as in other spirurids, and the intestine is typically a simple tube. One of the most characteristic features of filarids is the presence of microfilariae filling the uterus. There are many species of filaria that infect animals, and several examples will serve to illustrate the group.

D. immitis, the dog heartworm, is well recognized for the disease it produces in canines, felines, and humans. The adult worms live in the circulatory system, typically in the chambers and great vessels of the heart. The worms, as just stated, are large; have a thick, multilayered but smooth cuticle; have prominent coelomyarian/polymyarian muscles; have broad lateral cords; have a weak intestine; and, in the female, have paired uteri filled with microfilariae (Figure 6-97). Many other dirofilarias, such as *Dirofilaria repens* of the dog and *Dirofilaria tenuis* of the raccoon, live in subcutaneous locations and are distinctive in that the cuticle has prominent longitudinal ridges marked with transverse striations,

giving the external surface a beaded or corn-row appearance (Figure 6-98).

The genus *Onchocerca,* another common filarial infection of domestic animals, provides a good example of specific filarial anatomy in section. Adult female *Onchocerca* organisms are thin and extremely long, and have distinctive cuticular structures. These worms possess external circular ridges and striae in the inner layer of the cuticle (Figure 6-99). These ridges and striae are not only specific to the genus *Onchocerca,* but the number of striae per ridge has been shown to have great value in distinguishing various species within the genus. Also distinctive of adult female *Onchocerca* organisms are the muscle cells, which often appear to be weak and poorly developed, and a prominent amount of hypodermal tissue, even underlying the muscle cells (Figure 6-100). As far as it is known, adult *Onchocerca* organisms inhabit dense connective tissue, are tightly coiled, and, in some species, form distinct fibrous nodules.

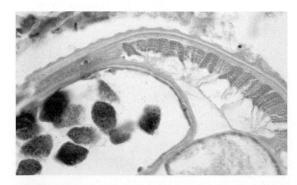

FIGURE 6-98   High power cross section through a portion of *Dirofilaria tenuis* in the subcutaneous tissues of a raccoon (×220). The longitudinal ridges on the surface of the cuticle are evident.

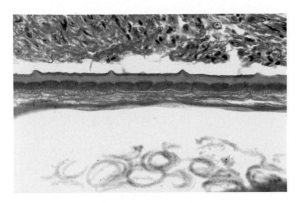

FIGURE 6-99 Female *Onchocerca cervicalis* in the nuchal ligament of a horse (× 560). The outer circular cuticular ridges and striae in the inner layer of the cuticle are evident. In *O. cervicalis,* there are four striae per ridge, one directly under and three between each ridge.

Enoplida
Trichinelloidea

This group contains the trichinelloids, the trichuroids, the capillarids, and the trichosomoids. In this group, the most characteristic feature, both grossly and in section, is the esophagus, a small cylindrical tube surrounded by individual stichocytes that compose the stichosome. The other distinctive feature of these

worms in section is the presence of a bacillary band(s). The bacillary band is a specialized section of the cuticle and hypodermis, including specialized hypodermal gland cells. In *Trichuris,* there is a single bacillary band in the esophageal region (Figure 6-101), whereas in *Trichinella* and *Capillaria,* there are two bacillary bands that run the length of the worm. In addition, the female reproductive tract is a single tube, the anus is usually terminal, the muscles are coelomyarian/polymyarian, and the eggs typically have bipolar prominences (plugs) and are frequently in an unembryonated state when passed or seen in tissues. Occasionally, eggs may develop and hatch in utero, as in the case of *Trichinella.* The first-stage larva is typically the infective stage for the definitive host. Most worms in this group display a high order of site specificity and, with the exception of *Trichinella,* a high order of host specificity as well. The host-organ listings should prove helpful in dealing with this group of parasites.

Adult Trichuris, as their common name *whipworm* suggests, have a whip-shaped body. The thin "whiplash" anterior portion is threaded through the epithelium of the large intestine, whereas the stout "handle" portion normally lies free in the lumen. Immature *Trichuris* lie entirely within the mucosa and are of uniform diameter. In an unusual case of *Trichuris vulpis* infection marked by persistent diarrhea, entire worms were found to lie in the submucosa (Figure 6-102).

Adult *Trichinella* are found threaded in the mucosa of the small intestine (Figure 6-103), and in tissue section, the adults resemble *Strongyloides,*

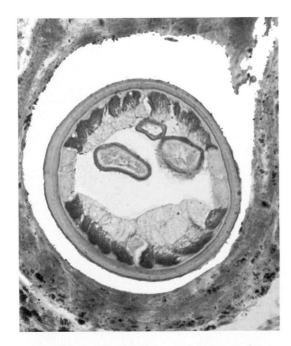

FIGURE 6-100 Cross section of female *Onchocerca cervicalis* in the nuchal ligament of a horse (× 340). The thick cuticle, prominent hypodermal tissue between the cuticle and muscle layers, and the whispy muscle cells are all prominent, as is the paired uteri and small intestine.

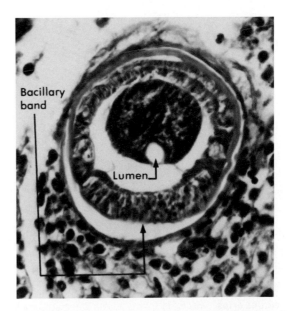

FIGURE 6-101 Cross section of the esophageal region of *Trichuris discolor* in the cecum of a heifer (×500).

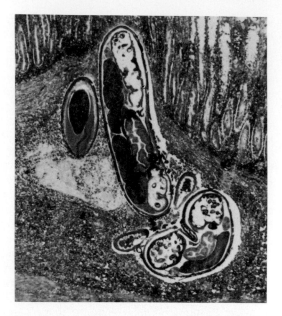

FIGURE 6-102 *Trichuris vulpis* in the submucosa of the large intestine of a dog (×33).

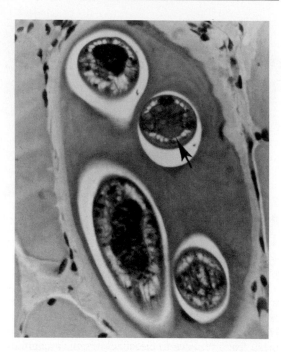

FIGURE 6-104 *Trichinella spiralis* first stage larvae in a skeletal muscle fiber showing a cross section of the stichosome esophagus (arrow) (×425).

except that they have a tubular esophagus embedded in the stichosome, male worms exist, and in female worms the uterus contains prelarvae instead of segmenting eggs. *Trichinella* larvae are found characteristically coiled in a "nurse cell" (Figure 6-104) in striated muscle, and they are characterized by stichocytes surrounding the esophagus (see Figure 3-139). Capillarids infecting the intestinal mucosa are somewhat larger than *Trichinella* and have eggs with bipolar plugs in their uteri.

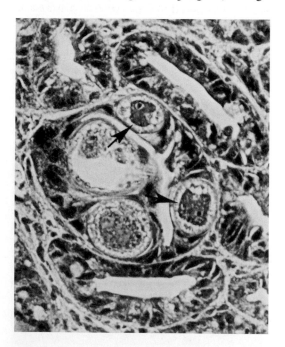

FIGURE 6-103 *Trichinella spiralis* adult in the mucosa of the small intestine of a rat (×480). Two cross sections of stichosome esophagus (arrows) are visible.

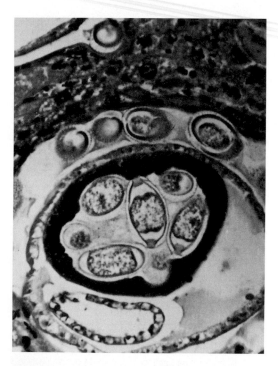

FIGURE 6-105 *Calodium* (= *Capillaria*) *hepaticum* in the liver of a rat (×360). Eggs with bipolar plugs are visible in the uterus.

The presence of single-celled eggs with bipolar plugs in the uterus is the best criterion for identifying capillarids in tissue sections (Figure 6-105). *Trichuris* spp. have larger eggs and are found only in the large intestine of mammals, practically the only epithelium in which capillarids will not be found.

Other common but less frequently seen members of this group include *Anatrichosoma* in the nasal mucosa of primates and marsupials and *Trichosomoides* in the bladder of rats. Both have larvated eggs with bipolar plugs (see Figure 3-142), and two or one bacillary band, respectively.

Acanthocephalans

Acanthocephalans, commonly called *thorny* or *spiny-headed worms,* are intestinal parasites of all vertebrates. The body may appear flattened in situ, but is actually cylindrical (see Figure 3-143). This worm has a body cavity, considered to be a pseudocoelom. The body wall is thick and multilayered but differs from the body wall of nematodes, and these features serve to clearly distinguish acanthocephalans in sections. It consists of an outer tegument, which is thick and divided into several layers; a middle layer of circular muscles; and an inner layer of longitudinal muscles (Figure 6-106). The outer

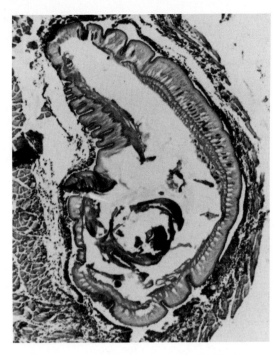

FIGURE 6-107   Cystacanth of *Macracanthorhynchus ingens* in skeletal muscle of a golden hamster (*Mesocricetus auratus*) (×66)
(Specimen provided by Dr. G.R. Fahnestock.)

tegument includes an outer plasma membrane and three fibrous layers: a thin outer layer; a thick, feltlike middle layer; and a very thick, fibrous inner layer. The inner layer includes holes or channels that make up the lacunar system (Figures 6-106 and 6-107). Between the inner layer of the tegument and the muscle layers is a thin layer of tissue that is

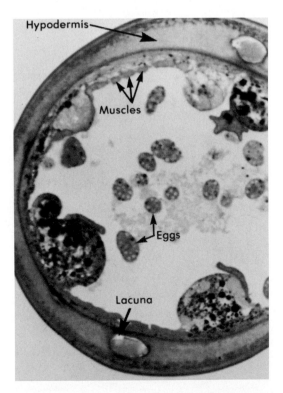

FIGURE 6-106   Cross section of a female acanthocephalan, *Neoechinorhynchus* (×240). "Eggs" are actually clusters of oogonia called ovarian balls that float free in the body cavity.

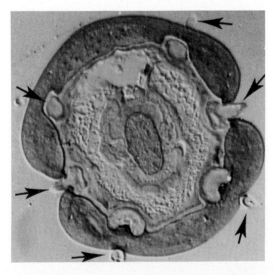

FIGURE 6-108   Cross section through the proboscis of *Neoechinorhynchus* showing hooks *(arrows)* ((×320).

referred to as the *dermis*. These parasites do not have a digestive tract, and their anterior end has an armed proboscis (Figure 6-108; see Figure 3-148) that is retracted by organs called *lemnisci*. In section, the lemnisci are large eosinophilic muscular bodies.

The acanthocephalans have separate sexes, and the reproductive system occupies the pseudocoelom. The female may have one or two ovaries, which typically break up into fragments also known as *ovarian balls*. These free-floating fragments are seen only in the mature female. The male has two testes enclosed in the ligament sac. Mature acanthocephalan eggs have a characteristic thick striated shell containing a partially developed larva called an *acanthor* (see Figure 3-145). The acanthor is infective to other animals such as fish or amphibians, where it develops to the cysticanth stage. The cysticanth stage is occasionally encountered in tissues of animals (see Figure 6-107), and although immature without a well-developed reproductive system, does have many features of an acanthocephalan.

■ **REFERENCES**

Binford CH, Connor DH, editors: *Pathology of tropical and extraordinary diseases,* vol 1 & 2, Washington, D.C., 1976, A.F.I.P.

Chitwood MB, Lichtenfels JR: Identification of parasitic metazoa in tissue sections, *Exp Parasitol* 32:407–519, 1972.

Connor DH, Chandler FW, Schwartz DA, Manz HJ, and Lack EE: *Pathology of Infectious Diseases,* vol 1 & 2, Stamford, CT, 1997, Appleton & Lange.

Gardiner CH, Fayer R, and Dubey JP: *An atlas of protozoan parasites in animal tissues,* Washington, D.C., 1988, AFIP, American Registry of Pathology.

Gutierrez Y: *Diagnostic Pathology of Parasitic Infections with Clinical Correlation,* Phildelphia, 1990, Lea & Febiger.

Meyers WN, Neafie RC, Marty AM, Wear DJ: *Pathology of Infectious Diseases,* vol 1, *Helminthiases.* Washington, DC, 2000, American Registry of Pathology, A.F.I.P.

Orihel TC, Ash LR: *Parasites in Human Tissues,* Chicago, Ill, 1995, ASCP.

Toft JD, Eberhard ML: Parasitic diseases. In Taylor BT, Abee CR, Henrickson R, editors: *Nonhuman primates in biomedical research: diseases,* San Diego, 1998, Academic Press, pp 111–206.

Appendix
ANTIPARASITE PRODUCTS BY SPECIES

TABLE A-1 ■ Equine Parasiticides

Active ingredient (dose)	Example trade name	Parascaris	Strongylus	Strongylus tissue stages	Cyathostomes	Encysted cyathostomes	Oxyuris equi	Triodontophorus	Trichostrongylus	Strongyloides	Onchocerca	Habronema	Draschia	Dictyocaulus	Anoplocephalids	Gasterophilus
piperazine (110 mg/kg PO)	Wonder Wormer for Horses	+	+		+		+									
pyrantel pamoate (6.6 mg/kg PO)	Strongid T	+	+		+										*	
pyrantel tartrate (2.64 mg/kg; daily as top dress)	Strongid C	+	+		+		+								*	
penbendazole (5.0 mg/kg PO)	Panacur	+	+	+	+		+									
fenbendazole (10.0 mg/kg PO)†	Panacur Paste 10% Powerpac	+	+	+	+	+	+									
oxibendazole (10.0 mg/kg PO)	Anthelcide EQ Equine Wormer	+	+		+		+	+		‡						
oxfendazole (10 mg/kg PO)	Benzelmin	+	+		+		+	+	+							
moxidectin (0.4 mg/kg PO)	Quest	+	+		+	+						+	+			+
ivermectin§ (0.2 mg/kg PO)	Eqvalan	+	+		+		+	+	+	+	+	+	+	+		+

FDA-approved labeling has been relied on for most of the drugs listed. For a comprehensive listing of off-labeled usage, see Chapter 5 and/or current literature.

*Takes increased amounts of pyrantel; pyrantel tartrate seems to work.

†10.0 mg/kg also recommended for foals with *Parascaris*.

‡15.0 mg/kg PO for *Strongyloides*.

§Please note that some generic preparations of ivermectin are not labelled for *Oxyuris equi* or *Triodontophorus*.

TABLE A-2 ■ Canine Parasiticides

Active Ingredient (Dose)	Example Trade Name	Roundworms		Hookworms			Trichuris	Dirofilaria	Tapeworms			Arthropods			
		Toxocara	Toxascaris	A. caninum	A. braziliensise	Uncinaria	Trichuris	Dirofilaria	Taenia	Dipylidium	Echinococcus	Ticks	Fleas	Otodectes	Sarcoptes
piperazine (55 mg/kg PO)	Pipfuge (and others)	+	+												
pyrantel pamoate (5 mg/kg PO)	Nemex	+	+	+	+	+									
dichlorvos (11 mg/kg PO)	Task Tabs	+	+	+	+										
dichlorophene (220 mg/kg PO)	Happy Jack Tapeworm Tablets								*	*	*				
toluene/dichlorophene (264 mg and 220 mg, resp/kg PO)	Happy Jack Trivermicide	+	+	+		+			*	*	*				
fenbendazole (50 mg/kg × 3 days PO)	Panacur	+	+	+	+	+	+		+						
praziquantel (5.0 to 7.5 mg/kg PO, SC, or IM)	Droncit								+	+	+				
epsiprantel (5.5 mg/kg PO)	Cestex								+	+					
praziquantel/pyrantel/febantel (5-12 mg, 5-12 mg, 25-62 mg/kg PO)	Drontal Plus	+	+	+	+	+	+		+	+	+				
diethylcarbamazine (6.6 mg/kg daily PO)	Filaribits	+						†							
diethylcarbamazine (55-110 mg/kg PO)	Filaribits (high dose)	+	+												
diethylcarbamazine/oxibendazole (6.6 mg + 5 mg., resp/kg daily PO)	Filaribits Plus	+	+	+	+	+	+	†							
ivermectin (0.006 mg/kg monthly PO)	Heartgard	+	+	+	+	+		†							
ivermectin + pyrantel (0.006 +5 mg, resp/kg monthly PO)	Heartgard Plus	+	+	+	+	+		†							
milbemycin (0.5 mg/kg monthly PO)	Interceptor	+	+	+			+								

Continued

TABLE A-2 ■ Canine Parasiticides—cont'd

Active Ingredient (Dose)	Example Trade Name	Roundworms		Hookworms			Trichuris	Dirofilaria	Tapeworms			Arthropods			
		Toxocara	Toxascaris	A. caninum	A. braziliensise	Uncinaria	Trichuris	Dirofilaria	Taenia	Dipylidium	Echinococcus	Ticks	Fleas	Otodectes	Sarcoptes
milbemycin/lufenuron (0.5 mg + 10 mg, resp/kg monthly PO)	Sentinel	+	+	+	+			†							
selamectin (6 mg/kg monthly topical)	Revolution							†				+/-	+		
moxidectin (0.003 mg/kg monthly PO)	ProHeart							†							
moxidectin (0.17 mg/kg 6 month injectable; at least 6 months old)	ProHeart 6			+				†							
lufenuron (10 mg/kg monthly PO)	Program												+		
nitenpyram (1 mg/kg as needed PO)	Capstar												+		
imidacloprid (9 to 24 mg/kg topical)	Advantage												+		
fipronil (topical)	Frontline											+	+		
melarsomine (2.5 mg/kg IM)	Immiticide							‡							

FDA-approved labelling has been relied on for most of the drugs listed. For a comprehensive listing of off-labelled usage. see Chapter 5 and/or current literature.
*Old efficacy data, current efficacy unclear.
†Preventive.
‡Adulticide.

TABLE A-3 ■ Feline Parasiticides

Active ingredient (dose)	Example trade name	Roundworms		Hookworms			Dirofilaria	Tapeworms			Arthropods		
		Toxocara	Toxascaris	A. tubaforme	A. braziliensise	Uncinaria	Dirofilaria	Taenia	Dipylidium	Echinococcus	Ticks	Fleas	Otodectes
piperazine (55 mg/kg PO)	Pipfuge		+										
pyrantel pamoate (10 to 20 mg/kg PO)*	Nemex	+	+	+	+	+							
dichlorvos (11 mg/kg PO)	Task Tabs	+	+	+		+							
toluene/dichlorophene (264 mg and 220 mg, resp/kg PO)	Happy Jack Trivermicide	+				+		+†	+†	+†			
praziquantel (5 to 10 mg/kg PO, SC, or IM)	Droncit							+	+	+			
epsiprantel (2.8 mg/kg PO)	Cestex							+	+				
praziquantel/pyrantel (5 mg +20 mg, resp./kg PO)	Drontal	+		+				+	+	+			
ivermectin (0.024 mg/kg monthly PO)	Heartgard for Cats			+	+		+						
milbemycin (2.0 mg/kg monthly PO)	Interceptor	+		+			+						
selamectin (6 mg/kg monthly topical)	Revolution	+		+			+					+	+
lufenuron (30 mg/kg monthly PO)	Program											+	
nitenpyram (1 mg/kg daily as needed PO)	Capstar											+	
imidacloprid (9 to 24 mg/kg topical)	Advantage											+	
fipronil (topical)	Frontline										+	+	
milbemycin (0.25 mg/ear topical)	Milbemite												+
ivermectin (0.05 mg/ear topical)	Acarexx												+

FDA-approved labeling has been relied on for most of the drugs listed. For a comprehensive listing of off-labeled usage, see Chapter 5 and/or current literature.

*Commonly used in cats, although not FDA approved for use in cats.

†Old efficacy data; current efficacy unclear.

TABLE A-4 ■ Bovine Parasiticides

Active ingredient (dose)	Example trade name	Withholding period in days		Helminths													Arthropods							
		Milk	Meat	Oesophagostomum	Ostertagia	Trichostrongylus	Nematodirus	Haemonchus	Cooperia	Dictyocaulus	Bunostomum	Strongyloides	Trichuris	Thelazia	Fasciola	Moniezia	Chorioptes	Sarcoptes	Psoroptes	Sucking lice	Damalinia	Haematobia	Hypoderma	Coccidia
morantel tartrate (10 mg/kg PO)	Rumatel	0	14	+	+	+	+	+	+															
levamisole (6 mg/kg SC or bolus; 8 mg/kg in feed; 10 mg/kg pour-on)	Tramisol Injectable	NFD*	2-9	+	+	+	+	+	+	+	+													
oxfendazole (4.5 mg/kg PO)	Synanthic	NFD	7-11	+	+	+	+	+	+	+	+					+								
fenbendazole (5 mg/kg PO)	Safe-Guard	0†	8-16	+	+	+	+	+	+	+	+					‡								
albendazole (10 mg/kg PO)	Valbazen	NFD	27	+	+	+	+	+	+	+	+				+	+								
ivermectin (0.2 mg/kg SC)	Ivomec Injection	NFD	35	+	+	+	+	+	+	+	+							+	+	+			+	
ivermectin (0.5 mg/kg Pour-on)	Ivomec Pour-on	NFD	48	+	+	+	+	+	+	+	+							+	+	+	+	+	+	
ivermectin (5.7 mg/kg SR—bolus)	Ivomec SR Bolus	NFD	180	+	+	+	+	+	+	+	+	+	+					+	+	+			+	
eprinomectin (0.5 mg/kg Pour-on)	Ivomec Eprinex Pour-on	0	0	+	+	+	+	+	+	+	+	+	+				+	+		+	+	+	+	
moxidectin (0.5 mg/kg Pour-on)	Cydectin Pour-on	0	0	+	+	+	+	+	+	+	+	+	+	+			+	+	+	+	+	+	+	
doramectin (0.2 mg/kg SC or IM)	Dectomax Injectable	NFD	35	+	+	+	+	+	+	+	+	+	+					+	+	+			+	
doramectin (0.5 mg/kg Pour-on)	Dectomax Pour-on	NFD	45	+	+	+	+	+	+	+	+	+	+	+			+	+	+	+	+	+	+	
clorsulon (7.0 mg/kg PO)	Curatrem	NFD	8												+									

Continued

TABLE A-4 ■ Bovine Parasiticides—cont'd

Active ingredient (dose)	Example trade name	Withholding period in days Milk	Meat	Oesophagostomum	Ostertagia	Trichostrongylus	Nematodirus	Haemonchus	Cooperia	Dictyocaulus	Bunostomum	Strongyloides	Trichuris	Thelazia	Fasciola	Moniezia	Chorioptes	Sarcoptes	Psoroptes	Sucking lice	Damalinia	Haematobia	Hypoderma	Coccidia
ivermectin/clorsulon (0.2 and 2.0 mg/kg SC)	Ivomec Plus Injection	NFD	49	+	+	+	+	+	+	+	+				+			+	+	+			+	
amprolium (prevention 5 mg/kg PO; 10 mg/kg treatment PO)	Corid	NFD	1																					+
lasalocid (100 to 360 mg/head/day PO)	Bovatec	0	0																					+
decoquinate (0.5mg/kg day PO)	Deccox	NFD	0																					+
monensin (50 to 360 mg/head/day PO)	Rumensin 80	NFD	0																					+
sulfaquinoxaline (9 to 66 mg/kg/day PO)	Sulfa-Q 20%	NFD	10																					+
sulfamethazine (330 mg/kg SR bolus)	Bovazine SR Cattle Bolus	NFD	8																					+

Helminths · Arthropods

FDA-approved labeling has been relied on for most of the drugs listed. For a comprehensive listing of off-labeled usage, see Chapter 5 and/or current literature.
*NFD, Not for dairy cattle.
†Mineral and suspension formulations not for dairy cattle (NFD).
‡Not all formulations are successful.

TABLE A-5 ■ Porcine Parasiticides

Active ingredient (dose)	Example trade name	Withholding period in days	Ascaris	Ascarops	Oesophagostomum	Metastrongylus	Strongyloides	Stephanurus	Hyostrongylus	Trichuris	Haematopinus	Sarcoptes
piperazine base (110 mg/kg PO)	Wazine	21	+		+							
pyrantel tartrate (in feed 800g/ton for treatment; 96 g/ton for continuous control)	Banminth 48	1	+		+							
hygromycin B (in feed 12 g/ton)	Hygromix 8	15	+		+					+		
dichlorvos (12.5 mg/kg PO)	Atgard Swine Wormer	0	+	+	+					+		
levamisole (8 mg/kg PO)	Levasole	3	+		+	+	+	*				
fenbendazole (9 mg/kg for 3 to 12 days PO)	Safe-Guard EZ scoop	0	+		+	+	+	+	+	+		
ivermectin (0.30 mg/kg SC; 1.8 grams (starters, growers, and finishers) or 9 grams (adult)/ton in feed)	Ivomec	18	+	†	+	+	+	+	+		+	+
doramectin (0.30 mg/kg IM)	Dectomax Injectable solution	24	+		+	+	+	+	+		+	+

FDA-approved labeling has been relied on for most of the drugs listed. For a comprehensive listing of off-labeled usage, see Chapter 5 and/or current literature.
*Levamisole premix is effective against Stephanurus.
†Ivermectin premix is effective against Ascarops.

TABLE A-6 ■ Ovine Parasiticides

Active ingredient (dose)	Example trade name	Withholding period in days Milk	Meat	Oesophagostomum	Ostertagia	Trichostrongylus	Nematodirus	Marshallagia	Haemonchus	Cooperia	Dictyocaulus	Bunostomum	Chabertia	Strongyloides	Trichuris	Monieza	Thysanosoma	Fasciola hepatica	Fascioloides magna	Oestus ovis	Coccidia
levamisole (4.0 mg/Kg PO)	Levasole sheep wormer	0	3	+	+	+	+		+	+	+	+	+								
albendazole (7.5 mg/Kg PO)	Valbazen	NFMS	7	+	+	+	+	+	+	+	+	+	+			+	+	+	+		
ivermectin (0.2 mg/Kg PO)	Ivomec sheep drench	NFMS	11	+	+	+	+		+	+	+	+	+	+	+					+	
lasolocid (15 to 70 mg/head/day PO)	Bovatec	0	0																		+
decoquinate (0.5 mg/Kg daily for > 28 days PO)	Deccox	NFMS	0																		+

FDA-approved labeling has been relied on for most of the drugs listed. For a comprehensive listing of off-labeled usage, see Chapter 5 and/or current literature.
NFMS, Not for milking sheep.

INDEX

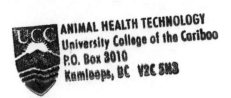

ANIMAL HEALTH TECHNOLOGY
University College of the Cariboo
P.O. Box 3010
Kamloops, BC V2C 5N3